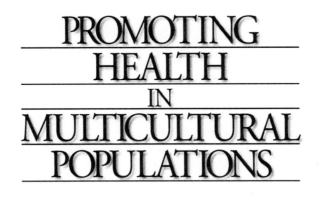

PROMOTING HEALTH IN MULTICULTURAL POPULATIONS

To Kathryn, Eric, and Erin
—R. M. H.

This book is lovingly dedicated to Anita and Elyse (z"l)
—M. V. K.

Robert M. Huff   Michael V. Kline

PROMOTING
HEALTH
IN
MULTICULTURAL
POPULATIONS

A HANDBOOK
FOR PRACTITIONERS

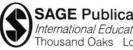

SAGE Publications
International Educational and Professional Publisher
Thousand Oaks   London   New Delhi

For information:

SAGE Publications, Inc.
2455 Teller Road
Thousand Oaks, California 91320
E-mail: order@sagepub.com

SAGE Publications Ltd.
6 Bonhill Street
London EC2A 4PU
United Kingdom

SAGE Publications India Pvt. Ltd.
M-32 Market
Greater Kailash I
New Delhi 110 048 India

Printed in the United States of America

Library of Congress Cataloging-in-Publication Data

Main entry under title:

Promoting health in multicultural populations: A handbook for practitioners / edited by Robert M. Huff and Michael V. Kline.
    p. cm.
  Includes bibliographical references and index.
  ISBN 0-7619-0182-5 (cloth: acid-free paper)
  ISBN 0-7619-0183-3 (pbk.: acid-free paper)
    1. Minorities—Medical care—United States.   2. Health promotion—United States.   3. Transcultural medical care—United States.   I. Huff, Robert M.   II. Kline, Michael V.
  RA448.4 .P76 1998
  362.1'089'00973—ddc21   98-25455

This book is printed on acid-free paper.

99 00 01 02 03 04 05 7 6 5 4 3 2 1

Acquiring Editor:	Dan Ruth
Editorial Assistant:	Anna Howland
Production Editor:	Sanford Robinson
Editorial Assistant:	Stephanie Allen
Designer/Typesetter:	Christina M. Hill
Cover Designer:	Candice Harman
Indexer:	Janet Perlman

Contents

PART 1: FOUNDATIONS

PART 5: ASIAN AMERICAN POPULATIONS

PART 6: PACIFIC ISLANDER POPULATIONS

Foreword

Nations, states, communities, and institutions seeking to create multicultural societies in which equity stands as a central value face a series of paradoxes. One is that multiculturalism by definition strives to maintain a respect for differences, and differences conspire against equity. People cannot be simultaneously different and equal on all counts of living. This paradox forces a definition of equity that must distinguish it from notions of equality, uniformity, and sameness. It also forces limitations on the range of living conditions and lifestyles to which the concept of equity or equality can be applied.

A second paradox is that the only way in which to achieve equity in the face of inherited social, economic, and political inequalities and inequitable societal forces is to treat people or populations differently. The provinces of British Columbia and Ontario, for example, must pay higher taxes to subsidize the Canadian commitment to equity through revenue sharing and income transfers to the poorer provinces in the Maritimes. Rich people must pay higher taxes to subsidize essential societal services to the poor. Whole classes and regions, then, must be treated unequally in the name of equity. The only alternative to this strategy is to limit the concept of equity more severely to include equality of economic opportunity and to ignore history, political traditions, prejudice, catastrophic illness, and conditions of birth and inheritance that give people unequal circumstances and starting points in availing themselves of their otherwise equal economic opportunities.

These two paradoxes force a third paradox for individuals in a multicultural society. Each of us must act toward other people of different ethnic origins with recognition and respect for their differences while treating them equally in every other way. But where do we draw the line in our behavior between differences and equality to achieve equity? In what ways should we be equal, and what are the "every other" ways? We face this daily in our relations between genders in the workplace. Affirmative action in hiring, building ramps for disabled people to have equal access, avoiding sexual harassment in gender relations between teachers and students or between colleagues, and recognizing the disadvantages an employee, a client, or a student had at the beginning of a professional encounter all reflect our efforts to reconcile these paradoxes.

These instances of societal adjustments to inherent differences while seeking to achieve equity hold lessons for the health professions and other sectors seeking to promote health in multicultural populations. Cultural differences related to health can be obvious or subtle, malleable or rigid, prescribed or proscribed, or dictated by religious or secular traditions, edicts, norms, customs, or ideologies. Thus, these differences can be treated as partial guides in the planning, implementation, and evaluation of health promotion programs. Beyond these partial guides, those involved in multicultural health care efforts cannot and should not claim science as their compass. Some combination of philosophical commitment, cultural knowledge, human sensitivity, and open communication must be brought to bear in achieving the balance and proper trade-offs between equality and distinctiveness that multiculturalism and equity demand.

This book presents the experiences of health promotion professionals in their work with various ethnically and culturally identified populations. Each chapter can be read for the lessons it may hold for other professionals working with the same population. Each can be read with some greater caution for the lessons it may hold for working with other populations. Generalizability might be the least appropriate scientific construct to be brought to bear in multicultural health promotion. Even within the culturally identified categories used in the chapter titles such as Latino, African American, American Indian, Alaska Native, Asian American, and Pacific Islander, one finds vastly varied populations. One must exercise similar caution in generalizing from these categories to their counterparts living under national conditions other than the United States. The American Indian and Alaskan Native counterpart "First Nations" populations of Canada and Aboriginal populations of Australia, for example, have some common heritage, genealogy, economic disadvantage, and cultural characteristics vis-à-vis their respective majority neighbors. But each has distinct features and circumstances that would make some generalization from the American experiences in this book misguided, if not hazardous, for health promotion professionals working cross-culturally in other countries.

These cautions aside, the authors of the chapters in this anthology of multicultural experiences offer a wealth of insight and a treasure of stories that can enlighten the cultural knowledge and awaken the cultural sensitivity of practitioners everywhere. As a handbook for practitioners, this volume promises to serve health promotion well.

If I were compelled to draw one overriding lesson, principle, or prediction from the multicultural experiences reflected in this handbook, it would be that promoting health in multicultural populations ultimately must be from within the cultures, that collaboration between the population and the professional practitioners from other cultures can be helpful and productive, but that such collaboration must be in the spirit of participatory research. Why participatory research? Because the health promotion task in every community is first to understand itself, second to communicate that understanding with consistency and credibility, and third to produce action from the understanding and commitment mobilized by its communication. These are the three elements of participatory research: systematic investigation or self-study, learning, and action. Practitioners working cross-culturally can participate in the self-study, learning, and action process effectively only if the population affected by the issues is actively engaged in all three of these elements.

LAWRENCE GREEN
Director, Institute of Health Promotion Research
Professor of Health Care and Epidemiology
University of British Columbia, Vancouver, Canada

Acknowledgments

The editors thank all those who helped in the preparation of this book. We especially thank our Sage editor, Dan Ruth, for his guidance, support, and many helpful suggestions for the organization and development of this book. We also acknowledge the assistance of Darleen Schuster, who spent countless hours in the library researching articles on multicultural health promotion and disease prevention and who also provided helpful comments in reviewing several of the chapters; our editorial board members for their many insights and suggestions that helped clarify points made in the chapters; and our many colleagues in the field who provided the impetus for the writing of this book. We especially thank Anthony Alcocer, Jayne Brechwald, and Matiana Grogan for reviewing the book and providing many helpful suggestions. Finally, we thank our families for their support, encouragement, and patience during the preparation of the book.

Preface

Health educators and other health practitioners have become increasingly challenged to effectively design and initiate culturally specific activities for promoting health. These activities include working with and around physical handicaps, language, culture, gender, age, religion, and a variety of other demographic, social, cultural, and health-related factors. If ignored, these factors can seriously affect the ability of a health promotion program to achieve its objectives. Fortunately, there is a growing body of literature describing theory and practice in health promotion and disease prevention (HPDP). However, it is difficult for many health professionals to obtain access to this voluminous body of literature because it is scattered throughout a variety of professional journals, monographs, reports, books, and related materials. The magnitude of this literature also leaves most readers overwhelmed and confused with respect to identifying and applying theories, models, and interventions for promoting health in various situations.

Health practitioners have little time to sift through this large corpus of literature looking for answers, directions, or models for designing, implementing, and evaluating HPDP programs for populations and target groups of special interest to them. Most practitioners would like to be able to access and readily employ this type of information in their day-to-day activities but generally have little opportunity to do so.

An intensive review of the health promotion literature and conversations with health practitioners in the field revealed the need to bring together in one book the current thinking and practice issues related to promoting the health of people in their communities regardless of their backgrounds, ages, ethnicities, or health issues. Furthermore, practitioners note that it is becoming much more demanding in all communities to effectively initiate and facilitate systematically designed and culturally specific activities for promoting health in special populations where issues of ethnicity, nontraditional health beliefs and practices, and other factors are encountered with increasing frequency. Many health practitioners are little prepared to address these issues in their work settings and communities.

The primary aim of this book is to provide in-depth specialized coverage of current theory, intervention models, and other information and considerations related to promoting health and preventing disease within a variety of special population groups. To achieve this aim, the chapters intensively discuss "special populations" including what is meant by this designation. Population characteristics with regard to health issues and problems and the special considerations inherent in working with special population groups in HPDP also are presented. Thus, this book reviews and presents in simple, practical, and understandable terms the most current theoretical models and strategies being employed to promote health and prevent disease in a variety of multicultural community and health care settings. Finally, we hope that the book will help health practitioners improve their understanding, skills, and effectiveness in planning HPDP programs regardless of their situations or settings.

The editors and chapter authors recognize that ethnicity is a rather broad way in which to examine special populations. However, categorization by ethnicity does make it possible to focus on the unique characteristics of ethnic groups with respect to their cultural values, beliefs, and mores and how these may affect programs addressed to improving their health and well-being. Regardless of the special populations being treated, we recognize that with the passage of time, many of these special populations have produced second generations of native-born children of native-born parents. In most instances, they straddle two or more cultures and face the challenges of living in both while seeking their own identities and lifestyle patterns. In addition, the number of recent and new immigrants coming from myriad countries has brought forth a variety of old and new health problems and issues that must now be addressed. These problems and needs will require health care practitioners to think and act in new ways to effectively address the health care needs of these special population groups. There are, obviously, a number of difficulties associated with defining special population groups that will present some challenges to a book such as ours. These include issues such as gender and age differences as well as generational differences in which adoption of Western health practices might be in conflict with more traditional practices. The editors and chapter authors also recognize that special populations can be defined on the basis of shared similarities, including chronic or acute health problems, disabilities, sexual orientation, and almost anything else one might consider when trying to categorize people. It is not the aim of this book to try to address all of these issues. Rather, we seek to combine theory, practice, and ethnic considerations that address the broad range of special population characteristics in the belief that, through this approach, practitioners can adapt these to their particular needs and issues.

This book is grounded in the premise that working within multicultural settings to promote health and prevent disease requires an understanding of the basics of program planning and an in-depth understanding of the cultural group being targeted, that is, an awareness of who these people are, including variables such as their history and immigration patterns, cultural values and norms, cosmology and religious practices, social and political systems, health beliefs and practices, and other culture-specific demographic variables that characterize the population and/or subpopulations of interest. There is a need for health professionals to actively seek out, develop, and improve their skills as culturally competent and sensitive providers of health programs or services to populations different from their own.

This book, then, has been written for a variety of health practitioners representing the many disciplines of public health, medicine, psychology, sociology, and other helping professions who are in daily contact with culturally diverse population groups. It also has been written for students training in these professions to help them develop perspectives on cultural differences and on how these affect HPDP programs or services. The book is divided into seven major sections and is intended to be used as a handbook of concepts, methods, tips, and suggestions for working with multicultural peoples. The editors recognize that no single book can possibly present all of the issues related to multicultural HPDP but hope that the reader will find this book useful in helping to organize his or her thinking about working with culturally diverse populations.

The first section of the book seeks to establish a foundation for the sections that follow and presents five chapters that define and consider concepts of culture and cultural competence; traditional concepts of health and disease; an overview of current models, theories, and principles of HPDP; an overview of planning models, theory, and practice issues; and "tips" for the practitioner who is engaged in designing and implementing HPDP programs for multicultural groups.

The next five sections consider five specific multicultural groups: Hispanic/Latino, African American, American Indian and Alaska Native, Asian American, and Pacific Islander population groups. Each of these sections includes three chapters followed by a "tips" chapter. The first of these chapters presents an overview devoted to understanding this special population from a variety of perspectives and includes terms used to define the subgroups within the broader population, historical and demographic characteristics, immigration patterns, health and disease issues and concerns, and health beliefs and practices. The second chapter of each section is concerned with how to assess, plan, implement, and evaluate programs for each of the specific groups including tips, models, and suggestions for more effective program design. The third chapter in each section presents a case study to emphasize the points made in the overview and planning chapters.

The final section of the book begins by presenting a cultural assessment framework to help guide the practitioner in designing needs assessment activities that reflect a cultural perspective. This framework provides the health promoter with a series of categories and questions that can be included in needs assessment instruments and activities. Data from this type of assessment can help provide information critical to planning programs or services to multicultural population groups. The final chapter in this section seeks to consider where we are going with multicultural HPDP programs as we move into the 21st century and concludes with a discussion of the ethical dilemmas and concerns faced by the practitioner working with multicultural populations in a variety of health care settings.

ROBERT M. HUFF
MICHAEL V. KLINE

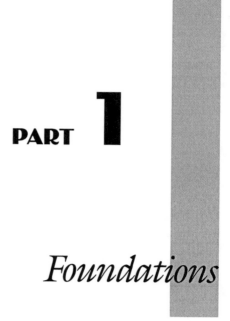

PART 1

Foundations

1

Health Promotion in the Context of Culture

ROBERT M. HUFF
MICHAEL V. KLINE

Activities for promoting health and preventing disease in any population, whether directed at individuals, groups, or communities, is a formidable task. Such endeavors require an organized effort characterized by an understanding that *cultural forces,* among other social forces, are powerful determinants of health-related behaviors. Culture, in any group or subpopulation, can exist as a total or partial system of interrelationships of human behavior guided and influenced by the organization and the products of that behavior. Indeed, the beliefs, ideologies, knowledge, institutions, religion, and governance, as well as nearly all activities (including efforts to achieve health-related behavior change), are affected by the forces of the culture that guides one's group or subgroup. Efforts to promote health and prevent disease within culturally different ethnic subgroups, as in any target group, will entail influencing the health behavior of individuals, families, groups, or communities. This will require identifying and changing those factors it is possible to modify that are associated with accomplishing the desired health-related behavior. Also, these efforts probably will require some type of sustained collaboration between the public and private sectors and the people most directly affected by a defined health concern or problem. Cultural considerations ultimately may determine whether a particular population or target group will choose to participate in health promotion and disease prevention (HPDP) programs. There will need to be a continuing communication between these stakeholders that establishes and maintains working relationships characterized by mutual understanding and respect.

There are many settings in the community where activities are conducted for promoting health or preventing disease in a population. These include myriad work sites, schools, health care program sites, and the community itself. Comprehensive health promotion activities at a work site consisting of a large, culturally diverse employee population may, for example, carry out employee health risk assessments (including screenings and appraisals) as well as establish and maintain an appropriate variety of educational programs, services, and activities to reduce or eliminate identified areas of health risk. In this setting, a work site must carry out culturally sensitive and effective interventions that meet the needs of the employees. This sensitivity must be carried over in the group as well as in one-to-one counseling or educational encounters. Awareness and sensitivity to cultural diversity, then, must be reflected in the planning, design, and implementation phases of such a complex undertaking.

HPDP efforts in multicultural populations are very demanding undertakings involving a combination of activities associated with achieving desired outcomes. There is, then, a need at the outset of this chapter to distinguish between the concepts of health promotion and health education and to briefly examine the implications and impact of culture at these two overlapping levels. This chapter also provides an overview of culture, particularly as cultural differences affect HPDP efforts, and discusses current paradigms that have been proposed to improve practitioner skills in working in multicultural health care settings (including the barriers to effective multicultural HPDP efforts).

HEALTH PROMOTION AND DISEASE PREVENTION

The terms *health promotion* and *disease prevention*, when used in this text, encompass a similar range of interests and concerns as expressed in the Joint Committee on Health Education Terminology (1991) report. The committee defined HPDP as "the aggregate of all purposeful activities designed to improve personal and public health through a combination of strategies, including the competent implementation of behavior change strategies, health education, health protection measures, risk factor detection, health enhancement, and health maintenance" (p. 102). Central to this conceptualization is the need to achieve different levels of outcomes (e.g., individual, family, group, organization, community) through a combination of health promotion and health education strategies and intervention activities. *Health promotion* has been defined as "any planned combination of educational, political, regulatory, and organizational supports for actions and conditions of living conducive to the health of individuals, groups, or communities" (Green & Kreuter, 1991, p. 432). Explicit in this definition is the need for interventions that respond to a broad level of community concern related to stimulating, establishing, and sustaining an appropriate combination of educational, organizational, and political supports needed to facilitate actions aimed at achieving desired community health outcomes. *Health education* has been defined as "any planned combination of learning experiences designed to predispose, enable, and reinforce voluntary behavior conducive to health in individuals, groups, or communities" (p. 432). Intervention efforts from this vantage point concentrate on facilitating the voluntary acquisition of specific health-related knowledge, attitudes, and practices associated with achieving specific health-related behavior changes. Health promotion emerged out of health education and designates a broader level of outcome than does health education. However, health education is considered a primary instrumentality for achieving health promotion outcomes. For example, the focus of health education interventions in a cervical cancer education and screening program targeting Latino women may be concerned with making educational programs more available and accessible to this group. Such programs can enable the target group to develop skills for carrying out defined voluntary screening behaviors related to reducing the risk of this life-threatening disease. The planning of interventions and related activities at this level, then, focuses on reaching only one target group among the many possible groups in need of specific educational programs. On the other hand, the planning of strategies and interventions at the health promotion level goes beyond a single cervical cancer education program focus. For example, interventions may focus on the need to establish and sustain a more accessible and equitably distributed system of women's health screening and education programs for enhancing the overall health of all poor and underserved women in that particular community. The complexity of health promotion program efforts requires a greater scope of coordination, participation, commitment, and expense than does the cervical cancer education and screening program aimed at a single target group. Indeed, many community participants representing a plethora of public, private, and voluntary agencies, organizations, and institutions will need to be involved in this endeavor. Health promotion efforts also may be conducted at a broader community level and may seek health and health-related behavior changes or social outcomes through ecological or environmental approaches intended to result in permanent structural changes or supports in the form of policies, regulations, and expanded access to resources affecting people where they work or live (Green & Kreuter, 1991; Green, Richard, & Potvin, 1996; McLeroy, Bibeau, Steckler, & Glanz, 1988; Richard, Potvin, Kishchuk, Prlic, & Green, 1996). Finally, whatever the focus of the HPDP effort is, it must of necessity include an awareness and sensitivity to culture and the many cultural differences reflected in the population to be targeted.

HEALTH PROMOTION AND CULTURE

What we see as science, the Indians see as magic. What we see as magic, they see as science. I don't find this a hopeless contradiction. If we can appreciate each other's views, we can see the whole picture more clearly. To heal ourselves or to help heal others, we need to reconnect magic and science, our right and left brains. (Hammerschlag, 1988, p. 14)

Promoting health and preventing disease is a noble goal that, to many, might seem straightforward, logical, and highly scientific. After all, we know about germ theory, diseases of lifestyle, medications, radiation, surgery, and other

Western approaches to preventing and/or diagnosing and treating health problems in the general population. What Hammerschlag (1988) is pointing out, however, is that this process is not always what it seems to be. Indeed, there are many different ways of perceiving, understanding, and approaching health and disease processes across cultural and ethnic groups with which health practitioners need to become better acquainted.

Cultural differences can and do present major barriers to effective health care intervention. This is especially true when health practitioners overlook, misinterpret, stereotype, or otherwise mishandle their encounters with those who might be viewed as different from them in their assessment, intervention, and evaluation planning processes.

There is not a day that goes by that we are not exposed to a variety of sights, sounds, and tastes reflecting influences coming at us from a multitude of sources including the news media, our work settings and contacts in the community, and the foods we choose to eat. From these, we form opinions, make judgments, and take actions perceived to be appropriate to the situations and settings in which we find ourselves. When these choices involve our efforts to improve the health of the many "publics" we encounter in our health care roles, our perceptions of how these publics relate and respond to our efforts may be colored by our own ethnocentric views of the world. In turn, we may be viewed by our publics in a similar manner. That is, whereas we might view a client as delusional if the individual comes to us for help and tells us that he or she has been seeing a traditional folk healer because the client believes that someone has put a hex on him or her, that client might view us as ignorant and inexperienced when we offer him or her counseling and medication as the treatment for the problem. In both cases, cultural beliefs and practices born out of years of enculturation and socialization in divergent worldviews have gotten in the way of the communication and treatment possibilities.

Brislin and Yoshida (1994) note that health care professionals' lack of knowledge about health beliefs and practices of culturally diverse groups and problems in intercultural communication has led to significant challenges in the provision of health care services to multicultural population groups. They also observed that the cultural diversity of the health care workforce itself can present problems that can disrupt the provision of services because of competing cultural values, beliefs, norms, and health practices in conflict with the traditional Western medical model. For example, Putsch (1985) describes a situation in which an elderly Navajo patient with mild senile dementia has returned for an outpatient visit after several long hospitalizations. He greets his physician in Navajo, shakes hands, and embraces him. He then turns to greet the nurse's aide, who will act as an interpreter, and extends his hand to her. She flees from the room visibly frightened. When later questioned about her behavior, she relates that she had been warned by her mother never to shake hands with gray-haired people because they might "witch you." She also notes that she knew about this man through her husband's family and that he was "no good" (p. 3346). In exploring cultural differences in more detail, a discussion of what we mean by *culture, ethnicity, acculturation,* and other related terms will help set the scene for how these may affect our ability to assess, plan, implement, and evaluate HPDP programs for a variety of multicultural population groups.

CULTURE

The term *culture* has been defined in many ways over the years and continues to be a concept that is hotly debated among anthropologists even today. In 1871, E. B. Tylor defined culture as "that complex whole which includes knowledge, belief, art, morals, law, custom, and any other capabilities and habits acquired by man as a member of society" (quoted in Bock, 1969, p. 17). Stein and Rowe (1989) define culture as "learned, nonrandom, systematic behavior that is transmitted from person to person and from generation to generation" (p. 4). Kagawa-Singer and Chung (1994) describe culture as "a tool which defines reality for its members" (p. 198) and note that within this perception of reality, the individual's purpose in life emerges through a process of socialization in which he or she learns the appropriate beliefs, values, and behaviors shared by society. Thus, culture is seen as both integrative and functional in that the beliefs and values transmitted to the individual provide a sense of identity as well as the rules the individual must follow to enable his or her culture to survive over time.

Slonim (1991) identifies five basic criteria for defining a culture: having a common pattern of communication, sound system, or language unique to the group; similarities in dietary preferences and preparation methods; common patterns of dress; predictable relationship and socialization patterns among members of the culture; and a common set of shared values and beliefs. No matter how it may be defined, culture can be seen as a dynamic template or framework a society uses to view, understand, behave, and pass on its culture to each succeeding generation. Culture helps to specify what behaviors are acceptable in any given society, when they are acceptable, and what is not acceptable. It also provides some guidance for dealing with the basic problems of life. Anderson and Fenichel (1989) caution, however, that this cultural framework is only a set of tendencies or possibilities for behavior and that individuals within any given society are essentially free to choose from all the available possibilities within this frame.

What do these issues have to do with HPDP? Consider, if you will, what possible barriers one might encounter if one were designing a health program for a community primarily composed of first-generation Hmong who were recent emigrants to the United States. Certainly, language could be a problem, but so too could the many cultural differences at nearly every level, from the basic nuances of communication to the significant differences in their worldview of what constitutes health and disease, from cause and prevention to treatment and cure. In fact, the Hmong health belief system is primarily based on the supernatural, and much of their traditional treatment is based on spiritual appeasement (Brainard & Zaharlick, 1989). A failure to understand and appreciate these "differences" would have serious implications for the success of any HPDP effort.

ETHNICITY

Ethnicity relates to the sense of identity an individual has based on common ancestry and national, religious, tribal, linguistic, or cultural origins. It generally implies that there are shared values, lifestyles, beliefs, and norms among those claiming affiliation to a specific ethnic group (Nunnally & Moy, 1989; Paniagua, 1994). Ethnic identity provides a sense of social belonging and loyalty for the individual and often is used by others outside the ethnic group to identify or label "differences" (Kagawa-Singer & Chung, 1994). Unfortunantly, ethnicity also is used to stereotype diversity in human populations and frequently leads to misunderstanding and/or distrust in all sorts of human interactions. In fact, the use of an ethnic label by someone outside the ethnic group may lead to a partial or complete shutdown of the learning curve for both parties to this process. For example, it can be seen that once the stereotype has been identified, one party (or both parties) often ceases to look beyond the stereotype to find out who each really is.

Slonim (1991) distingushes between culture and ethnicity but notes that they tend to overlap with respect to how they are defined and used. She notes that culture is concerned with symbolic generalities and universals about social and family groups, whereas ethnicity is concerned with one's sense of identification and belonging to a specific reference group within any given society. Ethnicity, then, helps shape the way in which we think, relate, feel, and behave within and outside our reference group and defines the patterns of behavior that provide an individual with a sense of belonging and continuity with his or her ethnic group over time.

Ethnicity is a word that often is used in the same breath as the word *race*. It is important, however, not to confuse ethnicity with race, the latter of which is a biological term used to describe ethnic groups on the basis of physical characteristics such as skin color or shape of the eyes, nose, and mouth (Montagu, 1964). Nelson and Jurmain (1988) note that *race* is an ancient concept that, in more recent times, has been used by scientists to place human populations into "racial" categories for purposes of classification. This form of classification, although convenient, ignores the issue of genetics, which is concerned with heredity and biological variation in all living things. Nelson and Jurmain regard the term *race* as a sociocultural concept rather than a biological one. Thus, people often are classified along racial lines regardless of their genetic traits, and these racial categories have long been used as a basis for promoting discrimination, hatred, and divisiveness among human groups all around the world. In this book, the term *race* is not used to describe the various multicultural groups discussed. The exceptions are where contributors report epidemiological data presented by federal, state, or local health agencies that gather and report health statistics using race as a variable. The terms *ethnic, multicultural,* and *culturally diverse* are preferred by the editors, who believe that these terms reflect a more accurate description of human populations. For the health practitioner, reframing the term *race* to *multicultural, ethnic,* or *culturally diverse* may serve to promote a greater sensitivity to the challenges, potentialities, and rewards of working with diverse cultural groups in HPDP activities.

ACCULTURATION AND ASSIMILATION

Acculturation is a term used to describe the degree to which an individual from one culture has given up the traits of that culture and adopted the traits of the dominant culture in which he or she now resides. Locke (1992) identifies four levels of acculturation: the "bicultural" individual, who can function equally well in his or her own culture and the dominant culture; the "traditional" individual, who holds on to most, if not all, of his or her traits from his culture of origin; the "marginal" individual, who seems not to have any real contact with traits from either culture; and the "acculturated" individual, who has given up most of his traits of origin for those of the dominant culture. Locke notes the importance of assessing the degree of acculturation when working in a multicultural setting because there is a natural tendency on the part of many culturally diverse individuals to resist acculturation. This resistance can lead to significant misunderstandings and the inability to establish meaningful and mutually beneficial working relationships between the health care practitioner and those he or she may be seeking to help or influence. An example might be the practitioner who encounters a Latina mother with a newborn who feels that the child is ill because of the *mal de ojo* (evil eye), that is, the belief that a sudden change in the emotional or physical health of an infant or young child is caused by the jealousy (or admiration) of a person with powerful eyes (De Paula, Lagana, & Gonzalez-Ramirez, 1996). A failure to recognize the significance of this problem for the patient, and the prescribing of a treatment that seems out of order in the mind of the mother, might result in her not following through or even engaging in an active way in the clinical encounter.

Assimilation is a closely related process to acculturation and is viewed as the social, economic, and political integration of a cultural group into a mainstream society to which it may have emigrated or otherwise been drawn (Casas & Casas, 1994). Generally, for assimilation to occur, there must be at least some minimal acculturation with respect to the language, values, laws, customs, and other major features of the dominant society. As Locke (1992) notes, however, there may be a genuine resistance and rejection of many of the values of the dominant culture with only a minimal level of cultural assimilation into mainstream society. Like acculturation, then, the level of an ethnically diverse client's assimilation into mainstream society might need to be assessed by a health practitioner to better understand and perhaps predict how well that person will accept and/or participate in HPDP recommendations and behaviors. One has only to pay a visit to areas of his or her city where recent immigrants have settled or where there is a long established but insular population characterized by the maintenance of the culture-of-origin behaviors, language, customs, food practices, and other social conventions that keeps its members isolated from mainstream society.

ASSESSMENT OF ACCULTURATION

The measurement of acculturation levels in the clinical setting has been the focus of a number of investigators studying a diversity of multicultural groups (Cuellar, Harris, & Jasso, 1980; Hoffman, Dana, & Bolton, 1985; Mendoza, 1989; Milliones, 1980; Ramirez, 1984; Smither & Rodriguez-Giegling, 1982; Suinn, Rickard-Figueroa, Lew, & Vigil, 1987). Paniagua (1994) comments on the variety of acculturation scales that can be used, depending on the ethnic group in which one is interested, and describes the Brief Acculturation Scale suggested by Burnam, Hough, Karno, Escobar, and Telles (1987). This scale employs three variables: generation in the United States, preferred language, and preferences for whom the individual most often socializes. The assumptions underlying these variables hold that (a) the longer the individual is exposed to the dominant culture or the younger the individual is at the time he or she enters this culture, the more the individual communicates in the language of the dominant culture, and (b) the more the individual socializes outside his or her primary cultural group, the more acculturated the individual is likely to become within the dominant society.

In general, assessment of acculturation has been used in clinical research settings rather than in health education or health promotion programs. Incorporating assessment of acculturation into the formative stages of HPDP program planning could prove quite valuable to the practitioner. For example, Ramirez, Cousins, Santos, and Supic (1986) devised and tested a four-item Media Acculturation Scale for use with Mexican Americans that focused on media and language preferences and were able to demonstrate that the instrument could identify subsets of their study group by their distinct media usage patterns and demographic characteristics. The ability to identify specific target group media preferences and sources is a much more efficacious way in which to reach one's audience than guessing at them and expending resources that might have little payoff. Marin and Gamba (1996) developed and validated a Bidimensional Acculturation Scale for use with Hispanics that they note works very well with Mexican Americans and Central Americans. They argue that acculturation is bidirectional in that as the individual is learning and taking on characteristics of the new culture, the individual is simultaneously doing the same within his or her culture of origin. Marin and Gamba note that understanding this process can help the practitioner be more aware of what Hispanics go through as they acculturate. It also would seem that the practitioner who is aware of where his or her target group is with respect to acculturation might be better able to tailor interventions that integrate health-promoting strategies into the learning that is occurring in both the culture of origin and the new culture as that acculturation process proceeds.

Although acculturation scales have been used primarily in research and clinical settings, what seems clear is that these scales have the potential to be included within needs assessment instruments used in the early stages of program plan development. For example, Castro, Cota, and Vega, in Chapter 7 of this book, present a scale they have found quite useful in a variety of settings working with Hispanics in health-promoting efforts. Thus, the use of acculturation scales for HPDP activities represents a relatively new and innovative tool the practitioner can employ to better understand the culturally diverse population groups with which he or she may be working.

ETHNOCENTRISM

Ethnocentrism is a concept that often plays a part in confusing an already difficult situation when working with ethnically diverse individuals or cultural groups. Ferguson (1991) describes ethnocentrism as the assumption an individual makes that his or her way of believing and behaving is the most preferable and correct one. She notes that often the health practitioner is unaware of his or her own ethnocentric behavior and that this can lead to dysfunctional treatment encounters. For example, the practitioner may directly or indirectly discount or ignore the client's cultural orientation and belief system, considering them unimportant, incorrect, or in conflict with the practitioner's own perceptions or worldview of how best to treat the client's health problem or issue. This can leave the client feeling angry, frustrated, and uncooperative. Of equal importance is the awareness that whereas the health care practitioner may be caught in his or her own ethnocentric dance, so too may the culturally diverse client the practitioner is serving. That is, the culturally diverse client may view the health professional as foreign, ignorant of illness or disease causality, or uneducated regarding proper social customs, forms of address, and nonverbal behaviors deemed appropriate by the client for dealing directly or indirectly with his or her health problem or concern. For example, Kramer (1992) notes that Native American elders find behaviors such as getting right down to business, speaking to strangers in a loud and confident tones, and frequently interrupting the speaker as intolerably rude. This, in turn, may lead to the withholding of important information the health professional needs for an accurate assessment and intervention plan.

One can argue, then, that there is a need for both the health professional and the culturally diverse client to develop a modicum of cultural sensitivity and cultural competence with respect to each other's values, beliefs, and health practices. This would be a major step forward in achieving a more balanced and respectful partnership in any health-related encounter.

CULTURAL COMPETENCE AND ETHNOSENSITIVITY

There is a large literature emerging from the social, behavioral, and health sciences promoting a philosophy of cross-cultural competence to which all persons working with multicultural groups should subscribe. Cross, Bazron, Dennis, and Isaac (1989), examining how health care agencies serve culturally diverse clients, view the process of cultural competence among these agencies on a continuum ranging from "culturally destructive" to "culturally competent." On this continuum, agencies that provide health care services may be seen as moving through a number of phases as they become increasingly more aware of how it is that they serve culturally diverse groups. Agencies that do not consider that culture is an important factor when delivering services can be seen as "culture blind," whereas agencies that accept, respect, and work with cultural differences can be seen as "culturally competent."

Campinha-Bacote (1994) defines cultural competence as "a process for effectively working within the cultural context of an individual or community from a diverse cultural or ethnic background" (pp. 1-2). She proposes a culturally competent model of health care that encompasses four levels: cultural awareness, cultural knowledge, cultural skill, and cultural encounter. *Cultural awareness* is concerned with the process of becoming more sensitive to differences manifest in culturally diverse clients and with the health professional's own biases and prejudices toward different cultural groups. *Cultural knowledge* is the process of gaining an understanding of different cultural groups including their beliefs, values, lifestyle practices, and ways of solving problems in their world. *Cultural skill* is concerned with the process of cultural assessment as the first step in designing treatment interventions for culturally diverse clients. Through this process, the practitioner seeks to identify his or her client's specific values, beliefs, and practices in an effort to include these in the planning of a mutually acceptable treatment plan. *Cultural encounter* is the final stage of the model and is the process of directly relating to culturally diverse groups in an effort to refine one's knowledge and skills for working in culturally diverse settings. The model reflects a process that is ongoing in that the health professional always should be on a continuous quest to increase and improve his or her abilities to work in a variety of cross-cultural settings.

In concert with cultural competence is the concept of *ethnosensitivity,* which is concerned with the process of becoming more sensitive and respecting of cross-cultural differences. Borkan and Neher (1991) describe a developmental model of ethnosensitivity that can be used to help train physicians to improve their cross-cultural communication and practice skills. Their model proposes a seven-stage developmental continuum that can be used to assess a health care provider's ethnosensitivity. These stages consist of fear or mistrust of different cultural groups, denial of cultural differences, feelings of superiority over other cultural groups, minimization of cultural differences, cultural relativism (acceptance and respect for differences), empathy, and cultural integration in which the practitioner becomes a multicultural person able to relate well to several different cultural groups. For example, once the developmental stage is identified, specific interventions can be tailored to help the physician move forward in the learning process. This is only one of a number of models being used in medical school and hospital-based training programs that hold promise for improving the cross-cultural skills of health care providers. For those interested readers, the following brief exercise is offered as a way in which to begin looking at one's own ethnosensitivities. Consider the last time you saw or interacted with someone you categorized as representing a particular ethnic group. How did you come to categorize that individual as representing a particular ethnic group? How have you come to your knowledge of the specific characteristics you employed to categorize that individual? How accurate do you think these characteristics are with respect to that specific individual? What do you actually know or not know about that specific individual in terms of his or her cultural heritage, lifestyle, and the like? What more did you seek to learn about that individual? How would you feel knowing that others may be categorizing you in similar ways? Your honest answers to these questions may provide a better understanding of how easy it is to stereotype or otherwise categorize people about whom you know little. Often, these categorizations are quite inaccurate and insensitive. As noted earlier, once they are employed, they generally decrease one's interest in learning much more about a particular individual or group.

The need to develop an awareness of one's own interpersonal and communication style is of equal importance in becoming competent and sensitive to cultural differences. These areas have been identified by a number of investigators as potential barriers to working with culturally diverse population groups. Bell and Evans (1981) discuss the need for the practitioner to become aware of the interpersonal style he or she is operating from when dealing with persons from other cultures. They note five interpersonal styles: overt hostility, covert prejudice, cultural ignorance, color blindness, and cultural liberation. The first four of these styles fail to respect or openly consider cultural differences in the health care consultation, whereas cultural liberation reflects a lack of fear of cultural differences, awareness of one's own attitudes toward different cultural groups, acceptance and encouragement of the client's expressions regarding the client's feelings about his or her ethnicity, and the ability to use these feelings as shared learning experiences.

It is easy for practitioners to quote models and recommendations, and it is even easier to pay "lip service" to their value in becoming more culturally competent and sensitive. However, if we are to improve our skills in these areas, then we must be willing to step out of our current frames of reference and take the risk of discovering our own biases and stereotypes and to open ourselves up to new and perhaps quite divergent points of view about the world in which we live. In taking these steps, we also will need to consider the challenge of learning to communicate across cultures.

CROSS-CULTURAL COMMUNICATION

Brislin and Yoshida (1994) comment that the typical Western medical model for communication in the health care encounter is the direct question-and-answer method, which seeks to quickly establish the facts of the case and often relies on the use of negative and double-negative questions, for example, "You don't want to get heart disease, do you?" For the culturally diverse individual (or family), this approach to the communication process might be seen as cold and too direct or otherwise in conflict with his or her more traditional beliefs, values, and ways of seeking, communicating, and receiving health care. For example, Kramer (1992) notes that there are significant differences in how Native Americans perceive the initial visit with a health care provider. They might expect the initial visit to begin with a brief light handshake rather than the typical firm handshake of the Westerner, which is seen as a sign of aggressiveness. Furthermore, behaviors such as staring, excessive eye contact, and direct questioning are considered rude and an invasion of privacy and dignity.

Northouse and Northouse (1992) define communication as a process of information sharing in which those involved in the communication share a common set of rules. These rules may prescribe how the communication will take place, through what channels, when it will occur, and even how feedback may or may not be provided between the message communicator and the message receiver. For example, in a traditional Japanese family, it is often the head of the household who will be the primary individual communicating with the health care practitioner in the event a family member needs medical care. Likewise, the head of the household is the one who will make the decisions about treatment options and even what the ill family member should be told about his or her medical condition. Northouse and Northouse further divide communication into two subsets: human communication and health communication. Human communication relates to the interactions between and among people through the use of common symbols and language. Health communication is human communication primarily concerned with health-related interactions and processes. Here the common symbols and language may be obscured by special professional jargon including the use of medical terms to describe the condition and treatment options available to a client or patient. All of these communication processes are dynamic, ongoing, and ever changing transactions that involve human feelings, attitudes, knowledge, and behavior. Thus, in an interaction between two or more individuals representing divergent cultural orientations and where different rules might govern the communication process, the opportunity for miscommunication is significant.

A review of the many models of interpersonal communication advanced over the past 40 to 50 years suggests that there are a variety of factors affecting communication in general and in cross-cultural encounters specifically. These factors include the communication skills, attitudes, knowledge, social systems, and culture of both the sender and receiver of communication transactions; the framing of the communication with respect to structure, content, and coding; the communication channel that will involve one or more of the five senses; "noise," which refers to auditory, perceptual, or psychological factors that can affect the communication anywhere along the channel; and feedback mechanisms, which ensure that all parties to the communication transaction heard and understood the communication as it was intended. In addition, human interaction factors including dominance-submission or love-hate relationships, communication transactions, and the contexts in which they occur have been identified as important to understanding and improving the communication process (Brislin & Yoshida, 1994; Kreps & Kunimoto, 1994; Northouse & Northouse, 1992).

Given the incredible diversity of multicultural populations in the world today, the potential for miscommunication in any human encounter is staggering.

For the health professional seeking to develop an increased sense of cultural competence and sensitivity as well as improved communication skills, the task might seem daunting. However, patience and persistence are the keys to unlocking these skills, and many recommendations have been posited in the literature for improving the entire cross-cultural experience in health care. Among these are a series of recommendations made by Kreps and Kunimoto (1994). They urge that health professionals develop a genuine interest in and respect for cultural differences including the development of communication attitudes and skills that demonstrate an appreciation for and sensitivity to cultural differences. This process can begin by reading about other cultural groups, learning a new language, attending multicultural events, or spending time in communities representative of the cultural or ethnic group of interest. Kreps and Kunimoto also recommend that health professionals become aware of the many different interpretations of reality that exist in the world, especially where health and health care issues are concerned. Here again, a patient's interpretation of what might be causing his or her problem (e.g., a witch, a ghost, fate) might run totally counter to what the health care professional thinks is going on. Reading about different cultures and talking with willing members of the group of interest can provide valuable insights into these multiple realities. Finally, the practitioner should be ready and willing to endure uncertainty and discomfort when working in cross-cultural health care settings. It is, after all, those times when we are most uncomfortable that we have the greatest opportunity for learning and growth. We just have to be open to that possibility.

BARRIERS TO MULTICULTURAL HEALTH PROMOTION AND DISEASE PREVENTION

As is no doubt evident to the reader by this time, there are a multitude of factors that can act as barriers or impediments to successful HPDP efforts. For purposes of this discussion, a *barrier* is defined as any obstacle that might interfere with the ability of the health practitioner or his or her culturally diverse client (to whom the practitioner is intending to provide interventions) to be able to fully achieve the intended assessment, intervention, or evaluation objectives. The range of potential barriers is extensive and not necessarily easily categorized, although some attempt will be made here to cluster some of these variables for purposes of discussion. Figure 1.1 presents a partial listing of demographic, cultural, and health care systems barriers that have been identified in the literature as having the potential to impede HPDP efforts.

As can be seen in Figure 1.1, there are a variety of demographic factors that can play a role in impeding multicultural health-promoting efforts, and no doubt the reader can add many more items to this list. It is important to recognize that many of the barriers identified heretofore will be mediated by the degree of

Demographic Barrier	Cultural Barrier	Health Care System Barrier
Age	Age	Access to care
Gender	Gender, class, and family dynamics	Insurance or other financial resources
Ethnicity	Worldview/perceptions of life	
Primary language spoken	Time orientation	Orientation to preventive health services
Religion	Primary language spoken	Perceptions of need for health care services
Educational level and literacy level	Religious beliefs and practices	Ignorance and/or distrust of Western medical practices and procedures
Occupation, income, and health insurance	Social customs, values, and norms	Cultural insensitivity and competence
Area of residence	Traditional health beliefs and practices	Western vs. folk health beliefs and practices
Transportation	Dietary preferences and practices	Poor doctor-patient communications
Time and/or generation in the United States	Communication patterns and customs	Lack of bilingual and bicultural staff

Figure 1.1   Potential Barriers to Health Promotion and Disease Prevention

acculturation and assimilation of the client being targeted for health promotion interventions, and it is incumbent on the health practitioner to assess these levels before implementing programs. Although many of these barriers are fairly self-explanatory, a quick look at several of these might help to highlight the importance of demographics when working with or planning health promotion programs and services for the culturally diverse. For example, gender may become an issue when seeking to provide health promotion services such as screening mammography. Mo (1992) describes the problems in providing this type of service to Chinese women and notes that cultural values associated with modesty and sexuality, coupled with institutional barriers such as the unavailability of educational materials written in Chinese and a lack of female physicians, played a significant role in the low number of women in her study who accessed breast health services. Ohmans, Garrett, and Treichel (1996) recognize that social class can be a significant barrier, particularly for new immigrants whose social status or class distinction may have been radically altered since leaving their country of origin. They caution that we should be particularly careful with health education and not assume that immigrant or refugee status equates with poverty or lack of education. Kramer (1992) comments that older Native Americans report a fear of non-Native American health professionals, expect to be treated unfairly by them, and anticipate negative contact experiences when they do encounter these health professionals. Uba (1992) reports that many Southeast Asians have difficulties in accessing health care services (even if they know about them) because of language difficulties associated with making appointments or even understanding the process. Furthermore, they often lack health insurance benefits because many of these people are poor and are working in low-paying jobs. Geographic factors including a lack of hospitals or private physician offices in their communities, as well as difficulties in accessing public transportation or getting a driver's license, also complicate their access problems. By now, the reader may have noticed how these demographic factors cross over into the other categories identified in Figure 1.1. There are, in fact, many shades of gray to be considered when looking at barriers, and this makes the process that much more difficult to understand.

Cultural barriers include a number of factors of importance to the HPDP process. Like the demographic barriers, some of these seem readily understandable, whereas others need clarification. For example, Uba (1992) notes that many Southeast Asians are reluctant to seek health care services because of their attitudes regarding the nature of life and the inevitability of suffering. She comments that suffering and illness are seen as an unavoidable part of life, so seeking health care services early may be considered inappropriate. She cites the Hmong as an example of a cultural group that believes that life is predetermined, so life-saving medical intervention is worthless. With respect to communication patterns and customs, Ramakrishna and Weiss (1992) describe nonverbal communication patterns among East Indian patients where the patient might not know how to respond to the American physician's social smiles or might use lateral motions of the head to indicate a positive affirmation. In India, smiles are exchanged only between social equals, and East Indians use head shaking to denote *yes,* which might confuse a Western physician.

Health beliefs and practices are the subject of Chapter 2, but a few brief comments might be of value here. Uba (1992) comments that many Southeast Asians view disease and illness etiology as arising from a variety of possible sources. These include organic problems, an imbalance between the "yin" and "yang," an obstruction of chi (life energy), failure to be in harmony with nature, a curse from an offended spirit, and a punishment for immoral behavior. Riser and Mazur (1995) discuss folk illnesses among Hispanics and comment that the most common ailment in their study population was *mal ojo.* This folk illness was attributed to someone with "strong eyes" looking at a child (often unintentionally). The result of this "look" was felt to heat up the child's blood and lead to inconsolable crying, fever, diarrhea, vomiting, and gassy stomach. They also described *empacho,* a folk illness attributed to certain foods such as swallowed gum, grape skins, and poorly mixed powdered milk or formula that sticks in the intestines. Obviously, there are significant differences in perception of disease causality and treatment that must be understood and worked with if health-promoting efforts are to be effective. In addition, there are a variety of common but divergent values among multicultural groups that the health promotion practitioner might find to be useful in his or her practice efforts. Schilling and Brannon (1986) developed a list of these common values, which are presented in Figure 1.2.

Anglo-American	Other Ethnocultural Groups
Mastery over nature	Harmony with nature
Personal control over the environment	Fate
Doing/activity	Being
Time dominates	Personal interaction dominates
Human equality	Hierarchy/rank/status
Individualism/privacy	Group welfare
Youth	Elders
Self-help	Birthright inheritance
Competition	Cooperation
Future orientation	Past or present orientation
Informality	Formality
Directness/openness/honesty	Indirectness/ritual/"face"
Practicality/efficiency	Idealism
Materialism	Spiritualism/detachment

Figure 1.2   Comparison of Common Values From Dominant and Nondominant Perspectives
SOURCE: Adapted from Schilling and Brannon (1986).

It is obvious that the practitioner engaged in health promotion efforts is likely to be confronted by any number of divergent viewpoints regarding the nature of life and social interaction. As May (1992) notes, this will require the practitioner to be flexible in his or her design of programs, policies, and services to meet the needs and concerns of the diverse cultural groups he or she is likely to encounter.

Health care system variables present yet another level of potential barriers that the health promotion practitioner will need to be aware of when working in multicultural contexts. As Figure 1.1 demonstrates, access to health care services, access to insurance or financial resources, and other demographics play a role in health care systems barriers, but as Mull (1993) comments, there are a number of other systems issues that need to be considered. For example, the concept of preventive health is not one that is well known or understood among peoples from developing countries. Although they might know about immunization, the rationale for Pap smears, mammography, and other screening procedures might elude them. In fact, they might not even perceive that there is a need for preventive or other health care services unless more traditional methods of care have been found to be ineffective in dealing with a health issue or problem. Fear of Western medical procedures including common practices such as drawing blood also can present as a barrier. Among people from Third World countries, the fear of loss of blood is quite real. They believe that this blood cannot be replaced and will result in weakening the body. Uba (1992) comments that among Southeast Asians such as rural Cambodians, there is a strong distrust of Western medicine that often is associated with death. This attitude can be traced to accessing health care services late in the course of an illness, often resulting in death at the point the patient enters the health care system for treatment. Uba also notes that services such as dietary counseling that discuss typical Western food choices will be considered irrelevant or inappropriate by many whose cultural or ethnic preferences conflict with the recommendations they may be given.

Given the number of potential barriers that may be encountered in HPDP efforts, what can be done to help overcome some of these impediments?

STRATEGIES TO OVERCOME BARRIERS

As noted in earlier sections of this chapter, improving one's cultural competence and sensitivity to differences can be a significant step forward in overcoming many of the problems that have been identified in this chapter. This includes learning about and practicing cross-cultural communication skills *and* adding questions to the usual assessment tools that seek to better understand the target group's orientation toward health, disease, and folk treatment practices; acculturation levels; and other related assessment items. (See Chapter 26 for questions and strategies that can be incorporated into the assessment process.) In addition, taking more time to explain Western concepts of health, disease, prevention, and treatment in terms that are culturally understandable and relevant to the target group, designing and employing educational materials that are relevant and culturally appropriate to the target group, using well-trained bilingual/bicultural staff, employing indigenous health workers when working in and with diverse multicultural communities, and seeking ways in which to improve access to services for multicultural populations are but a few strategies that can be used to overcome barriers to HPDP efforts.

CHAPTER SUMMARY

The United States often has been described as a melting pot in which immigrants arrive, become acculturated, and assimilate into American society and culture. As May (1992) points out, however, this blending is a very inaccurate and potentially destructive way in which to view American culture and society. A more accurate metaphor would be to view America as a rich and complex tapestry of colors, backgrounds, and interests. Having an understanding of this tapestry and its implications on health and disease patterns can enable the health promotion practitioner to be much more effective in reducing morbidity and mortality among the many multicultural population groups residing in the United States and elsewhere in the world.

This chapter has not sought to provide a comprehensive overview of culture; rather, it has sought to provide insights into the complex nature of culture with respect to the potential impact of cultural diversity on HPDP efforts. Culture was defined as a template or framework that a society uses to make sense of and to organize its world. A variety of terms including *acculturation, assimilation, ethnocentrism, cultural competence, ethnosensitivity,* and *cross-cultural communications* were defined and discussed to make overt the implications of these factors on HPDP practices. Barriers to promoting health among multicultural populations were described, and a number of recommendations were made for improving the efficacy of health-promoting efforts when working with multicultural population groups.

REFERENCES

Anderson, P. P., & Fenichel, E. S. (1989). *Serving culturally diverse families of infants and toddlers with disabilities.* Washington, DC: National Center for Clinical Infant Programs.

Bell, P., & Evans, J. (1981). *Counseling the black client.* Center City, MN: Hazelden Education Materials.

Bock, P. K. (1969). *Modern cultural anthropology: An introduction.* New York: Knopf.

Borkan, J., & Neher, J. (1991). A developmental model of ethnosensitivity in family practice training. *Family Medicine, 23,* 212-217.

Brainard, J., & Zaharlick, A. (1989). Changing health beliefs and behaviors of resettled Laotion refugees: Ethnic variation in adaptation. *Social Science and Medicine, 29,* 845-852.

Brislin, R. W., & Yoshida, T. (Eds.). (1994). *Improving intercultural interactions: Modules for cross-cultural training programs.* Thousand Oaks, CA: Sage.

Burnam, M. A., Hough, R. L., Karno, M., Escobar, J. I., & Telles, C. A. (1987). Acculturation and lifetime prevalence of psychiatric disorders among Mexican Americans in Los Angeles. *Journal of Health and Social Behavior, 28,* 89-102.

Campinha-Bacote, J. (1994). Cultural competence in psychiatric mental health nursing: A conceptual model. *Nursing Clinics of North America, 29*(1), 1-8.

Casas, J. M., & Casas, A. (1994). The acculturation process and implications for educational services. In A. C. Matiella (Ed.), *The multicultural challenge in health education.* Santa Cruz: ETR Associates.

Cross, T. L., Bazron, B., Dennis, K. W., & Isaac, M. R. (1989). *Towards a culturally competent system of care.* Washington, DC: Georgetown University Child Development Center, CASSP Technical Assistance Center.

Cuellar, I., Harris, L. C., & Jasso, R. (1980). An acculturation scale for Mexican American normal and clinical populations. *Hispanic Journal of Behavioral Sciences, 2,* 199-217.

De Paula, D., Lagana, K., & Gonzalez-Ramirez, L. (1996). Mexican Americans. In J. G. Lipson, S. L. Dibble, & P. A. Minarik (Eds.), *Culture and nursing care: A pocket guide.* San Francisco: UCSF Nursing Press.

Ferguson, B. (1991). Concepts, models and theories for immigrant health care. In B. Ferguson & E. Browne (Eds.), *Health care and immigrants: A guide to the helping professions.* Sydney, Australia: MacLennan & Petty.

Green, L. W., & Kreuter, M. W. (1991). *Health promotion planning: An educational and environmental approach.* Mountain View, CA: Mayfield.

Green, L. W., Richard, L., & Potvin, L. (1996). Ecological foundations of health promotion. *American Journal of Health Promotion, 10,* 270-281.

Hammerschlag, C. A. (1988). *The dancing healers: A doctor's journey of healing with Native Americans.* San Francisco: Harper.

Hoffman, T., Dana, R., & Bolton, B. (1985). Measured acculturation and MMPI-168 performance of Native American adults. *Journal of Cross-Cultural Psychology, 16,* 243-256.

Joint Committee on Health Education Terminology. (1991). Report of the 1990 Joint Committee on Health Education Terminology. *Journal of Health Education, 22,* 97-108.

Kagawa-Singer, M., & Chung, R. (1994). A paradigm for culturally based care in ethnic minority populations. *Journal of Community Psychology, 22,* 192-208.

Kramer, B. J. (1992). Health and aging of urban American Indians. *Western Journal of Medicine, 9*(157), 281-285. (Special issue)

Kreps, G. L., & Kunimoto, E. N. (1994). *Effective communication in multicultural health care settings.* Thousand Oaks, CA: Sage.

Locke, D. C. (1992). *Increasing multicultural understanding: A comprehensive model.* Newbury Park, CA: Sage.

Marin, G., & Gamba, R. (1996). A new measurement of acculturation for Hispanics: The Bidirectional Acculturation Scale for Hispanics (BAS). *Hispanic Journal of Behavioral Sciences, 18,* 297-316.

May, J. (1992). Working with diverse families: Building culturally competent systems of health care delivery. *Journal of Rheumatology, 19*(33), 46-48.

McLeroy, K. R., Bibeau, D., Steckler, A., & Glanz, K. (1988). An ecological perspective on health promotion programs. *Health Education Quarterly, 15,* 351-377.

Mendoza, R. H. (1989). An empirical scale to measure type and degree of acculturation in Mexican-American adolescents and adults. *Journal of Cross-Cultural Psychology, 20,* 372-385.

Milliones, J. (1980). Construction of a black consciousness measure: Psychotherapeutic implications. *Psychotherapy: Theory, Research and Practice, 17,* 175-182.

Mo, B. (1992). Modesty, sexuality, and breast health in Chinese-American women. *Western Journal of Medicine, 9*(157), 260-264. (Special issue)

Montague, A. (Ed.). (1964). *The concept of race.* London: Collier Books.

Mull, J. (1993). Cross-cultural communication in the physician's office. *Western Journal of Medicine, 159,* 609-613.

Nelson, H., & Jurmain, R. (1988). *Introduction to physical anthropology* (4th ed.). St. Paul, MN: West.

Northouse, P. G., & Northouse, L. L. (1992). *Health communications: Strategies for health professionals* (2nd ed.). Norwalk, CT: Appleton & Lange.

Nunnally, E., & Moy, C. (1989). *Communication basics for health service professionals.* Newbury Park, CA: Sage.

Ohmans, P., Garrett, C., & Treichel, C. (1996). Cultural barriers to health care for refugees and immigrants: Providers' perceptions. *Minnesota Medicine, 5*(79), 26-30.

Paniagua, F. A. (1994). *Assessing and treating culturally diverse clients: A practical guide.* Thousand Oaks, CA: Sage.

Putsch, R. W., III. (1985). Cross-cultural communication: The special case of interpreters in health care. *Journal of the American Medical Association, 254,* 3344-3348.

Ramakrishna, J., & Weiss, M. G. (1992). Health, illness, and immigration: East Indians in the United States. *Western Journal of Medicine, 9*(157), 265-270. (Special issue)

Ramirez, A. G., Cousins, J. H., Santos, Y., & Supic, J. D. (1986). A media-based acculturation scale for Mexican-Americans: Application to public health programs. *Family and Community Health, 9*(3), 63-71.

Ramirez, M. (1984). Assessing and understanding biculturalism-multiculturalism in Mexican-American adults. In J. L. Martinez & R. H. Mendoza (Eds.), *Chicano psychology.* Orlando, FL: Academic Press.

Richard, L., Potvin, L., Kishchuk, N., Prlic, H., & Green, L. W. (1996). Assessment of the ecological approach in health promotion programs. *American Journal of Health Promotion, 10,* 318-328.

Riser, A., & Mazur, L. (1995). Use of folk remedies in a Hispanic population. *Archives of Pediatric and Adolescent Medicine, 149,* 978-981.

Schilling, B., & Brannon, E. (1986). *Strategies for working with culturally diverse communities and clients.* Bethesda, MD: Association for the Care of Children's Health, Maternal and Child Health Bureau.

Slonim, M. (1991). *Children, culture, and ethnicity: Evaluating and understanding the impact.* New York: Garland.

Smither, R., & Rodriguez-Giegling, M. (1982). Personality, demographics, and acculturation of Vietnamese and Nicaraguan refugees to the United States. *International Journal of Psychology, 17,* 19-25.

Stein, P. L., & Rowe, B. M. (1989). *Physical anthropology* (4th ed.). New York: McGraw-Hill.

Suinn, R. M., Rickard-Figueroa, K., Lew, S., & Vigil, S. (1987). The Suinn-Lew Asian Self-Identity Acculturation Scale: An initial report. *Educational and Psychological Measurement, 47,* 401-407.

Uba, L. (1992). Cultural barriers to health care for Southeast Asian refugees. *Public Health Reports, 107,* 545-548.

2

Cross-Cultural Concepts of Health and Disease

ROBERT M. HUFF

Health is one consequence of the balance between the "yin" and "yang" energy forces that rule the world, and an imbalance between these two forces can result in illness (Seidel, Ball, Dains, & Benedict, 1995). So begins one explanation for health and disease that characterizes traditional Chinese beliefs about disease causation. As this explanation implies, the relationship of culture to health beliefs and practices is highly complex, dynamic, and interactive. Often, these explanations involve family, community, and/or supernatural agents in both cause, effect, placation, and treatment rituals to prevent, control, or cure illness across a variety of multicultural groups. By contrast, the Western biomedical model explains illness in terms of the presenting pathophysiology. Sickness often is reduced to disease, and the focus is on the body rather than on the whole person within the context of his or her culture.

This chapter seeks to expand on the concept of culture presented in the previous chapter but with a focus on health-related cultural concepts as defined by the "explanatory models" that different multicultural groups use to describe and make sense of health, illness, and disease. A brief discussion of health beliefs associated with traditional peoples living in the United States and elsewhere is included. The author recognizes that trying to cover these issues in a few pages is an impossible task but hopes that the brief sketches provided will present a glimpse of some of the traditional concepts of health and disease held by those peoples who are being addressed in this book.

CONCEPTS OF HEALTH AND DISEASE

Landrine and Klonoff (1992) note that many multicultural groups in the world view health and illness as fluid and continuous manifestations of the long-term and changing relationships and dysfunctions the individual has with his or her family, community, and environment. They observe that the health concepts of many of these cultural groups involve macrolevel, interpersonal, and supernatural agents of illness and disease causality. Many of those holding these views may choose not to seek Western medical treatment procedures because they do not view their illnesses or diseases as coming from within themselves. In fact, Dimou (1995) observes that among many Eastern cultures and other cultures in the developing world, the locus of control for disease causality often is centered outside the individual, whereas in Western cultures, the locus of control tends to be more internally oriented. That is, in Eastern cultures, the illness or disease may be perceived as retribution coming from an angry spirit for some transgression or violation of one's role within his or her family or social group rather than recognizing that one's illness may be due to his or her lifestyle choices and associated behaviors over which the person has some control. Landrine and Klonoff (1992) note that if the more traditionally entrenched person does seek Western medical treatment, he or she might be labeled as a *poor historian,* a *difficult patient,* or a mentally ill *somaticizer* because this person cannot provide or describe his or her symptoms in precise terms that the Western medical practitioner can readily treat. This person also might not follow through with the treatment recommendation because he or she perceives the medical encounter as a negative, and perhaps even hostile, experience.

Kleinman (1980) describes a process for explicitly distinguishing the explanations that individual patients and health care practitioners have about health and disease causality. He calls these "explanatory models" and defines them as "the notions about an episode of sickness and its treatment that are employed by all those engaged in the clinical process" (p. 105). He comments that the explanatory models of patients and health practitioners are important in helping us to understand how each player perceives, understands, and treats illness and can help illuminate the real or potential problems that might occur in a clinical or other health care communication encounter. Kleinman also distinguishes explanatory models from general beliefs about sickness and health care, noting that general health beliefs are part of the health ideology of the patient, whereas explanatory models, although they draw from the basic health ideology, are much more specific to a particular episode of an illness. He distinguishes five major concerns that explanatory models seek to answer for illness episodes. These include the etiology, the time and mode of onset of symptoms, the pathophysiology of the illness, and the course of the illness including severity, sick role behaviors, and treatment. Kleinman comments that Western health care practitioner models tend to answer all or most of these questions, whereas patient or family models address only the most important concerns for them. Paying attention to these patient explanations can help to disclose the significance of the illness for the patient (or family) including the desired treatment goals.

Pachter (1994) notes that most clinical encounters can be viewed as an interaction between two cultures, that is, the culture of the patient and the culture of medicine. Both are likely to have divergent perceptions, knowledge, attitudes, behaviors, and communication styles relative to the illness or health issue as a result of their explanatory models of health, disease, causality, and treatment. An individual's model is generally a conglomeration of his or her ethnocultural beliefs and values; personal beliefs, values, and behaviors; and understanding of bio-medical concepts. In fact, Pachter suggests that there is a range or spectrum of illness beliefs, with one end encompassing illnesses defined within the Western biomedical model. Here also can be found lay/popular explanatory models, which are more closely aligned with Western models (e.g., cancer as an abnormal growth). In this case, the sickness episode is acknowledged by both systems, and there is high potential for a good exchange of ideas between the systems with regard to mutually acceptable treatment options. In the middle of this spectrum are other illness categories in which the incompatibility between lay/popular beliefs and biomedical beliefs is much wider (e.g., high blood pressure caused by too much blood). On the far end of the spectrum can be found the illness explanations, which are the most widely discrepant between the lay/popular beliefs and the biomedical model. These illnesses often are classified as folk illnesses commonly recognized or associated with specific cultural groups such as the illness "empacho" (e.g., food sticking to the inside of the stomach or intestines) among Latino population groups. Obviously, the more widely disparate the differences between the biomedical model and the lay/popular explana-tory model, the greater the potential for encountering resistance to Western medical assessment, treatment, and adherence to treatment recommendations. Thus, it would seem appropriate for the health promoter to take the time in his or her initial needs assessment efforts to explore the explanatory models of the cultural or ethnic group with which the health promoter will be working. This can serve to uncover potential barriers to the programs and services the health promoter is planning and even to suggest intervention approaches more accept-able to his or her target audience.

TRADITIONAL CONCEPTS OF ILLNESS CAUSALITY

Helman (1984) describes folk illnesses as syndromes that individuals from particular cultural groups claim to have and from which they define the etiology, diagnostic procedures, prevention methods, and traditional healing/curing prac-tices. He notes that folk illnesses are more than just a cluster of signs and symptoms the patient experiences; they also have symbolic meaning to the individual and culture from which the folk illness arises. These meanings may be moral, social, or psychological, and they often link the illness of the patient to changes in the natural world or the workings of the supernatural realm. Helman offers a caveat to all those working with different cultural groups. He ob-serves that folk illnesses can be, and often are, learned. For example, the child who sees and learns to respond to a range of illness symptoms (e.g., physical, social, emotional) in culturally patterned ways will, over time, come to exhibit these in response to specific episodes of illness. Thus, the health practitioner working with diverse cultural groups must make himself or herself aware of how these groups acquire, display, and typically define and treat their traditional folk illnesses.

A number of researchers (Buchwald, Panwala, & Hooton, 1992; Helman, 1984; Jack, Harrison, & Airhihenbuwa, 1994; Landrine & Klonoff, 1992; Seidel et al., 1995; Spector, 1991; Uba, 1992) have sought to place illness causality into a series of categories as a way of helping to make sense of and classify lay theories of illness. Helman (1984) describes four categories: the patient, the natural world, the social world, and the supernatural world. He notes that lay illness explanatory models may arise from any one or combination of these. At the patient level, illness may result from malfunctions of the body as a result of factors such as diet or behavior over which the person has some control. This is a common explanation used in Western societies, where illnesses associated with health behaviors such as smoking, drinking, and lack of exercise are commonly cited as personal choices the individual makes and for which he or she might have to pay a health-related price over time. This category also recognizes hereditary, social, economic, and other personality factors that may play a role in illness causality and response. Here it is important to determine the individual's locus of control to determine whether the person will take responsibility for his or her own health or see it as lying outside of the person.

The natural world includes both animate and inanimate factors thought to cause illness. For example, causality might be attributed to microorganisms such as bacteria or viruses (e.g., flu, tuberculosis), parasitic infections such as pinworms, and injuries caused by animals, birds, or fish. Other factors include environmental irritants such as smog, pollens, and poisons; natural disasters where physical injury may occur such as earthquakes, floods, and fires; and climatic conditions such as extremes of heat, cold, wind, rain, or snow.

The social world is concerned with interpersonal conflicts that include physical injuries inflicted by people on others (i.e., personal assaults resulting from gang violence, war, or other similar causes). Stresses resulting from conflicts with family, friends, or employment also are part of this social causality. In more traditional non-Western cultures, illness often is ascribed to sorcery or witchcraft in which certain people have the power to cast spells, create potions, or carry out rituals that can result in illness or death for individuals against whom the sorcerer or witch has a personal vendetta.

The supernatural world includes ancestral and other spirits and gods who can directly intercede in human life and cause personal difficulties, illness, and death. Illnesses inflicted from the supernatural world include things such as spirit possessions, spirit aggression, and soul loss as retribution for behavioral lapses (e.g., sinful behavior such as getting drunk, offending a particular ancestor's spirit, or breaking a particular social taboo). Where supernatural causes of illness are suspected, neither traditional home remedies nor a Western medical practitioner are considered useful in treating and curing the illness. Such situations call for repentance, prayer, and intercession of a shaman, priest, or other spiritual adviser or healer. As Helman (1984) observes, however, most cases of lay illness have multiple causalities and may require several different approaches to diagnosis, treatment, and cure. For the health promoter, an awareness of how the cultural or ethnic group perceives and defines disease causality and the appropriate treatment interventions can help him or her to tailor programs, services, and/or medical treatment recommendations that consider and incorporate these cultural differences in the health promoter's planning and intervention processes.

TRADITIONAL MODELS OF HEALTH CARE DELIVERY

Folk illnesses, which are perceived to arise from a variety of causes, often require the services of a folk healer who may be a local curandero, shaman, native healer, spiritualist, root doctor, or other specialized healer. These traditional healers are thought to be capable of prescribing specific teas, ointments, and compresses to cure illness. They also may be consulted to carry out spiritual rituals and ceremonies or other magical practices to promote health and prevent or cure disease. Murray and Rubel (1992) discuss practices that fall under the rubric of alternative medicine and identify five categories of practitioners who may be found practicing alternative medicine. The first category is the "spiritual and psychological" practitioners including religious faith healers, psychics, and mystics who may use a variety of psychological techniques to heal or cure their patients. The second category is "nutritional" and includes those persons who use herbal remedies and special diets for healing. The third category includes "drug and biological" specialists who employ various chemicals, drugs, and vaccines to cure or prevent disease. The fourth category includes those who employ treatment with physical forces and devices (e.g., chiropractors, massage therapists). The fifth category includes those who use other techniques that do not seem to fit the other categories of healers (e.g., aroma therapists, iridologists). The uses of these traditional or alternative models of health care delivery are widely varied and may come into conflict with Western models of health care practice. An understanding of these differences may help the health promoter be more sensitive to the special beliefs and practices of his or her target group when planning a program for a particular multicultural population group. It goes without saying that the health practices of any population group will be mediated by a variety of factors including level of acculturation, socioeconomic status, education, and access to Western health care services. With these thoughts in mind, the following discussion explores some of the traditional health beliefs, practices, and folk healers used by the population groups described in this book.

Latino Americans

Within the traditional Latino American community, with its highly diverse population groups, the explanatory models for health and illness are generally associated with the social, psychological, or physical domain. For example, among Brazilians, illnesses may be attributed to divine intervention or fate. They also may result from changes in temperature, food ingestion, activity, or very strong emotions (Hilfinger Messias, 1996). Among Central Americans (e.g.,

Guatemalans, Salvadorans, Nicaraguans), illness may be the result of an imbalance between the individual and his or her environment (thus a concern with hot, cold, weak, and strong forces), extremes of emotion, and outside sources including evil eye, ghosts, a witch's curse, and other similar agents (Boyle, 1996). For Cubans, the concept of equilibrium and balance between the individual and his or her environment and the germ theory of disease are well accepted as explanations for illness, although other causes such as stress, extreme nervousness, evil spells, and voodoo-type magic also are included in their explanatory models (Lassiter, 1995; Varela, 1996). Mexican Americans also view ill health as an imbalance between the individual and his or her environment, with variables such as emotions, social, physical, and spiritual factors accounting for sickness (De Paula, Lagana, & Gonzales-Ramirez, 1996). For Puerto Ricans, illness may be attributed to heredity, lack of personal attention to health, punishment from God for a sin, or evil or negative environmental forces (Juarbe, 1996). In general, these belief systems comprise a folk medical system called *curanderismo.*

Curanderismo as a system has evolved from a variety of elements drawn from spiritualistic, homeopathic, Aztec, Spanish, and other Western scientific foundations (Kiev, 1968; Lassiter, 1995; Roeder, 1988; Spector, 1991). Within this system, the folk healer can be either male or female and may arrive at his or her calling by being born into it, serving an apprenticeship, or being called to it through a vision, trance, or dream. De Paula et al. (1996) and others (Kiev, 1968; Roeder, 1988) identify a number of different types of folk healers within the curanderismo system. These include the *curandero* or *curandera,* who generally uses rituals, prayers, pledges, and herbal baths to affect healing; the *yerbalista,* who employs herbal prescriptions that are brought home by the patient (or family) and brewed into a broth or tea; the *sobador* or *sobadora,* who uses massage and may manipulate bones and joints if no physician is available; the *partera* (midwife), who is a woman skilled in pregnancy care and delivery; the *tendor* or *tendora,* who is a birth assistant who holds or supports the woman in labor; *brujas, brujos,* and *hechiceros* (witches, warlocks, and sorcerers), who practice black magic and who may be asked to counteract it; and *espiritistas* and *espiritualistas* (spiritualist and spiritist mediums), who go into trances and may call on the assistance of a well-known deceased healer (e.g., don Pedro Jaramillo) to effect a cure.

Although illness causality has many explanations among Latino population groups, one major concept within the system that is important to recognize is that of "hot" and "cold" illnesses and remedies. That is, it is believed that certain illnesses are hot and must be treated with a cold remedy to restore balance (e.g., tonsillitis is a hot illness that would be treated with cold tomatoes). Cinnamon (a hot food) is used to treat respiratory infections, which are cold illnesses. Also, certain foods should not be mixed because they might bring about an imbalance in the body and cause illness, such as eating fish and drinking milk (Roeder, 1988).

As might be expected, those who use the curanderismo system might be less inclined to volunteer information about their beliefs in this system of care unless a high degree of trust has been established between themselves and their health care providers. The degree of acculturation also plays a role in how often or how much the system is used in the United States today, although in personal interviews Latinos who are at least third generation have confided that they still remember and occasionally use folk medical treatments before seeking, or in concert with, Western medical services.

Spector (1991) notes that when compared to the Western medical approach to healing with its more formal, expensive, and business-like approaches, the curandero or other specialized healer is generally less expensive, shares the worldview of his or her patient, maintains a more informal and friendly relationship with the family, and will come to the patient's home in the day or night. Suarez and Ramirez (Chapter 6, this volume) provide a more comprehensive overview of the health beliefs and practices of Latino population groups and observe that folk medicines and practices continue to be important cultural features that must be considered and evaluated when working with this diverse ethnic group.

African Americans

Among African American communities, the use of folk healers and folk remedies continues to be carried on in place of, or in a complementary manner with, Western treatment modalities. Lassiter (1995) observes that beliefs about health and health practices vary widely and are highly dependent on the degree of adherence to traditional ideas, geographic locale, education, scientific orientation, and socioeconomic status. She also observes that most African Americans retain a holistic philosophy of health and perceive the mind and body as inseparable, with balance and harmony in one's life central to maintaining health. Jack et al. (1994) comment that folk-healing practices among African Americans is centuries old and that the use of folk healers in modern society might be a reflection of their greater emotional, physical, and financial accessibility. They note that traditional African American healers include spiritualists who rely on prayer, ritual, magic, or other related practices and herbalists who may prescribe teas, herbs, and warm medicated compresses to heal or cure. These practitioners may be chosen for their calling by being born with "veils" over their faces (the amniotic sacs that surround the babies during pregnancies), or they may be apprenticed to folk healers, from whom they learn the secrets of the trade (Haskins, 1990; Hopp & Herring, Chapter 10, this volume). Those born with the veils are thought to be able to summon spirits or communicate with the dead.

Voodoo, a belief system directly traceable to West Africa and that is associated with the practice of white or black magic, still is thought to have some influence among some African Americans today (Spector, 1991). *Hoodoo,* a term thought to be derived from the term *juju* (to conjure), refers to both complex magical practices and simple medicinal procedures and superstitions associated with African American life that has evolved since the time slavery was first introduced into North America (Haskins, 1990). Haskins provides a number of examples to demonstrate the differences between voodoo and hoodoo, although the boundary between them still seems quite gray. For example, a hoodoo procedure might involve placing a charm or hiding an object in someone's yard to bring about or ward off evil, or it might involve reading a sign such as a bird that has gotten into the house (which can portend the death of an immediate family member, often within a week's time). A voodoo procedure might involve casting a spell or hex on an enemy to cause trouble or even to bring death to the enemy. For example, practices such as the burning of different colored candles (black candles to cause a slow death or red to cause an accidental death) or the brewing of a special concoction to harm would reflect the dark side of voodoo. Haskins (1990) observes that the distinctions between voodoo and hoodoo have become blurred and are frequently used interchangeably. He comments that voodoo practitioners want to get away from the images of dolls stuck with pins and serpent rites and prefer to use the term *spiritualist* in referring to themselves. He also notes that modern practitioners of hoodoo and voodoo are not easily identified in the black community and might only be known by observing the numbers of visitors going into and out of their homes each day.

Hopp and Herring, in Chapter 10, provide an excellent overview of African American health beliefs and practices. They note that Blacks tend to attribute illness to one of two major categories: natural or unnatural. Within the natural category are illnesses caused by stress; drinking or eating too much; fighting with friends or neighbors; impurities in air, food, or water; cold air or winds; and other related factors. Natural illnesses can occur at any time and often are viewed as a punishment from God visited directly on the persons or their children. Unnatural illnesses are caused by evil influences that may have been induced by witchcraft and are not amenable to self-treatment or the usual traditional or Western treatment modalities. In this situation, a voodoo practitioner is required to remove the spell, curse, or hex.

In general, traditional models of health care delivery (faith and root healers) often are used in conjunction with Western approaches, although the use of folk healers might not be readily shared with the Western health care practitioner (Hopp & Herring, Chapter 10, this volume; Locks & Boateng, 1996). Lassiter (1995) points out that prayer often is the first treatment method employed to counter a health problem. This often is followed by a folk health treatment and then the professional health care system, if necessary. As Hopp and Herring (this volume) also observe, it is important to understand that folk healers often are the only health care providers available to low-income blacks.

Asian Americans

Among Southeast Asians, illness may arise from physical, metaphysical, or supernatural forces and may require the services of a shaman, a spirit medium, an astrologer, a herbalist, an acupuncturist, a Buddhist monk, or another specialist to effect a cure or healing. Chan (1992) discusses the evolution of ancient Chinese medicine and notes that it is an extremely well-organized medical system that has had an impact on the medical concepts of a number of Asian peoples, including Koreans, Japanese, and other Southeast Asians. Underlying traditional Chinese medicine is the concept of *Tao* (the harmony between heaven and earth), the forces of yin and yang, and the five elements (i.e., wood, fire, earth, metal, water). Following the Tao (the way or path) helps the individual to be in balance with the laws of nature and the universe. Yin and yang represent the dualism of the universe and can be seen as opposite ends of a mutually complementary and interacting system. Yin represents the passive or negative female force (i.e., moon, earth, water, poverty, sadness) that produces cold, darkness, and emptiness. Yang is the active male force (i.e., sun, heaven, fire, goodness, wealth) and is reflected in warmth, light, and fullness (Chan, 1992). To be healthy, the individual must seek to adjust himself or herself completely within the environment (the five elements) and balance the forces of yin and yang. A violation of this harmony can lead to chaos, one manifestation of which is illness.

Spector (1991) elaborates on these Chinese concepts, noting that various parts of the body correspond to the principles of yin and yang. That is, the inside of the body is yin, whereas the outside is yang. The front side of the body is yin, whereas the back side is yang. The five elements correspond to the liver, heart, spleen, lungs, and kidneys and are considered yin, whereas the gallbladder, stomach, large intestine, small intestine, and bladder are considered yang. The diseases of winter and spring are considered yin, whereas those of summer and fall are considered yang. For example, yin conditions include cancer, pregnancy, and postpartum care and are treated with yang foods (e.g., chicken, beef, eggs, spicy foods). Yang conditions include infections, hypertension, and venereal diseases and are treated with yin foods (e.g., pork, fish, fresh fruits and vegetables). Chan (1992) comments that for the traditional Chinese, the hot or cold classification of disease is a means for diagnosing and treating illness.

In addition to the hot-cold polarity, there are several other concepts relating to health and disease that are important to understand. The first is the concept of breath (*hay*), which resides in the respiratory system and provides resistance, strength, and freedom from illness. Next is the concept of blood, which may be weak or strong and, based on how well it is circulating, can contribute to atherosclerosis and hypertension. Finally, wind (*foong*) is associated with being bloated, passing gas, and having foam in the sputum. *Foong* is used to describe illnesses that have a fast onset and questionable outcomes (Lassiter, 1995). For the Chinese, a variety of healing methods may be used including acupuncture, acupressure, meditation, acumassage, moxibustion, cupping, coining, herbology, shamanistic rituals, and Western medicine, if necessary (Chan, 1992; Lassiter, 1995; Spector, 1991).

Among other traditional Southeast Asian population groups, illness may arise from a variety of causes, some of which closely parallel those of the Chinese. For the Hmong, mild illnesses are generally attributed to organic causes, whereas more serious illnesses are caused by supernatural forces including spirit attacks, soul loss, and other metaphysical manifestations that can be treated only by a shaman using a variety of ritualistic ceremonies and practices such as tying strings around the wrists in a *baci* ceremony to symbolically keep protective spirits within one's body (Brainard & Zaharlick, 1989; Johnson, 1996; Livo & Cha, 1991; Uba, 1992).

Livo and Cha (1991) observe that with the resettlement of many Hmong in the United States and in other areas of the world, many of their traditional habits and practices are changing. They do note that the more traditional Hmong peoples continue to hold to animistic beliefs (i.e., beliefs that spirits inhabit rocks, ponds, rivers, valleys, etc.) and to use the shaman (*tu-au-neng*), who is a combination of a medical doctor, a psychologist, a holy man, a spiritual healer, and an adviser. Typical shamanic healing practices may involve the use of rattles, gongs, finger bells, pieces of buffalo horn, and herbs and plants to restore patients to psychic balance and health. Livo and Cha also comment that some Western medical practices such as surgery and autopsy frighten the traditional Hmong and that other practices such as "coining" (vigorously rubbing the edge of a coin against the skin, which leaves bruises) with sick children also are avoided because they might be interpreted as child abuse by Western medical practitioners and could lead to the shaman's arrest.

The Vietnamese perceive magic, ancestors or natural spirits, and natural organic causes as agents of illness. Western biomedical explanations involving "germs" also may be accepted. Treatment for illness may require offerings and prayers to the spirits, the involvement of a powerful sorcerer, the use of treatment modalities derived from the Chinese medical system, or Western biomedical interventions (Brainard & Zaharlick, 1989; Chan, 1992; Farrales, 1996; Spector, 1991). Laotians and Cambodians also attribute illness to natural organic causes and to supernatural agents. Like other Southeast Asian population groups, the use of magic, prayer, medicinal potions, charms, and herbal remedies all have their place in Laotian and Cambodian health belief systems (Chan, 1992; Kulig, 1996). Brainard and Zaharlick (1989), in a study of Laotian, Cambodian, Vietnamese, and Hmong refugees in the United States, observe that Laotian refugees tended to move away from traditional healing practices to Western biomedicine, whereas Cambodians seemed to show no preference between traditional and Western approaches. Vietnamese refugees tended to use traditional methods first, with Western health care accessed only when these methods were unsuccessful. Hmong refugees were the least likely to use Western medical approaches and did so only when all other methods had failed.

As can be seen from this brief overview, illness causality and treatment methods are quite diverse, and the choice of the type of healer that may be used often will depend on the problem that has presented. Among traditional Southeast Asian groups, the perception of what constitutes a "good" health care provider or healer often is based on who intrudes on the body the least. That is, traditional healers generally employ four basic methods of diagnosis: looking, listening, inquiring, and feeling the pulse. Abdominal palpation also may be included in the diagnostic process (Chan, 1992). By contrast, Western health care diagnostic procedures often involve invasive procedures including removal of blood and other body fluids and extensive X-ray and related diagnostic procedures along with patient history taking and tracking of symptomology. Thus, the Western approach to medicine and health care may be perceived by some Southeast Asians as unnecessary, irrelevant, and rather excessive. It is important, however, to note that, as with the other population groups discussed in this section, the degree of acculturation, education, and socioeconomic status can play a significant role in how these groups perceive and access preventive and/or curative health care services.

Native Americans

Health beliefs and practices among American Indians and Alaskan Natives are extremely varied, although all seem to share a common belief that health is closely linked to spirituality. That is, there is an interconnectedness of all things, both living and nonliving, and humans are but one small piece of the fabric of the universe (Joe & Malach, 1992). Traditional American Indian medicine is holistic and focuses on the need to maintain a balance among the physical, mental, spiritual, and emotional (Jack et al., 1994; Kramer, 1992). Within this frame-work, illness is viewed as an imbalance resulting from natural or supernatural forces, and healing may require rituals and traditional medical practices carried out by an accepted native healer (Jack et al., 1994). Natural causes include disturbances in the equilibrium of the individual resulting from accidents not brought on by witchcraft, lifestyle choices, and the breaking of a cultural taboo or other violation against the natural or spiritual laws. Supernatural causes of illness include witchcraft, ghosts, spirit loss, spirit intrusion, spells, and other unnatural events (Joe & Malach, 1992; Lake, 1993; Levy, Neutra, & Parker, 1995; Lyon, 1996).

Native American traditional healing practices encompass a holistic and well-ness-oriented approach to treating the individual. As Kramer (1992) observes, the focus is on behavior and lifestyle and on seeking to reestablish harmony in one's physical, mental, spiritual, and personal life. These approaches may involve a combination of methods including prayer and chanting, dancing rituals, puri-fication ceremonies, prescribing botanical medicines, diagnosing disharmony, and/or performing physical manipulations (Hultkrantz, 1992; Lyon, 1996; Sorrell & Smith, 1993). While carrying out these methods, the traditional healer (who may be a man or a woman) may play the role of psychiatrist/psychologist, doctor, arbitrator, diviner, and/or religious consultant.

A review of the traditional health beliefs and practices of Alaskan Native populations revealed that these groups, like other Native American tribal groups, relate their religious beliefs and health practices to the environments in which they live, that is, a belief system that perceives the world as filled with spirits who inhabit the land, water, animals, and sky and who require respectful treatment (Jorgensen, 1990). Chance (1990) observes that despite the heavy influence of Western religious practices, some Alaskan Native populations continue to hold beliefs about spirit people who inhabit their environments, including monsters and other supernatural beings. He notes that among these peoples, the universe is seen as a place where the various supernatural forces are largely hostile toward humans. Through the use of ritual and magic, these forces can be influenced for the benefit of the people (e.g., improving the weather and food supply, seeking protection from illness, curing illness when it strikes). Explanatory models for illness among Alaskan Natives include both Western and traditional health beliefs and practices (Chance, 1990; Jorgensen, 1990; Lantis, 1947; Lyon, 1996; Minority Rights Group, 1994). Although many of the traditional beliefs and rituals have disappeared since the arrival of the first whites, there still are those who rely on native healers and shamans to cure illnesses, some of which are thought to arise from causes such as soul loss and the intrusion of foreign objects into the body. Traditional healing practices may include prayer, chants, dancing, divination, sucking of foreign objects from the body, physical manipulation (laying on hands), or plant and animal remedies (Chance, 1990; Fienup-Riordan, 1991; Jorgensen, 1990; Lyon, 1996).

A number of researchers and native healers have observed that many American Indians and Alaskan Natives see no conflict in the use of both Western and traditional medical practices (Chance, 1990; Fienup-Riordan, 1991; Kramer, 1992; Lake, 1993; Sorrell & Smith, 1993). In fact, in recent years there has been a movement toward combining traditional and Western therapies within the hospital and other clinical settings. Hodge and Fredericks, Duran and Duran, and Fredericks and Hodge, in Chapters 14, 15, and 16, respectively, observe that most Native American and Alaskan Native tribes continue to practice traditional ceremonies tied to maintaining balance and harmony and that it is not uncommon for both Western and traditional medicine to be practiced together. The interested reader is encouraged to review these chapters for a more detailed discussion of American Indian and Alaskan Native health promotion and disease prevention (HPDP) issues.

Pacific Islanders

Pacific Islanders comprise a diverse population group representing three major geographic locales in the Pacific: Melanesia, Micronesia, and Polynesia. The two most populous of these groups residing in the United States are the Native Hawaiians and the Samoans (Mokuau & Tauili'ili, 1992). For this reason, these two groups are the focus of this brief overview of health beliefs and practices among Pacific Islanders.

Casken, in Chapter 22, observes that traditional health beliefs among native Hawaiians were focused on the spiritual aspect of illness and its relationship to the breaking of rules for how one was to live and relate to both the spiritual and physical worlds, including family, neighbors, and community. Sickness was thought to be a punishment imposed directly or indirectly by the gods for having broken their *kapus* (taboos, prohibitions, or rules) and resulted in loss of *mana* (spiritual power) and in physical illness (Bushnell, 1993). Thus, healing of the body could occur only after the sick spirit was restored, and then only if the gods were so inclined. These beliefs have carried down to the present and also have come to incorporate germ theory as another cause of ill health (Casken, Chapter 22, this volume; Loos, Chapter 23, this volume; Mokuau & Tauili'ili, 1992).

According to Mokuau and Tauili'ili (1992), medical care in historical times often was left to the *Kahuna Lapa'au* (medical experts), who used prayers, physical massage, and medicinal plants and herbs. King (1987) comments that the term *kahuna* refers to someone who has mastered the secrets of some field of knowledge and that the term is used rather indiscriminately in modern Hawaii to denote someone who could be a priest, minister, sorcerer, psychic, healer, or shaman. Lyon (1996) describes seven types of kahunas including the *Kahuna*

Lapa'au, who conducted healing ceremonies with the support of his helping spirit (*Akua*), to which prayers and a sacrifice had been made. Sweat baths and herbs also could be used for treatment. Diagnosis of illness was done by a *Kahuna ha ha,* who felt the patient to determine what was wrong and made referrals based on whether the illness was of a spiritual cause or another cause. The *Kahuna Lomilomi* was a master of massage who was skilled at manipulating sore and stiff muscles to bring relief. The *Kahuna Kahea* was a master of psychotherapy and used prayer and the power of suggestion to cure. In addition, there were a variety of sorcerers who might be consulted if the illness was diagnosed as having been caused by an evil spirit or sorcery and requiring their intercession to effect a cure. In precontact Hawaii, religious beliefs were centered on the natural environment and ancestor worship, and despite the heavy influence of Christianity, there still exists a tendency to invoke ancestral guardian spirits and to practice religious beliefs related to the individual's relationship to nature and the gods. In fact, Mokuau and Tauili'ili (1992) observe that there has been a revival of these traditional beliefs and practices among Native Hawaiians in recent years.

In Samoa, there are two coexisting medical systems: traditional and Western. Depending on whether the illness is considered indigenous (*ma'i samoa*) or foreign (*ma'i palagi*), either system or both systems might be consulted (Casken, Chapter 22, this volume; Ishida, Toomata-Mayer, & Mayer, 1996; Mokuau & Tauili'ili, 1992). Traditional Samoan health beliefs are holistic (i.e., mind, body, and spirit all interconnected), with illness viewed as a consequence of one's actions toward the living or dead (Ishida et al., 1996). Although Samoans have strong beliefs in the Christian God, they also believe in supernatural powers and attribute the events of life to these powers. Thus, they feel that they have very little control over their own destinies (Mokuau & Tauili'ili, 1992). Ishida et al. (1996) comment that because of the holistic belief system of Samoans, healing practices are directed at restoring balance in the mind-body-spirit dimensions, which might require traditional or Western healing approaches or a combination of both to effect a cure. They also note that the concept of preventive health is not well established among Samoan population groups, an observation that Loos (Chapter 23, this volume) echos when he comments that Samoans view health as something that cannot be promoted and sickness as something that cannot be prevented. Mokuau and Tauili'ili (1992) observe that the use of Western medical facilities can be linked with Samoan religious beliefs in that God is seen as working through hospital care or medications. If persons "do right" before God, then they will be cured. They do note, however, that preference for traditional care and treatments or advice from relatives or a pastor will take precedence over Western health care services.

Zane, Takeuchi, and Young (1994), in discussing the health issues of Asians and Pacific Islanders, comment that both of these groups are affected by the same barriers to health care as are other segments of society, that is, high costs for services, fragmentation of the health care system, and inadequate health care facilities in urban and rural areas. In addition, socioeconomic factors (e.g., poverty, unemployment, lack of health insurance, lack of education, illiteracy) also are critical variables. They also perceive that the lack of cultural competence with respect to traditional health and healing practices has created significant conflict between native peoples and the Western biomedical health care system.

PROMOTING HEALTH ACROSS CULTURES

In the Western biomedical model, illness is explained in terms of a patient's presenting pathophysiology. Sickness often is reduced to disease, and the focus is on the patient's body rather than on the whole person, where illness can be seen as the person's experience of being sick and is reflected in the person's thoughts, feelings, and altered behaviors (Weston & Brown, 1989). Weston and Brown observe, "To understand a patient's experience of illness, a physician must attempt to enter the patient's world, to understand the patient's beliefs about what is wrong, why it happened, and what should be done" (p. 80). Their point is well taken and has application to any situation in which efforts to promote health and prevent disease are undertaken.

An equally important concept when working in culturally diverse settings is the need for the health promoter to suspend his or her personal biases and judgments about those for whom he or she may be planning HPDP activities. As Perrone, Stockel, and Krueger (1989) comment, if one is to understand healing traditions in other cultures, then one must be open to the possibility of encountering unfamiliar beliefs and concepts about health and disease and be willing to cast out personal bias. As has been discussed in this chapter, the range and variety of health beliefs and practices associated with humankind is staggering. Not seeking to understand, respect, and work with these differences might be the greatest error any health promoter can make.

CHAPTER SUMMARY

This chapter has sought to provide a brief overview of the explanatory models that different cultural groups use to explain and make sense of health and disease. Explanatory models were considered by Kleinman (1980) to be the notions people have about sickness episodes and how these were to be treated by those engaged in the clinical process. It was noted that explanatory models often differ significantly between the Western health care provider and more traditional peoples and that these models must be considered and respected when planning HPDP programs and activities.

Folk illnesses, or syndromes that define how a culture perceives, diagnoses, and treats illness, were reviewed broadly, and it was noted that these tend to be classified under four general headings: the patient, the natural world, the social world, and the supernatural world. Thus, illness causality could be the result of malfunctions of the body, microorganisms, injuries, environmental factors, interpersonal conflicts, sorcery or witchcraft, ancestral or other spirits, or malevolent gods who send sickness as a retribution for violations of taboos, rules, and laws of the culture.

Finally, a discussion of traditional versus Western approaches to the diagnosis and treatment of illness was described for the five major multicultural groups presented in this book. It was noted that all of these groups and the diverse subgroups within them employ traditional healers and healing methods for dealing with illness including the use of medicinal plants and herbs, physical manipulation of the body through massage and other methods, acupuncture, acupressure, coining, cupping, moxibustion, prayer, chants, incantations, divining, sorcery, and other related practices. Traditional healers tend to be specialists in different aspects of the healing tradition and often are seen and used by traditional peoples as the first step in diagnosing and treating a sickness episode. It also was observed that many cultural groups have adopted Western medical approaches where these seem appropriate or complementary to the treatment of illness and disease, but that it is critical to be culturally competent when seeking to promote health and prevent disease among diverse cultural groups. Finally, a recommendation was made that the health promoter be willing to suspend his or her judgments with respect to perceptions of how others different from the health promoter perceive and deal with health and disease. A failure to respect and work within these differing frameworks is likely to contribute to conflict, confusion, indifference, and poor health care outcomes for all of those involved in the HPDP encounter.

REFERENCES

Boyle, J. S. (1996). Central Americans. In J. G. Lipson, S. L. Dibble, & P. A. Minarik (Eds.), *Culture and nursing care: A pocket guide*. San Francisco: UCSF Nursing Press.

Brainard, J., & Zaharlick, A. (1989). Changing health beliefs and behaviors of resettled Laotion refugees: Ethnic variation in adaptation. *Social Sciences and Medicine, 29*, 845-852.

Buchwald, D., Panwala, S., & Hooton, T. M. (1992). Use of traditional health practices by Southeast Asian refugees in a primary care setting. *Western Journal of Medicine, 156*, 507-511.

Bushnell, O. A. (1993). *The gifts of civilization: Germs and genocide in Hawaii*. Honolulu: University of Hawaii Press.

Chan, S. (1992). Families with Asian roots. In E. W. Lynch & M. J. Hanson (Eds.), *Developing cross-cultural competence: A guide for working with young children and their families*. Baltimore, MD: Paul H. Brookes.

Chance, N. A. (1990). *The Inupiat and Arctic Alaska: An ethnography of development*. New York: Holt, Rinehart & Winston.

De Paula, T., Lagana, K., & Gonzales-Ramirez, L. (1996). Mexican Americans. In J. G. Lipson, S. L. Dibble, & P. A. Minarik (Eds.), *Culture and nursing care: A pocket guide*. San Francisco: UCSF Nursing Press.

Dimou, N. (1995). Illness and culture: Learning differences. *Patient Education and Counseling, 26*, 153-157.

Farrales, S. (1996). Vietnamese. In J. G. Lipson, S. L. Dibble, & P. A. Minarik (Eds.), *Culture and nursing care: A pocket guide*. San Francisco: UCSF Nursing Press.

Fienup-Riordan, A. (1991). *The real people and the children of thunder*. Norman: University of Oklahoma Press.

Haskins, J. (1990). *Voodoo and hoodoo: The craft as revealed by traditional practitioners*. New York: Scarborough House.

Helman, C. H. (1984). *Culture, health and illness*. Bristol, UK: John Wright.

Hilfinger Messias, D. K. (1996). Brazilians. In J. G. Lipson, S. L. Dibble, & P. A. Minarik (Eds.), *Culture and nursing care: A pocket guide*. San Francisco: UCSF Nursing Press.

Hultkrantz, A. (1992). *Shamanic healing and ritual drama: Health and medicine in Native North American religious traditions*. New York: Crossroad.

Ishida, D. N., Toomata-Mayer, T. F., & Mayer, J. F. (1996). Samoans. In J. G. Lipson, S. L. Dibble, & P. A. Minarik (Eds.), *Culture and nursing care: A pocket guide*. San Francisco: UCSF Nursing Press.

Jack, L., Jr., Harrison, I. E., & Airhihenbuwa, C. O. (1994). Ethnicity and the health belief systems. In A. C. Matiella (Eds.), *The multicultural challenge in health education*. Santa Cruz, CA: ETR Associates.

Joe, J. R., & Malach, R. S. (1992). Families with Native American roots. In E. W. Lynch & M. J. Hanson (Eds.), *Developing cross-cultural competence: A guide for working with young children and their families*. Baltimore, MD: Paul H. Brookes.

Johnson, S. (1996). Hmong. In J. G. Lipson, S. L. Dibble, & P. A. Minarik (Eds.), *Culture and nursing care: A pocket guide*. San Francisco: UCSF Nursing Press.

Jorgensen, J. G. (1990). *Oil Age Eskimos*. Berkeley: University of California Press.

Juarbe, T. (1996). Puerto Ricans. In J. G. Lipson, S. L. Dibble, & P. A. Minarik (Eds.), *Culture and nursing care: A pocket guide*. San Francisco: UCSF Nursing Press.

Kiev, A. (1968). *Curanderismo: Mexican-American folk psychiatry*. New York: Free Press.

King, S. (1987). The way of the adventurer. In S. Nicholson (Ed.), *Shamanism: An expanded view of reality*. Wheaton, IL: Theosophical Publishing House.

Kleinman, A. (1980). *Patients and healers in the context of culture*. Berkeley: University of California Press.

Kramer, B. (1992). Health and aging of urban American Indians. *Western Journal of Medicine, 157*, 281-285. (Special issue)

Kulig, J. C. (1996). Cambodians (Khmer). In J. G. Lipson, S. L. Dibble, & P. A. Minarik (Eds.), *Culture and nursing care: A pocket guide*. San Francisco: UCSF Nursing Press.

Lake, M. G. (1993). *Native healer: The path to an ancient healing art*. New York: Harper Paperbacks.

Landrine, H., & Klonoff, E. A. (1992). Culture and health-related schemas: A review and proposal for interdisciplinary integration. *Health Psychology, 11*, 267-276.

Lantis, M. (1947). *Alaskan Eskimo ceremonialism*. New York: J.J. Augustin.

Lassiter, S. M. (1995). *Multicultural clients: A professional handbook for health care providers and social workers*. Westport, CT: Greenwood.

Levy, J. E., Neutra, R., & Parker, D. (1995). *Hand trembling, frenzy witchcraft, and moth madness: A study of Navaho seizure disorders*. Tucson: University of Arizona Press.

Livo, N. J., & Cha, D. (1991). *Folk stories of the Hmong: Peoples of Laos, Thailand, and Vietnam*. Englewood, CO: Libraries Unlimited.

Locks, S., & Boateng, L. (1996). Black/African Americans. In J. G. Lipson, S. L. Dibble, & P. A. Minarik (Eds.), *Culture and nursing care: A pocket guide*. San Francisco: UCSF Nursing Press.

Lyon, W. S. (1996). *Encyclopedia of Native American healing*. Santa Barbara, CA: ABC-CLIO.

Minority Rights Group. (1994). *Polar peoples: Self-determination and development*. London: Minority Rights Publications.

Mokuau, N., & Tauili'ili, P. (1992). Families with Native Hawaiian and Pacific Island roots. In E. W. Lynch & M. J. Hanson (Eds.), *Developing cross-cultural competence: A guide for working with young children and their families*. Baltimore, MD: Paul H. Brookes.

Murray, R. H., & Rubel, A. J. (1992). Sounding board: Physicians and healers—Unwitting partners in health care. *New England Journal of Medicine, 326*(1), 61-64.

Pachter, L. M. (1994). Culture and clinical care: Folk illness beliefs and behaviors and their implications for health care delivery. *Journal of the American Medical Association, 271*, 690-694.

Perrone, B., Stockel, H. H., & Krueger, V. (1989). *Medicine women, curanderas, and women doctors*. Norman: University of Oklahoma Press.

Roeder, B. A. (1988). *Chicano folk medicine from Los Angeles, California*. Berkeley: University of California Press.

Seidel, H. M., Ball, J. W., Dains, J. E., & Benedict, G. W. (1995). *Mosby's guide to physical examination* (3rd ed.). St. Louis, MO: C. V. Mosby.

Sorrell, M. S., & Smith, B. A. (1993). Navajo beliefs: Implications for health professionals. *Journal of Health Education, 24*, 336-338.

Spector, R. E. (1991). *Cultural diversity in health and illness* (3rd ed.). Norwalk, CT: Appleton & Lange.

Uba, L. (1992). Cultural barriers to health care for Southeast Asian refugees. *Public Health Reports, 107,* 545-548.

Varela, L. (1996). Cubans. In J. G. Lipson, S. L. Dibble, & P. A. Minarik (Eds.), *Culture and nursing care: A pocket guide.* San Francisco: UCSF Nursing Press.

Weston, W. W., & Brown, J. B. (1989). The importance of patients' beliefs. In M. Stewart & D. Roter (Eds.), *Communicating with medical patients.* Thousand Oaks, CA: Sage.

Zane, N. W. S., Takeuchi, D. T., & Young, K. N. J. (1994). *Confronting critical health issues of Asian and Pacific Islander Americans.* Thousand Oaks, CA: Sage.

3

Models, Theories, and Principles of Health Promotion With Multicultural Populations

C. JAMES FRANKISH
CHRIS Y. LOVATO
WILLIAM J. SHANNON

Cultural influences have become more prominent in contemporary theories explaining the factors that determine health. Historically, theories applied in health promotion focused on individual determinants of health. More recently, this focus has expanded to social and cultural influences. It is clear from experience accumulated over the past two decades that to address health problems effectively, we must examine cultural factors and understand beliefs about health within a context that is relevant to the population of interest.

Cultural sensitivity in health promotion programs refers to planning interventions that are relevant and acceptable within the cultural framework of the population to be reached. Although the role of culture has long been acknowledged in widely used theories of late, culture has not been a central focus. For the health educator, developing a culturally sensitive program demands moving outside the paradigm of the dominant culture.

There are many different definitions of *theory*. In this chapter, the authors address theory from the perspective of the health promotion practitioner. The authors examine theories based on their utility in helping the practitioner to understand the determinants of health behaviors and develop interventions that will influence change. The chapter provides an overview of relevant theories of behavior change as they relate to health promotion with multicultural populations or groups. Information is provided regarding the rationale for the use of theory by health promotion practitioners and policymakers. Next, important theories are reviewed. This overview leads to the articulation of principles of health education that apply across theoretical perspectives. Finally, some practical concluding comments are made.

RATIONALE FOR USING A THEORETICAL FRAMEWORK

A theoretical framework provides researchers and program developers with a perspective from which to organize knowledge and to interpret factors and events. All programs are built on assumptions; however, these may or may not be well articulated. Identification and classification of elements of programs or interventions and their linkages (e.g., associative-causal, explanatory-predictive, direct-indirect) facilitate informed attempts at identifying and replicating promising parts of multicultural interventions and programs and the development of creative potential solutions to unsolved problems.

> By telling us about the what, how, when, and why, theories can inform programs in health education. . . . The what tells us the elements we should consider as the targets for the intervention. . . . The why tells us about the processes by which changes occur in the target variables. The when tells us about the timing and sequencing of our interventions in order to achieve maximum effects. The how tells us the methods or ways we should focus our interventions; it includes the specific means of inducing changes in the explanatory variables. (Glanz, Lewis, & Rimer, 1990, p. 21)

The first step in choosing an appropriate theory is clarifying the purpose or goals of the proposed program or intervention. The explicit goals of the program or intervention provide the marker for identifying classes of theories that might be applicable. Theories often are specific to targets of intervention or units of practice. For example, some theories address individual behavior change, whereas others address organizational change. Within the class of behavior change theories, some explain and predict solely volitional behaviors, whereas others generalize to addictive behaviors. If a multicultural program needs to incorporate aspects that address an addictive behavior, then it should not be based on a theory that addresses only voluntary behavior (Cheung, 1993). Likewise, a program that has the goal of behavior maintenance should not be based on a theory that explains only initial behavior change. Identifying the specific target and goals of the program will narrow the field of applicable theories. However, even once this guideline has been followed, there often are many theories from which to choose. "The next step is to identify the relevant theories and evaluate the evidence for each of them" (van Ryn & Heaney, 1992, p. 320).

DISTINGUISHING THEORIES, MODELS, AND FRAMEWORKS

When concepts and constructs are related to each other and purposely combined to form a unit, the resulting entity may be labeled a "framework," a "model," or a "theory." There is considerable controversy regarding the boundaries or limits defining and circumscribing each of these creations. Generally speaking, a framework is a planning tool (e.g., the PRECEDE model). It can incorporate theories or models or parts thereof, and it allows for organization of a large and unspecified number of potentially predictive or explanatory variables. A model is a grouping of a set number of selected variables that, taken together, act as an explanatory or a predictive indicator of behavior; the interrelationships among the variables are not definitively specified. A theory is, likewise, a set number of selected factors or variables; however, the hypothesized relationships among the variables are specified, as are the circumstances under which the relationships do or do not occur.

An example of a framework used in planning prevention health promotion interventions is the PRECEDE/PROCEED framework (Green & Kreuter, 1991). Using this framework, potentially important variables from a wide conceptual domain may be identified and targeted for intervention. These categories of variables include those identifying relevant quality of life, health, behavioral, environmental, organizational, and administrative concerns.

An example of a model frequently used in designing health surveys and interventions is the health belief model (Rosenstock, 1974). It is composed of four constructs: perceived severity, perceived susceptibility, perceived benefits of action, and perceived barriers to action. The constructs are said to be related multiplicatively, but researchers using the model generally do not combine them in this way.

An example of a theory used in elicitation research and intervention planning is the theory of reasoned action (Ajzen & Fishbein, 1980). Here the relationships among the variables are explicitly set out in directional and mathematical terms. In much of the literature, the terms *theory* and *model* are used interchangeably and/or without specification. This chapter reflects that pattern of usage to reflect the literature as accurately as possible.

VALUES AND THEORIES

Competing contemporary theories of health, the reductionist (purportedly value-free) and the relativist (purportedly value-based) theories, both rest on an understanding of value as grounded in desiring—a subjective state (Sade, 1995). Sade notes that both can be classified as subjectivist theories. An alternative set of theories, those resting on an understanding of value as grounded in desirability (or goodness) of an objective goal, can be classified as objectivist theories. Whatever one's theoretical perspective, the health promotion practitioner and program planner must be cognizant of their own values while at the same time respecting the values of the various cultural communities with whom they work (Smaje, 1996).

THEORIES AND MODELS OF RELEVANCE

In the field of health (e.g., health behavior, health promotion, illness prevention), many theories have been developed during the past 40 to 50 years. Some of these theories have been used to try to understand determinants of health as well as to maintain and improve health, by both behavioral and environmental change. These theories can be divided into groups according to the scope of their focus (e.g., intrapersonal, interpersonal, and group levels of interaction). Group-level theories include organizational change, diffusion of innovation, community organization, media advocacy, and social marketing. Theories also can be organized according to their style of focus (e.g., cognitive, behavioral, social, environmental).

Leviton (1989) discusses five relevant "families" of theories:

- *Cognitive and decision-making theories* including the theory of risk communication, the health belief model, and the theory of reasoned action
- *Learning theories* including the theory of operant conditioning, social learning theory, and subtheories of self-efficacy, relapse, and self-regulation
- *Theories of motivation and emotional arousal* including theories of fear and fear-arousing communications, helplessness, and coping strategies
- *Theories of interpersonal relations* including social influence, reactance, and group processes
- *Theories of communication and persuasion*

The theories underlying multicultural health promotion include the health belief model (Brunswick & Banaszakholl, 1996; Rosenstock, 1974); sick role behaviors (Kasl & Cobb, 1966); locus of control (Wallston & Wallston, 1978); physician-patient relationships (Haynes, Taylor, & Sackett, 1979); self-regulation theory (Leventhal, Meyer, & Gutmann, 1980); communications theory (Garrity, 1980); attribution, control, and decision theory (Janis & Rodin, 1979); grounded theory (Mullens & Reynolds, 1978); ecological theory (Stokols, 1992); family and systems theories (Becker & Maiman, 1975); communication-behavior model of behavior change (Matarazzo, Miller, Weiss, Herd, & Weiss, 1984); social learning theory (Bandura, 1986); hierarchy of learning model (Ray, 1973); self-control theory (Kanfer, 1975); attitude change model (Ajzen & Fishbein, 1980); and models of social problem solving (Goldfried & D'Zurilla, 1969). These theories and others have formed the foundation for the major health education, health promotion, and behavior modification programs (Bruhn, 1983) in North America. A summary of the basic concepts and constructs of each of these theories and models is given in the following.

Social Learning Theory

The three major constructs in social learning theory (also called social cognitive theory or social influence theory) are behavioral capacity (having the skills necessary for the performance of the desired behavior such as active living), efficacy expectations (beliefs regarding one's ability to successfully carry out a course of action or perform a behavior), and outcome expectations (beliefs that the performance of a behavior will have desired effects or consequences) (van Ryn & Heaney, 1992).

The leading concept in social learning theory is that of "reciprocal determinism." This means that behavior is determined by the interaction among three elements: the person, the person's behavior, and the environment. This approach is highly consistent with the view of living as a dynamic process and experience involving the reciprocal interaction of personal, social, and environmental factors. The person's actions contribute to creating the environment, and the actions and environment contribute to the person's cognitions or "expectancies." Expectancies are of three types: beliefs about how events are connected, beliefs about the consequences of one's own actions (outcome expectations), and beliefs about one's competence to perform the behavior needed to influence the outcomes (efficacy expectations). "Incentives" also contribute to behavior; incentive or reinforcement is the value of a particular outcome to a person. Behavior is regulated by its consequences, "but only as those consequences are interpreted and understood by the individual" (Maiman, Becker, & Liptak, 1988, p. 774).

The three important explanatory factors of social learning or social cognitive theory can be defined as follows.

> SLT [social learning theory] is useful to program development because, in addition to describing the important influences on behavior change, it describes the processes through which these influences can be modified. Thus, behavioral capacity or skill level can be modified through both direct experience or practice and observing someone else modeling the desired behavior. Both outcome and efficacy expectations can be modified by four different processes. Performance accomplishments refer to performing the behavior or close approximations of the behavior. Successful performance can increase a person's sense of confidence (self-efficacy) in being able to perform the behavior again. If the behavior leads to a desirable outcome, then that person's outcome expectations become more positive as well. (Bandura, 1988, p. 391)

A second important influence on expectations is observational learning or vicarious experience. Through seeing others who are similar to themselves behave in certain ways and succeed in bringing about desired effects, people modify their expectations about their own behavior.

The third influence, verbal persuasion, refers to attempts to change expectations by providing new or newly motivating information. People develop their sense of efficacy in part from how distressed, anxious, and tense they feel when faced with the need to perform the behavior. Efforts to decrease this emotional arousal may directly enhance efficacy expectations. When there are satisfactory levels of self-efficacy, the motivation to perform a particular behavior can be increased through the expectation that the behavior will lead to a desirable outcome (outcome expectation) and through incentives (rewards). Reward expectations can be influenced by observing others receiving rewards (vicarious reward) or by being rewarded oneself (direct reward). Rewards may come from external sources, such as awards, promotions, and professional recognition, or they may come from internal sources, such as the self-satisfaction a health educator might feel after implementing an effective intervention (van Ryn & Heaney, 1992).

Perceived self-efficacy is defined by Bandura (1988) as "people's judgments of their capabilities to organize and execute courses of action required to attain designated types of performances. It is concerned not with the skills one has but with judgments of what one can do with whatever skills one possesses" (p. 391).

It should be noted that self-efficacy refers to beliefs about performing specific actions in specific settings; it cannot refer to global situations or personality traits (Costa & Metter, 1994). Perceived self-efficacy is concerned with people's beliefs that they can exert control over their motivation, behavior, and social environment. People's beliefs about their capabilities affect what they choose to do, how much effort they mobilize, how long they will persevere in the face of difficulties, and whether they engage in self-debilitating or self-encouraging thought patterns. When lacking a sense of self-efficacy, individuals do not manage situations effectively, even though they know what to do and possess the requisite skills. Self-inefficacious thinking creates discrepancies between knowledge and action.

Numerous studies have been conducted linking perceived self-efficacy to health-promoting and health-impairing behavior. Feelings of self-efficacy derive from four sources: performance attainments, vicarious experience, verbal persuasion, and physiological feedback. For example, Sennott-Miller (1994) found differences in perceived self-efficacy among Hispanics and whites. Perceived self-efficacy and perceived difficulty were related to adoption and maintenance of cancer prevention activities.

As can be seen, self-efficacy is strongly linked to attribution theory. Attribution theory informs us that for change to occur and be maintained, it is necessary that the person feel in control of his or her own behavior. High self-efficacy can assist a person undergoing a relapse to see it as temporary. Under conditions of success, stable, global, and internal causal attributions for desirable outcomes should be reinforced. Under conditions of failure, unstable, specific, uncontrollable, and external attributions should be reinforced. Social learning theory and its variants are the most extensively applied psychosocial theories.

Self-efficacy is a person's ability to cope with a given situation. This capacity is strongly influenced by the person's perceived belief in his or her capacity to mobilize motivational and cognitive resources and actions needed to meet situational demands. Gonzalez, Geoppinger, and Lorig (1990) identify four empirically verified ways in which to enhance self-efficacy: reinterpretation of signs and symptoms, skills mastery, modeling, and persuasion. When judging a person's capabilities, one source of information that the person relies on is information from his or her physiological state. For example, a person may learn to reinterpret the symptoms associated with specific health behaviors (e.g., physical effort). Reinterpretation of symptoms may, in some cases, improve an individual's sense of self-efficacy; however, it also may lead to inappropriate maintenance of risky behaviors.

Optimism also is closely related to the concept of self-efficacy. Scheier and Carver (1992) review longitudinal and prospective research examining the beneficial effects of optimism on psychological and physical well-being. Their article identifies potential mechanisms that produce the beneficial effects of optimism and focuses on how optimism may lead a person to cope more adaptively with stress. Data also suggest that optimists are more likely than pessimists to engage in positive health habits. Similarities are noted between conceptualizing optimism versus pessimism in terms of general expectancies for good versus bad outcomes and approaches that conceptualize optimism versus pessimism in terms of attributional style or self-efficacy. Optimism also varies across cultural groups (Zhang & Schwarzer, 1995). Chang (1996) also recently reported cultural differences between Asian American and Caucasian American students. Asian Americans were found to be more pessimistic than Caucasian Americans. Asian Americans also were found to use more problem avoidance and social withdrawal coping strategies than Caucasian Americans.

The most effective way in which to enhance self-efficacy is through the mastery of skills. The acquisition of healthy behavior and skills is facilitated by self-identification of goals, breaking down of tasks into small and manageable units, and programming for success by sequencing subtasks according to level of difficulty or ordered learning objectives. Both the goals and consequences of health behaviors must be clear, consistent, and doable. Gonzalez et al. (1990) argue that contracting and feedback are such important aspects of health education that 30% of efforts should be directed toward these aspects.

Modeling is another effective way in which to enhance health behaviors (Bandura, 1986). The principle of modeling underlies the development of self-help groups. Modeling can be achieved through mutual aid, the use of lay instructors, and the use of age-appropriate models in educational materials such as videos and pamphlets.

The final way in which to enhance self-efficacy is through the use of persuasion. Although persuasive arguments on the part of health educators are a ubiquitous aspect of education, there is strong evidence that persuasion, in and of itself, is a relatively ineffective strategy. The use of persuasion in multicultural health promotion can be made more effective by delivering such arguments in the context of supportive small-group settings. People also should be persuaded to make small, incremental behavior changes rather than all-or-nothing efforts.

Reference Group-Based Social Influence Theory

Social influence (normative and informational) can be a significant predisposing factor (direct or indirect) for group members' behavior, either in health-enhancing or non-health-enhancing directions. Fisher (1988) presents a model showing effects of social networks and reference groups on AIDS risk and preventive behavior, according to whether the social network's values and norms are of high or low consistency with preventive behaviors. Krohn and Thornberry (1993) also provide a network theory model for understanding drug abuse among African American and Hispanic youths.

If preventive behavior is consistent with social norms, then the cultural network will be likely to exert social influence and exposure for supportive information facilitative of preventive behavior and sanctions for the lack of it.

Likewise, if preventive behavior is inconsistent with a group's norms and values, then the group is likely to exert pressure against participation in preventive behavior.

Group norms and values can be specific (e.g., against smoking) or general (e.g., in favor of exercise). Cultural groups can exert pressure on their members to conform to the status quo (normative social influence) and wield their power by means of sanctions (e.g., rejection or perceived future rejection) for nonconformity. There are a number of factors that may moderate the intensity of the network's response in protecting the status quo. These include the centrality of a value or behavior to the core of a group's assumptive world, the level of trust the group has for the person who is proposing change, and the network's previous history of remaining intact while being able to integrate previously inconsistent values (Fisher, 1988).

In addition to exerting normative influence, cultural groups exert informational influence by being open or closed to information relevant to a particular topic. Group members serve as models for each other; they may provide exposure for members to general and specific information and may influence members' perceptions of personal vulnerability to negative outcomes.

Various factors may moderate group members' reactions to cultural, network-based social influence. These include the size of the network (larger being more influential), cohesiveness of the reference group (more cohesive being more influential), enmeshment of the individual with the reference group (higher being more influential), non-unanimity of group opinion (lessening pressure to conform), and perception that group opinion is changing (lessening pressure to conform).

Cohesive, homogeneous cultural networks can provide difficulty for group members who attempt to initiate new behaviors. Reference groups attempt to protect their norms and values (status quo) from assault by both outsiders and insiders. Possible reasons for a network to resist change from within include "the fact that change that is inconsistent with the group's values may threaten the perceived veracity of group beliefs, the way the group views itself, the correctness of its behavior, or even the relations between group members" (Fisher, 1988, p. 916).

Social influence strategies include the use of slightly older peers to model and influence norms and the use of video representations of respected persons and tangible rewards. Awareness of social pressures and resistance training (i.e., identify pressures, examine motivation behind pressures, respond to pressures, develop skills to resist), also known as psychological inoculation, is an application of social influence theory that is of relevance to multicultural health promotion. For example, Walter, Vaughan, and Cohall (1993) compared three theoretical models of substance use among urban minority high school students. The socialization model of substance use was much more powerful than either the stress/strain or disaffiliation models in explaining past-year use of alcohol, cigarettes, and marijuana. However, certain variables derived from the stress/strain and disaffiliation models were important risk factors for the frequent use of these substances. Walter et al.'s findings suggest the need for further elucidation of the social influence process and for development, implementation, and evaluation of intensive programs for high-risk youths.

Coping Theory

Lazarus and Folkman (1984) define *coping* as the person's constantly changing cognitive and behavioral efforts to manage specific external and/or internal demands that are appraised as taxing or exceeding a person's resources. Gonzalez et al. (1990) identify several potential coping strategies of relevance to multicultural health promotion including confronting, distancing, self-control, seeking social support, accepting responsibility, escape avoidance, positive reappraisal (Lazarus & Folkman, 1984), activity, distraction, and self-talk (Rosensteil & Keefe, 1983).

Direct confrontation has limited suitability for use with multicultural health promotion. In certain limited and specific situations, confrontation may be useful and necessary in focusing a person's attention. However, confrontation clearly is not the strategy of first choice and should be cautiously employed in concert with education on other coping strategies.

Distancing involves the person separating himself or herself from a stressful situation. By definition, some degree of risk in life is unavoidable. The person may learn to distance himself or herself from the triggers or environmental conditions that increase risk for uncomfortable episodes. Again, distancing should be viewed as a secondary coping strategy in that avoidance strategies are largely ineffective in addressing the pervasive nature of opportunities for healthy behavior. Avoidance also may lead to a limiting of social interaction that can contribute to a "rebound" attraction to risky behaviors.

Perhaps more so than the other coping strategies, escape avoidance can be either useful or counterproductive. Whereas a person may wish to avoid triggers for problematic behaviors, this avoidance may manifest as escape behavior. Engaging in this pattern of responses may undermine the person's overall sense of coping and negatively influence his or her cultural and social relations. One key in behavior change is to frame the avoidance of risk as a positive coping strategy rather than as weakness on the part of the person.

Self-control is a strategy that often is highly recommended by educators. It involves an active interest in taking responsibility for health behavior and for corrective actions. Self-control may play a positive and important role, for example, in supporting people's efforts to engage in healthy living. However, people also need to distinguish between those situations they can influence and those over which they have no control.

Seeking social support also is put forward frequently as a means of coping. Recently, it has become clearly evident that any positive impact of social supports varies widely across people, cultural groups, and circumstances. The support network also must be matched to the person's individual characteristics (Grant & Ostrow, 1995; Orshan, 1996; Picot, 1995).

In an interesting article, Hill, Hawkins, Raposo, and Carr (1995) examine relations among coping strategies of African American mothers, their exposure to community violence, and their interpersonal victimization. Their findings suggest that coping strategies are used differentially as a function of the amount of violence within the sociocultural context and the education and financial resources of the mothers. In their study, mothers with college educations who live in lower violence areas preferred activism as a coping strategy, whereas those with comparable incomes and educations in higher violence areas preferred reliance on prayer and instituting safety practices. Coping strategies differed based on whether mothers had been physical victims of or witnesses to violence or had no personal experience with violence. This study provides important evidence of the interactions that exist among intrapersonal, interpersonal, and environmental factors and coping behaviors.

The question of accepting responsibility is a key question, particularly in the context of multicultural health promotion. Acceptance of responsibility for behavior should not degenerate into victim blaming of those who "fail," nor should it be used as a means of health service providers and legislators abrogating their responsibility for making environmental or policy changes to support behavior change.

Problem solving is perhaps one of the most effective coping strategies. However, most health promotion programs deliver content-focused interventions but fail to teach general problem-solving skills that could generalize to deal with broader health-related concerns (Gonzalez et al., 1990).

Positive reappraisal also is a strategy that has been used by many people to cope successfully with health issues. The potential for a strong beneficial impact from such an approach can be seen in the use of cognitive structuring strategies for the reappraisal of the meaning of particular life situations (Chavez, Hubbell, McMullin, Martinez, & Mishra, 1995).

Activity as a coping strategy has many positive features. It can be used as a coping strategy to change health-related behaviors such as diet and smoking. Generally, in coping with health issues, doing something is better than doing nothing. Distraction works on the principle that the average person cannot focus on two activities simultaneously. Distraction may be of limited utility with respect to coping with health issues in that it might only help primarily hypervigilant people who are overly attentive to possible prodromal signs of problems. Self-talk is a variant of cognitive restructuring, the premise of which lies in the power of positive thinking. Positive self-talk can be employed by people to deal with the maintenance of self-management skills and to cope with the periodic setbacks that inevitably occur.

In spite of theoretical recognition regarding the role of coping skills and strategies as moderators of stress, empirical findings indicate that they have only a modest effect. Spitzer, Bartal, and Golander (1995) examine the moderating effect of demographic variables on coping effectiveness, active cognitive coping, avoidance coping, and active behavioral coping. Their findings suggest that demographic variables do play an important and somewhat surprising role in the effectiveness of coping strategies to temper psychological distress. Of the various demographic variables studied, marital status was found to have a significant effect on active cognitive coping and avoidance coping, and adherence to a religious belief system was found to have a significant effect on avoidance coping. Acculturation strain also has been related to drug use behavior among Cuban and other Hispanic youths (Vega, Zimmerman, Gil, Warheit, & Apospori, 1993).

Negy (1995) recently explored Diaz-Guerrero's (1967) hypothesis that Anglo-Americans differed from Mexicans along a dimension of active versus passive coping styles. Specifically, Diaz-Guerrero postulated that Anglo-Americans preferred to engage in other-modification (active coping), whereas Mexicans preferred to engage in self-modification (passive coping), in response to stressful events. Negy (1995) found that socioeconomic status may be more related to active coping than is culture.

Learned Helplessness Theory

Learned helplessness theory grew out of the works of Seligman, Teasdale, and Abrahamson. Simply stated, the theory states that a person who is faced with an "insurmountable" task will, on occasion, appear to behave in a manner consistent with a feeling of helplessness, depression, and a sense of failure. Although learned helplessness theory does not suggest specific strategies for coping, it may suggest a possible sequencing of interventions (Clark, Gotsch, & Rosenstock, 1993). For certain people, it might be appropriate to emphasize cognitive or emotional aspects (related to perceptions of helplessness) before the presentation of behavioral and skills-oriented educational approaches.

Singhal and Kanungo (1996) recently examined the nature of learned helplessness as cognitive disposition among university students, using representative samples from one Canadian university and two Indian universities. The results revealed some generalizability of predictions derived from the model across the two cultures. Some unique cultural differences also were found.

Social Support Theory

Cohen and Wills (1985) examined whether the positive association between social support and well-being is attributable more to an overall beneficial effect of support (director model) or to a process of support protecting persons from potentially adverse effects of stressful events (buffering model). A review of studies was organized according to whether a measure assesses support structure (the existence of relationships) or function (the extent to which one's interpersonal relationships provide particular resources).

Evidence for the buffering model was found in relation to the social support measure and the perceived availability of interpersonal resources that are responsive to the needs elicited by stressful events. Evidence for a direct effect also was found in terms of a person's degree of integration in a large social network. Both conceptualizations of social support are correct in some respects, but each represents a different process through which social support may affect well-being. Taken together, the preceding evidence suggests that people would benefit greatly not only from social resources that can be accessed in times of need but also from a high degree of ongoing integration into a large cultural or social network.

Expectancy Value Theory

It is with the purpose of persuasion in mind that researchers have turned to models and theories in attempting to create and implement effective preventive interventions. Research has shown that attitude changes produced by learning techniques, including careful thinking through of information and creation of appropriate values, reinforced by inoculation or practice in refuting attacks on newly formed attitudes, are more stable, resistant to contrary forces, and likely to be translated into action than are those acquired on the basis of more superficial stimuli by or identification with a cue (e.g., using a celebrity as a "change agent") (Gleicher & Petty, 1992). Theories and models based on these premises are called by the name "expectancy value" and are the major type of theories and models to have been applied to date in some areas of prevention research. In expectancy value theories,

> behaviour is viewed as the end point of a chain of psychological events that begins with an evaluation of the possible consequences associated with each action under consideration. On the basis of this evaluation, an action is chosen and becomes the course that the decision maker intends to follow. Subsequent events permitting, this intention is carried out by performance of the chosen action. . . . Modern expectancy theories have evolved from two areas of research: social-psychological investigations of the relationships between attitudes, beliefs, and behaviours, and from behavioural decision theory. (Carter, Gayle, & Baker, 1992, p. 1070)

Leviton (1989) comments on the increasing likelihood of succeeding in getting persuasive messages across:

> Messages will be differentially effective depending on the positive or negative nature of the arguments or appeals. Threats will produce more compliance, but positive appeals are recalled better and behavior change is more likely in the longer term. If health threats are involved, a negative approach tends to prompt coping with fear or stress . . . while a positive approach tends to prompt coping with the danger. Message clarity, use of metaphors, drawing explicit conclusions, sticking to one's strongest arguments, dealing with the opposing arguments, and doing so early in a persuasive attempt all enhance persuasiveness. (p. 44)

Results of studies on some presentation and content issues are mixed because some psychological processes are competing against others. Persuasion increases with the first few repetitions of an argument, but attention and interest decline with further repetitions, and overloading the audience with information impedes persuasion. Presenting information at or below the reading level of the target group will help, and even highly educated people appreciate simple messages (Leviton, 1989).

Health Belief Model

The health belief model, a cognitive theoretical model developed during the 1950s, is a set of interrelated variables that, when accurately measured and multiplicatively correlated, suggests why people might be motivated to engage in health-seeking behavior. It was developed by social psychologists influenced by the theoretical work of Kurt Lewin. A major contributing construct from Lewin's work was the view that an individual exists in a life space composed of regions positively, negatively, or neutrally valued (valenced). Illness would be considered a negative event to be avoided or escaped from; people would try to remain in positive or neutral life spaces. It was later realized that this view was too simplistic; some illnesses may have positive payoffs, and addictions that may lead to future illness might provide gratification in the present that seems impossible to resist. The term *value expectancy* arose from this concept and describes expectations of the future value (potential outcome), having considered perceived benefits and costs, of taking certain actions in relation to future health and well-being.

The psychological orientation of the creators of the health belief model caused them to perceive that the inner world of a person determines his or her actions, with environment influencing the situation only insofar as it would influence a person's inner perceptions. Their orientation was ahistorical; they saw the past exerting an influence only as it is represented in present dynamics (Rosenstock, 1974). The health belief model is composed of four constructs: perceived personal susceptibility (to a negative health condition), perceived severity of the condition, perceived benefits of taking a particular action against the threat, and perceived barriers to taking that action. A concept labeled "cues to action" was tentatively incorporated into the model during its early years but has been dropped because it was found to be too difficult to measure. Derivative models also have been developed (Facione, 1993).

The construct of "self-efficacy" has been added to the health belief model. Rosenstock, Strecher, and Becker (1988) argue,

> For behavioral change to succeed, people must (as the HBM [health belief model] theorizes) have an incentive to take action, feel threatened by their current behavioral patterns, and believe that change of a specific kind will be beneficial by resulting in a valued outcome at acceptable cost, but they must also feel themselves competent (self-efficacious) to implement that change. A growing body of literature supports the importance of self-efficacy in helping to account for initiation and maintenance of behavioral change. (p. 179)

However, recent results with African Americans suggest an inverted causal sequence from what the model assumes—risk behavior leading to or predicting perceptions.

Another delineation of the components of the health belief model hypothesized to be necessary determinants of a decision to take a health-related action is as follows:

- The existence of sufficient motivation (or health concern) to make health issues salient or relevant
- The belief that one is susceptible (or vulnerable) to a serious health problem or to the sequelae of that illness or condition (often termed *perceived threat*)
- The belief that following a particular health recommendation would be beneficial in reducing the perceived threat and at a subjectively acceptable cost, with cost referring to perceived barriers that must be overcome to follow the health recommendation (including, but not restricted to, financial outlays) (Rosenstock et al., 1988)

Different measures from the health belief model (perceived susceptibility, perceived severity, self-efficacy, social support, and perceived barriers) have been used to predict the incidence of a variety of "safer sex" behaviors among multicultural adolescents (Steers, Elliott, Nemiro, Ditman, & Oskamp, 1996). Perceived susceptibility, self-efficacy, and social support predicted many safer sex behaviors. Although the health belief model predicted more safer sex behaviors for Euro-American students than for Hispanic American, African American, and Asian American students, the data also indicated few differences in behavior across these ethnic groups.

Yep (1993) also examined the predictive utility of the health belief model in relation to prevention of HIV infection among Asian American college students. Three hypotheses proposed positive relationships among perceived susceptibility, severity, and benefits, and HIV-preventive behavior, whereas a fourth hypothesis postulated a negative relationship between perceived barriers to prevention and actual HIV-preventive behaviors. Severity and barriers were significant predictors of adoption of preventive behaviors among Asian Americans. Severity was a significant predictor of becoming more careful about selection of intimate partners, reducing the number of sexual partners, and generally positive changes toward safer sexual behavior. Barriers were predictive of becoming more selective of intimate partners and ensuring that partners are not infected. It also appeared that cultural factors, such as beliefs about HIV, illness prevention, sexuality, and homosexuality, need to be better incorporated into the model to enhance its predictive power.

Theory of Reasoned Action

The theory of reasoned action (Ajzen & Fishbein, 1980) is a highly specific theory outlining cognitive and attitudinal determinants of behavior. Attitudes and subjective norms determine a person's intentions, which are predictive of behavior; the shorter the time span between "intentions" and "behavior," the more likely the behavior will follow the stated intentions. "An overview of research based on the theory of reasoned action indicates that correlations between behavioral intentions and behavior are usually between .6 and .9" (Petosa & Jackson, 1991, p. 466). Questions using this theory are very specific; it often is used for elicitation research to determine which variables to target when introducing a program or an intervention. Attitudes are composed of two beliefs: to what extent the participant believes a certain behavior will lead to a certain consequence and whether or not the participant values the consequence. Social norms also are measured by using two constructs: the participant's perception of his or her referent group's desires and the participant's predilection to conform to the referent group's desires.

Closely related to the theory of reasoned action is the theory of planned behavior (Jemmott, Jemmott, & Hacker, 1992). Jemmott et al. found that attitudes and subjective norms predicted intentions to use condoms and that, consistent with the theory of planned behavior, perceived behavioral control added a significant increment. African American adolescents' perceptions of their friends' approval of condom use was unrelated to their intentions, but their behavioral beliefs about the effects of condoms on sexual enjoyment, normative beliefs regarding partners' and mothers' approval, and control beliefs regarding technical skill at using condoms were associated with such intentions.

It also is possible to combine one or more theoretical perspectives. Norris and Ford (1995) used structural equation modeling to evaluate gender and ethnic differences in a theoretical model of condom use. Their sample consisted of urban, low-income, African American, and Hispanic males and females. Their model incorporated concepts from the health belief model, theory of reasoned action, and construct accessibility model. A new theoretical concept, condom predisposition, emerged as a predictor of condom use in all four groups. This concept combines attitude, partner norms, and accessibility of condom-related constructs. These results underscore the importance of investigating gender differences within ethnic groups and the benefits of integrating different theoretical perspectives.

Cognitive-Behavioral Approaches

The cognitive-behavioral approach to health promotion and disease prevention is based on the premise that many people engage in (or fail to engage in) health behaviors, not because they lack relevant information but rather because they lack cognitive and behavioral skills necessary to use information.

Learning responsible healthy behavior, for example, is best understood as a four-step process. People need access to relevant information on which to base decisions and behavior. They must perceive, comprehend, and store this information accurately. They must personalize and use information in making effective decisions. Finally, they need behavioral skills to implement these decisions in social situations. Each step in this sequence is important; all four steps must be emphasized in any program attempting to influence health behaviors. To make decisions, individuals first must relate available facts to their own beliefs, attitudes, and values. Relating specific facts to one's own life, or "relational thinking," is the process by which information becomes part of an individual's everyday reality. Operationally, relational thinking means transforming facts such as "Active living is healthy" into self-statements or thoughts such as "Every time I exercise, I become more healthy."

St. Lawrence et al. (1995) provide an example of a cognitive-behavioral intervention to reduce African American adolescents' risk for HIV infection. It consisted of either an educational program or an 8-week intervention that combined education with behavior skills training including correct condom use, sexual assertion, refusal, information provision, self-management, problem solving, and risk recognition. Skill-trained participants reduced unprotected intercourse, increased condom-protected intercourse, and displayed increased behavioral skills to a greater extent than did participants who received information alone. The results indicated that youths who were equipped with information and specific skills lowered their risk to a greater degree, maintained risk reduction changes better, and deferred the onset of sexual activity to a greater extent than did youths who received information alone.

Communication and Persuasion Theory

Health promotion messages to various multicultural groups will be differentially effective, depending on the positive or negative nature of the arguments or appeals. Threats will produce more compliance, but positive appeals are recalled better, and behavior change is more likely in the longer term (McGuire, 1988).

If health threats are involved, then a negative approach tends to prompt coping with fear or stress, as described earlier, whereas a positive approach tends to prompt coping with the danger. Message clarity, use of metaphors, drawing explicit conclusions, sticking to one's strongest arguments, dealing with the opposing arguments, and doing so early in a persuasive attempt all enhance persuasiveness (McGuire, 1988). Results of studies on some presentation and content issues are mixed because some psychological processes are competing against others. Persuasion increases with the first few repetitions of an argument, but attention and interest decline with further repetition, and overloading the audience with information impedes persuasion. Presenting information at or below the reading level of the target group will help, and even highly educated people appreciate simple messages.

Social Marketing Theory

Social marketing theory employs a consumer orientation, audience analysis and segmentation, and aspects of exchange theory in seeking to increase the acceptability of a behavior in a target group. An example is Project LEAN (Low-Fat Eating for America Now), a national campaign whose goal was to reduce dietary fat consumption to 30% of total calories through public service advertising, publicity, and point-of-purchase programs in restaurants, supermarkets, and school and work-site cafeterias (Samuels, 1993). Project LEAN successfully demonstrated the use of the media, market segmentation, effective spokespersons, and successful partnerships.

Diffusion of Innovation Theory

A special case of communication/marketing theory is the diffusion of innovation theory (Rogers & Storey, 1987), which examines the process by which an innovative idea or practice gains acceptance. Changes in health behavior among specific cultural groups or populations (e.g., initiation of active living) may be viewed as the adoption of an innovative behavior. Innovation theory identifies several key components:

- *Compatibility:* If innovations are consistent with the economic, sociocultural, and philosophical value system of the adopter, then adoption is more likely to take place.
- *Flexibility:* Innovations that can be unbundled and used as separate components will be applicable in a wider variety of user settings.
- *Reversibility:* If, for any reason, the adopting individual (or organization) wants to revert to his or her (or its) previous practices, then it is desirable that an innovation be capable of termination. Innovations that are not, are less likely to be adopted.
- *Relative advantage:* If an innovation appears to be beneficial when compared to current and previous methods, then adoption is more likely.
- *Complexity:* Complex innovations are more difficult to communicate and understand and are, therefore, less likely to be adopted.
- *Cost efficiency:* For an innovation to be considered desirable, its perceived benefits, both tangible and intangible, must outweigh its perceived costs (Lilley & Jackson, 1990).
- *Risk:* The degree of uncertainty introduced by an innovation helps to determine its potential for adoption. Innovations that involve higher risk are less likely to be adopted (Orlandi, Landers, Weston, & Haley, 1990).

Transtheoretical (Stages of Change) Model

Another model useful in planning behavioral intervention programs is the transtheoretical model (Prochaska & DiClemente, 1983). According to this conceptual model, health behavior change is a gradual, continuous, and dynamic process. People do not move directly from old to new behaviors; rather, they progress through a sequence of five discrete stages:

- *Precontemplative:* Individuals in this stage have no intention to change their behavior. They are unaware of the risk, deny the adverse outcome could happen to them, or are aware of the risk but have made a decision not to change their behavior.
- *Contemplative:* People in this stage have formed intentions to change but have no specific plans to change in the near future.
- *Preparation:* People in this stage have plans to change their behavior in the immediate future and might have taken some initial actions.
- *Action:* People in this stage have begun changing their behavior, but the behavior change is relatively recent and might be inconsistent.
- *Maintenance:* These people have maintained consistent behavior change for an extended period of time. The newly acquired behavior has become a part of their lives.

The model postulates that individuals engaging in a new behavior move through the stages of precontemplation, contemplation, preparation, action, and maintenance. Movement through these stages does not always occur in a linear manner; it also may be cyclical, as many individuals must make several attempts at behavior change before their goals are realized. The amount of progress people make as a result of intervention tends to be a function of the stage they are in at the start of treatment.

The stages are consistent with predisposing, enabling, and reinforcing factors in the PRECEDE model and represent a time course for examining when shifts in attitudes, intentions, and behaviors occur. Another aspect of the transtheoretical model is its delineation of processes of change. These reflect how shifts in behavior occur (Prochaska, DiClemente, & Norcross, 1992) and relate to enabling or skill-related factors. Processes of change are both covert and overt activities. Change may involve multiple techniques, methods, and interventions. Change processes identified by the authors of the model include the following:

- *Consciousness raising:* Increasing information about self and problem
- *Self-reevaluation:* Assessing how one feels and thinks about oneself with respect to a problem
- *Self-liberation:* Choosing and committing to act or believing in ability to change
- *Counterconditioning:* Substituting alternatives for problem behaviors
- *Stimulus control:* Avoiding or countering stimuli that elicit problem behaviors
- *Reinforcement management:* Rewarding one's self or being rewarded by others for making changes
- *Helping relationships:* Being open and trusting about problems with someone who cares
- *Dramatic relief:* Expressing feelings about one's problems and solutions
- *Social liberation:* Increasing alternatives for nonproblem behaviors available in society; derived from a wide range of psychosocial theories (Prochaska et al., 1992)

As an example, the Pawtucket Heart Health Project employed stages of change theory in designing a social marketing campaign, IMAGINE ACTION, which was designed to get residents to exercise more frequently. Planners matched the intervention to the different stages of changes (precontemplation, contemplation, preparation, and action) with respect to exercise behavior. The results indicated that most participants moved to a higher stage in the process. For example, two thirds of individuals in the contemplation stage of preparation groups became more active.

Schorling (1995) also used the stages of change model with rural African American smokers. That study identified smokers who were in various stages of readiness to quit and provided support for applying a stages-of-change model to different cultural groups. Many of the predictors of the stage of change are the same as those found in other populations.

Common-Sense Model of Illness Representation

Diefenbach and Leventhal (1996) recently reviewed the most commonly used approaches in the study of health behaviors (e.g., medical model, health belief model, theory of reasoned action) and presented the common-sense model as an alternative. By presenting evidence across a wide range of illness domains, they demonstrated the potential usefulness of a common-sense, self-regulatory approach. The common-sense model requires further exploration but holds promise for health research among minorities.

PRINCIPLES OF HEALTH EDUCATION AS APPLIED TO MULTICULTURAL HEALTH PROMOTION

The foregoing theories of behavior change and health share a number of common elements. These elements can be distilled into several principles of behavior change and health education (e.g., educational diagnosis, hierarchy, cumulative learning, participation, situational specificity, multiple methods, individualization, relevance, feedback, reinforcement, facilitation) that can usefully inform the design and evaluation of multicultural health promotion programs.

- *Principle of educational diagnosis:* This involves identification of the causes of health behavior in specific cultural groups.
- *Principle of hierarchy:* There is a natural order in the sequence of factors influencing health behavior.
- *Principle of cumulative learning:* Experiences must be planned in a sequence that takes into account the person's prior learning experiences and the concurrent incidental learning experiences or opportunities to which people may be exposed.
- *Principle of participation:* Changes in health behavior will be greater if people have identified their own need for change and have actively selected a method or an approach that they believe will enable them to change.
- *Principle of situational specificity:* There is nothing inherently superior or inferior about any method of intervention, but the effectiveness and efficiency of any multicultural health promotion program will depend on the circumstances and the characteristics of the person and/or the change agent (e.g., peer, teacher).
- *Principle of multiple methods:* Comprehensive multicultural health promotion programs should employ different methods or components in consideration of the interaction of person-specific and situation-specific factors.
- *Principle of individualization:* Individualization or tailoring of educational interventions applies the principles of participation, situational specificity, and cumulative learning in producing interventions that are both person relevant and situation relevant.
- *Principle of relevance:* The more relevant the contents and methods used are to the person's (learner's) circumstances and interests, the more likely the learning and behavior change process will be successful.
- *Principle of feedback:* Provision of feedback allows the person to adapt both the learning process and the resultant responses to his or her own situation and pace.
- *Principle of reinforcement:* Healthy behavior that is rewarded tends to be repeated.
- *Principle of facilitation:* This involves the degree to which an intervention either provides the means for people to take action or reduces the barriers to health

behaviors. As such, this principle is closely tied to the foregoing discussion of enabling factors. Application of this principle includes the development of skills to apply behavioral techniques for self-management. These skills may include avoiding risk behavior, "triggers," or risky environments; devising alter-responses to unavoidable triggers; pairing new behaviors with a natural cue; adjusting to suit the people's reality; and learning requisite skills and identifying sources of support to overcome barriers to maintaining adequate healthy behaviors in different environments (e.g., home, school, work, outdoors).

Principle of Educational Diagnosis

The first task in changing a behavior is to determine its causes. This is referred to as the diagnostic principle of changing behavior (Green, Eriksen, & Schor, 1989). Just as the physician must diagnose an illness before it can be properly treated, so too must a behavior be diagnosed before it can be properly changed. "Properly" in this context refers to interventions that are educational rather than manipulative or coercive. If the causes of unhealthy behaviors can be understood, then health professionals can intervene with the most appropriate combination of health education, training, resource development, support, and rewards to influence the factors that predispose, enable, or reinforce healthy behaviors. An intervention linked to a diagnosed problem and an understanding of the social and cultural contexts has the greatest chance of success.

Principle of Hierarchy

The second principle of behavior change can be called the hierarchical principle. This principle states that there is a natural order in the sequence of factors influencing health behaviors. Predisposing factors must be dealt with before attempting to influence enabling factors, which in turn must be dealt with before focusing on reinforcing factors. The principle then suggests that the beliefs of people should be addressed prior to intervening to provide skills or training and that changes in beliefs and abilities must precede an examination of those factors that serve to reinforce attitudinal or behavioral changes.

Evidence exists that it is inefficient and difficult to attempt to train a person in skills to enable behavior when he or she lacks prior motivation. Unless a belief in the potential efficacy of preventive actions and sense of competence or ability to engage in such action exists, there is little point in attempting to train a person in preventive or health promotion skills. Similarly, attempts to reinforce or reward active living behavior that is not predisposed or properly enabled are likely to fail (Green et al., 1989).

In reality, the principle of hierarchy often is violated for two reasons. First, a single intervention may address several factors at once. Second, the limited occurrence of opportunities for intervention may demand that predisposing, enabling, and reinforcing factors be dealt with simultaneously.

Principle of Cumulative Learning

The principle of cumulative learning is closely related to the principle of hierarchy. To maximally influence health behavior, learning experiences must be planned in a sequence that takes into account the person's prior learning experiences and the concurrent incidental learning experiences or opportunities to which the person may be exposed (Chavez & Oetting, 1995). Behavior responds to the cumulative learning experiences of the person, including those experiences that were incidental to, or preceded, the individual's participation in a planned health education or behavior change program. (It also must be recognized that behavior is strongly influenced by the social and cultural determinants of health.)

Principle of Participation

The prospects for success in any attempt to change health behavior will be greater if the person has identified his or her own need for change and has actively selected a method or an approach that the person believes will enable him or her to change (Young & Klingle, 1996). No principle of behavior change has greater generalizability than the principle of participation (Green, 1986; Uhl, 1989). In fact, this principle forms the foundation of the definition of health promotion (Green & Kreuter, 1991; World Health Organization [WHO], 1986, 1992). The Ottawa Charter for Health Promotion defines health promotion as "the process of enabling people to increase control over, and to improve, their health" (WHO, 1986, p. 3). Health promotion defined more operationally is "any combination of educational, organizational, economic, and environmental supports for actions conducive to health" (Green & Kreuter, 1991, p. 432).

Howell, Flaim, and Lung (1992) note that an effective program does not consist of a passive transfer of information. Rather, it involves the participants in an interactive manner with an emphasis on skill building that is enhanced by effective communication and frequent feedback. They note further that the process requires valid observations, use of good judgment, and appropriate decision making. Participation, in turn, relates to the principle of "ownership," that is, that people have a sense of responsibility for and control over promoting changes in their behavior and health status. Rifkin, Muller, and Bichmann (1988) note that participation cannot be divorced from equity and that it is crucial that professionals see the benefits of people's participation to allocate the necessary time and resources to developing an approach to empowering people.

Principle of Situational Specificity

The principle of situational specificity argues against the notion of the "magic bullet" approach and holds instead that there is nothing inherently superior or inferior about any method of intervention that attempts to achieve change in health behavior. The effectiveness and efficiency of any multicultural health promotion program will depend on the circumstances, the characteristics of the people or target audience, and the characteristics of the change agent (e.g., teacher).

New methods of education or intervention may appear to be superior to "traditional" methods, but this advantage typically fades when the method loses its novelty. Green and Kreuter (1991) note that the field of health education is strewn with failed approaches. The key to successful intervention appears to lie in the strategic application of a given intervention to the right audience, at the right time, in the right way. Efforts to change people's behavior should rely more on the diagnostic principle and the principle of participation than on the development of "novel" approaches.

Principle of Multiple Methods

Insofar as multiple causes will invariably be found for any given person's behavior, the principle of multiple methods is relevant. Simply stated, this principle suggests that a different method or component of a comprehensive multicultural health promotion program must be provided for each of the different predisposing, enabling, and reinforcing factors. This principle is akin to the multitrait-multimethod matrix approach in personality psychology, which suggests that behavior change results from a complex interaction of person-specific and situation-specific factors.

Principle of Individualization

The individualization or tailoring of health promotion interventions applies the principles of participation, situational specificity, and cumulative learning. It argues for an interactive approach to learning in which people are actively involved in the learning experience. Programmed instruction, exit interviews in which people's expectations can be clarified or questions can be answered, and follow-up contacts with people after completion of a program are examples of techniques that incorporate this principle. The provision of written or audiovisual materials in combination with personal communication from a health professional may enhance a person's ability to engage in successful health behaviors. The principle of multiple methods suggests that a combination approach may have a greater likelihood of success. However, health professionals must not mistake the simple provision of multiple forms of information for an effective intervention. They also should resist the temptation to substitute the pamphlet approach for more time-consuming, but effective, personal interactions with people.

West and Aiken (1993) review the strengths and weaknesses of designs and analyses of multicomponent intervention programs. Their analysis is useful in answering questions that assess (a) whether each of the individual components contributes to the outcome, (b) whether the program is optimal, and (c) which processes of the components of the program are achieving their effects. Given that "tailoring" suggests the adaptation of learning experiences for each person, such an approach may become impossible in a large-scale program. The difficulties inherent in designing person-specific interventions may lead to the development of simplistic "lowest common denominator" approaches to interventions.

Principle of Relevance

Closely related to the principle of individualization is the principle of relevance. The principle of relevance states that the more relevant the contents and methods used are to the person's (learner's) circumstances and interests, the more likely the learning process will be successful. The more interested the person is in learning, the more likely that information pertaining to specific health behaviors will be retained and that appropriate action (self-care) will be taken. Gregg and Curry (1994) provide evidence to this effect in their study of explanatory models for cancer among African American women and the implications for a cancer screening program.

Principle of Feedback

Given the preceding principles, the principle of feedback is crucial in designing health promotion efforts. It ensures that the person obtains direct and immediate feedback on his or her progress and the effects of the health behaviors. The provision of feedback allows the person to adapt to both the learning process and the behavioral responses within the person's own situation and at his or her own pace. When comprehension of a specific regimen is the goal, feedback can take the form of asking questions to determine the amount of information that has been acquired or retained. For long-term regimens, any method that makes progress visible to the person can provide the necessary supportive feedback. The principle of feedback is relevant to both program participants and health professionals or caregivers.

Principle of Reinforcement

A fundamental principle of human behavior is that behaviors that are rewarded tend to be repeated. Nonrewarded behaviors tend to be extinguished or to disappear. Application of the principle of reinforcement involves any activity (other than feedback) that is designed to reward a person for health behavior. Reinforcement may be intrinsic or extrinsic in nature.

THEORETICAL TRENDS INFLUENCING HEALTH PROMOTION

The use of theory in the planning, implementation, and evaluation of multicultural health promotion programs also must be considered with the broader contextual trends. Three such trends are the movement toward the so-called population health perspective, the emerging social ecology approach, and the importance of community participation in all aspects of health planning and decision making.

Population Health Promotion

The term *population health* refers to a perspective suggesting that to improve the health of people, action must be taken on a broad range of factors that determine health. These determinants acknowledge the diversity of the population's health on the basis of specific factors including age, sex, economic status, and culture as leading to differences in health status that cannot be changed by medical care alone. The underlying assumption is that by improving the health of individuals, the health of the entire population will be improved.

There are many similarities among population health, health promotion, public health, and community health; for example, each of them addresses the health of the larger public. *Population health* is a more contemporary term that describes an approach based on a synthesis of the available evidence regarding key factors and conditions that determine health status. These factors are identified in strategies for population health (Health Canada, 1994) as follows:

- *Income and social status:* The relative distribution of wealth is a key factor that determines health status. Social status also affects health by determining the degree of control individuals have over life circumstance and their capacity to take action.
- *Social support networks:* Support from families, friends, and communities helps people deal with difficult circumstances in their lives and maintain a sense of mastery over the circumstances they encounter.
- *Education:* Education provides people with knowledge and skills for living, enables them to participate in their community, and increases opportunities for employment.
- *Employment and working conditions:* Meaningful employment, economic stability, and a healthy work environment are associated with health.
- *Physical environment:* Air and water quality, housing, and community safety all play a role in determining health.
- *Biology and genetic endowment:* Inherited genetic factors also play an important role in determining health.
- *Personal health practices and coping skills:* Personal health practices can play a major role in preventing disease, and coping skills can enable people to be self-reliant, solve problems, and make choices that enhance health.
- *Healthy child development:* Prenatal and early childhood experiences have a significant effect on later health.
- *Health services:* The availability of preventive and primary care services is important in determining health.

To implement a population health promotion model requires identifying one of the health determinants listed, the action strategy to be used (e.g., strengthen community action, build healthy public policy, create supportive environments, develop personal skills, reorient health services), and the level of action to be taken (e.g., society, a specific sector/system, community, family, individual). By using this approach, program planning can move toward addressing a more comprehensive range of actions related to health.

Social Ecology

The dominant theoretical models used in health education today are based on social psychology. These theories have increasingly acknowledged the role of social and cultural influences in health behavior (Freudenberg et al., 1995) by adopting an ecological perspective. Complementary to the population-based approach, social ecology involves understanding health problems within the broader context of society. It strives to move away from an emphasis limited to individual determinants and toward a broader perspective that considers social, economic, organizational, and political environments as potential points of intervention. By considering both the individual and the sociocultural context in which he or she lives, the potential for achieving and sustaining meaningful behavioral and environmental changes is maximized (Green, Richard, & Potvin, 1996; Richard, Potvin, Kishchuk, Prlic, & Green, 1996).

Stokols (1992, 1996) offers a social ecological analysis of health-promoting environments, emphasizing the transactions between individual or collective behavior and the health resources and constraints that exist in specific environmental settings. He argues that health promotion programs often lack a clear theoretical foundation or are based on narrow conceptual models. For example, lifestyle programs typically emphasize individual behavior change strategies while neglecting the environmental underpinning of health and illness. Whereas each of the behavioral, environmental, and social ecological models has its key strengths and limitations, the models are complementary and can be used to derive practical guidelines for designing and evaluating multicultural programs. Murry (1996) provides a systematic ecological framework for examining sexual activity patterns of African American adolescents. Sasao and Sue (1993) propose a research framework called the "cube" model. This model aims to assist community psychologists working in ethnic-cultural communities. It helps to make appropriate decisions on conceptual and methodological issues from a culturally anchored, ecological-contextualist perspective.

Community Participation

The concept of community participation is closely tied to the population health and ecological approaches. The past decade has seen a clear trend from intervention approaches that are technology and institution based toward a more people-based approach that involves citizens in a more direct way. This trend places the health education professional in a different role. Rather than being the initiator, developer, implementor, and decision maker, he or she acts more as the consultant, advocate, mediator, and supporter (Green & Raeburn, 1990).

The basic premise underlying this approach is that communities themselves can act as their own change agents to achieve social and behavioral outcomes. Program planning, implementation, and evaluation require early involvement and ongoing participation of leaders and community members, thus creating owner-ship and enhancing program maintenance. Underlying this perspective is an emphasis on the social forces that influence behavior, that is, the idea that behavior is formed and influenced by cultural factors (Green & Raeburn, 1990). It is through community participation that these cultural influences are examined and incorporated into the program approach.

INTEGRATING THEORY IN HEALTH PROMOTION WITH MULTICULTURAL POPULATIONS

It has been observed by many that the practitioner does not seem to use theory. Others commonly regard the use of theory as unrealistic and inapplicable (Hochbaum, Sorenson, & Lorig, 1992). Theory is difficult to apply to the real world because the real world is much more complex than anything we can anticipate. After all, theory is by definition only a reified and hypothetical explanation of the way in which the world operates. Health promotion theories cannot tell a practitioner specifically how to plan a program or what interventions to use. Theories are merely instruments that guide our thinking as to the most promising approaches to planning intervention strategies (Hochbaum et al., 1992).

It also has been acknowledged that although the training of health promotion practitioners emphasizes the use of theory, it often is taught from an academic perspective that makes application difficult and elusive. In applying theory to a practical situation, D'Onofrio (1992) suggests that the health educator should be an active consumer who questions and analyzes the utility of theory by, first, dismantling the myth of theory as the almighty standard; second, acknowledging the limitations of theory in practice; and third, exerting leadership by directly identifying and openly discussing issues confronted in practice. For example, she suggests the following questions as useful issues to consider in making planning decisions:

- What dimensions of the problem does the theory concern?
- How does the theory explain this portion of the problem?
- What additional information does the theory suggest you should gather?
- How accurately does the theoretical explanation coincide with your own under-standing of the problem?
- What important aspects of the problem does the theory fail to consider?
- What would an educational program based on the theory be like?
- How effective do you expect the program would be in reducing the problem? Why?
- If the program did result in change, then how would the theory explain it?
- If you were guided by theory, what questions would you ask in program evaluation?
- In your own judgment, how helpful is the theory in working with the problem? What are the limitations?

Whatever theoretical perspective program planners or policymakers may adopt, they need to somehow integrate such theories into some broader frameworks. The most widely applied framework in health promotion and health education is the PRECEDE-PROCEED model of Green and Kreuter (1991) that has nearly 500 published applications, many with multicultural groups. More recently, the PEN-3 model developed by Airhihenbuwa (1995) provides a practical approach to ensuring the cultural relevance of a health promotion intervention. Similar frameworks addressing the ecological validity and cultural sensitivity of psycho-social treatments also have been offered recently (Bernal, Bonilla, & Bellido, 1995).

These approaches challenge professionals to address health issues at the macro level as well as at the micro level. It is based on the assumption that any program should be anchored in a participatory approach that involves a dialog among members of the targeted culture to address cultural sensitivity and appropriate-ness. The model is appealing in that it incorporates existing models or theories and frameworks of health education and reflects theory and application in cultural studies. There are three primary dimensions of health beliefs and behaviors to consider: health education, educational diagnosis of health behavior, and cultural appropriateness of health behavior. Within each of these dimensions are three categories.

The first dimension, the process of health education, is focused simultaneously at three levels.

- *Person:* Health education is committed to the health of all. Individuals should be empowered to make informed health decisions that are appropriate to their roles in their families and communities.

- *Extended family:* Health education is concerned not only with the immediate nuclear family but also with extended kin.

- *Neighborhood:* Health education is committed to promoting health and preventing disease in neighborhoods and communities. Involvement of community members and their leaders becomes critical in providing culturally appropriate programs.

The second dimension relates to the diagnosis or assessment of the health behavior and the factors that influence individual, family, or community health actions. This dimension is based on the health belief model, the theory of reasoned action, and the PRECEDE-PROCEED framework; however, it differs in that culture plays a central role in PEN-3.

- *Perceptions:* These include knowledge, attitudes, values, and beliefs, within a cultural context, that may facilitate or hinder personal, family, and community motivation to change.

- *Enablers:* These include cultural, societal, systematic, or structural influences or forces that may enhance or be barriers to change such as the availability of resources, accessibility, referrals, employers, government officials, skills, and types of services.

- *Nurturers:* These represent the degree to which health beliefs, attitudes, and actions are influenced and mediated or nurtured by extended family, kin, friends, peers, and the community.

The third dimension, cultural appropriateness, is the most critical component of the model and is pivotal to the development of a culturally sensitive health education program.

- *Positive behaviors:* These are behaviors that are based on health beliefs and actions that are known to be beneficial and must be encouraged.
- *Existential behaviors:* These are cultural beliefs, practices, and/or behaviors that are indigenous to a group and have no harmful health consequences and, thus, need not be targeted for change and should not be blamed for program failure simply because they are not understood.
- *Negative behaviors:* These are behaviors based on health beliefs and actions that are known to be harmful to one's health.

Taken together, the examined theories have demonstrated relevance to the work of practitioners, program planners, and policymakers who work in multicultural settings. Theories can

help us understand the nature of health behaviors. They can explain the dynamics of the behavior, the processes for changing behavior, and the effects of external influences on the behavior. Theories can help us identify the most suitable targets for programs, the methods for accomplishing change, and the outcomes for evaluation. Theories and models *explain* behavior and suggest ways to achieve behavior *change*. (Glanz & Rimer, 1995, p. 9, emphases in original)

REFERENCES

Airhihenbuwa, C. O. (1995). *Health and culture: Beyond the Western paradigm.* Thousand Oaks, CA: Sage.

Ajzen, I., & Fishbein, M. (1980). *Understanding and predicting social change.* Englewood Cliffs, NJ: Prentice Hall.

Bandura, A. (1986). *Social foundations of thought and action.* Englewood Cliffs, NJ: Prentice Hall.

Bandura, A. (1988). *Social foundations of thought and action* (2nd ed.). Englewood Cliffs, NJ: Prentice Hall.

Becker, M., & Maiman, L. (1975). Sociobehavioral determinants of compliance with health and medical recommendations. *Medical Care, 13,* 10-24.

Bernal, G., Bonilla, J., & Bellido, C. (1995). Ecological validity and cultural sensitivity for outcome research: Issues for the cultural adaptation and development of psychosocial treatments with Hispanics. *Journal of Abnormal Child Psychology, 23,* 67-82.

Bruhn, J. (1983). The application of theory in childhood asthma self-help programs. *Journal of Allergy and Clinical Immunology, 72,* 561-578.

Brunswick, A. F., & Banaszakholl, J. (1996). HIV risk behavior and the health belief model: An empirical test in an African-American community sample. *Journal of Community Psychology, 24*(1), 44-65.

Carter, W. B., Gayle, T. C., & Baker, S. (1992). Behavioral intervention and the individual. In K. K. Holmes, P. A. Mardh, P. F. Sparling, & P. J. Wieser (Eds.), *Sexually transmitted diseases* (pp. 1069-1074). New York: McGraw-Hill.

Chang, E. C. (1996). Cultural differences in optimism, pessimism, and coping: Predictors of subsequent adjustment in Asian-American and Caucasian-American college students. *Journal of Counseling Psychology, 43,* 113-123.

Chavez, E. L., & Oetting, E. R. (1995). A critical incident model for considering issues in cross-cultural research: Failures in cultural sensitivity. *International Journal of the Addictions, 30,* 863-874.

Chavez, L. R., Hubbell, F. A., McMullin, J. M., Martinez, R. G., & Mishra, S. I. (1995). Structure and meaning in models of breast and cervical cancer risk factors: A comparison of perceptions among Latinas, Anglo women, and physicians. *Medical Anthropology Quarterly, 9*(1), 40-74.

Cheung, Y. W. (1993). Beyond liver and culture: A review of theories and research in drinking among Chinese in North America. *International Journal of the Addictions, 28,* 1497-1513.

Clark, N., Gotsch, A., & Rosenstock, I. (1993). Patient, professional, and public education on behavioral aspects of asthma: A review of strategies for change and needed research. *Journal of Asthma, 30,* 241-255.

Cohen, S., & Wills, T. (1985). Stress, social support, and the buffering hypothesis. *Psychological Bulletin, 98,* 310-357.

Costa, P., & Metter, J. (1994). Personality stability and its contribution to successful aging. *Journal of Geriatric Psychiatry, 27*(1), 41-59.

Diaz-Guerrero, R. (1967). Sociocultural premises, attitudes, and cross-cultural research. *International Journal of Psychology, 2,* 79-87.

Diefenbach, M. A., & Leventhal, H. (1996). The common-sense model of illness representation: Theoretical and practical considerations. *Journal of Social Distress and the Homeless, 5*(1), 11-38.

D'Onofrio, C. N. (1992). Theory and the empowerment of health education practitioners. *Health Education Quarterly, 19,* 385-403.

Facione, N. C. (1993). The Triandis model for the study of health and illness behavior: A social behavior theory with sensitivity to diversity. *Advances in Nursing Science, 15*(3), 49-58.

Fisher, J. (1988). Possible effects of reference group-based social influence on AIDS risk behavior and AIDS prevention. *American Psychologist, 43,* 914-920.

Freudenberg, N., Eng, E., Flay, B., Parcel, G., Rogers, T., & Wallerstein, N. (1995). Strengthening individual and community capacity to prevent disease and promote health: In search of relevant theories and principles. *Health Education Quarterly, 22,* 290-306.

Garrity, T. (1980). Medical compliance and the patient-provider relationship. In R. Haynes (Ed.), *Patient compliance to antihypertensive medications.* Washington, DC: National Institutes of Health.

Glanz, K., Lewis, M., & Rimer, B. K. (1990). *Health behavior and health education: Theory, research and practice.* San Francisco: Jossey-Bass.

Glanz, K., & Rimer, B. K. (1995). *Theory at a glance: A guide for health promotion practice.* Washington, DC: National Institutes of Health.

Gleicher, F., & Petty, R. (1992). Expectations of reassurance influence: The nature of fear stimulated attitude change. *Journal of Experimental Social Psychology, 28*(1), 86-100.

Goldfried, M., & D'Zurilla, T. (1969). A behavior analytic model for assessing competence. In L. Spielberger (Ed.), *Current topics in clinical and community psychology.* New York: Holt, Rinehart & Winston.

Gonzalez, V., Geoppinger, J., & Lorig, K. (1990). Four psychosocial theories and their application to patient education and clinical practice. *Arthritis Care and Research, 3*(3), 132-143.

Grant, L. M., & Ostrow, D. G. (1995). Perceptions of social support and psychological adaptation to sexually acquired HIV among white and African-American men. *Social Work, 40,* 215-224.

Green, L. W. (1986). The theory of participation: A qualitative analysis of its expression in national and international policies. *Advances in Health Education and Promotion, 1A,* 211-236.

Green, L. W., Eriksen, M., & Schor, E. (1989). Preventive practices by physicians: Behavioral determinants and potential interventions. *American Journal of Preventive Medicine, 4*(Suppl.), 101-107.

Green, L. W., & Kreuter, M. (1991). *Health promotion planning: An educational and environmental approach.* Mountain View, CA: Mayfield.

Green, L. W., & Raeburn, J. (1990). Contemporary developments in health promotion: Definitions and challenges. In N. Bracht (Ed.), *Health promotion at the community level.* Newbury Park, CA: Sage.

Green, L. W., Richard, L., & Potvin, L. (1996). Ecological foundations of health promotion. *American Journal of Health Promotion, 10,* 270-281.

Gregg, J., & Curry, R. H. (1994). Explanatory models for cancer among African-American women at two Atlanta neighborhood health centers: The implications for a cancer screening program. *Social Science and Medicine, 39,* 519-526.

Haynes, R., Taylor, D., & Sackett, D. (1979). *Compliance in health care.* Baltimore, MD: Johns Hopkins University Press.

Health Canada. (1994). *Strategies for population health: Investing in the health of Canadians.* Ottawa: Minister of Supply and Services.

Hill, H. M., Hawkins, S. R., Raposo, M., & Carr, P. (1995). Relationship between multiple exposures to violence and coping strategies among African-American mothers. *Violence and Victims, 10*(1), 55-71.

Hochbaum, G. M., Sorenson, J. R., & Lorig, L. (1992). Theory in health education practice. *Health Education Quarterly, 19,* 295-313.

Howell, J., Flaim, T., & Lung, C. (1992). Patient education. *Pediatric Clinics of North America, 39,* 1343-1361.

Janis, I., & Rodin, J. (1979). Attribution, control and decision-making. In G. Stone (Ed.), *Health psychology.* San Francisco: Jossey-Bass.

Jemmott, J. B., III, Jemmott, L. S., & Hacker, C. I. (1992). Predicting intentions to use condoms among African-American adolescents: The theory of planned behavior as a model of HIV risk-associated behavior. *Ethnicity and Disease, 2,* 371-380.

Kanfer, F. (1975). Self-management methods. In F. Kanfer & A. Goldstein (Eds.), *Helping people change: A textbook of methods.* Elmsford, NY: Pergamon.

Kasl, S., & Cobb, S. (1966). Health behavior, illness behavior, and sick-role behavior. *Archives of Environmental Health, 12,* 246-250.

Krohn, M. D., & Thornberry, T. P. (1993). Network theory: A model for understanding drug abuse among African-American and Hispanic youth. *NIDA Research Monograph, 130,* 102-128.

Lazarus, R., & Folkman, S. (1984). *Stress, appraisal and coping.* New York: Springer.

Leventhal, H., Meyer, D., & Gutmann, M. (1980). The role of theory in the study of compliance. In R. Haynes (Ed.), *Patient compliance to antihypertensive medications.* Washington, DC: National Institutes of Health.

Leviton, L. (1989). Can organizations benefit from worksite health promotion? *Health Services Research, 24*(2), 159-189.

Lilley, J., & Jackson, L. (1990). The value of activities: Establishing a foundation for cost-effectiveness—A review of the literature. *Activities, Adaptation and Aging, 14*(4), 5-20.

Maiman, L., Becker, M., & Liptak, G. (1988). Improving pediatricians' compliance enhancing practices. *American Journal of Disorders in Childhood, 142,* 773-779.

Matarazzo, J., Miller, N., Weiss, S., Herd, J., & Weiss, S. (1984). *Behavioral health: A handbook of health enhancement and disease prevention.* New York: John Wiley.

McGuire, M. (1988). *Ritual healing in suburban America.* New Brunswick, NJ: Rutgers University Press.

Mullens, P., & Reynolds, R. (1978). The potential for grounded theory in health education research. *Health Education Research, 6,* 280-285.

Murry, V. M. (1996). An ecological analysis of coital timing among middle-class African-American adolescent females. *Journal of Adolescent Research, 11,* 261-279.

Negy, C. (1995). Coping and culture: A research note on Diaz-Guerrero's theory. *Psychological Reports, 76,* 680-682.

Norris, A. E., & Ford, K. (1995). Condom use by low-income African-American and Hispanic youth with a well-known partner: Integrating the health belief model, theory of reasoned action, and the construct accessibility model. *Journal of Applied Social Psychology, 25,* 1801-1830.

Orlandi, M. A., Landers, C., Weston, R., & Haley, N. (1990). Diffusion of health promotion innovations. In K. Glanz, M. Lewis, & B. K. Rimer (Eds.), *Health behavior and health education: Theory, research and practice* (pp. 288-313). San Francisco: Jossey-Bass.

Orshan, S. A. (1996). Acculturation, perceived social support, and self-esteem in Primigravida Puerto Rican teenagers. *Western Journal of Nursing Research, 18,* 460-473.

Petosa, R., & Jackson, K. (1991). Using the health belief model to predict safer sex intentions among adolescents. *Health Education Quarterly, 18,* 463-476.

Picot, S. J. (1995). Rewards, costs, and coping of African-American caregivers. *Nursing Research, 44*(3), 147-152.

Prochaska, J. O., & DiClemente, C. C. (1983). Stages and processes of self-change of smoking: Toward an integrated model of change. *Journal of Consulting and Clinical Psychology, 51,* 390.

Prochaska, J. O., DiClemente, C. C., & Norcross, J. C. (1992). In search of how people change: Applications to addictive behaviors. *American Psychologist, 47,* 1102-1114.

Ray, M. (1973). Marketing communication and the hierarchy of effects. In P. Clarke (Ed.), *New models for mass communication research.* Beverly Hills, CA: Sage.

Richard, L., Potvin, L., Kishchuk, N., Prlic, H., & Green, L. W. (1996). Assessment of the integration of the ecological approach in health promotion programs. *American Journal of Health Promotion, 10,* 318-328.

Rifkin, S., Muller, F., & Bichmann, W. (1988). Primary health care: On measuring participation. *Social Science and Medicine, 26,* 931-940.

Rogers, E. M., & Storey, J. D. (1987). Communication campaigns. In C. Berger & S. Chaffee (Eds.), *Handbook of communication science.* Newbury Park, CA: Sage.

Rosensteil, A., & Keefe, F. (1983). The use of coping strategies in chronic low back pain. *Pain, 17,* 33-40.

Rosenstock, I. M. (1974). Historical origins of the health belief model. *Health Education Monographs, 2,* 328-343.

Rosenstock, I. M., Strecher, V. J., & Becker, M. H. (1988). Social learning theory and the health belief model. *Health Education Quarterly, 15,* 175-183.

Sade, R. M. (1995). A theory of health and disease: The objectivist-subjectivist dichotomy. *Journal of Medicine and Philosophy, 20,* 513-525.

Samuels, S. (1993). Project LEAN: A national campaign to reduce dietary fat consumption. *American Journal of Health Promotion, 4,* 435-440.

Sasao, T., & Sue, S. (1993). Toward a culturally anchored ecological framework of research in ethnic-cultural communities. *American Journal of Community Psychology, 21,* 705-727.

Scheier, M., & Carver, C. (1992). Effects of optimism on psychological and physical well-being: Theoretical overview and empirical update. *Cognitive Therapy and Research, 16,* 201-228.

Schorling, J. B. (1995). The stages of change of rural African-American smokers. *American Journal of Preventive Medicine, 11*(3), 170-177.

Sennott-Miller, L. (1994). Using theory to plan appropriate interventions: Cancer prevention for older Hispanic and non-Hispanic white women. *Journal of Advanced Nursing, 20,* 809-814.

Singhal, S., & Kanungo, R. N. (1996). Learned helplessness among university students: A bi-national test of the attributional model. *Psychologia, 39*(1), 42-49.

Smaje, C. (1996). The ethnic patterning of health: New directions for theory and research. *Sociology of Health and Illness, 18*(2), 139-171.

Spitzer, A., Bartal, Y., & Golander, H. (1995). The moderating effects of demographic variables on coping effectiveness. *Journal of Advanced Nursing, 22,* 578-585.

Steers, W. N., Elliott, E., Nemiro, J., Ditman, D., & Oskamp, S. (1996). Health beliefs as predictors of HIV-preventive behavior and ethnic differences in prediction. *Journal of Social Psychology, 136,* 99-110.

St. Lawrence, J. S., Brasfield, T. L., Jefferson, K. W., Alleyne, E., O'Bannon, R. E., III, & Shirley, A. (1995). Cognitive-behavioral intervention to reduce African-American adolescents' risk for HIV infection. *Journal of Consulting and Clinical Psychology, 63,* 221-237.

Stokols, D. (1992). Establishing and maintaining healthy environments: Toward a social ecology of health promotion. *American Psychologist, 47,* 6-22.

Stokols, D. (1996). Translating social ecological theory into guidelines for community health promotion. *American Journal of Health Promotion, 10,* 282-298.

Uhl, J. (1989). International networking: Coordinating health promotion strategies with multiple interventions. *Annals of the Academy of Medicine, 18,* 280-285.

van Ryn, M., & Heaney, C. (1992). What's the use of theory? *Health Education Quarterly, 19,* 315-330.

Vega, W. A., Zimmerman, R., Gil, A., Warheit, G. J., & Apospori, E. (1993). Acculturation strain theory: Its application in explaining drug use behavior among Cuban and other Hispanic youth. *NIDA Research Monograph, 130,* 144-166.

Wallston, B., & Wallston, K. (1978). Locus of control and health. *Health Education Monographs, 6,* 107-115.

Walter, H. J., Vaughan, R. D., & Cohall, A. T. (1993). Comparison of three theoretical models of substance use among urban minority high school students. *Journal of the American Academy of Child and Adolescent Psychiatry, 32,* 975-981.

West, S., & Aiken, L. (1993). Probing the effects of individual components in multiple component prevention programs. *American Journal of Community Psychology, 21,* 571-605.

World Health Organization. (1986). *The Ottawa Charter for Health Promotion.* Ottawa: Health and Welfare Canada.

World Health Organization. (1992, November 20). *AIDS: "A Community Commitment" is the theme of World Aids Day* (Press Release WHO/19). Geneva, Switzerland: Author.

Yep, G. A. (1993). HIV prevention among Asian-American college students: Does the health belief model work? *Journal of American College Health, 41*(5), 199-205.

Young, M., & Klingle, R. S. (1996). Silent partners in medical care: A cross-cultural study of patient participation. *Health Communication, 8*(1), 29-53.

Zhang, J. X., & Schwarzer, R. (1995). Measuring optimistic self-beliefs: A Chinese adaptation of the General Self-Efficacy Scale. *Psychologia, 38*(3), 174-181.

4

Planning Health Promotion and Disease Prevention Programs in Multicultural Populations

MICHAEL V. KLINE

Deaths from breast cancer have been increasing for the past several years among Latino women living in a large metropolitan community. The local health jurisdiction, private providers, and voluntary agencies are very concerned and want to reduce the number of deaths drastically. There are severe financial limitations on initiating any new programs. Although increased screening, referral, and treatment programs are critically needed, monies will be available for providing health education programs only to selected target groups of women. Who will the target groups be, and which should have priority? What are the specific health education or health promotion needs, and how will they be identified? What types of breast cancer education and screening resources currently are available and accessible, and are they being used? Is one large program or a series of educational programs needed? What should be the objectives of the programs? What cultural considerations does the planner need to be aware of when selecting the programs' educational intervention strategies? If programs are implemented, then how will the administrator know whether the programs are having any effect on the problem?

This planning scenario unfolds in a large community setting involving the need for health promotion activities targeted at Latino women at risk for breast cancer. The scenario could have considered any ethnic population and been located within another community, work site, school, or health care program setting. The special needs posed by the target population and the particular setting and health problem are the types of challenges confronting the health promotion program planner in urban and rural communities, in inner cities, and on reservations. Planning in these settings must be a collaborative effort involving the planner, participants, governmental officials, and staff or workers involved in carrying out the program. All must be heard and represented in the decision-making processes. All who are expected to function effectively in multicultural planning must be aware and accepting of cultural differences, should be culturally knowledgeable about the target group, should be able to carry out a process of cultural self-assessment, and should possess skills that aid in adapting to diverse situations (Cross, Bazron, Dennis, & Isaacs, 1989).

The purpose of this chapter is to provide health practitioners with basic foundations for planning health promotion and health education programs in multicultural populations. The intent of the chapter is to serve as a general primer for the health promotion program planning process. Topics related to current health promotion planning models, specific elements of the planning process, and selected multicultural planning issues and concerns are covered here. This chapter serves as a prelude to Chapters 7, 11, 15, 19, and 23, which illustrate the application of program planning principles in several different ethnic populations.

Planning health promotion and disease prevention (HPDP) programs in multicultural populations is a dynamic and challenging process that requires systematic identification and selection of a particular course of action. These programs may concentrate on facilitating the voluntary acquisition of specific health-related knowledge, attitudes, and practices to achieve behavior related to improving or promoting health where people live and work. They also may seek social or environmental changes (supportive structures) in the form of policy changes, regulations, and new or increased organizational arrangements for encouraging, enabling, and reinforcing the practice of certain health-related behaviors (Green & Kreuter, 1991). Health promotion professionals also are involved in the development of ecological models that can be used for assisting the planner in better understanding the effect of the environment on behavior and vice versa (Bronfenbrenner, 1979; Green, Richard, & Potvin, 1996; McLeroy, Bibeau, Steckler, & Glantz, 1988; Richard, Potvin, Kishchuk, Prlic, & Green, 1996; Sallis & Owen, 1997; Stokols 1996; Syme, 1986). The application of these concepts will enable those working in community programs to develop further approaches for encouraging health-promoting and health-protecting behaviors.

The planning process also requires the planner and participants to define the level of change sought as a result of their program—at the health education or health promotion level. It is at the health education level, given the realities of financial support in most communities, where most current planning activities will occur and where the majority of those reading this chapter will function in their communities. Although planning processes and concepts are similar regardless of the level of program focus, this chapter operates more heavily from a health education vantage point. Health promotion encompasses health education, but health education is a primary instrumentality for achieving health promotion outcomes. Nevertheless, the program planning outcomes at each level of program focus will depend on the particular scope of objectives and the strategies and intervention activities for achieving the objectives. For example, the focus of health education interventions for a breast cancer education and screening program for Latino women is to make specific types of educational resources more available and accessible for enabling them to develop knowledge, attitudes, and skills for carrying out defined voluntary behaviors related to reducing the risk of a life-threatening disease. The planning of interventions and related activities in this instance focuses on reaching only one of the many possible target groups in need of a specific educational program. On the other hand, the planning of strategies and interventions at the health promotion program level goes beyond a single breast cancer screening program focus. Planning efforts at this level may be focused on putting in place a more accessible and equitably distributed system of women's health programs (including breast cancer education and screening programs, among other services) for enhancing the overall health of all poor and underserved women in that particular community. Intervention activities on this level will require the establishment of an appropriate combination of educational, organizational, and political supports in the community needed to stimulate, develop, and sustain the actions needed for achieving the desired outcome. The complexity of the community-level health promotion program effort requires a greater scope of coordination, agency, and citizen participation, commitment, and expense than does the breast cancer education and screening program that was aimed at a single target group.

Current Health Promotion Program
Planning Models as Guides to Practice

The formidable task of developing and implementing a health promotion program requires the planner and participants to work together to accomplish a complex range of activities including (a) assessing needs, problems, and resources of the target population; (b) developing appropriate goals and objectives; (c) devising strategies and interventions that consider the peculiarities of the settings; (d) implementing and monitoring the interventions; (e) evaluating the results; and (f) refining approaches toward greater program effectiveness and efficiency. Owing to the scope and complexity of the planning process, practitioners need to operate from some rational planning framework or model rather than solely on the basis of pragmatic, empirical, or expediency considerations. Program planning models provide organizing frameworks that encourage a more systematic approach to the development of health promotion programs for specific target groups. There are no perfect health education or health promotion planning models because none offers a predictable relationship between means used and ends achieved in the planning process. In spite of this limitation, several of the traditional health education planning models have been widely used over time and serve as well-established frameworks for planning. It is a limitation of the models that the planner must be able to adapt them to fit the needs of the planning situation and the cultural characteristics of the target group, setting, and health problem. Therefore, if the models are used in multicultural health promotion planning situations, then the planner must be extremely conscious of and sensitive to the need for building a cultural assessment component into the planning process. With these caveats, then, what planning models are available to the health promotion planner? Health education or health promotion planning models generally are grounded in some universally accepted principles of planning and health planning. Some of the health education or health promotion planning models that have served as the old "stand-bys" through the years include the model for health education planning (Ross & Mico, 1980), the comprehensive health education model (Sullivan, 1977), and the health education/promotion planning model (Dignan & Carr, 1992). These models follow a traditional planning approach and generally divide planning activities into three major parts: planning the program, implementing the program, and evaluating the program. Several subactivities usually are carried out in a similar sequence to operationalize the major activities. The frameworks vary in depth and perspective, but most are intended to help move the planner and participants systematically through the planning process regardless of target group or program setting. Each advocates the need to consider the cultural aspects of the planning situation but, as already noted, does not furnish in-depth instructions.

Another health education or health promotion planning framework, PRE-CEDE-PROCEED, needs to be discussed separately from the preceding models owing to its broad acceptance and use in the field (Green & Kreuter, 1991; Green, Kreuter, Deeds, & Partridge, 1980). The PRECEDE model originated in the 1970s and is an acronym standing for *Predisposing, Reinforcing, and Enabling Constructs in Educational Diagnosis and Evaluation*. Unlike the other models, the initial focus of the planner is on the desired final outcomes of the planning effort, and the planner tries to identify what will cause the desired outcome. The five-step framework requires the planner to systematically diagnose all of the important factors (e.g., social, epidemiological, behavioral, environmental, educational) that *precede* the desired outcomes prior to designing the program intervention (Green & Kreuter, 1991). The PROCEED (*Policy, Regulatory, and Organizational Constructs in Educational and Environmental Development*) segment of the framework, added in 1991, includes four more steps for converting the plan developed under PRECEDE into health education interventions, policy, organization, and regulation. The PROCEED component seeks to go beyond only considering the level of educational activities for changing unhealthy behaviors and moves into the political arena where policy and environmental supports can be put in place for affecting health of the entire population (Green & Kreuter, 1991). The nine phases of the PRECEDE-PROCEED planning process clearly guide the planner in a sequential manner. The framework, from the earliest stage, emphasizes the need to collect explicit diagnostic information necessary to progress systematically through the steps of health promotion program planning. In this regard, PRECEDE does encourage the collection of culture-specific information about the target group that assists in understanding its members' behaviors. The planner needs to understand the complexity of the model and the fact that it is based on the proposition that health behaviors are very complex, multidimensional, and influenced by a variety of factors (Gielen & McDonald, 1997). Also, over its 30-year history, it has been applied in a wide variety of health settings—multicultural and otherwise—focusing on many different health problem areas and target groups. A further indication of the model's theoretical robustness derives from the hundreds of published applications of the model demonstrating its utility for planning, implementation, and evaluation of health promotion and health education programs (Green et al., 1996). The model has been the single most frequently used health education planning framework in developing individual-level interventions (Steckler et al., 1995). Gielen and McDonald (1997) note that potential users of PRECEDE-PROCEED should recognize that the model is heavily dependent on data and that, depending on the situation, its application might require more funding and human resources than are available. It is a valuable framework, however, because many of its diagnostic components may be used by planning groups regardless of the planning model followed. Space considerations have allowed only cursory description of the framework and conceptual foundations.

There are other health education or health promotion planning models that can serve as useful frameworks for practitioners. The PATCH (Planned Approach To Community Health) framework was developed in the mid-1980s by the federal Centers for Disease Control and Prevention in partnership with state and local health departments and community groups (Kreuter, 1992; U.S. Department of Health and Human Services, 1996). The planning framework consists of five distinct phases for helping communities establish health promotion teams, collect and use local data, set health priorities, and design and evaluate interventions. PATCH is a bottoms-up approach initiated at the grassroots level. It uses the diagnostic planning principles of PRECEDE and emphasizes local ownership of planning and health promotion programs (Green & Kreuter, 1991, 1992; Kreuter, 1992). Tremendous amounts of data and information are collected during this planning process, so the planner must be culturally sensitive to the need for separating out cultural and socioeconomic variables during the data collection activities that can better define target groups and their specific program needs. Orenstein, Nelson, Speers, Brownstein, and Ramsey (1992) report on four evaluations that were conducted on PATCH between 1988 and 1991 and note that coordinators involved in the process of planning needed substantial training in the following areas: "PATCH planning process, leadership techniques, coalition building and maintenance, fund-raising, grant writing, media relations, legislative advocacy, volunteer management, intervention planning, and maintenance and institutional of PATCH" (p. 190). Another planning model with a different focus, the PEN-3 (Person, Extended family, Neighborhood) model, grew out of the need to develop a more culturally appropriate planning framework for health promotion programs in Africa and for African Americans (Airhihenbuwa, 1995). Planning issues involving cultural appropriateness and cultural sensitivity are made explicit in PEN-3. The model urges that culture should have a central role in the process of educational diagnosis and should be incorporated as a formal component when planning health promotion programs for any target group.

Also, the planner is in the beginning stages of applying ecological concepts and approaches for achieving and encouraging health-promoting and health-protecting behaviors (Green et al., 1996; McLeroy et al., 1988; Stokols, 1996). For example, these activities have had a profound effect on changing behaviors as to where and when smoking is permitted at work. In some instances, smoking has been banned in workplace environments as a result of local or state regulations. In general, the ecological models of health behavior will help the health promotion program planner identify and better understand the roles that intrapersonal, social/cultural, and physical environment variables have in affecting behavior, the interactions among these variables, the levels on which they operate, and their relationship to changing behaviors (Sallis & Owen, 1997).

A final important point needs to be addressed. Conceptually and practically speaking, a program planning model is not and should not be confused with an intervention strategy model (Steckler et al., 1995). They are not the same, do not serve the same purpose, and should not be used as synonymous concepts or organizing frameworks. The health education intervention strategy is a specific component of the program planning model. It is based on one or another of the theoretical models underlying the development of individual, group, or community interventions. These models, it should be noted, have their roots in the behavior and social sciences and educational theory. However, planning models, such as the PRECEDE-PROCEED and PATCH models, can provide the overall framework for helping practitioners to identify and apply intervention strategies for achieving change at the individual, group, community, or organizational level (Green & Kreuter, 1991).

Health Promotion and Disease Prevention Programs in Multicultural Populations: A Planning Framework

The framework conceptualized in Figure 4.1 depicts a traditional and detailed sequence of planning activities. The intent of the framework is to help practitioners visualize the health education or health promotion planning process as systematically as possible. Another intent is to provide an uncomplicated framework that can be used, at specific points of chapter discussion, for relating and applying various approaches and methods suggested by other planning models. The planning framework in Figure 4.1 identifies three major tasks, each with related subtasks. Each of these areas is discussed in this chapter. The sequence of the tasks and subtasks may vary, depending on the circumstances. Also, there are many different meanings and definitions for "community." For the purposes of this chapter, "community" refers to a group of people (a *target population*) who share a common ethnic background and identity as well as common values, norms, and communication channels and who occupy an area (geographical or otherwise) within which their health-related problems and needs can be defined and dealt with. The term *target groups* indicates aggregates of individuals selected from the target populations after the planning process identifies the relationships among their needs, problems, and resources (or resource gaps) and after priorities are defined and understood. Target groups constitute the focus of planning efforts.

Task 1: Planning the Program

Subtask A:	Involving those affected by the problem
Subtask B:	Assessing the needs of the community
Subtask C:	Diagnosing health-related concerns (problems and needs) in the community
Subtask D:	Prioritizing and selecting the target populations, problems, and settings
Subtask E:	Assessing the specific needs of the target group
Subtask F:	Developing appropriate target group goals and objectives
Subtask G:	Selecting health promotion program intervention activities that consider the peculiarities of the target group, health problem, and setting

Task 2: Implementing the Program

Subtask A:	Pre-implementation preparation
Subtask B:	Program implementation
Subtask C:	Implementation administration and monitoring

Task 3: Evaluating the Program

Subtask A:	Assessing the immediate impact of the program (impact evaluation)
Subtask B:	Assessing the long-term target group health and social outcomes (outcome evaluation)
Subtask C:	Assessing the quality of program inputs during the development and implementation phases (process/formative evaluation)

Figure 4.1   Planning Framework

TASK 1: PLANNING THE PROGRAM

Subtask A: Involving Those Affected by the Problem

Health education planners always have been encouraged to involve in the planning process those who are affected by the health-related problem. Their participation should occur from the time the problem is first felt but not well defined to the time it is well documented and ultimately serves as a basis for writing objectives, developing strategies, and implementing and evaluating the program. All of the planning models discussed earlier recognize the importance of this quality of participation. Figure 4.1 identifies the need to involve those affected by the problem as the first formal step of the program planning process. This principle of participation might well be the most important ingredient of program development (Gielen & McDonald, 1997; Green & Kreuter, 1991; Minkler, 1990; Ross & Mico, 1980; Sullivan, 1977). The planners needs to recognize the needs, the interests, and the social, cultural, and economic settings in which participants live. They should have a part in the planning, thus making the situation one in which there is planning *with* and not just *for* the people. Participants involved in the planning and those participating in the program's activities should likewise participate in its evaluation (Ross & Mico, 1980). The planner must identify the many possible points of involvement and understand that there are many ways and reasons for how and why people become involved.

Collaboration between the planner and participants is possible only if each understands the other's values, has mutual respect for the agenda to be accomplished, and accepts the other as integral to the approach to the problem.

The planner and participants need to be "culturally competent" as they interact and work together in the overall HPDP planning process (Huff & Kline, Chapter 26, this volume). Unlike common conceptions of cultural competence where the onus is on the health care professional to acquire such competence, it needs to be a two-way process between the planner and participants. Both must be sensitive to their own patterns and styles of interaction with other cultures, particularly as these styles could reflect biases or prejudices that could seriously disrupt the planning process. The planner and participants must avoid imposing their beliefs, values, and patterns of behavior on another culture (Campinha-Bacote, 1994; Leininger, 1978). Participants also must be prepared or trained to ultimately assume control over their own programs and planning processes.

Subtask B: Assessing the Needs of the Community or Target Population

The establishment of the need for a health promotion program for a specific target group or population should be based on the study of factual information and not on the hunches or biases of politicians, the planner, or participants. The scope of the assessment activity will depend on how complex the problems and needs of a target population are. In some instances, understanding of the problem will be very limited, and assessment must begin with an intensive multilevel study of the community. In other instances, the assessment will be more focused, and governmental or private grant monies may become available with instructions that precisely identify the setting, target group, health issue, and program intervention. Another situation could involve the authorization of funds for assessing some area of employee health risk at a designated work site to substantiate the need for a program to reduce employee health risk and employer costs. Furthermore, assessments are required to verify the magnitude of need related to providing legally mandated, tax-supported programs to some target group. At some level, then, an assessment of need must be conducted to identify the problems and needs of a target population and to identify and measure gaps between what is and what ought to be (Butler, 1997; McKenzie & Jurs, 1993; Timmreck, 1995; Windsor, Baranowski, Clark, & Cutter, 1984). Dignan and Carr (1992) view the needs assessment process as consisting of two related parts. The first segment, "community analysis," involves the collection of extensive information for investigating social and health-related problems, needs, and program resources of the community. "Community diagnosis" is the second segment and uses the information gathered in the first segment to identify specific health problems and resources that exist within specific target populations and HPDP programs to meet those needs. A process involving a more focused target group diagnosis is conducted later (in Subtask E).

If the planning situation requires a thorough assessment at the community level, then comprehensive data for defining target populations and their health-related problems and needs will have to be collected. Because an enumeration of the complete range of community assessment information to be collected would be too extensive, Table 4.1 is used to list obvious and available categories of information and examples of types of information. Several good texts are available for helping practitioners develop needs assessment formats including discussion of methods and techniques for collecting information (Dignan & Carr, 1992; Gilmore & Campbell, 1996; Green & Kreuter, 1991; Green et al., 1980). The several categories of community assessment data presented in Table 4.1 can provide the planner and participants with the information needed to be synthesized and analyzed at the diagnosis stage.

Subtask C: Diagnosing Health-Related Concerns (Problems and Needs) in the Community

The planner and participants need to take this segment of the needs assessment process very seriously. Sometimes, the problem definition is easy, and collected information may disclose obvious issues that require no protracted period of study. In these instances, of course, one still should verify the accuracy of the finding (McKenzie & Jurs, 1993). More often, the plethora of information constitutes a giant puzzle in need of time-consuming study, synthesis, interpretation, and verification to make sense out of all the pieces.

The diagnosis process should provide the planner with at least the following information: (a) objective description of the health- and non-health-related problems and where they are concentrated as well as their nature, extent, and trends and how they contribute to the problem; (b) identification of specific target groups within target populations that are affected; (c) understanding why the target population or group is affected (e.g., as a result of taking or not taking specific personal health actions if those actions would prevent or ameliorate the problem); (d) identification of necessary health behaviors needed to be taken by the target population to prevent, ameliorate, or eliminate the health-related problem; (e) identification of specific environmental interventions needed to prevent, ameliorate, or eliminate the health-related problem within the target population; (f) identification and understanding of the degree of control the target population or agencies or institutions in the community actually have to prevent, ameliorate, or eliminate the health-related problem; (g) understanding whether and how the problem was dealt with in the past; and (h) identification of the scope and adequacy, availability, and accessibility of resources necessary to deliver health and health promotion services to the target population related to preventing, ameliorating, or eliminating the health-related problem.

The PRECEDE-PROCEED model requires the planner to approach this diagnostic segment of the planning process in a systematic fashion and provides an excellent methodological format to follow (Green & Kreuter, 1991; Green et al., 1980). Phase 1 activities of the models are involved with performing a social diagnosis for assessing the quality of life as defined by social problems in the target population. An epidemiological diagnosis also is performed (Phase 2) and seeks to identify specific health- and non-health-related problems and their contributing roles in the social and health problems identified. Once these types of problems are identified and prioritized, decisions can be made as to which of the problems will be dealt with by the programs. The process of diagnosis

TABLE 4.1 Examples of Needs Assessment Information

Category of Information	Types of Information
1. "Eyeball" information for getting to know the physical-spatial character of the community (urban/inner city, rural, reservation)	Neighborhood pride, transportation, physical terrain, geographical isolation, parks, population density, physical condition of neighborhoods, traffic, congestion
2. General information about who lives in the community	Demographic data: age, sex, sex ratios, marital status, income, employment status, types of jobs, condition of housing, level of education, religion, nationality, generational information, poverty, in-/out-migration, family and household characteristics; vital events: births, deaths, marriages, divorces, mobility, dependency ratios, immigration status
3. General information about the community	Governmental structure (city, county, reservation, federal), political and power structure, quality of life, stress indicators (homicides, suicides, drunk driving, robberies, assualts, education and recreation facilities and resources), access to drugs, alcohol beverage outlets, gang problems, school dropout rate, self-esteem, spousal and child abuse, alienation, discrimination, feelings of hope and despair, feelings of anger, civic pride, gatekeepers, community leadership, communication channels, opinion leaders, local economy, industry
4. Information about the state of health of the people who live in the community	Morbidity (illness) and mortality (death): total numbers/percentages by age, race/ethnicity, sex, cause, geographical area of occurrence; incidence and prevalence rates of chronic diseases and communicable diseases: distribution, intensity, duration; risk factors: disability by cause, days of work lost; occupational risks and diseases: mental illness, alcohol and drug problems, immunization levels
5. Information about health care and social services system in the community	Health facilities: numbers, types, location, adequacy (hospitals, emergency facilities, outpatient/urgent walk-in care, mental health alcohol/drug treatment programs, nursing homes), acessibility and availability of services, adequacy of numbers of trained public health and private health personnel, number covered by health insurance (Medicare, Medicaid, private insurance, Supplemental Security Income), adequacy of local welfare programs in covering basic needs, scope and adequacy of local health department services, scope and adequacy of local voluntary health, operational health promotion programs (work sites, schools, community, health providers)
6. Preliminary baseline health education-related information gathered from community target populations	Level of health knowledge, health attitudes, and health behaviors/skills; identification of health risks, knowledge about location and availabilty of promotion/education programs and resources, patterns of using health promotion and health education resources

ultimately provides the important foundations for deriving program objectives and for the ultimate selection of the strategies and methods to be used to accomplish the objectives (Steuart, 1969).

Subtask D: Prioritizing and Selecting the Target Population or Group, Health Problem, and Setting

Communities do not possess the capacity to deal with all of the health problems and target group issues identified in the needs assessment and diagnosis phases. The planner and participants must establish priorities in a rational manner concerning the problems, target groups, and program needs. Techniques and approaches for prioritizing needs range from simple discussion and concensus using nominal group process techniques to qualitative ranking procedures (Blum, 1974; Gilmore & Campbell, 1996; Timmreck, 1995). The PATCH planning model proponents recommend that, prior to setting priorities related to which target group and health problem should be tackled first, the planner and participants should complete the following tasks:

- Set criteria, examine community data, and develop a list of health problems
- Assess the community's capacity to address the health problems
- Determine the changeability and importance of priority health problems
- Assess social, political, [and] economic issues that might influence the ability to address the health problems
- Identify community programs and policies already addressing the health problems (U.S. Department of Health and Human Services, 1996, p. CG4-1)

It also is useful for the planner to employ several basic questions raised in Phase 2 of the PRECEDE-PROCEED model that can help prioritize health problems or goals. Some of these questions are concerned with the following: Which problem has the greatest impact in terms of death, disease, days lost from work, and cost to the community? Which subpopulation is at specific risk? Which problem would be most amenable to program intervention? Which problem, when appropriately addressed, has the greatest potential for resulting in improved health status, economic savings, and the like? (Green & Kreuter, 1991).

Priorities selected must be based on the importance of the identified health problem to the community and on the community's ability to realistically do something about the problem. The planner and participants should seriously consider selecting the fewest number of health problems and target groups to focus on so that resources can be allocated in the most effective manner. It is at this priority-setting stage, well before the implementation stage (which is discussed later under Task 2), that issues need to be addressed related to the monies and other resources needed and the probable political, social, and psychic obstacles to ultimate initiation of a priority program.

Subtask E: Assessing the Specific Health Promotion Needs of the Target Group

Assessment, diagnosis, and prioritization activities assist the planner in under-standing and focusing on the specific health problems and on who is affected. The planner will use this information as a starting point for detailed investigation of the status of health-related knowledge, attitudes, and behaviors of target groups and its relationship with the identified problems (Dignan & Carr, 1992). Planning efforts must now initiate a more focused cultural, behavioral, and educational analysis and diagnosis of the target group and program needs identified as priorities. This segment of the program planning process is referred to as the "targeted assessment" phase (Dignan & Carr, 1992). The challenge to the planner at this point is to identify those target group behaviors, cultural factors, and/or environmental factors that are contributing to the health problem. The next challenge is to identify the factors that are amenable to change through health promotion programs.

McLeroy et al. (1995) observe that the problem of defining target populations of older adults and diverse cultural groups may derive from the substantial heterogeneity within groups in terms of culture, racial/ethnic background, social norms, and generational and acculturation differences. They further note that intraethnic audience segmentation, as used in the application of social marketing approaches, has disclosed heterogeneity within racial/ethnic classifications. The work of Chen and Hawks (1995) indicates that the model healthy Asian American/Pacific Islander stereotype is a myth. This is partly attributed to the practice of data collection systems to clump these ethnically heterogeneous populations into one or two broad categories (Asian Americans and Pacific Islanders) that, in effect, masks their true health status. The planner, in these instances, should collect ethnically specific data and avoid aggregation of Asian American and Pacific Islander data (Chen & Hawks, 1995). Interventions may fail miserably if the planner is not attentive to the need for differentiating among ethnic subgroups including their generational differences. Williams and Flora (1995) demonstrate the value of disaggregating ethnic groups.

In assessing differences among Hispanic subgroups (e.g., education, income, health practices, communication channels), the researchers found that they constituted different audience segments warranting different messages in a com-munication campaign. Also, Padilla (1980) strongly encourages the need to consider *acculturation* as an important cultural variable by which to segment intraethnic groups. Balcazar, Castro, and Krull (1995) provide the planner with a methodology for assessing key factors such as acculturation and educational status in various subgroups of Hispanics. Such an assessment can identify information to help plan more culturally appropriate cancer risk reduction programs. Marin et al. (1995) believe that health education programs need to target and consider the unique conditions experienced by underserved groups. If the program is targeted only to the needs of the general population, then it might not reach the underserved groups or might not be effective in achieving the desired behavioral changes within these groups. In light of the preceding findings, the planner needs to consider the inclusion of an intensive cultural assessment component within the targeted assessment process.

The cultural assessment framework developed by Huff and Kline, in Chapter 26, this volume, provides practitioners with an assessment approach and a framework for better understanding the similarities and differences between the mainstream culture and the specific cultural/ethnic group targeted for intervention. It seeks to provide guidelines for the identification of the major areas that should be considered when assessing individual patients in the clinical setting. These guidelines also have application to the small group, community, and organizational levels of assessment, and they provide practitioners with major suggestions pertinent to identifying important demographics, epidemiological factors, cosmology, general and specific cultural characteristics, general and specific health beliefs and practices, environmental and biocultural factors, and organizational variables. To some degree, assessment of these factors should be part of any basic formative evaluation process conducted to determine baseline characteristics of a population being targeted for a HPDP program. It is again stressed that there is a need to formally include a cultural assessment as a routine component of any needs assessment process that includes a multicultural population within the target group to be addressed by a program plan.

The PRECEDE model provides a detailed approach that the planner can follow in conducting a behavioral and educational assessment and diagnosis of the target group, and the planner is encouraged to use the PRECEDE texts as the guide (Green & Kreuter, 1991; Green et al., 1980). The "behavioral and environmental diagnosis" phase (Phase 3) is concerned with identifying and prioritizing specific lifestyle behaviors and environmental factors that may place the target group at risk for the health problem. The planner also is encouraged to consider the role of nonbehavioral factors such as gender, age, and family history of a specific disease as well as how these may contribute to the health problem even though these factors cannot be changed through a health promotion program (Gielen & McDonald, 1997). For example, a breast cancer screening program targeted at Latino women should be very concerned with reaching those who are at high risk owing to family history of breast cancer. The behavioral and environmental diagnosis also should try to identify the role of environmental factors external to the individual and within the social, biological, and physical environments as they contribute to the problem. Some of these factors often are found to be beyond the control of the individual, but some can be identified and modified to support the behavior or to influence the health outcome. For example, undetected breast cancer among many in the hypothesized target group of Latino women may be a function of not seeking routine screening examinations (behavioral factor), which in turn is affected by the absence of available screening programs in their community (environmental factor) (Gielen & McDonald, 1997). After the planner identifies each of the behavioral and environmental factors, he or she must carefully rank each factor in terms of its importance or relationship to the health problem. Then, the planner should rate each factor in terms of the degree to which it can realistically be changed through program intervention. Awareness of needs for program effectiveness and efficiency is a consideration in rating which factors are most important and most changeable. This gives the planner and participants greater capability to select specific behavioral and environmental targets for intervention. Then, the planner formulates measurable objectives that define the desired behavioral or environmental change sought.

After the behavioral and environmental targets have been selected, PRECEDE moves the planner to further identify specific factors and the role they play as they can influence the initiation or maintenance of the targeted health behavior. Phase 4, the "educational and organizational diagnosis" phase, helps the planner to identify these factors by grouping them into one of three types: predisposing factors, enabling factors, or reinforcing factors. *Predisposing factors* (e.g., knowledge, attitudes, beliefs, values, cultural mores, personal preferences, existing skills, self-efficacy beliefs) function to motivate a person or target group to take action or carry out a desire behavior. For example, an important predisposing factor to be considered in the Latino women's target group would be their existing knowledge and concern about having family histories that place them at high risk and whether this knowledge may encourage the women to go for routine breast screening examinations. *Enabling factors* could include the new skills acquired by the target group and other resources that enable (allow) the woman or target group to perform the desired behavior. To acquire the new skills might further depend on other enabling factors such as the availability and accessibility of community breast screening and health care programs that are necessary for the earlier defined behavioral and environmental outcomes to be realized. *Reinforcing factors* provide the incentives or rewards for the individual or target group to maintain the desired health-related behavior. They could include the social support and encouragement for obtaining a mammogram provided by the family or significant others. Peer support and influence, supportive feedback from physicians or other health providers, and support from the neighborhood healer also could serve as reinforcing factors. As in the previous diagnostic step of the PRECEDE framework, these three types of factors must be identified and ranked in terms of importance and changeability. Targets are then prioritized and selected for intervention. Finally, measurable objectives based on predisposing, enabling, and reinforcing factors are written in the form of learning and resource objectives.

Subtask F: Developing Appropriate Goals and Objectives

The planners and participants are ready to establish health promotion and health education program goals and objectives when they more clearly understand the relationships between (a) the health problems, environment, and antecedent target group behaviors and (b) the role of predisposing factors, enabling factors, and reinforcing factors as they influence those target group behaviors. Program goals and objectives exist in a hierarchical relationship to each other. Those at the top represent the major overall outcome a program strives to achieve. Objectives at the lowest level of the hierarchy must be achieved first to achieve the objectives at the next highest level. Achievement then ascends up the hierarchy until the overall program objective is achieved. Goals and objectives, therefore, must be

Program Goal

Latino women in the target population age 55 years or over will increase their participation in mammography screening programs made available by the local health jurisdiction

Educational Goal

Latino women in the target population age 55 years or over will:

1. Learn the importance of early detection and breast cancer survival
2. Learn the importance of family history and breast cancer
3. Actively participate in community mammography screening clinics

Figure 4.2 Example of Program Goal and Educational Goal for a Breast Cancer Education and Detection Program

written coherently and must specify the various levels of program (and target group) activity and accomplishment. The quality of the ultimate evaluation of the program will depend on how careful the program's goals and objectives were formulated. It also is at this stage that the planner should begin developing the program's evaluative approaches.

Goals and objectives are related, but their difference lies in the precision with which they measure program accomplishment. *Goals* are formulated to tell the planner and participants what should happen as a result of the program. They usually *are not measurable,* but they are attainable, identify a desired future state or condition, are stated as occurring in the longer term rather than in the shorter term, and lack a specific deadline for accomplishment (Butler, 1997; Dignan & Carr, 1992; McKenzie & Jurs, 1993; Timmreck, 1995). It is useful for the planner to formulate at least two types of goals: those for the overall program and those for educational services to be delivered as part of the overall program. This is helpful in clearly establishing the role of education in the program needed to achieve the program goals (Dignan & Carr, 1992). Figure 4.2 provides examples of a *program goal* and a related *educational goal.*

Objectives, unlike goals, are written in measurable, time-bound, and realistic terms; are derived from the earlier detailed assessment of the target group; and stipulate the tasks needed for program and educational goal accomplishment. They also specify the magnitude and direction of the change sought (in terms of increasing knowledge, attitudes, or behavior or decreasing the occurrence of certain behavior or activity) within a certain time period. In this way, objectives serve as roadmaps for systematically reaching the goals. Behavioral outcomes of target group performance are the most concrete and sought-after targets of the health promotion program's educational interventions (discussed in Subtask G subsection). Well-written health promotion and education program plans should include a formal hierarchy of objectives. This hierarchy should include (a) the overall health promotion program outcome objectives, (b) the overall health education target group program objectives, (c) the health education (knowledge, attitude, and behavior) target group objectives, and (d) the health education instructional learning objectives (see Figure 4.3). The overall health education program objectives are generally stated in behavioral terms. The instructional

Overall Health Promotion Program Outcome Objective

The target population of Latino women age 55 years or over obtaining mammography screening at local clinics will show an increase of __% within 2 years of program implementation

The number of breast cancer education programs for Latino women in the target group will increase by __% within 2 years of program implementation

Overall Health Education Program Objectives

Educational: To increase the number by __% of Latino women in the target group attending breast cancer education programs who obtain screening at a community mammography clinic by the end of fiscal year 19__

Resource: To increase the number by __% of breast cancer education programs for Latino women in the target group by the end of fiscal year 19__

Health Education Target Group Objectives

To increase the number by __% of women in the target group who carry out *appropriate behaviors* related to obtaining a mammogram at a community clinic by _____ (date)

To increase the number by __% of women in the target group who possess *favorable attitudes* related to obtaining a mammogram at a community clinic by _____ (date)

To increase the number by __% of women in the target group who possess *appropriate knowledge* related to the need to obtain a mammogram at a community clinic by _____ (date)

Health Education Instructional Learning Objectives

Knowledge   By the end of the program, 80% of the Latino women in the target group:
1. Will identify at least four risk factors associated with breast cancer
2. Can state that familial history of breast cancer is a risk factor associated with breast cancer
3. Will identify mammograms as necessary for detecting breast cancer
4. Can state that free mammograms are available at the clinic

Attitudes   By the end of the program, 70% of the Latino women in the target group:
1. Will express the feeling that the consequences of breast cancer can be very serious
2. Will express the feeling that if one's mother or other close relative had breast cancer, then there is a risk of having breast cancer
3. Will express the feeling that they can take action leading to the early detection and treatment of breast cancer

Skills   By the end of the program, 70% of the Latino women in the target group:
1. Will be able to call the mammography screening clinic and make appointments
2. Will be able to arrange transportation to the mammography screening clinic to keep their appointments

Reinforcing   By the end of the program, 90% of the Latino women in the target group:
1. Will have verbally encouraged women in their target group to make appointments for mammography screening at the clinic
2. Will have verbally encouraged women in their target group to keep their appointments for mammography screening at the clinic

Figure 4.3   Examples of a Hierarchy of Program Objectives for a Breast Cancer Education and Detection Program

learning objectives are concerned with the predisposing, enabling, and reinforcing factors identified earlier and are necessary for effecting target group behavior change (Green & Kreuter, 1991). Figure 4.3 shows examples of each type and level of objective in the hierarchy.

Subtask G: Selecting Health Promotion Program Intervention Activities That Consider the Peculiarities of the Target Group, Health Problem, and Setting

Now, decisions must be made related to formulating the most appropriate target group strategies and interventions for achieving the change specified in the goals and objectives. Windsor et al. (1984) define an *intervention* as "a planned and systematically applied combination of program elements designed to produce cognitive, affective, skill, behavior, or health status changes among individuals exposed at a specific site and during a specified period" (p. 4). Green et al. (1980) consider a health education *strategy* as including one or more of a combination of interventions made up of methods and activities "that may be used to affect the predisposing, reinforcing, and enabling factors which directly or indirectly influence behaviors" (p. 86).

There is no foolproof way in which to select the right combination of interventions that will ensure the most effective results. The planner cannot expect that the same health education program found to be effective in one underserved population will be equally effective in another (Marin et al., 1995). Furthermore, the background factors that characterize a particular target group may affect its capability to participate in a program (e.g., knowledge, attitudes, beliefs, values, generational differences, language, socialization and family roles, acculturation and assimilation, societal inequities) and must be considered when planning any health education intervention (Marin et al., 1995). Regardless of the target group, the health problem, or the setting, the selection of the intervention and educational activities should be based on a sound rationale that considers the relationship between the cultural characteristics of the target group and the health behaviors or changes sought.

The planner also will have greater capacity to base his or her health promotion and health education interventions and methods on a sound rationale if the planner understands the roles and relationships of predisposing factors, enabling factors, reinforcing factors, and environmental support needs as well as how these can affect behavior (Green & Kreuter, 1991). The earlier scenario helps to illustrate how these factors are involved and how the grouping of these factors according to the specific features of the situation can suggest the types of alternative program approaches to be explored. The hypothetical assessment disclosed that the target group does not have appropriate knowledge about the risk factors of breast cancer or about the availability of mammography screening in the community (predisposing factors). Perhaps its members also do not know or believe that they need to obtain routine mammograms or that the practice of such behavior can help in the early detection of breast cancer (predisposing factors). So, they do not obtain routine mammograms (the behavior). Furthermore, the women's families and their neighborhood folk healers, owing to concepts of health and disease within the cultural milieu, might view breast cancer fatalistically (fatalismo) or as a source of embarrassment and shame (negative reinforcing factors). This view might discourage the women from obtaining routine mammograms. Even if the health education program helps them to recognize the need to obtain screening, there still will be a need for the behavior to be positively rewarded and supported by their peers, families, family physicians, and neighborhood folk healers (positive reinforcing factors) who constitute yet another important target group in this scenario. Also, the situation is worsened if there are no education programs in the community to serve as a resource where the women can gain accurate knowledge or the skills required to obtain screening (enabling factor and a source of environmental need). Thus, there also are program needs for making program resources available and accessible (enabling factor). The preceding information can help the planner to systematically identify alternative intervention strategies that new programs need to develop as the most appropriate means for enabling the target group to carry out the needed actions. From this scenario, the more obvious types of interventions needed might include (a) educational sessions to strengthen the *predisposing factors* related to assisting the target group in acquiring appropriate knowledge and positive attitudes concerning the need to obtain routine mammogram screening and to recognize that the practice of such behavior can help them in the early detection of breast cancer; (b) indirectly working with physicians, peers, clergy, neighborhood healers, families, and others to strengthen the *reinforcing factors;* and (c) target group skills training related to strengthening the various *enabling factors* such as making and keeping clinic appointments for mammograms, political intervention within the community health service system/community organizations/voluntary agencies, cultural competence training for physicians and other health professionals, and including the development of environmental support resources (Green & Kreuter, 1991).

The planner needs to consider several questions that are involved in the rational selection of a program approach in multicultural populations. Will the interventions be based on an appropriate theory? What individual-level theories are important to consider? Frankish, Lovato, and Shannon, in Chapter 3 of this volume, provided a comprehensive treatment of health behavior theories and issues to consider in the selection and development of program interventions that can be integrated into the planning framework at this stage. All target groups do not react the same way to the same intervention. This should encourage the planner to ask the following questions: Is the intervention appropriate for the demographics (age, gender, and socioeconomic status), knowledge, skills, and behavior of the target population? Do the intervention activities fit the purpose of the program (McKenzie & Jurs, 1993)? The PRECEDE-PROCEED planning framework also can help the planner to understand the complexity of the influence of behavioral and environmental factors on health and to consider the use of carefully planned multiple strategies for influencing those factors (Green & Kreuter, 1991). The PATCH approach encourages the use of multiple strategies in intervention activities at three levels of action: governmental, organizational, and individual (U.S. Department of Health and Human Services, 1996).

The rationale for the selection of an approach can be strengthened by studying interventions that have been successful in particular settings and target groups. Steckler et al. (1995) note that despite the range of methodological limitations in many studies of individual-level health education interventions, some of the well-designed studies can provide the planner with valuable information about the efficacy of different approaches. They cite four common elements in successful individual-level interventions. First, *the intervention is grounded in a "clearly operationalized underlying theoretical perspective . . . generally derived from the behavioral and social sciences and educational theory"* (p. 310, emphasis added) such as Bandura's (1986) theory of social learning and self-efficacy, Lazarus and Folkman's (1984) theory of coping, Cassel's (1976) theory of social support, and Seligman and Maier's (1967) theory of learned helplessness. Second, *the intervention uses "a wide range of educational and behavioral strategies suggested by the theoretical perspectives"* (Steckler et al., 1995, p. 310) such as cognitive behavioral strategies including shaping and guided practice, reinforcement control, behavioral contracting, commitment strategies, goal setting, and self-control strategies. Third, *the intervention incorporates the element of social support* (Israel, 1985). Fourth, *the intervention combines diverse strategies including multiple-component interventions* such as the successful Morisky, DeMuth, Field-Fass, Green, and Levine (1987) study of health education for hypertensive patients using a combination of three strategies: interviewing following the visit to increase understanding of and compliance with the medical regimen, a home visit to encourage a family member to reinforce and support the patient, and small group sessions with the patient to help better self-manage his or her problems.

Interventions also need to incorporate the use of target group-specific educational methods and techniques. Pasick, D'Onofrio, and Otero-Sabogal (1996) cite the need to differentiate between the terms *tailoring* and *targeting*. Targeting implies the need to clearly identify the specific population subgroup that will be exposed to the intended intervention. The planner must be acutely aware of the group's and subgroup's diversity in history, cultural practices including health beliefs and practices, language, socioeconomic status, and generational differences. Each subgroup may represent varying degrees of acculturation and assimilation in its current country of residence. Once the planner has targeted, he or she also needs to be able to tailor. Tailoring, as espoused by Pasick et al. (1996), implies the need for the planner to be able to adapt the intervention and/or total design to "fit the needs and characteristics of a target audience" (p. S145). *Cultural tailoring,* then, urges the planner to develop the interventions, strategies, methods, messages, and materials to be adaptable to the specific cultural characteristics of the target group (Pasick et al., 1996). In short, the health promotion planner cannot tailor until he or she has correctly targeted.

Green et al. (1980) provide a useful framework to help the planner select educational strategies according to the characteristics of the health problem. They also consider the use of three broad categories of methods: (a) "communication" methods such as lecture-discussion, individual counseling or instruction, media techniques (mass media, audio-visual aids, educational television, and programmed learning); (b) training methods such as skills development, simulations and games, inquiry learning, small-group discussions, modeling, and behavior modification; and (c) organizational methods such as community development, social action, social planning, and organizational development. Ross and Mico (1980) also provide practitioners with a useful listing and description of methods for health education that should be of practical use. McKenzie and Jurs (1993), in their planning text, describe and discuss categorization of nine specific types of intervention activities: traditional educational activities or methods, activities based on behavior modification, environmental change activities, regulatory activities, community participation activities to influence public policy, activities affecting organizational culture, communication activities, economic and other incentives, and social intervention activities.

TASK 2: IMPLEMENTING THE PROGRAM

Implementation is the behind-the-scenes processes and activities required to put the health promotion and education program plan into action and then guide it toward achievement of the defined outcomes in the most effective and efficient manner. The plan should set forth a clear statement of the problem, needs, and priorities; the identification of the target group and the particular problem in need of change; an explicit statement of goals and objectives at all levels of the program; an explicit delineation of the strategies and interventions; and an accompanying description of planned activities and methods to be employed to achieve the objectives. Implementation is concerned with initiating the activity, providing assistance to it and its participants, and problem-solving issues that may arise including reporting (or documenting) on progress (Ross & Mico, 1980). It also is described as the process of bringing programs into reality and includes "staff selection and training; the procurement of facilities, materials, and teaching aids; and the recruitment of learners (students, clients) into the program" (Greene & Simons-Morton, 1990, p. 33). Other planners have observed that implementation begins when the monies are allocated, authorization is given, administrative sanctions are established, and the management system required for project execution is in place (Timmreck, 1995). Still others view implementation as occurring in a series of five interrelated phases: gaining acceptance for the program, specifying program tasks and estimating resource needs, developing plans for progam activities, establishing a system for program management, and putting plans into action (Dignan & Carr, 1992).

Implementation is viewed differently, but the commonality of perspective, if any, concentrates on the need for administrators and staff to carry out a necessary range of activities for mobilizing the program, keeping the program operational, and keeping it focused on accomplishment of its objectives. It is useful to divide program implementation activities into at least three subtask areas related to the different foci in the development and operation of the program: pre-implementation preparation, program implementation, and implementation administration and monitoring. Some of the activities occur early in the program's developmental stages prior to initiation, some during the operational phases of the program, and some throughout the life of the program. Only a brief discussion will be devoted to the topic of implementation, owing to the great variations in the scope, size, objectives, and interventions of health promotion

Identification, contact, development, and maintenance of support (including financial: fees, grants, gifts) and sponsorship for the program by community power bases

Identification, contact, development, and maintenance of support (including financial: fees, grants, gifts) and organizational sponsorship for the program by the professional, political, and administrative power bases

Identification of staffing needs and specific program tasks to be performed (e.g., planning, identifying resources, advertising, marketing, conducting the program, evaluating the program, making arrangements for space and program materials, handling clerical work, keeping records for sign-up/collection of fees/attendance/budgeting)

Identification of space needs and procurement of program facilities

Identification and acquisition of program supplies and equipment

Program curricula ready for instructional use; preparation of other related cultural-specific instructional/educational support materials acquired

Preparation and preliminary field testing of evaluation instruments

Development and initiation of media and marketing activities for getting the word out and for recruitment of participants

Provision of troubleshooting, consultation, and/or technical assistance to planners and staff on as-needed basis to keep pre-implementation activities on track

Figure 4.4   Listing of Pre-Implementation Preparation Activities

and health education programs. A selected listing of major activities that should take place within each area is presented in Figures 4.2, 4.3, and 4.4. Readers also are encouraged to seek greater coverage on specific aspects of the topic from the texts cited here (Dignan & Carr, 1992; Greene & Simons-Morton, 1990; McKenzie & Jurs, 1993; Ross & Mico, 1980).

Subtask A: Pre-Implementation Preparation

A program must have formal administrative (and community) support in the form of necessary capital and operating budgets. This support is needed early because many of the activities within this task area begin well before the initiation of the program including selecting and training staff (e.g., cultural competency training); marketing and publicity activities for recruiting participants; identifying, purchasing, or acquiring cultural-specific educational and other materials; identifying space needs and acquiring program facilities; and acquiring equipment. The planner needs to think about all of the factors critical for effective program initiation. Timmreck (1995) advises administrators and staff to mentally walk through all of the steps and activities needed to implement the program project including the order of the activities and staffing needs and responsibilities. A selected listing of the scope of activities to be undertaken or completed within this phase is found in Figure 4.4.

Continuing contact, development, and maintenance of support (including financial: fees, grants, gifts) and sponsorship for the program by community power bases and administrative power bases

Continuing review and needed modifications concerning all program activities, staff, and program participants

As-needed maintenance of publicity, advertising, and marketing activities to encourage continuing involvement of participants

Conducting the program; evaluating the program; continuing review of appropriateness of instructional curricula and preparation of other needed cultural-specific instructional/educational support materials

Continuing refinement of evaluation instruments

Provision of continuing and as-needed troubleshooting, consultation, and/or technical assistance activities to keep implementation activities on track

Figure 4.5   Listing of Program Implementation Activities

Subtask B: Program Implementation

Implementation occurs after the program has been planned, publicized, and marketed and its initially required resources have been identified and allocated. Health education and promotion programs can be implemented in one of three ways: using a pilot or demonstration approach, phasing in the program over a specific period, or implementing the total program immediately (Parkinson & Associates, 1982). Pilot approaches are used to determine the feasibility of implementing on a larger scale and can be combined with either of the other two approaches. This also is a period of "working the bugs out" of the program through formative evaluation activities. A selected listing of the scope of activities to be undertaken or completed within this phase is found in Figure 4.5.

Subtask C: Implementation Administration and Monitoring

Administration and monitoring activities related to implementation begin prior to initiation and continue through completion or continuation. These activities keep the program operational and promote the program to stakeholders and community through the routine preparation and dissemination of progress and performance reports. This subtask area also involves program managerial control functions. A myriad of activities are conducted including staff and volunteer supervision, maintenance of program records, program fee collection, monitoring of attendance, preparation of budgets, and providing emotional and intellectual support to the program. Green and Kreuter (1991) observe the critical need, prior to and during implementation, for the program to operate compatibly with the policies, regulations, and organization under which it is expected to

Initiation and maintenance of the program's evaluation activities

Development of overall implementation plan (including the specific time lines by event, anticipation of problems, and barriers to implementing according to schedule)

Timely and continuing review such as facilitation of needed modifications of the overall implementation plan (including the specific time lines by event, anticipation of and dealing with problems and barriers to implementing according to schedule)

Development of a system for program management

Recruitment, selection, hiring, and training of full-time and part-time program staff and volunteers

Continuing review of needs related to recruitment, selection, hiring, and training of full-time and part-time program staff and volunteers

Supervision of full-time and part-time program staff and volunteers

Continuing coordination activities related to reducing duplication and achieving maximum efficiency in use of staff and materials

Continuing review of space needs and procurement of program facilities as needed

Continuing review of needs related to acquisition of program materials, supplies, and equipment

Training for all staff and volunteers related to understanding legal concerns inherent in the program (e.g., informed consent, negligence)

Provision of continuing and as-needed consultation and/or technical assistance activities on as-needed basis to keep implementation activities on track

Preparation of written and oral reports related to documenting and promoting the program; dissemination of reports to stakeholders and policymakers

Figure 4.6   Listing of Administration and Monitoring Activities

function. Figure 4.6 presents a selected listing of additional activities to be maintained within this phase.

TASK 3: EVALUATING THE PROGRAM

Did the program make a difference? The planner, program administrators, and program staff want to know what their programs accomplish without being influenced by subjective judgments or political motives. Breckon, Harvey, and Lancaster (1985) stress that administrators and educators should "feel obligated to determine what has been accomplished as a result of their efforts" (p. 213). Evaluation cannot be treated as an afterthought because the planner needs to learn what was achieved and what could have been improved. Evaluation is of critical importance to the continuation of program support and to account for how program funds were spent.

Health promotion and education program evaluation requires (a) an explicit description of the problem, (b) a clear description of the program focus, (c) an explicit statement of goals and objectives at all program levels, (d) a clear determination of the information needed, (e) the establishment of a clear basis for proof of effectiveness, (f) a determination of data collection methods required, (g) developiment and testing of instruments, (h) organization of the database, (i) analysis of results, and (j) modification of the program (Mico & Ross, 1980). Israel et al. (1995) provide a useful update of health education program-related evaluation issues. They note the complexities of evaluation issues associated with the conceptual design of the approaches and their limitations, and they stress the need to be aware of the different foci of health promotion and education programs and the implications for evaluation. There are some good texts that can assist the reader in gaining more in-depth information about the following important evaluation-related issues: selection of the evaluation study design and its limitations, issues of instrument design and development, issues and conduct of evaluation-related data collection activities, and issues of measurement precision involving reliability and validity (Dignan, 1989; Dignan & Carr, 1992; Green & Kreuter, 1991; Green & Lewis, 1986; Mohr, 1992; Sarvela & McDermott, 1993; Suchman, 1967; Windsor et al., 1984).

Practitioners should be able to apply at least three dimensions of evaluation in their program if they understand the concept, limitations, and relationship of each: impact evaluation, outcome evaluation, and process evaluation. Each level is used to answer different questions about the program. The levels of impact and outcome include direct measures associated with achieving the program's stated goals and objectives. Process evaluation constitutes a more indirect way of assessing a program and examines the quality by which specific program inputs are produced as they are thought to be associated with achieving certain target group outcomes. Process evaluation is conducted during the development and implementation stages of the program and seeks ways in which to improve the overall program and its educational component. Any one of the levels may be used exclusively under certain conditions, but it will yield only limited information. When all three are used together, they form a fairly comprehensive approach to evaluation. Each level is based on specific assumptions that need to be understood before making any judgments about program effectiveness. These three levels are briefly described next and, where appropriate, specific caveats are offered.

Subtask A: Assessment of the Immediate Impact of the Program (Impact Evaluation)

By the end of the breast cancer education and screening program, how many in the target group of high-risk Latino women made appointments or obtained scheduled mammograms? Impact evaluation examines the immediate or short-term impact of the program (or the methods and activities used) on changes in target group knowledge, attitudes, and behavior as well as predisposing, enabling, and reinforcing factors (Green et al., 1980). This is the level of evaluation used by most health education program planners because it is amenable to measurement and can be used for reporting concrete results about the designated target group at different periods of time. *The program objectives formulated earlier serve as the basis for this level of measurement.* The standards or criteria for accomplishment and for purposes of measurement are clear. When using this level of evaluation, one must be very careful not to assume that the knowledge, attitude, or behavior changes that occur, whether positive or negative, are necessarily and directly attributable to the effect of the program. It is simply too difficult to control all of the possible conditions and variables to which the changes might be attributed. If care was observed in aspects of instrument design, data collection protocol, and efforts to build in reliability and validity, then one can make inferences more safely about program effect. If the program did not accomplish the objectives, then it is useful to go back and review aspects of the program at the process level (discussed later).

Subtask B: Assessment of the Long-Term Target Group Health and Social Outcomes (Outcome Evaluation)

Does the target group of Latino women (at high risk owing to familial history of breast cancer) routinely obtain mammograms at 6 months, 1 year, and 5 years after completing the program? Of those in the target group attending the program who were diagnosed and treated early, how many survived for 1, 5, or 10 years? Are there increased numbers of new programs in place that are available and accessible for breast cancer education and routine mammography screening?

Outcome evaluation is concerned with examining health or social benefits over time. The planner again must use his or her objectives formulated earlier that contain the explicit criteria for measuring longer-term and overall performance at the outcome level. The outcome level, unlike the assessment of impact, usually reports program accomplishment at the end of a longer time period. It is more difficult to evaluate health and social benefits because trends or events are not discernible for long periods of time, and most populations do not remain stable or geographically in place over long periods (Green et al., 1980). Thus, to evaluate the long-term effect of the community program in terms of a legitimate increase or decrease in cancer mortality, a greater level of funding and resources, a larger target group of program participants, and the capability of spending more time in follow-up would be required. *When using this level of evaluation, one also must be careful not to assume that the positive long-term behavioral, structural, or mortality changes related to the target group that occur are directly attributable to the effects of the program.* As in impact evaluation, all of the possible conditions and variables to which the changes might be attributed cannot ever be completely controlled.

Subtask C: Assessment of the Quality of Program Inputs During the Development and Implementation Phases (Process Evaluation)

How well is the breast cancer education and screening program being developed and implemented? Are the educational activities provided to the target group of Latino women *designed* in an appropriate manner and sequence to assist them in acquiring the knowledge, attitude, and skills related to obtaining mammograms at the clinic? Are the educational activities provided to the target group *implemented* in an appropriate manner and sequence to assist them in acquiring the knowledge, attitude, and skills related to obtaining mammograms at the clinic? Are the educational activities appropriately related to achieving the program's objectives? During the educational sessions, does the program staff achieve the desired *quality of interaction* with the target group for appropriately discussing and conveying required techniques related to obtaining mammograms at the clinic? Are the educational activities designed and implemented in the appropriate sequence for enabling "significant others" to acquire the knowledge and attitudes necessary to perform supportive roles for encouraging and reinforcing the target group behavior (obtaining mammograms at the clinic)? *Process evaluation, as viewed in the context of these questions, is based on the assumption that if certain elements are present in the program in the appropriate fashion (usually as defined by the planning participants), the program will have greater capability to achieve the desired outcome* (Donabedian, 1966). Process evaluation is a more indirect way in which to assess the quality of the program elements that have been put in place. It is strongly desirable to base the measures on predetermined and accepted practices related to what are thought to be the most appropriate inputs for achieving certain program outcomes. This requires evaluators to specify, as far as possible, the relevant dimensions, values, and standards to be used in the assessment of the development and implementation of the educational program. Owing to the assumption on which this level is based, it is important to be able to identify as clearly as possible what represents the value or "standard" of measurement. Many times, the "standard" may end up being a rule-of-thumb judgment arrived at through negotiation with the planner, participants, staff, and implementers. Process evaluation, with its limitations, could be used to identify and examine the qualitative and quantitative aspects of the educational segment. Evaluators could look at, for example, the degree to which the rationale relating to the design and implementation of the educational segment is based on appropriate theoretical and programmatic foundations. Evaluators also could examine process variables related to the qualitative aspects of how and by whom the educational program is implemented, the appropriateness of the strategies and interventions selected in terms of their expected effects, staff and target group interaction and performance during the sessions, and the levels of necessary and expected target group participation. The CATCH (Child and Adolescent Trial for Cardiovascular Health) study, funded under the federal National Heart, Lung, and Blood Institute (main trial initiated in 1991), was conducted in school-based settings. It provides a useful model for practitioners to design and use evaluation concepts in other health education program settings (McGraw et al., 1994).

Information from process evaluation activities also can identify areas in which program changes, adjustments, or refinements might be needed to help the planner anticipate or prevent problems before the program starts and during program implementation. *Formative evaluation,* a type of process evaluation, is conducted early in the program's developmental stages and continues to operate through implementation to provide immediate feedback about program performance and program dynamics (Herman, Morris, & Fitz-Gibbon, 1987; Sarvela & McDermott, 1993). Formative evaluation information can be obtained through focus group interviews, observations, surveys, and audits and could be used to answer the following types of questions: Are the breast cancer education and screening programs for the target group located at accessible sites? Is the number of programs scheduled adequate in terms of the expected numbers of participants? Are program staff appropriately trained to teach the educational classes? Are there adequate numbers of (Spanish-speaking and culturally competent) trained staff for conducting the sessions? Does the program have sufficient and appropriate equipment and culturally specific educational materials for conducting the planned activities? Have the educational materials been tested for appropriate content and readability? Are participants attending the educational sessions (making appointments to obtain mammograms) at the times they have been scheduled? How satisfied are the program participants with the program staff, the curriculum, and the educational materials? Are the educational sessions and screening clinics held at appropriate times for the target group? Does the program furnish transportation to those in the target group who need these services to reach and participate in the educational and screening programs? Do the program recipients truly represent the target group as it was identified in the targeted assessment phase of the needs assessment?

CHAPTER SUMMARY

Planning in multicultural HPDP settings must be a collaborative effort involving the planner and participants. The formidable task of developing and implementing a health promotion program requires the planner and participants to work together to accomplish a complex range of activities including (a) assessing the needs, problems, and resources of the target population; (b) developing appropriate goals and objectives; (c) devising strategies and interventions that consider the peculiarities of the settings; (d) implementing and monitoring the interventions; (e) evaluating the results; and (f) refining approaches toward greater program effectiveness and efficiency. All must be heard and represented in the decision-making processes. All who are expected to function effectively in multicultural planning must be aware and accepting of cultural differences and should be culturally knowledgeable about the target group.

Owing to the scope and complexity of the planning process, practitioners need to operate from some rational planning framework or model rather than solely on the basis of pragmatic, empirical, or expediency considerations. Program planning models provide organizing frameworks that encourage a more systematic approach to the development of health promotion programs for specific target groups. The planner must be able to adapt these models to fit the needs of the planning situation and the cultural characteristics of the target group, setting, and health problem. In addition, the planner must be extremely conscious of and sensitive to the need for building a comprehensive cultural assessment component into the planning process. Regardless of the target group, the health problem, or the setting, the selection of the intervention and educational activities must be based on a sound rationale that considers the relationship between the cultural characteristics of the target group and the health behaviors or changes sought.

REFERENCES

Airhihenbuwa, C. O. (1995). *Health and culture: Beyond the Western paradigm*. Thousand Oaks, CA: Sage.

Balcazar, H., Castro, F. G., & Krull, J. L. (1995). Cancer risk reduction in Mexican American women: The role of acculturation, education, and health risk factors. *Health Education Quarterly, 22,* 61-84.

Bandura, A. (1986). *Social foundations of thought and action: A social cognitive theory*. Englewood Cliffs, NJ: Prentice Hall.

Blum, H. (1974). *Planning for health: Development and application of social change theory*. New York: Human Sciences Press.

Breckon, D. J., Harvey, J. R., & Lancaster, R. B. (1985). *Community health education: Settings, roles, and skills*. Rockville, MD: Aspen.

Bronfenbrenner, U. (1979). *The ecology of human development*. Cambridge, MA: Harvard University Press.

Butler, J. T. (1997). *Principles of health education and health promotion*. Englewood, CO: Morton.

Campinha-Bacote, J. (1994). Cultural competence in psychiatric mental health nursing: A conceptual model. *Nursing Clinics of North America, 29,* 1-8.

Cassel, J. (1976). The contribution of social environment to host resistance. *American Journal of Epidemiology, 104,* 107-123.

Chen, M. S., & Hawks, B. L. (1995). A debunking of the myth of healthy Asian Americans and Pacific Islanders. *American Journal of Health Promotion, 9,* 261-268.

Cross, T. L., Bazron, B. J., Dennis, K. W., & Isaacs, M. R. (1989). *Towards a culturally competent system of care* (Vol. 1). Washington, DC: CASSP Technical Assistance Center, Georgetown University Child Development Center.

Dignan, M. B. (Ed.). (1989). *Measurement and evaluation of health education* (2nd ed.). Springfield, IL: Charles C Thomas.

Dignan, M. B., & Carr, P. A. (1992). *Program planning for health education and promotion*. Philadelphia: Lea & Febiger.

Donabedian, A. (1966). Evaluating the quality of medical care. *Milbank Memorial Fund Quarterly, 44,* 166-203.

Gielen, A. C., & McDonald, E. M. (1997).The PRECEDE-PROCEED planning model. In K. Glantz, F. M. Lewis, & B. K. Rimer (Eds.), *Health behavior and health education: Theory, research, and practice*. San Francisco: Jossey-Bass.

Gilmore, G. D., & Campbell, M. D. (1996). *Needs assessment strategies for health education and health promotion*. Madison, WI: Brown & Benchmark.

Green, L. W., & Kreuter, M. W. (1991). *Health promotion planning: An educational and environmental approach*. Mountain View, CA: Mayfield.

Green, L. W., & Kreuter, M. W. (1992). CDC's planned approach to community health as an application of PRECEDE and an inspiration for PROCEED. *Journal of Health Education, 23,* 140-147.

Green, L. W., Kreuter, M. W., Deeds, S. G., & Partridge, K. B. (1980). *Health education planning: A diagnostic approach*. Mountain View, CA: Mayfield.

Green, L. W., & Lewis, F. M. (1986). *Measurement and evaluation in health education and health promotion*. Mountain View, CA: Mayfield.

Green, L. W., Richard, L., & Potvin, L. (1996). Ecological foundations of health promotion. *American Journal of Health Promotion, 10,* 270-281.

Greene, W. H., & Simons-Morton, B. G. (1990). *Introduction to health education*. Prospect Heights, IL: Waveland.

Herman, J. L., Morris, L. L., & Fitz-Gibbon, C. T. (1987). *Evaluator's handbook*. Newbury Park, CA: Sage.

Israel, B. A. (1985). Social networks and social support: Implications for natural helper and community level interventions. *Health Education Quarterly, 12,* 65-80.

Israel, B. A., Cummings, K. M., Dignan, M. B., Heaney, C. A., Perales, D. P., Simons-Morton, B. G., & Zimmerman, M. A. (1995). Evaluation of health education programs: Current assessment and future directions. *Health Education Quarterly, 22,* 364-389.

Kreuter, M. (1992). PATCH: Its origin, basic concepts, and links to contemporary public health policy. *Journal of Health Education, 23,* 135-139.

Lazarus, R. S., & Folkman, S. (1984). *Stress appraisal and coping*. New York: Springer.

Leininger, M. (1978). *Transcultural nursing: Concepts, theories and practices*. New York: John Wiley.

Marin, G., Burhansstipanov, L., Connell, C. M., Gielen, A. C., Helitzer-Allen, D., Lorig, K., Morisky, D. E., Tenney, M., & Thomas, S. (1995). A research agenda for health education among underserved populations. *Health Education Quarterly, 22,* 346-363.

McGraw, S. A., Stone, E. J., Osganian, S. K., Elder, J. P., Perry, C. L., Johnson, C. C., Parcel, G. S., Webber, L. S., & Luepker, R. V. (1994). Design of process evaluation within the Child and Adolescent Trial for Cardiovascular Health (CATCH). *Health Education Quarterly, 2*(Suppl.), S6-S26.

McKenzie, J. F., & Jurs, J. L. (1993). *Planning, implementing, and evaluating health promotion programs: A primer.* New York: Macmillan.

McLeroy, K. R., Bibeau, D., Steckler, A., & Glantz, K. (1988). An ecological perspective on health promotion programs. *Health Education Quarterly, 15,* 351-377.

McLeroy, K. R., Clark, N., Simons-Morton, B., Forster, J., Connell, C. M., Altman, D., & Zimmerman, M. A. (1995). Creating capacity: Establishing a health education research agenda for special populations. *Health Education Quarterly, 22,* 390-405.

Minkler, M. (1990). Improving health through community organization. In K. Glantz, F. M. Lewis, & B. K. Rimer (Eds.), *Health behavior and health education: Theory, research, and practice*. San Francisco: Jossey-Bass.

Mohr, L. B. (1992). *Impact analysis for program evaluation*. Newbury Park, CA: Sage.

Morisky, D. E., DeMuth, N. M., Field-Fass, M., Green, L. W., & Levine, D. M. (1987). Evaluation of family health education to build social support for long-term control of high blood pressure. *Health Education Quarterly, 73,* 153-162.

Orenstein, D., Nelson, C., Speers, M., Brownstein, J. N., & Ramsey, D. C. (1992). Synthesis of the four PATCH evaluations. *Journal of Health Education, 23,* 187-192.

Padilla, A. M. (1980). *Acculturation: Theory, models and some new findings*. Boulder, CO: Westview.

Parkinson, R. S., & Associates. (1982). *Managing health promotion in the workplace: Guidelines for implementation and evaluation*. Mountain View, CA: Mayfield.

Pasick, R. J., D'Onofrio, C. N., & Otero-Sabogal, R. (1996). Similarities and differences across cultures: Questions to inform a third generation for health promotion research. *Health Education Quarterly, 23*(Suppl.), S142-S161.

Richard, L., Potvin, L., Kishchuk, N., Prlic, H., & Green, L. W. (1996). Assessment of the ecological approach in health promotion programs. *American Journal of Health Promotion, 10,* 318-328.

Ross, H. S., & Mico, P. R. (1980). *Theory and practice in health education*. Mountain View, CA: Mayfield.

Sallis, J. F., & Owen, N. (1997). Ecological models. In K. Glantz, F. M. Lewis, & B. K. Rimer (Eds.), *Health behavior and health education: Theory, research, and practice*. San Francisco: Jossey-Bass.

Sarvela, P. D., & McDermott, R. J. (1993). *Health education evaluation and measurement: A practitioner's perspective*. Madison, WI: Brown & Benchmark.

Seligman, M., & Maier, S. (1967). Failure to escape traumatic shock. *Journal of Experimental Psychology, 75,* 1-9.

Steckler, A., Allegrante, J. P., Altman, D., Brown, R., Burdine, J. N., Goodman, R. M., & Jorgensen, C. (1995). Health education intervention strategies: Recommendations for future research. *Health Education Quarterly, 22,* 307-328.

Steuart, G. W. (1969). Planning and evaluation in health education. *International Journal of Health Education, 2,* 65-76.

Stokols, D. (1996). Translating social ecological theory into guidelines for community health promotion. *American Journal of Health Promotion, 10,* 282-298.

Suchman, E. A. (1967). *Evaluative research: Principles and practice in public service and social action programs.* New York: Russell Sage.

Sullivan, D. (1977). *Educating the public about health: A planning guide* (DHEW Publication No. [HRA] 78-14004). Washington, DC: Public Health Service.

Syme, L. (1986). Strategies for health promotion. *Preventive Medicine, 15,* 492-507.

Timmreck, T. (1995). *Planning, program development, and evaluation: A handbook for health promotion, aging, and health services.* Boston: Jones & Bartlett.

U.S. Department of Health and Human Services. (1996). *PATCH: Planned Approach to Community Health—Guide for the local coordinator.* Washington, DC: Centers for Disease Control and Prevention.

Williams, J. E., & Flora, J. A. (1995). Health behavior segmentation and campaign planning to reduce cardiovascular disease risk among Hispanics. *Health Education Quarterly, 22,* 36-48.

Windsor, R. A., Baranowski, T., Clark, N., & Cutter, G. (1984). *Evaluation of health promotion and education programs.* Mountain View, CA: Mayfield.

5

Tips for the Practitioner

MICHAEL V. KLINE
ROBERT M. HUFF

The intent of the previous four chapters was to provide health promotion and education practitioners with general foundations, definitions, key terms, concepts, and theories that underlie the five sections to follow. They were concerned with assisting practitioners in better understanding the processes, issues, and challenges to be faced in the development of health promotion and disease prevention (HPDP) activities targeted at particular ethnic/cultural target populations. The chapters that follow use these foundations and provide information for practitioners working in the areas of multicultural HPDP. This short "tips" chapter summarizes some of the more important ideas and concepts from these earlier chapters. These tips should not be viewed as mutually exclusive of one another; rather, they should be used as building blocks and skill anchor points for developing multicultural HPDP activities.

HEALTH PROMOTION IN THE CONTEXT OF CULTURE

The health practitioner needs to be aware that cultural forces, among other social forces, are powerful determinants of health-related behaviors in any group or subpopulation. The beliefs, ideologies, knowledge, institutions, religion, governance, and nearly all activities (including efforts to achieve health-related behavior change) are affected by the forces of the culture that dominates one's group or subgroup. The practitioner will need to identify the cultural factors that can be modified to facilitate the desired health-related behavior change. Thus, awareness and sensitivity to cultural diversity must be reflected in the planning, design, and implementation of health promotion programs. With these suggestions in mind, the HPDP practitioner should keep the following in mind:

► Be aware of the many ways of perceiving, understanding, and approaching health and disease processes across cultural and ethnic groups and that cultural differences can and do present major barriers to effective health care intervention.

► Be careful in the assessment, intervention, and evaluation planning processes not to overlook, misinterpret, stereotype, or otherwise mishandle encounters with those who might be viewed as different from yourself.

► Be aware of the perceptions target groups might hold about your agency or planning group because these may impede the health promotion process.

► Recognize that the cultural diversity of the groups targeted for intervention may present problems that can disrupt the provision of services because of competing cultural values, beliefs, norms, and health practices in conflict with the traditional Western medical model (Brislin & Yoshida 1994).

► Learn and understand the concepts of culture, ethnicity, acculturation and ethnocentrism in terms of how these may affect your ability to assess, plan, implement, and evaluate HPDP programs for a variety of multicultural population groups.

► Be aware that ethnicity often is used to stereotype diversity in human populations and frequently can lead to misunderstanding and/or distrust in all sorts of human interactions. Once a stereotype has been identified, one party or both parties might cease to look beyond the stereotype to find out who the other party really is.

► Reframe the term *race* to *multicultural, ethnic,* or *culturally diverse* to promote a greater sensitivity to the challenges, potentialities, and rewards of working with diverse cultural groups in HPDP activities.

► Assess the degree of acculturation in the target group when working in a multicultural setting because there is a natural tendency on the part of many culturally diverse individuals to resist acculturation.

► Be aware of the possible barriers that might be encountered if the program is targeted to a community primarily composed of first-, second-, or even third-generation people. Acculturative processes affect these groups in different ways.

► Recognize that there are a variety of acculturation scales that can be used for assessment, depending on the ethnic group being targeted. These can assist in tailoring interventions that integrate health-promoting strategies into the learning that is occurring in both the culture of origin and the new culture (Castro, Cota, & Vega, Chapter 7, this volume; Marin & Gamba, 1996; Ramirez, Cousins, Santos, & Supic, 1986).

► Be careful not to become caught in your own ethnocentrism, because culturally diverse target groups may view you as foreign; ignorant of illness or disease causality; or uneducated to proper social customs, forms of address, and nonverbal behaviors deemed appropriate by the groups for dealing directly or indirectly with their health problems or concerns.

▶ Seek to become more culturally competent and sensitive. The process is ongoing, and the you always should be striving to increase and improve your abilities to work in a variety of cross-cultural settings.

▶ Be willing to step out of your current frames of reference and take the risk of discovering your own biases and stereotypes and opening yourself up to new and perhaps quite divergent points of view about the world in which you live.

▶ Become aware of the interpersonal and communication style from which the target group is operating when dealing with persons from other cultures including factors such as overt hostility, covert prejudice, cultural ignorance, color blindness, and cultural liberation (Bell & Evans, 1981).

Cross-Cultural Communication

▶ Be acutely aware that in an interaction between two or more individuals representing divergent cultural orientations, the rules governing the communication process may be different and the opportunity for miscommunication is significant.

▶ Remember that the typical Western medical model for communication in the health care encounter seeks to quickly establish the facts of the case and often relies on the use of negative and double-negative questions. This approach to the communication process may be seen as cold, too direct, or otherwise in conflict with a target group's more traditional beliefs, values, and ways of communicating and of seeking and receiving health care (Brislin & Yoshida, 1994).

▶ Remember that those involved in the process of communication should share a common set of rules prescribing how the communication will take place and through what channels, when it will occur, and even how feedback may or may not be provided between the message communicator and the message receiver (Northouse & Northouse, 1992).

▶ Seek to develop improved communication skills, and be aware that patience and persistence are the keys to unlocking these skills.

▶ Recognize that health care system variables (e.g., access to health care services, insurance or financial resources, other demographics) can present potential barriers that you will need to consider when working in multicultural settings.

▶ Consider using strategies that have been demonstrated to be effective in overcoming barriers to HPDP efforts such as (a) taking more time to explain Western concepts of health, disease, prevention, and treatment in terms that are culturally understandable and relevant to the target group and (b) designing and employing educational materials that are relevant and culturally appropriate to the target group, using well-trained bilingual/bicultural staff, employing indigenous health workers when working in and with diverse multicultural communities, and seeking ways in which to improve access to services for multicultural populations.

TRADITIONAL CONCEPTS OF HEALTH AND DISEASE

When viewed across a variety of multicultural groups, explanations for health and disease that characterize many traditional beliefs about disease causation, treatment, and general health practices can be seen as highly complex, dynamic, and interactive. These explanations often involve family, community, and/or supernatural agents in cause and effect, placation, and treatment rituals to prevent, control, or cure illness. A failure to understand and appreciate these "differences" can have serious implications for the success of any HPDP effort. Thus, the practitioner should consider the following:

▶ Be aware that the health concepts held by many cultural groups may result in people choosing not to seek Western medical treatment procedures because they do not view the illness or disease as coming from within themselves.

▶ Be aware that in many Eastern cultures and other cultures in the developing world, the locus of control for disease causality often is centered outside the individual, whereas in Western cultures, the locus of control tends to be more internally oriented (Dimou, 1995).

▶ Remember that if the more traditional person does seek Western medical treatment, then that person might not be able to provide or describe his or her symptoms in precise terms that the Western medical practitioner can readily treat (Landrine & Klonoff, 1992).

▶ Recognize that individuals from other cultures might not follow through with health-promoting or treatment recommendations because they perceive the medical or other health-promoting encounter as a negative or perhaps even hostile experience.

▶ Acknowledge that many individual patients and health care practitioners have specific notions about health and disease causality and treatment called *explanatory models*. These models are generally a conglomeration of the respective cultural and social training, beliefs, and values; the personal beliefs, values, and behaviors; and the understanding of biomedical concepts that each group holds (Kleinman, 1980).

▶ Recognize that the more disparate the differences are between the biomedical model and the lay/popular explanatory models, the greater the potential for you to encounter resistance to Western HPDP programs.

▶ Be aware of the need to be flexible in the design of programs, policies, and services to meet the needs and concerns of the culturally diverse population groups that are likely to be encountered.

Traditional Concepts of Illness Causality

▶ Be aware that folk illnesses are generally learned syndromes that individuals from particular cultural groups claim to have and from which their culture defines the etiology, behaviors, diagnostic procedures, prevention methods, and traditional healing or curing practices.

▶ Remember that most cases of lay illness have multiple causalities and may require several different approaches to diagnosis, treatment, and cure including folk and Western medical interventions.

▶ Recognize that folk illnesses, which are perceived to arise from a variety of causes, often require the services of a folk healer who may be a local *curandero,* shaman, native healer, spiritualist, root doctor, or other specialized healer.

▶ Recognize that the use of traditional or alternate models of health care delivery is widely varied and may come into conflict with Western models of health care practice. Understanding these differences may help you to be more sensitive to the special beliefs and practices of multicultural target groups when planning a program.

MODELS, THEORIES, AND PRINCIPLES OF HEALTH PROMOTION WITH MULTICULTURAL POPULATIONS

The focus of health promotion has been expanding to include social and cultural influences. To address health problems effectively, we must examine cultural factors and understand beliefs about health within a context that is relevant to the population of interest. Practitioners who are culturally sensitive in health promotion programs must be able to plan interventions that are relevant and acceptable within the cultural framework of the population to be reached (Frankish, Lovato, & Shannon, Chapter 3, this volume). Therefore, HPDP practitioners should observe the following:

▶ Remember that there are a variety of theories, principles, and frameworks that can be used in planning health promotion and education programs. There is a need to take the time to determine which of these will have the best fit with respect to the cultural group, health issue, program setting, and intervention needed.

▶ Use a theoretical framework in designing programs because this can provide researchers and program developers with a perspective from which to organize knowledge and interpret factors and events. In choosing an appropriate theory, you must first clarify the purpose of the proposed program or intervention.

▶ Be aware that health promotion theories cannot tell you specifically how to plan a program or what interventions to use. They can guide your thinking as to the most promising approaches to planning intervention strategies (Hochbaum, Sorenson, & Lorig, 1992).

▶ Be aware that theories can be divided into groups according to the scope of their focus (e.g., intrapersonal, interpersonal, or group levels of interaction). Group-level theories include organizational change, diffusion of innovation, community organization, media advocacy, and social marketing. Theories also can be organized according to their style of focus, (e.g., cognitive, behavioral, social, environmental).

PLANNING HEALTH PROMOTION AND DISEASE PREVENTION PROGRAMS IN MULTICULTURAL POPULATIONS

Planning HPDP programs in multicultural populations is a dynamic and challenging process that requires systematic identification and selection of a particular course of action. Developing and implementing a health promotion program requires that planners and participants work together to accomplish a complex range of activities including (a) assessing needs, problems, and resources of the target population; (b) developing appropriate goals and objectives; (c) devising strategies and interventions that consider the peculiarities of the settings; (d) implementing and monitoring the interventions; (e) evaluating the results; and (f) refining approaches toward greater program effectiveness and efficiency. Given these guidelines, the practitioner should note the following:

▶ Be able to define the level of change sought as a result of your program (i.e., the health education level or the health promotion level).

▶ Remember that implementing a health promotion program on a community level requires that the planner identify specific health-related factors that affect health, the action strategy to be used (e.g., strengthen community action, build healthy public policy, create supportive environments, develop personal skills, reorient health services), and the level of action to be taken (e.g., society, a specific sector/system, community, family, individual) (Frankish et al., Chapter 3, this volume).

▶ Recognize that planners and participants need to be culturally competent as they interact and work together in the overall HPDP planning process (Huff & Kline, Chapter 1, this volume). Each must be sensitive to his or her own beliefs, values, patterns, and styles of interaction with other cultures, particularly as these styles could reflect biases or prejudices that could seriously disrupt the planning process.

Health Promotion Program Planning Models as Guides to Practice

▶ Be aware that planners must operate from some rational planning framework or model that can provide a systematic approach to the development of health promotion programs for specific target groups.

▶ Recognize that there are no perfect health education and health promotion planning models. You must adapt them to fit the needs of the planning situation and the cultural characteristics of the target group, setting, and health problem.

▶ Be aware that planning models, such as the traditional models and others including PRECEDE-PROCEED, PATCH, and PEN-3, can provide you with an overall framework for helping to identify and apply intervention strategies for achieving change at the individual, group, community, or organizational level.

Planning Health Promotion Programs

▶ Be aware that planning in multicultural settings must be a collaborative effort involving planners, participants, government officials, and staff/workers involved in carrying out the program. All must be heard and represented in the decision-making process.

▶ Remember that planners working in multicultural settings always must build in a cultural assessment component.

▶ Be aware that after target group priorities and program needs have been identified, health promotion planners must initiate a more focused behavioral, educational, and cultural analysis and diagnosis.

▶ Be aware of the need to identify those target group behaviors, cultural factors, and environmental factors that are contributing to the health problem and are amenable to change through health promotion and health education programs.

▶ Recognize that the substantial heterogeneity (with regard to culture; ethnic background; social norms; and generational, acculturation, and assimilation differences) within diverse cultural groups may increase the difficulty of defining target groups and tailoring interventions.

▶ Recognize that clumping ethnically heterogeneous populations into one or two broad categories might mask their true health status.

▶ Recognize that planners and participants can be ready to establish health promotion and health education program goals and objectives only when they clearly understand the relationships among (a) the health problems, the environment, and antecedent target group behaviors and (b) the role of predisposing, enabling, and reinforcing factors as these influence target group behaviors.

▶ Be aware that there is no foolproof way in which to select the right combination of interventions that will ensure the most effective results.

▶ Remember that regardless of the target group, the health problem, or the setting, the selection of the intervention and educational activities should be based on a sound rationale that considers the relationship between the cultural characteristics of the target group and the health behaviors or changes sought.

▶ Be aware that program evaluation methods should reflect an understanding of cultural or ethnic preferences, interests, and experiences to ensure adequate and appropriate data collection efforts.

CHAPTER SUMMARY

There are a great many issues and factors to consider in planning, implementing, and evaluating programs for multicultural target groups. Although it is not possible to identify all the variables that can affect these processes, this chapter has sought to identify some of the key points that the practitioner should have in mind as he or she prepares to design programs for diverse cultural and/or ethnic groups. Chief among these are the variables related to cultural competence and sensitivity including cross-cultural communication patterns, the explanatory models employed by all parties to a multicultural health promotion encounter, and the traditional health practices of the culturally diverse populations targeted for HPDP activities and services. In addition, the practitioner was reminded that the use of theories and models is critical to the planning of programs that will be relevant and acceptable to the target group being served. Finally, it was observed that planning HPDP programs for multicultural groups is a dynamic process requiring a systematic approach to the planning, implementation, and evaluation process and must include a comprehensive cultural assessment component. This can help ensure that the planner has an adequate understanding of the health issues, needs, interests, and potential barriers to a successful implementation of the program or services to be offered to the target group.

REFERENCES

Bell, P., & Evans, J. (1981). *Counseling the black client*. Center City, MN: Hazelden Education Materials.

Brislin, R. W., & Yoshida, T. (Eds.). (1994). *Improving intercultural interactions: Modules for cross-cultural training programs*. Thousand Oaks, CA: Sage.

Dimou, N. (1995). Illness and culture: Learning differences. *Patient Education and Counseling, 26,* 153-157.

Hochbaum, G. M., Sorenson, J. R., & Lorig, L. (1992). Theory in health education practice. *Health Education Quarterly, 19,* 295-313.

Kleinman, A. (1980). *Patients and healers in the context of culture*. Berkeley: University of California Press.

Landrine, H., & Klonoff, E. A. (1992). Culture and health-related schemas: A review and proposal for interdisciplinary integration. *Health Psychology, 11,* 267-276.

Marin, G., & Gamba, R. (1996). A new measurement of acculturation for Hispanics: The Bidirectional Acculturation Scale for Hispanics (BAS). *Hispanic Journal of Behavioral Sciences, 18,* 297-316.

Northouse, P. G., & Northouse, L. L. (1992). *Health communications: Strategies for health professionals* (2nd ed.). Norwalk, CT: Appleton & Lange.

Ramirez, A. G., Cousins, J. H., Santos, Y., & Supic, J. D. (1986). A media-based acculturation scale for Mexican-Americans: Application to public health programs. *Family and Community Health, 9*(3), 63-71.

PART **2**

Hispanic/Latino Populations

6

Hispanic/Latino Health and Disease

An Overview

LUCINA SUAREZ
AMELIE G. RAMIREZ

Plagued by an assortment of ethnic labels, the people who trace their origins to a single Spanish nation always have been an influential force in American society. Prior to the Hispanic/Latino identifier, the federal government recognized these people as *Mexican born* (1850 census), of *Mexican parentage* (1890 census), with *Spanish mother tongue* (1910 census), of the race of *Mexicans* (1930 census), *Spanish surnamed* (1950 census), and of *Spanish origin* (1970 census). The term *Hispanic* was introduced into the official government lexicon by the Office of Budget and Management in 1978, creating an ethnic category that included persons of Mexican, Puerto Rican, Cuban, Central American, South American, or some other Spanish origin (Trevino, 1987). This historical collection of ethnic labels refers to populations that are bound by a common ancestral language and cultural characteristics but that vastly differ in immigrant history and settlement in the United States. Members of this heterogeneous yet distinct population trace their roots back to Spain and its domination of the native populations of the southwestern United States, Mexico, Central America, South America, and the Caribbean Islands.

In the latter half of the 1980s, Hayes-Bautista and Chapa (1987) introduced the term *Latinos,* restricting the name to persons residing in the United States whose ancestries are from Latin American countries in the Western Hemisphere. Both terms enjoy wide use, depending on the region of the United States (e.g., Latino in California, Hispanic in Texas). The authors prefer to use identifiers that refer to country of origin (e.g., Mexican, Cuban, Guatemalan) because each group, although bound by a common language and history, will differ in behavior and customs—and, therefore, in health status. Because of the lack of health information on other Hispanic-origin groups, this overview is limited to the three largest Hispanic population groups in the United States: Mexican Americans, Cuban Americans, and Puerto Ricans.

The majority (61%) of the 22 million Hispanics in the United States are of Mexican origin (National Association of Hispanic Publications [NAHP], 1995; U.S Bureau of the Census, 1994). Three fourths of the Mexican American population live in Texas or California. The rest, for the most part, reside in Illinois, Colorado, New Mexico, or Arizona. The other two major Hispanic groups consist of 2.7 million Puerto Ricans and 1.0 million Cuban Americans living on the mainland. Approximately 40% of the mainland Puerto Ricans live in New York, and the remainder are concentrated in the eastern states such as New Jersey, Connecticut, Pennsylvania, and Florida. Fully 65% of the Cuban Americans reside in Florida. Recent immigration has increased the number of Central Americans (1.3 million) in the United States. In 1990, the U.S. Latin American population included 565,000 Salvadorans, 269,000 Guatemalans, 203,000 Nicaraguans, 520,000 Dominicans, and 379,000 Colombians (U.S. Bureau of the Census, 1993). High fertility rates and net immigration levels into the United States will increase the population of Hispanics to 41.0 million by the year 2010 (13% of the total U.S. population). By the next decade, the number of Hispanics will exceed that of African Americans to become the second largest racial/ethnic group in the country. The future health behavior of the growing Hispanic population will have a tremendous impact on the nation's health.

HISTORY OF HISPANICS IN THE UNITED STATES

Mexican Americans

Mexicans have lived in Texas, California, and other southwestern lands for generations. When the Treaty of Guadalupe Hidalgo transferred these territories to the United States in 1848, ending the Mexican War, tens of thousands of Mexican citizens became Americans, creating the Mexican American population. From this beginning, these Americans were treated as a race apart and often relegated to second-class status (Bean & Tienda, 1987; Hayes-Bautista & Chapa, 1987). Losing power, rights, and property, their society eventually was dominated by the Anglo population. Thus, Mexican Americans became a minority population in their native lands (Rosales, 1993). Since the early part of the century, there always has been a steady immigration, both legal and illegal, of Mexicans into the United States. Large influxes occurred during the 1910s, shortly after the Mexican revolution, and during the 1940s and 1950s, with the U.S. need for temporary workers. In terms of socioeconomic status and generational composition, this history has made the Mexican American population the most heterogeneous of all Spanish-origin groups (Bean & Tienda, 1987).

Puerto Ricans

The history of Puerto Ricans on the mainland began in 1898 when the United States gained the island from Spain after the Spanish-American war. In 1920, passage of the Jones Act granted Puerto Ricans U.S. citizenship. Most Puerto Ricans came to the mainland during World War II and during the 1950s for the promise of economic prosperity (Rosales, 1993). Because of economic and historical ties, Puerto Ricans migrated to New York City for employment in the manufacturing and service sectors (Bean & Tienda, 1987). When the island of Puerto Rico became a commonwealth of the United States in 1953, easier access to U.S. society should have secured a better economic position for Puerto Ricans. Yet, Puerto Ricans have met with social and economic discrimination, and often racial discrimination, leaving them at the bottom rung of the U.S. system. Part of the Puerto Rican experience is a continuous migration to and from the mainland and the island. This experience has made the assimilation process unique from that of Mexican or Cuban Americans. Puerto Ricans operate in two completely different societies: one Anglo dominant and one their own.

Cuban Americans

The Cuban American population in the United States came about from forces completely different from those that created the Puerto Rican and Mexican American populations (Bean & Tienda, 1987). The Cuban revolution of 1959 brought large-scale immigration of mainly European Cubans to the United States as political refugees seeking asylum from the Castro regime. Unlike immigration waves from Mexico and Puerto Rico, these immigrants were from the upper and middle class of Cuban society. Flow of Cubans to Florida continued until the early 1970s, creating a strong first-generation community with many advantages and resources provided by a federal government eager to antagonize a Communist regime. The Mariel incident in 1980 brought 125,000 more Cuban exiles to the United States. The newer arrivals were more reflective of all Cubans and came from working classes and were more African in origin (Rosales, 1993). Because of the nature of entry into the United States, Cuban Americans have been quick to integrate into the U.S. economic structure while still retaining a strong Cuban American identity.

Hispanic and Race

In the United States, nearly all Hispanics are classified as white race (96%), but some 2% are of African American race (del Pinal, 1992). The genetic background of Mexican Americans is distinct from those of Cuban Americans and Puerto Ricans and sprang from the intermixing of Spaniards and the Native American population over the course of history. Persons of Mexican origin are mestizo (mixed heritage), with the Amerindian admixture ranging from 15% to 45% (Diehl & Stern, 1989). Puerto Rican and Cuban ancestries are derived from the original Taino Indians, the Spanish, and the West Africans (Rosales, 1993).

Therefore, the racial admixture differs somewhat from that of Mexican Americans. A substantial proportion of Cubans and Puerto Ricans are of African race. Whereas Mexicans evolved from a balance of Native American and Spanish races, in Puerto Rico and Cuba, Africans and Europeans commingled with the few surviving natives to form the Spanish Caribbean mixture (Rosales, 1993). In the Caribbean, after the near annihilation of the indigenous people, the Spaniards brought slave labor from West Africa to work in their plantation systems. By the mid-1800s, Africans were 40% to 50% of the Cuban and Puerto Rican populations. The race distinctions are important, not only in having shaped the experience of each group in the United States but also in influencing social and economic positions for each group. These, in turn, affect health outcomes differentially for black Hispanics and white Hispanics (del Pinal, 1992; Trapido et al., 1995).

SOCIODEMOGRAPHIC FACTORS THAT AFFECT HEALTH

To understand the patterns of disease and health status of Hispanics, it is important to review the sociodemographic factors that may influence health. Many of the differences in health status of the different Hispanic groups can be explained by examining the differences in demographic characteristics. Hispanics are a young population. In 1992, the median age of Hispanics was 27 years, a decade younger than that of non-Hispanic whites (U.S. Bureau of the Census, 1994). Among the Hispanic groups, there is wide variation in the age structure. Of the three Hispanic groups in 1992, Mexican Americans were the youngest, with a median age of 25 years, followed closely by Puerto Ricans (27 years). Cuban Americans were nearly two decades older in median age (44 years). The difference in age structure will have an effect on the observed prevalence of chronic diseases such as cancer, cardiovascular disease, and diabetes, which are diseases of the elderly. About 5% of the Mexican American and Puerto Rican populations was age 65 years or over in 1992 (U.S. Bureau of the Census, 1994). However, 20% of the Cuban American population was age 65 years or older, so that the prevalence of the major killers mirrors that of non-Hispanic whites. Fully 38% of Mexican Americans and 37% of Puerto Ricans were under 18 years of age.

The economic status of Hispanics, and therefore their health status, is closely tied to education levels. Adult Hispanics lag behind other groups in education levels. Only about 50% of Hispanics age 25 years or over had completed high school educations in 1992, compared to 84% of their non-Hispanic white counterparts (U.S. Bureau of the Census, 1994). Again, there was significant variation in education levels among Mexican, Cuban, and Puerto Rican Americans. Mexican American adults were the least educated (only 46% had high school diplomas), whereas Puerto Ricans (60%) and Cubans (62%) were the most educated.

Economic status, the most critical factor that determines health care access, follows the same pattern as seen for education. The 1992 median income of Hispanic families was about $24,000, compared to $41,000 for non-Hispanic families (U.S. Bureau of the Census, 1994). That same year, the poverty rate among Hispanic families was nearly four times that of non-Hispanic whites (26% vs. 7%). Among Hispanic groups, Cuban Americans had the highest median income ($31,000), followed by Mexican Americans ($24,000) and Puerto Ricans ($20,000). At 33%, Puerto Ricans had the highest poverty rate among the three groups.

The family characteristics of Hispanic groups are noteworthy. Puerto Rican households in 1991 were much more likely to be headed by females (41%) than were Mexican or Cuban American families (19%) (U.S. Bureau of the Census, 1993). Although Mexican American families were larger in size and Cuban American families were smaller, the married-couple family structure was as common in both groups as it was among non-Hispanic white households. Given the higher rate of disrupted families among Puerto Ricans, they also were much more likely to receive public assistance than were Mexican or Cuban Americans (U.S. Bureau of the Census, 1993).

ASSIMILATION AND ACCULTURATION

Concepts important to the health status of Hispanics are "assimilation," the degree to which individuals integrate into the U.S. society, and "acculturation," the degree to which the dominant culture is adopted. Since 1850, the federal census has collected one or more standard assimilation measures such as place of birth, birthplace of parents, and language spoken.

Foreign Born

During the past four decades, the number and percentage of legal immigrants from Mexico and Latin America increased from 6% (150,000) to 37% (2.7 million) by the 1980s (NAHP, 1995). According to NAHP data, overall, 39% of the Hispanic population in the United States are foreign born, first generation in the United States. Because of Mexico's history with the United States, most Mexican Americans are U.S. born (64%). Approximately 71% of Cuban Americans were born in Cuba, and 39% of Puerto Ricans were born in Puerto Rico (NAHP, 1995). Even within a Hispanic group, there is likely to be considerable variation in generation status from city to city. From population surveys of older Mexican American women in Texas, the proportions born in Mexico were 61% in El Paso and Houston and 31% in San Antonio (McAlister et al., 1995; Suarez et al., 1997). Other population surveys among older Mexican American women show that the percentage born in Mexico might be higher in the border areas of California, for example, 84% in San Diego (En Accion, personal communication, July 1996). Assessing the generation status in the United States sometimes is useful to researchers because it is linked so closely to socioeconomic status, language, and other acculturation attributes.

Spanish Language

In the United States, Spanish is the dominant language of Hispanics; fully 78% of Hispanics report speaking Spanish at home (NAHP, 1995). But again, there is some variation among Mexican, Cuban, and Puerto Rican populations. The 1990 census reported that 39% of Mexican Americans do not speak English very well, compared to 34% of Puerto Ricans and 49% of Cuban Americans. The degree to which Spanish is the primary language varies with generation status, age, and gender. For example, among older low-income Hispanic women, 75% to 90% speak Spanish as a primary language (En Accion, 1993).

Acculturation

Acculturation, the degree to which Hispanics have adopted the attitudes, values, and behaviors of non-Hispanic whites or mainstream U.S. culture, is one of the most important factors that explain risk behavior and health status of Hispanics. Although acculturation often has been reduced to measurement of language use, it encompasses many dimensions. Studies have used a variety of indicators and measures to tap into the acculturation process. Besides language use, birthplace, or generation status (Cuellar, Harris, & Jasso, 1980; Delgado, Johnson, Roy, & Trevino, 1990), these include ethnic identity, value placed on preserving cultural origin, attitudes toward family, gender roles in the family, and social interaction with non-Hispanics (Hazuda, Stern, & Haffner, 1988).

Few studies of Hispanic health have examined other important acculturation dimensions that are characteristic of Hispanic culture. These attributes include *familismo, simpatia, respeto, fatalismo,* and religiosity. Strong attitudes toward *familismo* (family) is a core characteristic in the Hispanic culture (Alvarez, 1993; Sabogal, Marin, Otero-Sabogal, Marin, & Perez-Stable, 1987). Within the Hispanic culture, there is a strong identification with one's family and strong feelings of support from nuclear and extended family members. Embedded in the structure of *la familia* is the authority and protection of the father, the sacrificing nature of the mother's role, and the *respeto* (respect) that children must give to family members (Alvarez, 1993). A few studies have suggested that the degree to which Hispanics adhere to this core characteristic positively influences health behavior (Prislin, Suarez, Simpson, & Dyer, 1996; Suarez, 1994). Familism is independent of socioeconomic class or language use and is similarly held among different Hispanic groups (e.g., Mexican, Cuban, Central American) (Sabogal et al., 1987). For Hispanics, decisions about the use of medical care or preventive care or treatment are family based. In a Los Angeles study of four ethnic groups, Mexican Americans were more likely to hold a family-centered model of decision making than the patient autonomy model favored by African and European Americans (Blackhall, Murphy, Frank, Michel, & Azen, 1995).

Simpatia (being nice) is the Hispanic tendency to avoid conflict in social and personal encounters. Cultural value is placed on achieving harmony in interpersonal relationships. *Respeto* toward individuals is acknowledged and reciprocated and is based on age, sex, and social positions of authority. Survey research among Hispanics requires recognition of these two cultural values to be successful (Marin & Marin, 1991). Having an appropriate interviewer of a certain age or demeanor who can provide appropriate *respeto* will enhance the quality of data collected from Hispanic individuals. Marin and Marin (1991) suggest that *simpatia* may contribute to the low refusal rates among Hispanics in community surveys and also to the overreporting of socially desirable responses (e.g., use of preventive examinations).

Fatalism, the belief that an individual has little control over personal health outcomes, is a common theme in Hispanic attitudes (Hazuda, Stern, & Haffner, 1988; Perez-Stable, Sabogal, Otero-Sabogal, Hiatt, & McPhee, 1992). In a study of Latinos and Anglos, higher proportions of Latinos believed that cancer was a death sentence and God's punishment and that there was very little one could do to prevent cancer (Perez-Stable et al., 1992). There are measurable differences in fatalistic beliefs among Anglo, Black, less assimilated, and highly assimilated Mexican Americans. In one study, fatalism was highest among least assimilated Mexican Americans and lowest for Anglos (Neff & Hoppe, 1992). Among Mexican Americans living in San Antonio, Hazuda and colleagues found that fatalism and religiosity were strongly held, with almost no acculturation toward Anglo attitudes (Hazuda, Stern, & Haffner, 1988).

Several popular acculturation scales are available to researchers, although much work needs to be done to measure more dimensions of acculturation such as religiosity and fatalism. The original Cuellar scale taps into language use, ethnic identification, social interactions, generation status, contact with Mexico, and cultural pride (Cuellar et al., 1980). An abbreviated, mostly language-based version was used in the 1982-1984 Hispanic Health and Nutrition Examination Survey (HHANES) (Delgado et al., 1990). Many recent studies (Otero-Sabogal, Sabogal, Perez-Stable, & Hiatt, 1995; Perez-Stable et al., 1992) have used a strictly language-based acculturation scale developed by Marin, Sabogal, Marin, Otero-Sabogal, and Perez-Stable (1987). Items measured include proficiency and preference for speaking Spanish as a child, at home, while thinking, with friends, and at school or work. A more multidimensional scale is the Hazuda scale developed from a large Mexican American population in San Antonio (Hazuda, Stern, & Haffner, 1988). It has proven useful in identifying other cultural attributes that can have positive influences on health behavior (Suarez, 1994; Suarez & Pulley, 1995). Dimensions other than language measured by the scale include attitudes toward family and gender roles, social interaction, and cultural values (Hazuda, Stern, & Haffner, 1988).

A few comments about the long-term use of assimilation measures of generation status and language are offered here. Although easy to assess, birthplace and generation status will be poor indicators of the dynamic process of acculturation because they are unvaried for a given individual. Most researchers agree that birthplace or generation status inadequately measure acculturation level now that many multidimensional scales are available. Neff and Hoppe (1992) point out that generational status or nativity might fail to address the degree of integration into the dominant culture because it is possible that a first-generation Hispanic may be more acculturated than a second-generation individual due to differing influences, experiences, and circumstances. English language use measures functional integration into the U.S. mainstream but might fail to adequately measure cultural attitudes, particularly in settings where Spanish language is preferred but not necessary (e.g., El Paso, San Diego). Language use, or the ability to speak English, is highly correlated with socioeconomic status (Negy & Woods, 1992a, 1992b). To assess the influence of acculturation, it is important to separate out the effects due to economic status, a common determinant of health status in all populations.

EPIDEMIOLOGY OF DISEASE AMONG HISPANICS

In 1995, the life expectancy of Hispanics males was 75 years, one year longer than that of non-Hispanic white males and 10 years longer than that of non-Hispanic African American males (U.S. Bureau of the Census, 1995). Hispanic females had a life expectancy of 82 years, 2 years longer than that of non-Hispanic white females and 8 years longer than that of non-Hispanic African American females. Vital statistics information (National Center for Health Statistics [NCHS], 1996; Plepys & Klein, 1995) and cohort studies have consistently shown that Hispanics have a lower mortality from all causes than do non-Hispanic whites and blacks. This relative advantage is considerable and differs somewhat for men and women. Mortality is 20% to 26% lower for Hispanic men than for non-Hispanic men and is 18% to 25% lower for Hispanic women than for non-Hispanic women (NCHS, 1996; Sorlie, Backlund, Johnson, & Rogot, 1993). Mortality data for all Hispanic subgroups are sparse, but at least one study has indicated that the deficit in mortality from all causes is enjoyed by Mexican, Puerto Rican, and Cuban groups (Sorlie et al., 1993). This deficit in mortality is remarkable in light of the lower socioeconomic status of Hispanics compared to other groups. When income is taken into account, the relative risk of death for Hispanics is even lower (Sorlie et al., 1993). An examination of the specific causes of mortality has shown that Hispanics have much lower rates of the two leading causes of death, cardiovascular disease and cancer. However, Hispanics have higher death rates due to diabetes, the seventh leading cause of death in the country.

Cardiovascular Disease

Cardiovascular disease mortality clearly is lower among Hispanics, despite their higher risk profile for diabetes, obesity, and blood lipids. In 1992, the age-adjusted death rate from cardiovascular disease among Hispanics was 121 per 100,000, compared to 173 per 100,000 among whites and 265 per 100,000 among blacks (Plepys & Klein, 1995). Studies from Texas (Goff, Ramsey, Labarthe, & Nichaman, 1993; Stern et al., 1987) have shown that death rates from coronary heart disease are about 20% to 25% lower among Mexican American men than among their white counterparts. The relative advantage in coronary heart disease mortality is not shared by Mexican American women, who have rates equal to those of white women (Goff et al., 1993). This pattern has held for the past two decades (Goff et al., 1993). Much of the information known about the incidence of cardiovascular disease and related risk factors among Hispanics comes from the San Antonio Heart Study of Mexican Americans (Stern, Rosenthal, Haffner, Hazuda, & Franco, 1984) and the Puerto Rico Heart Health Program (Ramirez, 1991). Other than HHANES, there exist few studies that include Cubans and Puerto Ricans (Delgado et al., 1990; Ramirez, 1991). Studies have shown that, compared to non-Hispanic whites, the risk of coronary heart disease and the prevalence of myocardial infarctions is lower for Mexican American men but not for women (Mitchell, Haffner, Hazuda, Patterson, & Stern, 1992; Mitchell, Hazuda, Haffner, Patterson, & Stern, 1991b). This lower risk was not observed, however, among Hispanics living in Colorado, who have less Mexican ancestry than do populations in Texas (Rewers et al., 1993). Puerto Ricans living in Puerto Rico showed the same low rate of coronary disease compared to U.S. whites (Ramirez, 1991). Paradoxically, despite the low rates of heart attack and death, Mexican American men have angina pectoris at a rate twice that of non-Hispanic white men (Mitchell, Hazuda, Haffner, Patterson, & Stern, 1991a). Cardiovascular researchers speculate that the genetic makeup of Mexican Americans leaves them vulnerable to diseases such as angina and diabetes yet relatively invulnerable to the fatal outcomes. In other words, their hearts are too strong to die from these diseases.

Diabetes

Without question, diabetes is the major health problem among Hispanics. The San Antonio Heart Study has firmly established that Mexican Americans have a two- to threefold excess risk of non-insulin-dependent diabetes mellitus (Hazuda, Haffner, & Stern, 1988; Stern et al., 1984). Approximately 10% to 15% of Mexican American men and women have diabetes (Diehl & Stern, 1989). Hispanics have higher risks along the entire spectrum of disease, have higher levels of undiagnosed diabetes, have higher incidence of diagnosed diabetes, endure more severe complications from diabetes, and die more frequently from the disease than do non-Hispanic whites (Baxter et al., 1993; Diehl & Stern, 1989; Haffner et al., 1993; Hanis et al., 1983; Perez-Stable et al., 1989; Pugh, Stern, Haffner, Eifler, & Zapata, 1988; Samet, Coultas, Howard, Skipper, & Hanis, 1988). The risk appears to be correlated with the proportion of Native American genetic admixture (Diehl & Stern, 1989) and varies among Hispanic populations living in different regions of the country (Samet et al., 1988). The uncommonly high risk of non-insulin-dependent diabetes mellitus, in combination with high obesity rates and higher risks of gallbladder disease, may constitute a genetic syndrome derived from Native American ancestry (Diehl & Stern, 1989; Hanis et al., 1993; Weiss, Ferrell, & Hanis, 1984).

Acculturation into Anglo society appears to have a beneficial effect on the prevalence of diabetes and probably is mediated by acculturation effects on obesity (Hazuda, Haffner, & Stern, 1988). Hazuda and colleagues found that more-acculturated Mexican American women tend to be leaner than less-acculturated women, which would lessen the risk of diabetes (Hazuda, Haffner, & Stern, 1988). Aside from acculturation, a simple rise in socioeconomic status has a beneficial effect, indicating that the burden of this disease can be alleviated with better access to medical care. With diabetes so prevalent among Hispanics, the interventions needed seem obvious. Interventions should be geared toward educating and informing Hispanic diabetics to control this disease and to prevent severe outcomes. In addition, strategies are needed to help Hispanics reduce their fat intake and increase physical exercise to control obesity, which increases diabetes risk.

Cancer

Historically, Hispanic men and women have had consistently lower rates of cancer than have non-Hispanic whites and blacks. These low rates of cancer overall are due to the low rates of the leading types of cancer such as lung, breast, prostate, and colorectal cancer. Hispanics, however, tend to be at greater risk for stomach, gallbladder, liver, and cervical cancer.

Lung Cancer and Other Respiratory Cancers

Lung cancer incidence and mortality rates are 60% to 80% lower in all Hispanic groups including Mexican Americans, Cubans, and Puerto Ricans (Trapido et al., 1995). The lower rates of lung cancer are, of course, due to historically low rates of cigarette smoking among Hispanics, especially Hispanic women. Other smoking-related cancers (e.g., oral cavity, esophagus, bladder) also are consistently lower in Hispanics (En Accion, 1993; Perkins, Hoegh, Wright, & Young, 1993; Texas Department of Health, 1993; Wolfgang, Semeiks, & Burnett, 1991). The one exception to the low pattern of smoking-related cancers is esophageal cancer, which was found to be twice as high in Puerto Rican men than in their white counterparts in New York City (Wolfgang et al., 1991). The main risk factor for esophageal cancer is the combination of cigarette smoking and excessive alcohol consumption.

Breast, Prostate, and Colon Cancers

Cancer registry data from California, Texas, Florida, and New York show that breast cancer is 50% to 30% less frequent in Hispanic women (En Accion, 1993; Trapido et al., 1995). Because the disease is less common among Hispanic women, overall death rates from breast cancer also are lower. However, if a Hispanic woman gets breast cancer, she is less likely to be diagnosed at an early stage of the disease, that is, when treatment is more effective in preventing her death (En Accion, 1993). For men, prostate cancer is less frequent among Mexican Americans but not among Puerto Rican or Cuban men, who have rates comparable to those of non-Hispanic white men (En Accion, 1993; Perkins et al., 1993; Texas Department of Health, 1993; Trapido et al., 1995; Wolfgang et al., 1991). Although prostate cancer incidence is low among Hispanics, prostate cancer mortality rates in some border populations are equal to those of Anglos (Texas Cancer Registry, 1996). This suggests a problem with access to medical care or more late-stage diagnosis among prostate cancer patients, resulting in poorer rates of survival. Colon and rectum cancer rates also are consistently lower for all Hispanic groups in the United States (Trapido et al., 1995).

We have little understanding of why Hispanics are at low risk for these particular cancers. All three sites of cancer are thought to have a dietary association in which diets high in animal fat and low in fiber increase risks (Tomatis et al., 1990). A high socioeconomic status is associated with increased risk of breast, colon, and prostate cancers, possibly reflecting more Western diets (high fat, low fiber). Although no studies have been conducted, it follows that more acculturated Hispanics, who lose their traditional diets, apparently a protective factor, eventually will develop risks of these cancers comparable to those of whites. Both breast and prostate cancers also have a genetic component in their etiologies, and breast cancer has a strong reproductive etiology (Tomatis et al., 1990). The younger age at which Hispanic women have pregnancies, and the larger number of births, probably offers Hispanic women some protection against breast cancer because these factors are known to affect risk.

Cervical Cancer

Cervical cancer incidence is two to three times higher in Mexican American and Puerto Rican women as in Anglo women (En Accion, 1993). In addition, in most areas of the Southwest, the risk of dying from cancer of the cervix is twice as high in Mexican American women as in Anglo women (En Accion, 1993). The risk of cervical cancer and related death in Cuban American women is equivalent to that in non-Hispanic white women (Trapido et al., 1995). The higher risk of dying in Mexican American women clearly is related to late-stage diagnosis of this disease (Caplan, Wells, & Haynes, 1992; Suarez, Martin, & Weiss, 1991). Data from Texas show that about 50% of cervical cancer in Mexican Americans is found early, compared to 68% in non-Hispanic white women (Suarez et al., 1991). Screening programs to improve earlier diagnosis of cervical cancer should be implemented in Hispanic communities to reduce the death rate.

No one really knows why Mexican American women have higher risks of developing cervical cancer in the first place. Risk factors for the development of cervical cancer are well documented. These include sexual behavior (e.g., early onset of sexual activity, multiple sex partners, promiscuity of sex partners), exposure to sexually transmitted agents, socioeconomic factors, and cigarette smoking (Franco, 1991; Reeves et al., 1989). Recent studies have indicated a causal role for human papillomavirus (Bosch & Munoz, 1989; Koutsky et al., 1992). There are no studies of the prevalence of the human papillomavirus in Mexican American women or in any U.S. population (Franco, 1991). Although Mexican American women marry early, engage in sexual intercourse at an earlier stage, and have lower economic status, they have fewer sex partners and smoke less. One study has shifted attention away from the sexual behavior of the women as a risk factor and toward the sexual behavior of the Latino husbands.

Zunzunegui, King, Coria, and Charlet (1986) found that, among Mexican Americans, the larger the number of sex partners of the husband, the greater the risk for cervical cancer.

Stomach Cancer

Stomach cancer is very much a cancer of the poor, reflecting diets that lack fresh fruits and vegetables and a heavier dependence on salty, smoked, and preserved foods (Tomatis et al., 1990). With poverty as an indirect risk factor, it is not surprising that rates are high among Mexican Americans and Puerto Ricans. Among men, incidence rates of stomach cancer are twice as high in Mexican Americans as in non-Hispanic whites (En Accion, 1993). Rates in Mexican American women are three times higher than those in other women. Stomach cancer rates in Puerto Rican men and women are about 50% higher than those in non-Hispanic whites. Cuban Americans have rates 10% to 20% lower than those of non-Hispanic whites (Tomatis et al., 1990). The low rates of stomach cancer among Cuban Americans probably reflect their relatively higher socio-economic status compared to other Hispanic groups.

Gallbladder and Liver Cancer

Gallbladder and liver cancer are two extremely rare cancers but are of interest to Hispanic populations because of the excessive risks. Cancer of the gallbladder is about five times higher in Mexican American women than in white women. It also is higher in Mexican American men, but only twice as high. Mortality due to gallbladder cancer also is high. This excess in gallbladder cancer appears to be confined to the Mexican population and follows the general pattern (female preponderance and Native American ancestry) of high rates of gallbladder diseases (gallstones) among this population (Diehl & Stern, 1989; Hanis et al., 1993).

Liver cancer is excessive among all Hispanic groups, with the highest risk observed among Mexican American populations in Texas (En Accion, 1993; Suarez & Martin, 1987). In the United States, most liver cancer occurs in association with cirrhosis, but alcohol consumption is low, at least among Hispanic women. This leads to the consideration of environmental and occupational exposures. Other risk factors known to be associated with primary liver cancer are chronic Hepatitis B and exposure to aflatoxin. The prevalence of these risk factors, especially Hepatitis B, among Hispanics is generally unknown, but acute hepatitis has been shown to be high for some groups of Hispanics (Alter et al., 1990). Mexican diets tend to include corn and bean products, which may be a path of exposure for aflatoxin. The risk of liver cancer also might be related to occupational exposures to pesticides. Mexican Americans are more likely to be exposed to pesticides than are other groups because they constitute the majority of farmworkers in the Southwest. Geographic analysis of primary liver cancer shows the highest excess in counties along the U.S.-Mexico border, primarily an agricultural region. However, no studies have been able to establish a strong relationship between farmworking and exposures to agricultural chemicals and liver cancer (Suarez, Weiss, & Martin, 1989). Research is needed to assess the role of etiologic factors such as Hepatitis B infection and agricultural exposures in the development of primary liver cancer in Hispanics.

Tuberculosis and AIDS

After decades of decreasing prevalence, the nation is experiencing an increase in tuberculosis in many regions and demographic groups (Friedman, 1994). The most marked increase in cases of tuberculosis is occurring in the Hispanic population, which experienced a 72% increase in new cases from 1985 to 1991. The increase is largely due to more cases of tuberculosis among the foreign born and to the associated increase of HIV infections among young adult Hispanic males (Friedman, 1994). Overall, the incidence of tuberculosis is 23 per 100,000 for Hispanics, nearly six times the rate for white non-Hispanics (4 per 100,000). New immigrants from Latin America have higher rates of tuberculosis, about 50% higher than those of U.S.-born Hispanics (McKenna, McCray, & Onorato, 1995). Tuberculosis is a disease found among the poor and is readily transmitted in crowded conditions and in the undernourished. It is emerging as a major public health problem in the Hispanic community.

Related to this epidemic of tuberculosis is the high incidence of AIDS among the Hispanic population. Nationwide, the reported incidence of AIDS in 1992 was 53 per 100,000 for Hispanic-origin persons compared to 18 per 100,000 for whites and 104 per 100,000 for blacks (Plepys & Klein, 1995). About one third of the 100,000 AIDS cases reported to the Centers for Disease Control and Prevention (CDC, 1994a) are among Hispanics. The highest rates occur among Hispanics living in the Northeast, where the Puerto Rican population is concentrated. In the Southwest, AIDS rates for Hispanics (probably Mexican Americans) are lower than those for whites (CDC, 1994a).

RISK BEHAVIORS

Cigarette Smoking

Data from the HHANES conducted during the early 1980s showed that age-adjusted smoking rates were high for Mexican American (43%), Puerto Rican (40%), and Cuban American (42%) men (Haynes, Harvey, Montes, Nickens, & Cohen, 1990). Smoking was less prevalent in Hispanic women (24% in Mexican American, 30% in Puerto Rican, and 24% in Cuban women). Rates in Hispanic men were higher than those reported for whites, but rates in Hispanic women were about equal to (Cuban and Puerto Rican women) or lower than (Mexican American women) those in white women. The HHANES also showed that Puerto Rican and Cuban American men were more likely to be heavy smokers and that Mexican American men were more likely to be light smokers. For Mexican American women, acculturation, as measured by the Cuellar abbreviated language scale, tended to increase the level of smoking (Haynes et al., 1990).

More recent information from the CDC's Behavioral Risk Factor Surveillance System (BRFSS) shows that Hispanic women still smoke less than do white women (15% vs. 22%) (CDC, 1994b). Hispanic men appear to have rates slightly lower than those of white men (22% vs. 25%). No information from the BRFSS is available for the different Hispanic groups. The state of California conducted the most comprehensive population smoking surveys in its tobacco control efforts. Data for 1990-1991 in California showed the same smoking pattern for Mexican- and other-origin Hispanics, that is, lower smoking for women and rates equal to those of whites for men (California Department of Health Services, 1993). There has been recent speculation that young Hispanics might have started smoking more because of the tobacco industry's marketing focus on the Hispanic and young adult populations. However, there is no real evidence that young Hispanics smoke more than do other groups. In that same California survey, the smoking prevalence ratios (comparing Hispanics to non-Hispanic whites) among 18- to 24-year-olds were the same as those for older age groups. The 1991 national school-based Youth Risk Behavior Survey showed that white high school students still were more likely than Hispanic students to be frequent cigarette users (15% vs. 7%) (Kann et al., 1993). These observations are similar to what was reported for children 12 to 17 years of age in 1994 (11% vs. 6%) (NCHS, 1996). Otero-Sabogal, Sabogal, and Perez-Stable (1995) suggest that adolescent Latinas are protected from smoking because they tend to spend more of their free time with family than do non-Latina white adolescents.

Alcohol Consumption

Alcohol consumption among Hispanics is characterized by a gender difference (high among men, very low among women) and by a pattern among Hispanic men whereby drinking is infrequent, but high quantities are consumed at a given time (i.e., binge drinking) (Neff & Hoppe, 1992; Otero-Sabogal, Sabogal, Perez-Stable, & Hiatt, 1995). National survey data for 1990 showed that percentage current drinking among Hispanic men ages 18 to 44 years was 71%, compared to 80% among white non-Hispanics (NCHS, 1996). Among Hispanic women ages 18 to 44 years, 42% were current drinkers, compared to 65% among non-Hispanic white women. Only 28% of Hispanic women age 45 years or over currently drink. Heavy drinking was more frequent among Mexican American and Puerto Rican men than among Cuban American men (Marks, Garcia, & Solis, 1990), but this observation might be confounded by the age and socioeconomic differences among the groups. As with cigarette smoking, traditional Hispanic values do not permit alcohol consumption by women, but with assimilation, women adopt the higher alcohol use of mainstream members (Black & Markides, 1993; Neff & Hoppe, 1992). Among Hispanic males, the heavier drinking pattern is characteristic of least acculturated males; more acculturated males have lower but more frequent alcohol use, a pattern common among non-Hispanic white men (Neff & Hoppe, 1992; Otero-Sabogal, Sabogal, Perez-Stable, & Hiatt, 1995). The relationship between alcohol use and acculturation might have more to do with socioeconomic factors than with cultural attitudes (Neff & Hoppe, 1992) but also might reflect patterns of drinking common in

Latin American countries (Otero-Sabogol, Sabogal, Perez-Stable, & Hiatt, 1995).

Obesity

Studies of coronary risk factors among Hispanics consistently find that Mexican Americans are overweight (Diehl & Stern, 1989; Hazuda, Mitchell, Haffner, & Stern, 1991; NCHS, 1989; Samet et al., 1988; Stern et al., 1981). This ethnic difference between Mexican Americans and non-Hispanic whites is greater in women than in men (Hazuda et al., 1991; NCHS, 1996). In some populations of Hispanics, the proportion of Hispanics defined as overweight exceeds 50% (Hazuda et al., 1991; NCHS, 1989), depending on socioeconomic status and age group. Particularly for women, acculturation and socioeconomic status have pronounced effects on obesity levels; with increased acculturation and socioeconomic status, obesity levels decrease (Hazuda et al., 1991; Stern et al., 1984).

The prevalence of obesity among Hispanics was found to be intermediate between the rates for U.S. whites and those for Pima Indians (Stern et al., 1981). Furthermore, at least in Mexican American women, the level of obesity is correlated with the degree of Amerindian genetic admixture (Mitchell et al., 1993). Among Hispanics in New Mexico, who are considered by some to have less American Indian admixture and to be more European than Mexican Americans (Bean & Tienda, 1987), the prevalence of obesity was less than that among Mexican Americans in Texas but was more than that among U.S. whites (Samet et al., 1988). Thus, the pattern of obesity parallels the risk observed for diabetes and gallbladder disease. Still puzzling, however, is that the obesity burden does not seem to result in higher coronary disease, hypertension, or death (Diehl & Stern, 1989). The levels of hypertension and high serum cholesterol among Mexican Americans are comparable to those among Anglos (Franco et al., 1985; Mitchell et al., 1991a, 1992; Rewers et al., 1993). However, interventions that will help members of the Hispanic community reduce obesity will have a favorable impact on the risk for diabetes that is so highly prevalent in the Hispanic community.

HEALTH CARE USE PATTERNS

The success that Hispanics have in dealing with their unique pattern of disease will largely depend on access to medical care and participation in prevention practices. Access to medical care in the United States is determined by individual health insurance coverage. Trevino, Moyer, Valdez, and Stroup-Benham (1991) document that during the early 1980s, Hispanics were far less likely than whites to have any type of health insurance. The percentage uninsured also varied greatly among the three Hispanic groups. Approximately 35% of Mexican Americans were uninsured, compared to 22% of Puerto Ricans and 29% of Cuban Americans. One third of the Puerto Rican population was on Medicaid, whereas only about 6% of Mexican and Cuban Americans were on Medicaid. The difference in Medicaid coverage was likely due to the eligibility requirements (more Puerto Rican families, headed by females, qualify) and the restrictive policies that vary from state to state (e.g., Texas vs. New York). The latest information from the NCHS (1996) shows that not much changed by 1994; fully 33% of Hispanics were not covered by any type of health insurance, compared to 15% of non-Hispanic whites. The ethnic differences in uninsured rates among Mexican Americans, Puerto Ricans, and Cuban Americans remained almost exactly as they did a decade ago. The proportion of Mexican Americans on Medicaid increased from less than 10% in 1984 to 16% in 1994.

Lack of health insurance is the major barrier to preventive care for the Hispanic population. It makes for less likely participation in dental care, cancer screening, and prenatal care (NCHS, 1996). Less than half of Hispanics age 25 years or over had dental visits during the past year, compared to two thirds of non-Hispanic whites. To reduce the number of breast cancer deaths, a national initiative was begun to get more women to use mammography. Mammography was a relatively new tool during the 1980s; only about 20% of Hispanic women age 50 years or over had recently used mammography in 1987 (NCHS, 1996). The percentage of non-Hispanic white women who used mammography was 29%. All groups of women, including Hispanics, have greatly increased their participation in screening mammography. Although Hispanic women still lag behind, the percentage among those age 50 years or over who use mammography has risen to about 50%, compared to 60% among non-Hispanic white women (NCHS, 1996). Again, there is considerable variation among Hispanic groups and among specific age groups. Among women age 65 years or over, 36% of Hispanic women have had recent mammograms—far less than the 55% of other similarly aged women.

Regarding prenatal care, 82% of white mothers receive prenatal care in their first trimesters of pregnancy (NCHS, 1996). Mexican American and Puerto Rican mothers receive prenatal care less often (65% and 70%, respectively). Cuban American mothers receive prenatal care as often as do non-Hispanic white mothers (89%). Although slight increases have occurred in the past decade for all mothers, these ethnic differences are essentially the same as they were 15 years ago (NCHS, 1996). But again, paradoxically, Mexican American mothers, who are the least likely to receive prenatal care, have birth outcomes that are as healthy as those for white mothers. Of the four groups, only 5.8% of live births to Mexican American mothers are low birthweight, compared to 6.0% of those to non-Hispanic white mothers, 9.2% of those to Puerto Rican mothers, and 6.2% of those to Cuban American mothers (NCHS, 1996).

CHAPTER SUMMARY

The immigrant and settlement history of each Hispanic group in the United States has determined the socioeconomic characteristics, the age structure, and the assimilation and acculturation levels of the populations today. Cuban Ameri-

TABLE 6.1 Summary of Evidence on Relative Risk of Diseases and Risk Factors in U.S. Hispanic Men Compared to Non-Hispanic White Men

	Hispanic	Mexican American	Puerto Rican	Cuban
Disease				
Total mortality	−	−	=	−
Heart disease mortality	−	−	−	
Stroke mortality	−	+=	+	
Diabetes mellitus prevalence		++	++	
Total cancer incidence		−	−	−
Lung cancer incidence		−	−	−
Esophogeal cancer incidence		−	++	−
Prostate cancer incidence		−	=	=
Colon cancer incidence		−	−	−
Stomach cancer incidence		+	+	−
Gallbladder cancer incidence		++	=	++
Liver cancer incidence		++	++	+
Tuberculosis incidence	++	++		
AIDS incidence	++	−	++	++
Risk factor				
Cigarette smoking	−	=		
Alcohol use	=	=	=	=
Overweight		+	=	+
Hypertension		−=+		
Serum cholesterol		=		

NOTE: The relative risk (*RR*) is the ratio of the rate of Hispanic males to the rate of non-Hispanic white males, as follows: *RR* is greater than 2.0 (++), *RR* is between 1.1 and 2.0 (+), *RR* is between 0.9 and 1.1 (=), *RR* is between 0.5 and 0.9 (−), *RR* is less than 0.5 (—). Evidence is based on references cited in the text.

cans are an older population, whereas the Mexican American and Puerto Rican populations are much younger than non-Hispanic whites. Mexican Americans and Puerto Ricans are less educated and have lower incomes than Cuban Americans, but all groups lag behind non-Hispanic whites. Certain acculturation characteristics such as use of the Spanish language, family loyalty, and fatalistic attitudes toward life still are strongly held among all groups. Acculturation factors, some correlated with income and education, will affect health behavior in both positive and negative ways. Each factor has to be examined separately within each group and considered along with socioeconomic status.

Variability in social, economic, and assimilation characteristics has caused some differences in the general health status of Mexican Americans, Cuban Americans, and Puerto Ricans. Yet, for some health outcomes, there is consistency in risk among Hispanic groups. First, Hispanics have a longer life span than do non-Hispanic whites and African Americans, despite the social and economic disadvantages. The main reason for this is the lower death rates from the leading causes of death. Even taking into account their younger ages, Hispanics are less likely to die from heart disease and cancer, the two most common killers in the United States. Tables 6.1 and 6.2 summarize what is known about the relative risks for various diseases and risk factors among Hispanic men and women compared to those among non-Hispanic whites. Cancer is reduced in Hispanics because they smoke less than do Anglos and have not adopted more Westernized

TABLE 6.2 Summary of Evidence on Relative Risk of Diseases and Risk Factors in U.S. Hispanic Women Compared to Non-Hispanic White Women

	Hispanic	Mexican American	Puerto Rican	Cuban
Disease				
Total mortality	−	−	−	−
Heart disease mortality	−	=	−	
Stroke mortality	−	−=	=	
Diabetes mellitus prevalence		++	++	
Total cancer incidence		−	−	−
Lung cancer incidence		—	—	—
Breast cancer incidence		−	−	−
Colon cancer incidence		−	−	−
Cervical cancer incidence		++	++	+
Stomach cancer incidence		++	+	−
Gallbladder cancer incidence		++	+	+
Liver cancer incidence		++	+	+
Tuberculosis incidence	++	++		
Risk factor				
Cigarette smoking	−	−		
Alcohol use	−	−	−	—
Overweight		+	+	+
Hypertension		−=		
Serum cholesterol		=		

NOTE: The relative risk (*RR*) is the ratio of the rate of Hispanic males to the rate of non-Hispanic white males, as follows: *RR* is greater than 2.0 (+ +), *RR* is between 1.1 and 2.0 (+), *RR* is between 0.9 and 1.1 (=), *RR* is between 0.5 and 0.9 (–), *RR* is less than 0.5 (—). Evidence is based on references cited in the text.

diets high in animal fat and low in fiber. As for the lower risk of heart disease, some speculate that the genetic makeup of Mexican Americans in particular provides some protection against the lethal effects of cardiovascular risk factors. Diseases that are very high among Hispanics, particularly Mexican Americans, are diabetes, obesity, and gallbladder and liver cancers. These diseases may have a genetic component linked to the Native American admixture, and risks may be strongly enhanced by environmental factors. Lack of health insurance and less participation in medical and preventive care are factors in certain health outcomes such as higher risk of cervical cancer death, which can be completely prevented by routine Pap smears. Interventions that open access to the medical care system and emphasize positive cultural attributes of Hispanics would benefit all Americans.

REFERENCES

Alter, M. J., Hadler, S. C., Judson, F. N., Mares, A., Alexander, J., Hu, P. Y., Miller, J. K., Moyer, L. A., Fields, H. A., Bradley, D. W., & Margolis, H. S. (1990). Risk factors for acute non-A, non-B hepatitis in the United States and association with Hepatitis C virus infection. *Journal of the American Medical Association, 264,* 2231-2235.

Alvarez, R. R. (1993). The family. In N. Kanellos (Ed.), *The Hispanic American almanac: A reference work on Hispanics in the United States.* Detroit, MI: Gale Research.

Baxter, J., Hamman, R. F., Lopez, T. K., Marshall, J. A., Hoag, S., & Swenson, C. J. (1993). Excess incidence of known non-insulin-dependent diabetes mellitus (NIDDM) in Hispanics compared with non-Hispanic whites in the San Luis Valley, Colorado. *Ethnicity and Disease, 3,* 11-21.

Bean, F. D., & Tienda, M. (1987). *The Hispanic population of the United States.* New York: Russell Sage.

Black, S. A., & Markides, K. S. (1993). Acculturation and alcohol consumption in Puerto Rican, Cuban-American, and Mexican-American women in the United States. *American Journal of Public Health, 83,* 890-893.

Blackhall, L. J., Murphy, S. T., Frank, G., Michel, V., & Azen, S. (1995). Ethnicity and attitudes toward patient autonomy. *Journal of the American Medical Association, 274,* 820-825.

Bosch, F. X., & Munoz, N. (1989). Human papillomavirus and cervical neoplasia: A critical review of the epidemiological evidence. In N. Munoz, F. X. Bosch, & O. M. Jensen (Eds.), *Human papillomavirus and cervical cancer.* Lyon, France: World Health Organization, International Agency for Research on Cancer.

California Department of Health Services. (1993). *Tobacco use in California 1990-1991.* Sacramento: Author.

Caplan, L. S., Wells, B. L., & Haynes, S. (1992). Breast cancer screening among older racial/ethnic minorities and whites: Barriers to early detection. *Journals of Gerontology, 47,* 101-110. (Special issue)

Centers for Disease Control and Prevention. (1994a). AIDS among racial/ethnic minorities: United States, 1993. *Morbidity and Mortality Weekly Report, 43,* 644-646.

Centers for Disease Control and Prevention. (1994b). Prevalence of selected risk factors for chronic disease by education level in racial/ethnic populations: United States, 1991-1992. *Morbidity and Mortality Weekly Report, 43,* 894-899.

Cuellar, I., Harris, L. C., & Jasso, R. (1980). An acculturation scale for Mexican American normal and clinical populations. *Hispanic Journal of Behavioral Sciences, 2,* 199-217.

Delgado, J. L., Johnson, C. L., Roy, I., & Trevino, F. M. (1990). Hispanic Health and Nutrition Examination Survey: Methodological considerations. *American Journal of Public Health, 80*(Suppl.), 6-10.

del Pinal, J. H. (1992). *Exploring alternative race-ethnic comparison groups in current population surveys* (Current Population Reports, Special Studies, Series P23-182). Washington, DC: Government Printing Office.

Diehl, A. K., & Stern, M. P. (1989). Special health problems of Mexican Americans: Obesity, gallbladder disease, diabetes mellitus, and cardiovascular disease. *Advances in Internal Medicine, 34,* 73-96.

En Accion: National Hispanic Leadership Initiative on Cancer. (1993). *Report on cancer risk and behaviors among study populations of En Accion: Archival data from Brownsville-San Antonio, Miami, New York, San Francisco, and San Diego.* Unpublished report, University of Texas Health Science Center, San Antonio.

Franco, E. L. (1991). The sexually transmitted disease model for cervical cancer: Incoherent epidemiologic findings and the role of misclassification of human papillomavirus infection. *Epidemiology, 2,* 98-106.

Franco, L. J., Stern, M. P., Rosenthal, M., Haffner, S. M., Hazuda, H. P., & Comeaux, P. J. (1985). Prevalence, detection, and control of hypertension in a biethnic community: The San Antonio Heart Study. *American Journal of Epidemiology, 121,* 684-696.

Friedman, L. N. (Ed.). (1994). *Tuberculosis: Current concepts and treatment.* Boca Raton, FL: CRC Press.

Goff, D. C., Ramsey, D. J., Labarthe, D. R., & Nichaman, M. Z. (1993). Acute myocardial infarction and coronary heart disease mortality among Mexican Americans and non-Hispanic whites in Texas, 1980 through 1989. *Ethnicity and Disease, 3,* 64-69.

Haffner, S. M., Mitchell, B. D., Moss, S. E., Stern, M. P., Hazuda, H. P., Patterson, J., Van Heuven, W. A. J., & Klein, R. (1993). Is there an ethnic difference in the effect of risk factors for diabetic retinopathy? *Annals of Epidemiology, 3,* 2-8.

Hanis, C. L., Ferrell, R. E., Barton, S. A., Aguilar, L., Garza-Ibarra, A., Tulloch, B. R., Garcia, C. A., & Schull, W. J. (1983). Diabetes among Mexican Americans in Starr County, Texas. *American Journal of Epidemiology, 118,* 659-672.

Hanis, C. L., Hewett-Emmett, D., Kubrusly, L. F., Maklad, M. N., Douglas, T. C., Mueller, W. H., Barton, S. A., Yoshimaru, H., Kubrusly, D. B., Gonzalez, R., & Schull, W. J. (1993). An ultrasound survey of gallbladder disease among Mexican Americans in Starr County, Texas: Frequencies and risk factors. *Ethnicity and Disease, 3,* 32-43.

Hayes-Bautista, D. E., & Chapa, J. (1987). Latino terminology: Conceptual bases for standardized terminology. *American Journal of Public Health, 77,* 61-68.

Haynes, S. G., Harvey, C., Montes, H., Nickens, H., & Cohen, B. H. (1990). Patterns of cigarette smoking among Hispanics in the United States: Results from HHANES 1982-84. *American Journal of Public Health, 80*(Suppl.), 47-54.

Hazuda, H. P., Haffner, S. M., & Stern, M. P. (1988). Effects of acculturation and socioeconomic status on obesity and diabetes in Mexican Americans: The San Antonio Heart Study. *American Journal of Epidemiology, 128,* 1289-1301.

Hazuda, H. P., Mitchell, B. D., Haffner, S. M., & Stern, M. P. (1991). Obesity in Mexican American subgroups: Findings from the San Antonio Heart Study. *American Journal of Clinical Nutrition, 53*(Suppl.), S1529-S1534.

Hazuda, H. P., Stern, M. P., & Haffner, S. M. (1988). Acculturation and assimilation among Mexican Americans: Scales and population-based data. *Social Science Quarterly, 69,* 687-706.

Kann, L., Warren, W., Collins, J. L., Ross, J., Collins, B., & Kolbe, L. J. (1993). Results from the national school-based 1991 Youth Risk Behavior Survey and progress toward achieving related health objectives for the nation. *Public Health Reports, 108,* 47-55.

Koutsky, L. A., Holmes, K. K., Critchlow, C. W., Stevens, C. E., Paavonen, J., Beckman, A. M., DeRouen, T. A., Galloway, D. A., Vernon, D., & Kiviat, N. B. (1992). A cohort study of the risk of cervical intraepithelial neoplasia Grade 2 or 3 in relation to papillomavirus infection. *New England Journal of Medicine, 327,* 1272-1278.

Marin, G., & Marin, B. V. (1991). *Research with Hispanic populations* (Applied Social Research Methods series, Vol. 23). Newbury Park, CA: Sage.

Marin, G., Sabogal, F., Marin, B. V., Otero-Sabogal, R., & Perez-Stable, E. J. (1987). Development of a short acculturation scale for Hispanics. *Hispanic Journal of Behavioral Science, 9,* 183-205.

Marks, G., Garcia, M., & Solis, J. M. (1990). Health risk behaviors of Hispanics in the United States: Findings from HHANES, 1982-84. *American Journal of Public Health, 80*(Suppl.), 20-26.

McAlister, A. L., Fernandez-Esquer, M.-E., Ramirez, A. G., Trevino, F., Gallion, K. J., Villarreal, R., Pulley, L. V., Hu, S., Torres, I., & Zhang, Q. (1995). Community level cancer control in a Texas barrio: Part 2. Base-line and preliminary outcome findings. *Journal of the National Cancer Institute, 18,* 123-126.

McKenna, M. T., McCray, E., & Onorato, I. (1995). The epidemiology of tuberculosis among foreign-born persons in the United States, 1986 to 1993. *New England Journal of Medicine, 332,* 1071-1076.

Mitchell, B. D., Haffner, S. M., Hazuda, H. P., Patterson, J. K., & Stern, M. P. (1992). Diabetes and coronary heart disease in Mexican-American men. *Annals of Epidemiology, 2,* 101-106.

Mitchell, B. D., Hazuda, H. P., Haffner, S. M., Patterson, J. K., & Stern, M. P. (1991a). High prevalence of angina pectoris in Mexican-American men: A population with reduced risk of myocardial infarction. *Annals of Epidemiology, 1,* 415-426.

Mitchell, B. D., Hazuda, H. P., Haffner, S. M., Patterson, J. K., & Stern, M. P. (1991b). Myocardial infarction in Mexican American and non-Hispanic whites: The San Antonio Heart Study. *Circulation, 83,* 45-51.

Mitchell, B. D., Williams-Blangero, S., Chakraborty, R., Valdez, R., Hazuda, H. P., Haffner, S. M., & Stern, M. P. (1993). A comparison of three methods for assessing Amerindian admixture in Mexican Americans. *Ethnicity and Disease, 3,* 22-31.

National Association of Hispanic Publications. (1995). *Hispanics-Latinos: Diverse people in a multicultural society* (special report). Washington, DC: Author.

National Center for Health Statistics. (1989). *Vital and health statistics: Anthropometric data and prevalence of overweight for Hispanics—1982-84* (Series 11, data from National Health Survey No. 239, DHHS Publication No. [PHS] 89-1689). Hyattsville, MD: Public Health Service.

National Center for Health Statistics. (1996). *Health, United States, 1995.* Hyattsville, MD: Public Health Service.

Neff, J. A., & Hoppe, S. K. (1992). Acculturation and drinking patterns among U.S. Anglos, blacks, and Mexican Americans. *Alcohol and Alcoholism, 27,* 293-308.

Negy, C., & Woods, D. J. (1992a). The importance of acculturation in understanding research with Hispanic-Americans. *Hispanic Journal of Behavioral Sciences, 14,* 224-247.

Negy, C., & Woods, D. J. (1992b). A note on the relationship between acculturation and socioeconomic status. *Hispanic Journal of Behavioral Sciences, 14,* 248-251.

Otero-Sabogal, R., Sabogal, F., & Perez-Stable, E. J. (1995). Psychosocial correlates of smoking among immigrant Latina adolescents. *Journal of the National Cancer Institute Monographs, 18,* 65-71.

Otero-Sabogal, R., Sabogal, F., Perez-Stable, E. J., & Hiatt, R. A. (1995). Dietary practices, alcohol consumption, and smoking behavior: Ethnic, sex, and acculturation differences. *Journal of the National Cancer Institute Monographs, 18,* 73-82.

Perez-Stable, E. J., McMillan, M. M., Harris, M. I., Juarez, R. Z., Knowler, W. C., Stern, M. P., & Haynes, S. G. (1989). Self-reported diabetes in Mexican-Americans: HHANES 1982-84. *American Journal of Public Health, 79,* 770-772.

Perez-Stable, E. J., Sabogal, F., Otero-Sabogal, R., Hiatt, R. A., & McPhee, S. J. (1992). Misconceptions about cancer among Latinos and Anglos. *Journal of the American Medical Association, 268,* 3219-3223.

Perkins, C. I., Hoegh, H. J., Wright, W. E., & Young, J. L. (1993). *Cancer incidence and mortality in California, 1988-1990.* Sacramento: California Department of Health Services, Cancer Surveillance Section.

Plepys, C., & Klein, R. (1995). *Health status indicators: Differentials by race and Hispanic origin* (Healthy People 2000, Statistical Notes No. 10, DHHS Publication No. [PHS] 95-1237). Hyattsville, MD: Public Health Service.

Prislin, R., Suarez, L., Simpson, D. M., & Dyer, J. A. (1996). *When acculturation hurts: Immunization status of Hispanic children under the age of two.* Unpublished manuscript, San Diego State University.

Pugh, J. A., Stern, M. P., Haffner, S. M., Eifler, C. W., & Zapata, M. (1988). Excess incidence of treatment of end-stage renal disease in Mexican Americans. *American Journal of Epidemiology, 127,* 135-144.

Ramirez, E. A. (1991). Cardiovascular health in Puerto Ricans compared to other population groups in the United States. *Ethnicity and Disease, 1,* 188-199.

Reeves, W. C., Brinton, L. A., Garcia, M., Brenes, M. M., Herrero, R., Gaitan, E., Tenorio, F., De Britton, R. C., & Rawls, W. E. (1989). Human papillomavirus infection and cervical cancer in Latin America. *New England Journal of Medicine, 320,* 1437-1441.

Rewers, M., Shetterly, S. M., Hoag, S., Baxter, J., Marshall, J., & Hamman, R. F. (1993). Is the risk of coronary heart disease lower in Hispanics than in non-Hispanic whites? The San Luis Valley Diabetes Study. *Ethnicity and Disease, 3,* 44-54.

Rosales, F. A. (1993). A historical overview. In N. Kanellos (Ed.), *The Hispanic American almanac: A reference work on Hispanics in the United States.* Detroit, MI: Gale Research.

Sabogal, F., Marin, G., Otero-Sabogal, R., Marin, B. V., & Perez-Stable, E. J. (1987). Hispanic familism and acculturation: What changes and what doesn't? *Hispanic Journal of Behavioral Sciences, 9,* 397-412.

Samet, J. M., Coultas, D. B., Howard, C. A., Skipper, B. J., & Hanis, C. L. (1988). Diabetes, gallbladder disease, obesity, and hypertension among Hispanics in New Mexico. *American Journal of Epidemiology, 128,* 1302-1311.

Sorlie, P. D., Backlund, E., Johnson, N. J., & Rogot, E. (1993). Mortality by Hispanic status in the United States. *Journal of the American Medical Association, 270,* 2464-2468.

Stern, M. P., Bradshaw, B. S., Eifler, C. W., Fong, D. S., Hazuda, H. P., & Rosenthal, M. (1987). Secular decline in death rates due to ischemic heart disease in Mexican Americans and non-Hispanic whites in Texas, 1970-1980. *Circulation, 76,* 1245-1250.

Stern, M. P., Gaskill, S. P., Allen, C. R., Garza, V., Gonzales, J. L., & Waldrop, R. H. (1981). Cardiovascular risk factors in Mexican Americans in Laredo, Texas. *American Journal of Epidemiology, 113,* 546-555.

Stern, M. P., Rosenthal, M., Haffner, S. M., Hazuda, H. P., & Franco, L. J. (1984). Sex difference in the effects of sociocultural status on diabetes and cardiovascular risk factors in Mexican Americans: The San Antonio Heart Study. *American Journal of Epidemiology, 120,* 834-851.

Suarez, L. (1994). Pap smear and mammogram screening in Mexican American women: The effects of acculturation. *American Journal of Public Health, 84,* 742-746.

Suarez, L., & Martin, J. (1987). Primary liver cancer mortality and incidence in Texas Mexican-Americans, 1969-80. *American Journal of Public Health, 77,* 631-633.

Suarez, L., Martin, J., & Weiss, N. (1991). Data-based interventions for cancer control in Texas. *Texas Medicine, 87,* 70-77.

Suarez, L., & Pulley, L. (1995). Comparing acculturation scales and their relationship to cancer screening among older Mexican American women. *Journal of the National Cancer Institute Monographs, 18,* 41-47.

Suarez, L., Roche, R. A., Pulley, L., Weiss, N. S., Goldman, D., & Simpson, D. M. (1997). Why a peer intervention program for Mexican-American women failed to modify the secular trend in cancer screening. *American Journal of Preventive Medicine, 13,* 411-417.

Suarez, L., Weiss, N. S., & Martin, J. (1989). Primary liver cancer death and occupation in Texas. *American Journal of Industrial Medicine, 15,* 167-175.

Texas Cancer Registry. (1996). *Cancer incidence and mortality along the Texas-Mexico border.* Austin: Texas Department of Health.

Texas Department of Health. (1993). *Cancer Registry Division: Cancer incidence 1980-85.* Unpublished manuscript.

Tomatis, L., Aitio, A., Day, N. E., Heseltine, E., Kaldor, J., Miller, A. B., Parkin, D. M., & Riboli, E. (1990). *Cancer: Causes, occurrence and control* (IARC Scientific Publication No. 100). Lyon, France: World Health Organization, International Agency for Research on Cancer.

Trapido, E. J., Valdez, R. B., Obeso, J. L., Strickman-Stein, N., Rotger, A., & Perez-Stable, E. J. (1995). Epidemiology of cancer among Hispanics in the United States. *Journal of the National Cancer Institute Monographs, 18,* 17-28.

Trevino, F. (1987). Standardized terminology for Hispanic populations. *American Journal of Public Health, 77,* 69-71.

Trevino, F., Moyer, E., Valdez, R. B., & Stroup-Benham, C. A. (1991). Health insurance coverage and utilization of health services by Mexican Americans, mainland Puerto Ricans, and Cuban Americans. *Journal of the American Medical Association, 265,* 233-237.

U.S. Bureau of the Census. (1993). *Current Population Reports: Population characteristics* (Series P23-183). Washington, DC: Government Printing Office.

U.S. Bureau of the Census. (1994). *Current Population Reports: Population characteristics* (Series P20-475). Washington, DC: Government Printing Office.

U.S. Bureau of the Census. (1995). *Current Population Reports: Population projections of the United States by age, sex, race, and Hispanic origin—1995 to 2050* (Series P25-1130). Washington, DC: Government Printing Office.

Weiss, K. M., Ferrell, R. E., & Hanis, C. L. (1984). A New World syndrome of metabolic diseases with a genetic and evolutionary basis. *Yearbook of Physical Anthropology, 27,* 153-178.

Wolfgang, P. E., Semeiks, P. A., & Burnett, W. S. (1991). Cancer incidence in New York City Hispanics, 1982 to 1985. *Ethnicity and Disease, 1,* 263-272.

Zunzunegui, M. V., King, M.-C., Coria, C. F., & Charlet, J. (1986). Male influences on cervical cancer risk. *American Journal of Epidemiology, 123,* 302-307.

7

Health Promotion in Latino Populations

A Sociocultural Model for Program Planning, Development, and Evaluation

FELIPE G. CASTRO
MARYA K. COTA
SANTOS C. VEGA

In this chapter, the authors present a Hispanic/Latino[1] perspective on the development of health promotion programs for Latinos. Their aim is to provide the reader with scholarly and applied information that aids the program planner in designing health promotion programs that serve Latino populations. The perspective presented here emphasizes the role of cultural factors as critical components of a health promotion program that meets the needs of various Latino clients. Devoid of this perspective, many mainstream programs fail to attract, involve, and retain Latino clients. Many Latinos cannot relate to such health programs because they consider them impersonal, unresponsive, and ineffective. Motivating Latino client involvement and participation in health promotion programs is a major challenge. Programs that succeed in inspiring active Latino client participation are those that are *culturally relevant* in their content and activities. Designing such programs requires that the program planner understand the Latino cultural characteristics that make various Latinos "different" from the middle class mainstream U.S. population.

AUTHORS' NOTE: We thank Dr. Elizabeth Valdez and Luz Sarmina-Gutierrez for their insightful comments on an earlier version of this chapter.

IMPORTANCE OF CULTURAL COMPETENCE

A major reason why mainstream health promotion programs are ineffective in service delivery to Latino clients is because mainstream administrators, program planners, and service delivery staff lack the *cultural competence* for designing and implementing programs that appeal to members of a targeted Latino population. Unfortunately, some administrators and program planners regard "culture" as a vague intangible that is irrelevant to the delivery of health services and instead focus their administrative efforts on managing budgets, staff, and service delivery. However, when a health program for a minority population is designed without regard for cultural aspects, the program's effectiveness in meeting the health needs of members of that population will be markedly compromised.

Programmatic failure is inadvertently "designed into a program" that aims to serve Latinos when that program fails to consider several cultural factors. These include (a) the availability of health services in Spanish when needed, (b) hiring bilingual/bicultural staff and providing them with cultural competence training, (c) integrating Latino cultural aspects of interpersonal relations into the program's services (e.g., *la familia Latina, personalismo, respeto, simpatia*) (Marin & Marin, 1991), (d) adjusting the services offered to the *levels of acculturation* that exist within the targeted population, and (e) being sensitive to other aspects of the local Latino culture that would make the program *culturally operative* in the local community. A culturally operative program is defined as one that "works" by promoting healthy behavior change in a culturally relevant fashion. This involves the use or design of interventions that incorporate the existing *strengths* of the culture. This effort includes *health promotion research* to identify and understand the effects of *culturally specific factors,* those that are unique to a culture, because these may be targeted as possible *mediators* of healthy behavior change. All of these efforts enhance the cultural competence of the health promotion program.

Furthermore, incorporating cultural competence into the planning, design, and implementation of a community health promotion is a multistaged process that mobilizes people and resources for a common health promotion purpose (Castro et al., 1995). Here, culturally competent community programs use two important systems principles: the *principle of relevance* (starting where the people are) and the *principle of participation* (eliciting the participation of community residents), thus promoting their sense of ownership in the program while also fostering active learning through participation (Minkler, 1990).

Involving community residents and/or members of the targeted population in the initial conceptualization and design of a health promotion program is a core goal in minority health promotion. Doing so uses the principle of participation by eliciting community residents' "insider" views on the nature and extent of community health needs. This creates a *health partnership* while challenging health professionals to use their social, psychological, and medical knowledge to address the community's expressed needs. Such a health partnership aids in "grounding" the proposed health promotion program within the health context of the local community. The insights generated by such a health partnership aid in designing a health promotion program that is truly tailored to the most pressing needs of the local community.

STRATEGIES

Overview of Some Guiding Models

In the field of health promotion, a dynamic tension seems to exist over the approach used by various health professionals in program development and delivery. On the one hand, the *scholarly approach* features a model-driven, top-down strategy that emphasizes an organized plan of program design, delivery, and evaluation. By contrast, a *grassroots community approach* features an inductive, "design as you go" approach that tries to build a program from the bottom up, based on a sensitivity to current community needs. The strength of the scholarly approach is its organization and planning. Its weakness is its possible lack of fit with current local conditions and its potential insensitivity to unique but important and changing conditions in the local environment. By contrast, the strength of the grassroots community approach is its closeness and sensitivity to the current conditions within the local community. Its weakness seems to be potential inefficiency, lack of organization, and ambiguous programmatic thrust.

In the applied setting, many social service and health promotion programs are delivered based on a specific perceived or documented need and are driven by units of service delivered and/or by certain targeted outcomes. However, such programs seldom are governed by a well-specified conceptual model; they focus solely on the delivery of a service, with little effort to examine and understand the likely "causal" mechanisms that would make these services effective. By contrast, the contemporary scholarly approach to health promotion program planning features an array of relevant health promotion models. Among these, the most popular are the Health Belief Model (Becker, 1974; Hochbaum, 1958; Rosenstock, 1990), the Theory of Reasoned Action (Ajzen & Fishbein, 1980; Fishbein, 1967), Social Learning Theory (Bandura, 1986; Perry, Baranowski, & Parcel, 1990), Green's PRECEDE model (Green, Kreuter, Deeds, & Partridge, 1980), and Diffusion of Innovation (Orlandi, Landers, Weston, & Haley, 1990; Rogers, 1983).

A contemporary challenge in the health promotion field is to *integrate* the scholarly and grassroots approaches so that program planners and health educators use theory and models that guide their service delivery efforts and their understanding of the likely mechanisms that influence service delivery outcomes. By contrast, extant models must be modified or expanded to be "grounded" within the context of the local community. Nongrounded models will offer a poor fit with local community needs, thus yielding poor predictions and invalid inferences on local processes that influence health outcomes. These issues are

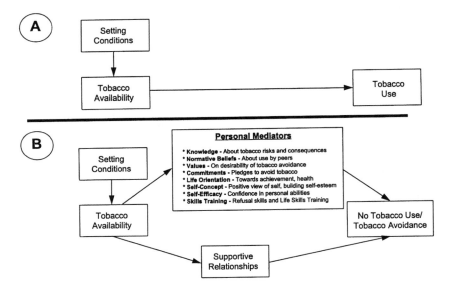

Figure 7.1   Basic Models of Tobacco Use and Avoidance

particularly relevant and acute for health promotion with minority populations because often the relevance and fit of the major models are not established and likely will require model expansions or modifications to enhance fit by making them culturally relevant to the needs of the local minority population.

The Concept of a Mediator

Contemporary health promotion programs emphasize the role of *mediators* as intermediate causal factors that operate as part of the "causal chain" of events that influence health behavior. To illustrate this, Figure 7.1 presents a simple model of how conditions in the *natural environment* can promote tobacco use. In this simple model (Panel A), the presence of various *setting conditions* and *tobacco availability* are presented as existing factors that prompt tobacco use. This model simplifies matters because several factors depicted here as setting conditions contribute toward prompting tobacco use, whereas tobacco availability clearly is another factor that operates as an *antecedent* (a prior condition) that can be classified as a *risk factor* for tobacco use.

A goal in *prevention* is to modify the antecedent factors that lead to disease and thus to reduce the risk of disease. Here, a direct public health intervention would be to restrict tobacco availability, for example, through taxes that increase the cost of tobacco products or through limiting public access of tobacco products by restricting the location or conditions of sale of tobacco products.

Panel B in Figure 7.1 presents a set of psychosocial *mediators* that can aid in preventing tobacco use. In a review of many studies (Tobler, 1986), these factors are identified as specific interventions used that aid in reducing alcohol, tobacco, and other drug use among adolescents and young adults (Hansen, 1992). The basic notion here is that one or more of these specific interventions (ideally several in an "intervention package"), when incorporated into a health promotion program, will operate to prevent alcohol, tobacco, or other drug use.

Accordingly, providing factual information on substance abuse will contribute (although not by itself) toward youth avoidance of alcohol, tobacco, and other drugs. Similarly, changing *normative beliefs* about the extent to which peers (i.e., other adolescents) use tobacco may change current misconceptions that tobacco use is a pervasive and desirable behavior. Also, changing *values* toward a view that tobacco use is not desirable and asking youths to make public *commitments* (pledges) are other interventions aimed at changing these mediators of tobacco use. Encouraging *life orientations* (e.g., sports activities) that compete with or are incompatible with tobacco use also can discourage tobacco use. Similarly, increasing a youth's *self-esteem* or changing his or her *self-concept* (self-image) as a "nonsmoker" also may discourage tobacco use. In addition, increasing *self-efficacy* in avoiding tobacco (i.e., increasing a youth's confidence that he or she can successfully avoid tobacco) also can discourage tobacco use. Finally, increasing skills in avoiding tobacco (e.g., refusal skills) also aids in promoting tobacco avoidance. Thus, a group's or population's overall capacity for tobacco avoidance can be increased by developing a health promotion prevention intervention that *builds capacity* in one or more of these psychosocial mediators of tobacco avoidance.

New frontiers in health promotion with minority populations involve community-based research to examine the effectiveness of these mediators individually or in some combination for effectively preventing tobacco or other substance use with various members of a targeted minority population. Here also, the frontier of health promotion in minority populations involves the identification and testing of *culturally specific* mediators, that is, the design of intervention activities that are specific or uniquely relevant to members of a targeted population. For Latinos, based on Latino cultural values, mediators such as *family traditionalism, ethnic identity* enhancement, teaching *indigenous cultural norms* and *biculturalism,* and using *Promotora* (peer health leader) activities may be effective in discouraging tobacco and other drug use.

The Role of Cultural Competence

This expressed importance of "culture" as an integral component of a health promotion program for Latinos prompts the need to fortify the cultural competence of program staff and of the intervention program. Generally, *cultural competence* refers to the capacity of health professionals or of health service delivery systems to understand and plan for the health needs of a specific cultural subgroup. From a public health perspective, enhancing the health of persons who are "culturally different" from mainstream U.S. society requires a clear *conceptualization* and *assessment* of their health needs. This involves taking a systems approach that uses a model to guide the conceptualization, design, implementation, and evaluation of health promotion programs that are effective with minority populations.

−3	1. Cultural Destructiveness • Avows the "superiority" of a dominant culture and the "inferiority" of other cultures
−2	2. Cultural Incapacity • Professes "separate but equal" treatment
−1	3. Cultural Blindness • Professes that all cultures and people are "alike and equal"
0	
+1	4. Cultural Openness (Sensitivity) • Has a basic understanding and appreciation of the importance of sociocultural factors in work with minority populations
+2	5. Cultural Competence • Has a capacity to work with more complex issues and with *cultural nuances*
+3	6. Cultural Proficiency • The highest capacity for work with minority populations with a commitment to excellence and proactive effort

Figure 7.2   Cultural Orientation Continuum
SOURCE: Kim, McLeod, and Shantzis (1992).

To address this challenge, health promotion with special populations requires a systemic adjustment of an existing health service delivery system to mobilize the resources, both staff and organizational, that are needed to meet this challenge. For Latinos, this effort should aim to reduce the persistent gap in health status observed among members of various Latino populations relative to the health status observed among members of the mainstream U.S. population (Council on Scientific Affairs, 1991).

Capacity for Cultural Competence

Building cultural competence begins with a clear conceptualization of what this is. Figure 7.2 presents various orientations toward culture that are organized according to progressive levels of *cultural capacity*. Thus, the capacity for cultural competence is shown to vary along a graded continuum. This concept of a *cultural competence continuum* has been proposed previously by various scholars (Cross, Bazron, Dennis, & Isaacs, 1989; Kim, McLeod, & Shantzis, 1992; Orlandi, Weston, & Epstein, 1992) and has been modified and expanded elsewhere (Castro, 1998).

On this cultural capacity continuum, the lowest level is *cultural destructiveness* (−3), which involves openly negative and destructive attitudes that emphasize the "superiority" of the dominant culture and the "inferiority" of the indigenous culture. Next on this continuum is *cultural incapacity* (–2), which refers to a professional or an organizational orientation that emphasizes the "separate but equal" treatment of clients. This incapacity is superseded by a *cultural blindness* (–1) orientation, which asserts that "all cultures and people are alike and equal." Beyond these negative orientations, the first level of true cultural capacity is *cultural openness (sensitivity)* (+1), which is characterized by the presence of a basic understanding and appreciation of the importance of cultural factors in the delivery of health services.

Beyond cultural sensitivity, *cultural competence* (+2) is an orientation that demonstrates a higher capacity to work with members of a given cultural group. Attaining cultural competence requires greater depth of skills and experience that allows the health professional to move beyond a superficial analysis of cultural features and by the capacity to understand and to work with *cultural nuances* (Figure 7.2).

Finally, *cultural proficiency* (+3) is the highest expression of cultural capacity. It serves as an ideal rather than as a state that is necessarily attained by a particular health professional. Cultural proficiency represents a state of *high mastery,* the capacity to design and deliver health services and health promotion programs that are truly responsive to the needs of members of a specific population (Castro & Gutierres, 1997) (Figure 7.2).

On the positive side of this continuum, the basic understanding of cultural issues known as cultural sensitivity as applied to Latinos is demonstrated by a health professional's basic understanding of the role of linguistic factors, inter-personal factors (e.g., *personalismo, respeto, confianza*) and of familial factors (e.g., *la familia Latina,* traditionalism, familism) as these influence the health-related behaviors of various Latinos. Cultural sensitivity also is demonstrated by a health professional's understanding of the *within-group variability* that exists for a given cultural group. For Latinos, this within-group variability (diversity) is moderated by *level of acculturation.*

Beyond cultural sensitivity, cultural competence is a more potent form of cultural capacity. Cultural competence is characterized by a health professional's clear understanding of cultural nuances, which allows the health professional to interpret the ethnic client's subtle communications and their meanings within the client's specific *cultural context.* Thus, the health professional is capable of planning culturally effective interventions that appeal to ethnic clients and elicit their participation while motivating their sustained involvement in the program. For example, among Latinos, a culturally competent program planner would understand various details of *personalismo,* the importance that Latinos give to interpersonal relationships. Thus, the program planner would incorporate *person-alismo* as a programmatic feature for initiating and maintaining client involvement in a given program.

Finally, cultural proficiency, the highest level of cultural skills and mastery, is characterized by a health professional's deep understanding of cultural issues and their nuances, that is, a health professional's capacity for leadership in the design of effective interventions for minority populations (Castro, 1998).

Origins of Health Promotion Programs

Health promotion programs originate under a variety of different "starting conditions" that determine a program's purpose, identity, and developmental trajectory. Among the many possible starting conditions, the most typical are (a) local epidemiological need, (b) a call for proposals, (c) conversion of an existing program, and (d) community demand.

The direct approach to the establishment of a health promotion program emphasizes program development based on *local epidemiologic need*. In this approach, a series of observed cases of disease will prompt the analysis of other cases using epidemiological data. For example, low rates of vaccinations among Latino children within a local community might emerge as a potential public health problem, based on the accumulation of several clinical observations. Then, the analysis of epidemiological data from the local public health department might confirm that this is a problem. Such data might show that, relative to a given reference group, the rates of preventable disease (e.g., the rates of rubella) are higher for the Latino children age 5 years or under who live within a given impoverished district. Under these starting conditions, the targeted population would be defined according to the observed problem, that is, Latino children age 5 years or under and their parents who live within a targeted district. Thus, the program's health promotion goal would be to develop a culturally relevant outreach intervention to mobilize Latino parents from this community by offering outreach and low-cost vaccinations.

A second approach that might have its roots in documented epidemiological need is the design of a health promotion program that is based on a *call for proposals*. Under this approach, a sponsoring agency (the federal government, a state or county health agency, or a private foundation) identifies a particular health problem, identifies a targeted population, and describes the relevant health promotion program that it seeks to fund.

For example, a request for applications or a request for proposals from the federal government might announce the availability of federal funds to support health promotion research or service delivery projects to provide mammography screenings to low-income populations such as low-acculturated Latino women (Latinas). The request for applications announces the available range of funding and presents basic guidelines for program design and development. Under these basic starting conditions, a team of researchers or interventionists could develop a health promotion program proposal that includes a rationale for the program, a proposed curriculum, an implementation design, a time line, and a budget. The sponsoring agency would review the proposals that are submitted for scientific and programmatic merit, and the best proposals would be funded based on sufficient merit as determined by a panel of expert reviewers.

A third mechanism for the origin of a health promotion program involves the *conversion of an existing program* into a newer or modified program. Under these starting conditions, the new program inherits aspects of the previous program, perhaps including its staff. For example, a community-based AIDS prevention program that has served Mexican Americans/Chicanos in five cities in the

Southwest might expand to include primarily Puerto Rican populations in the New England area and in Puerto Rico as well as Cuban populations in the greater Miami area of Florida. In this case, the targeted population would remain Hispanics, but an intervention originally designed for Mexican Americans would be expanded to serve Puerto Ricans and Cubans in other parts of the country. Here, cultural competence in program design would involve the modification of the prior AIDS prevention curriculum to address the somewhat differing local needs of the Puerto Rican and Cuban populations that this expanded program would purport to serve.

A fourth mechanism for initiating a health promotion program is *community demand*. Based on community organization and political action on the part of a local group of concerned citizens, this group may demand resources to solve a local public health problem. For example, a group of residents from an inner-city housing project that is ravaged by drug abuse and violence might lobby the city council for funds earmarked to address this problem. United as a local housing coalition, this group ultimately might procure funding for a 2-year project aimed at consolidating the citizens' coalition and at educating all housing project residents on strategies for drug and violence prevention.

In this case, the population targeted for this health promotion intervention would be restricted geographically to those who are residents of the local housing project. Then, after this project is funded, community experts from the local university and from local community-based social service agencies might be hired as consultants to further design, monitor, and evaluate the program. In this case, a general program plan would be funded, and experts acceptable to the local community subsequently would be hired to work out the details that aim to make the program successful.

These four types of starting conditions for health promotion programs that have been observed in various Latino communities illustrate the diversity of conditions that influence the identity and development of a given health promotion program. In each case, the deeper goal is to develop and implement a health promotion program that is effective in meeting the deep and pervasive health problems that affect members of the targeted Latino community.

ASSESSMENT

Key Factors in Initial Assessment of Health Needs

The growing diversity involving Latino consumers of health services in the United States has prompted the need for an expanded yet *clear conceptualization* of Latino health needs and for the design of health promotion programs that meet these needs. These needs are illustrated by statistics on the health status of Latino populations that document the lower health status of Latinos relative to members of the U.S. mainstream population (Carter-Pokras, 1994; Hale, 1992).

Unfortunately, many available statistics reflect national trends and give little information at the local level that would be useful to local program planners. To document local need and to ground a proposed program within the local community, the administrator, health educator, or other program planner must know the characteristics of the various subpopulations that reside within the proposed program's catchment area. Doing so requires access to existing data for the local community or the collection of data for a small representative sample of the targeted group. Such local sociocultural data, if available, can help generate a descriptive profile of clients from the targeted group or population.

Here, the design of new local population databases that are useful for designing culturally effective programs for Latinos should move beyond the use of conventional but global demographic variables such as "race," "ethnicity," and "income." Although useful at a broad level, these categorical variables fail to get at the deeper aspects of culture that characterize the lifestyles and health needs of Latinos and other ethnic groups. Although seldom the case for Latino populations, an improved and culturally relevant health needs database should include the mean (average) acculturation score for Latinos in the local community as well as the range of acculturation that exists among these members. It also would be useful to compute the group's mean and range (maximum and minimum values) for improved and more culturally relevant indicators of socioeconomic status (income and education).

Where a new survey can be designed and conducted, it also would be desirable to obtain data on various indicators of Latino *subjective culture* that relate to health needs (e.g., knowledge, beliefs, attitudes) and as these relate to the program's targeted health problem. Other important data concerns include information on *program access* such as the proportions of clients from the targeted group who have adequate health insurance, transportation, and so on. In sum, conducting a local survey of client characteristics and client health needs, especially with the inclusion of culturally relevant indicators of health needs, is an important investment for sound program development at the local level (Rossi & Freeman, 1989). Such data facilitate strategic program planning that aims to meet the specific health needs of members of various local subpopulations.

Acculturative Status

A major factor that describes the within-group variability that exists among Latinos/Hispanics is level of acculturation. For a Latino/Hispanic client, *acculturative status* refers to the client's cultural orientation and level of involvement in Latino culture (e.g., Mexican, Cuban). Here, it is noteworthy that most "acculturation scales" do not measure the *process* of acculturation (cultural change) but instead measure a current level of acculturative status as measured on a hypothetical dimension (continuum) that ranges from an identity that is very Mexican (or Hispanic) to an identity that is very Anglo-American.

Within the past two decades, several acculturation scales for Latinos have been developed. As summarized in Figure 7.3, the Cultural Orientation Continuum, recurring thematic content within these scales involves five factors: the partici-

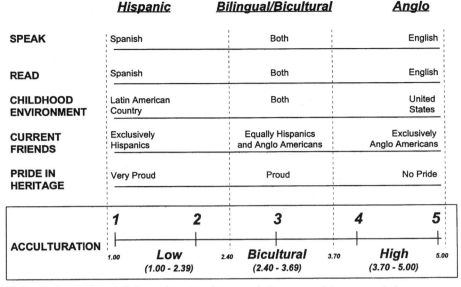

Figure 7.3 Cultural Orientation Continuum: A Conceptual Framework for a General Acculturation Index

SOURCE: © Felipe G. Castro, Hispanic Research Center, Arizona State University.

pant's linguistic capabilities in speaking English and Spanish, the participant's linguistic capabilities in reading English and Spanish, the participant's level of exposure to the Anglo-American (North American) and Mexican or native Latino cultures (e.g., Mexican, Puerto Rican, Cuban), the ethnic identity of the participant's current circle of friends (e.g., entirely Latino, from both, entirely Anglo or other), and the level of pride that the participant has toward his or her own cultural group.

As measured by a typical acculturation scale for Latinos, a prevailing concept in the literature on Latinos is that there are three basic levels of acculturative status: low acculturated, bilingual bicultural, and high acculturated (see Figure 7.3). In terms of the major sociocultural characteristics of members of these three subpopulations, low-acculturated clients are primarily Spanish speaking, have a strong bond with their native Latino culture, maintain primarily Latino friends, and express strong pride in their native cultural background. By contrast, high-acculturated Latinos are those who primarily or exclusively speak English, feel a closer bond to the Anglo-American culture, have primarily or exclusively Anglo-American friends, and have little or no pride in being from a Latino culture. Here also, some high-acculturated persons who are strongly oriented toward *assimilation* into the Anglo-American culture will deny any identification with Latino cultural activities. Such clients may self-identify as "white" or as "American."

Despite the limitations of a one-dimensional measurement of the acculturation variable (Rogler, Cortes, & Malgady, 1991), measuring this variable offers greater precision in describing the within-group variation that exists for a given Latino population. This is an improvement over demographic indicators that simply define a population as "Hispanic" or as "Mexican American." Level of acculturation can be measured by using one of various scales that have been developed (Barona & Miller, 1994; Cuellar, Arnold, & Maldonado, 1995; Cuellar, Harris, & Jasso, 1980; Marin, Sabogal, Marin, Otero-Sabogal, & Perez-Stable, 1987).

The present authors have developed and used a short scale in telephone survey research, in community-based studies, and in the clinical setting (see Appendixes A and B) (Balcazar, Castro, & Krull, 1995; Castro, 1988). The measured acculturation index (General Acculturation Index) can be used in conjunction with the Cultural Orientation Continuum (Figure 7.3) to describe a Latino client's level of acculturation. This index has exhibited sound psychometric properties (coefficient alpha $\geq$ .80) with various Latino populations and can be administered by self-report or by interview with Anglo-Americans as well as with Latinos (Balcazar et al., 1995; Castro & Gutierres, 1997).

Socioeconomic Status

Socioeconomic status is a frequently used composite indicator of social position. Within many Latino communities, low level of acculturation is correlated with low socioeconomic status. Indeed, with *upward social mobility*, as some Latinos acquire the skills for economic growth (e.g., education, language, social contacts) and advance upwardly in socioeconomic status within the mainstream American society, level of acculturation also tends to increase concurrently.

Thus, as observed at a population level, the association between level of acculturation and socioeconomic status typically is positive. For example, in one community survey involving more than 500 Latino women, among immigrant Latino women (Latinas), level of acculturation was positively correlated ($r = .22$) with these women's highest level of education in Latin America (Balcazar et al., 1995). Among U.S.-born Latinas, level of acculturation was positively correlated ($r = .21$) with these women's highest level of education in the United States (Balcazar et al., 1995). Also, in the total sample of women, level of acculturation was positively correlated with monthly household income ($r = .50$), underscoring the strength of association that often is observed between these two variables within a community sample of Latinas. However, it must be noted that for most Latinos at the individual level, this correlated process does not suggest the eventual occurrence of complete *assimilation,* which refers to an ethnic person's total immersion into the mainstream culture and that person's complete loss of identification with his or her native ethnic culture. In other words, at the population level, these correlations reflect the apparent movement of Latinos across the acculturation continuum as they rise in socioeconomic status, but this does not necessarily indicate that a given Latina or Latino is motivated by a desire to assimilate.

Identifying and Segmenting the Population:
A Basic Schema

Most descriptive accounts of the characteristics of Hispanics emphasize the fact that Hispanics are a heterogeneous population (Marin & Marin, 1991).

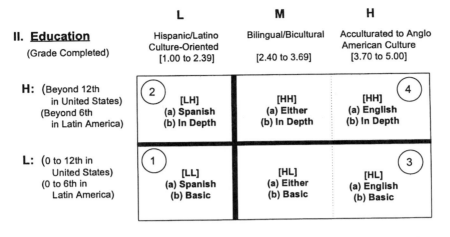

	L	**M**	**H**
II. Education (Grade Completed)	Hispanic/Latino Culture-Oriented [1.00 to 2.39]	Bilingual/Bicultural [2.40 to 3.69]	Acculturated to Anglo American Culture [3.70 to 5.00]
H: (Beyond 12th in United States) (Beyond 6th in Latin America)	② [LH] (a) Spanish (b) In Depth	[HH] (a) Either (b) In Depth	[HH] (a) English (b) In Depth ④
L: (0 to 12th in United States) (0 to 6th in Latin America)	① [LL] (a) Spanish (b) Basic	[HL] (a) Either (b) Basic	③ [HL] (a) English (b) Basic

(a) *Language of Intervention:* Whether English, Spanish, or Either
(b) *Depth of Coverage:* Detail in content and meaning: basic content or in-depth or more complex content.

L = Low, M = Medium, and H = High

Figure 7.4   A Two-Factor Schema for Health Promotion With Latino Populations

Indeed, the U.S. Hispanic population is really a cluster of related subpopulations, each of which can be identified in various ways such as by *nationality* (e.g., Mexican Americans, Puerto Ricans, Cubans, Dominicans) (Marin & Marin, 1991; U.S. Department of Commerce, 1993).

Although nationality identifies meaningful subgroups within the population, it does not necessarily yield distinct and meaningful subgroups in relation to health needs. Instead, health needs covary more meaningfully in relation to socioeconomic status and level of acculturation (Balcazar et al., 1995). The availability of a meaningful and easy-to-adapt method for segmenting the Latino population would be useful for the program planner who works with Latino populations.

As an assessment aid in population segmentation for health education program planning with Latinos, Latino client needs may be conceptualized in a combined fashion using level of acculturation and socioeconomic status in a 2 × 2 schema (Balcazar et al., 1995) (Figure 7.4). Level of acculturation, when segmented (for simplicity) into lower levels (mean = 1.00 to 2.39) and higher levels (mean = 2.40 to 5.00), identifies the need for health education and services as delivered in Spanish (for low-acculturated clients) and in English (for high-acculturated clients), respectively. A proxy but less accurate measure that approximates this segmentation is a client's self-report of whether he or she prefers to speak in English or Spanish.

These two levels of acculturation can then be cross-tabulated with a Latino client's lower or higher level of educational preparedness to comprehend programmatic information by using the client's highest level of education, which also is a component of the more complex variable of socioeconomic status. Here, *lower* educational level (6 years or less in Latin America or 12 years or less in the United

States) is distinguished from *higher* educational level. When cross-tabulated with level of acculturation as defined previously, this yields four distinct Latino sociocultural groups (in a 2 × 2 schema) that segment the general Latino population into distinct and more homogeneous subpopulations that have differing health and health educational needs (Figure 7.4) (Balcazar et al., 1995, p. 65).

Within this schema, the low-acculturated, low-educated group (Group 1) is the "least advantaged" Latino group, both socially and economically, and its members typically require more intense health promotion program planning to address their needs. By contrast, the high-acculturation, high-education group (Group 4) is the "most advantaged" group and will respond to a health promotion program that is much different in design and implementation. Here, it might be noted that Group 4 Latino clients would be able, both linguistically and by health needs, to participate in a health promotion program that is designed for middle-class Anglo-American clients, whereas Group 1 Latinos would not.

Facilitating Problem Conceptualization and Assessment

A major problem in health promotion program planning is the challenge of clearly conceptualizing the set of conditions that may lead to disease and, consequently, in further conceptualizing a proposed intervention approach that can arrest or counter a disease-inducing condition in the local environment. In other words, the problem of conceptualization in the assessment phase, "capturing the story" (modeling the causal process) to describe what is happening and what can be done to counter or prevent disease, has not been a simple task. The need exists for an intuitively simple yet meaningful framework that helps program planners and health educators think through the details of a process in a way that facilitates program design. Figure 7.5 presents a simple descriptive "causal model" framework to help health promotion program planners and health educators in thinking about (conceptualizing) and planning (designing) prevention interventions with a targeted group or population.

This descriptive causal model consists of two related parts: the descriptive disease risk model and the descriptive prevention intervention model. Also, it uses conventional sentence structure to help guide the program planner in formulating a plausible chain of events that describe a "likely causal process" that may occur within the local community. Part A, the descriptive disease risk model, describes a progressive disease process that, if left unmodified, would lead to disease outcomes. Part B, the descriptive prevention intervention model, presents a similar process while introducing a proposed prevention intervention that is aimed at countering the naturally occurring disease-inducing process. In other words, this model framework helps answer the following question: "What can be done programmatically in the design of a program for members of a targeted population to effectively counter a certain naturally occurring disease-inducing process?"

This model framework introduces a simplified format for thinking through a plausible disease-inducing process as it may occur naturally in the local environment. The process that is "modeled" may or may not be entirely correct, although

A. *Descriptive Disease Risk Model*

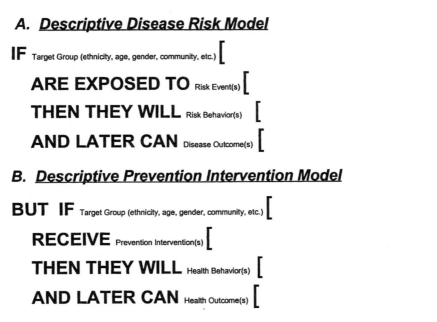

IF Target Group (ethnicity, age, gender, community, etc.) [   ]

    ARE EXPOSED TO Risk Event(s) [   ],

    THEN THEY WILL Risk Behavior(s) [   ]

    AND LATER CAN Disease Outcome(s) [   ].

B. *Descriptive Prevention Intervention Model*

  BUT IF Target Group (ethnicity, age, gender, community, etc.) [   ]

    RECEIVE Prevention Intervention(s) [   ],

    THEN THEY WILL Health Behavior(s) [   ]

    AND LATER CAN Health Outcome(s) [   ].

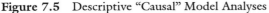

Figure 7.5   Descriptive "Causal" Model Analyses

the aim is to use theoretical and empirical health promotion knowledge and available local data to support the exposition of what may actually be happening in the local environment.

This set of descriptive models serves as an heuristic tool that has intuitive appeal for health providers and for other health promotion professionals. Its appeal is simplicity, with an aim toward effectiveness in bypassing "mental blocks" that occur among many health professionals and service delivery staff who find difficulty in describing the possible causal process that may operate in what it is that they do. Ideally, the present framework sharpens the conceptual skills of such health professionals in a manner that clarifies the chain of events that surround what they do and that helps them to generate more probing critiques for the purpose of enhancing the effectiveness of what they do.

This model serves as a conceptual template for hypothesis development. It is a hybrid of various existing model approaches. It uses conventional sentence structure to offer a logical and an intuitively simple progression regarding unhealthy and healthy events. It also builds on a variety of other model approaches such as the impact model (Rossi & Freeman, 1989), the PRECEDE model (Green et al., 1980), and the behavioral ABC (Antecedent, Behavior, Consequences) model used in behavior analysis (Watson & Tharp, 1989).

However, unlike prior models, this model system eliminates the ambiguity or confusion for many health professionals that seems to be imposed by the use of squares, circles, vectors, and other diagrammatic indicators of variables, factors, and causal effects. This systems model does not criticize prior approaches but does propose to offer various health professionals an intuitively appealing and user-friendly system that ideally complements the use of other existing models.

As shown in Figure 7.5, the descriptive disease risk model aims to describe a naturally occurring process in the local environment. Here, the sentence completion format prompts a description of a *targeted group* by describing the group's ethnicity, age, gender, community of residence, and perhaps other defining factors (e.g., Latino 10-year-old males from El Barrio). The *risk event* prompts information of events or conditions to which members of the targeted group are exposed (e.g., adult family members who smoke cigarettes, easy access to cigarettes). The subsequent *risk behavior* reflects a consequence of the risk event(s) as these youths would experiment with cigarette smoking. The future *disease outcome* could be that these youths could develop lung cancer and/or coronary heart disease.

Following the descriptive disease risk model analysis, under the descriptive prevention intervention model analysis, the program planner is challenged to identify a competing healthy causal process. Here, the targeted population would remain the same, so this item is automatically carried over as the starting point of the prevention intervention model. However, under this model, a prevention intervention is proposed. For these Latino 10-year-old males from El Barrio, this *prevention intervention* could consist of culturally relevant information and refusal skills training. The aim would be to promote a certain health behavior whereby these youths would learn how to avoid offers to smoke cigarettes. Accordingly, the desirable health outcome would be that these youths can avoid early lung and coronary heart disease as linked to cigarette smoking.

As a second example, the descriptive disease risk model could state the following: *If* adolescent Mexican American females (ages 12 to 16 years) from El Barrio *are exposed to* cooking practices that feature high-fat foods, *then they will* prepare high-fat meals for themselves and their families *and later can* develop obesity and non-insulin-dependent diabetes mellitus by 35 years of age. By contrast, the descriptive prevention intervention model might state the following: *But if* adolescent Mexican American females (ages 12 to 16 years) from El Barrio *receive* training in heart-healthy meal preparation, *then they will* prepare low-fat, high-fiber meals for themselves and their families *and later can* maintain normal weight and avoid the development of non-insulin-dependent diabetes mellitus.

Taking Stock of Resources: Financial and Staffing

In assessing a program's capacity for intervention or service delivery, a proposed health promotion program must establish a balance in program scope between two programmatic resources: (a) the available budget for program delivery and (b) the roster of staff available to deliver the intervention. Even for a specific health problem (e.g., weight management in obese Latino men and women), the health service needs of most indigent groups or populations and their lack of resources create conditions of overall need that far outweigh the programmatic resources available to meet those needs. Thus, it often is necessary to narrow the scope of the intervention to define "a feasible, manageable, affordable set of behaviors and outcomes to address and measure in a program" (Windsor, Baranowski, Clark, & Cutter, 1994, p. 83).

Limiting the amount of staff-client contact in terms of number of program sessions offered is one strategy to reconcile program offerings with available staff resources. By contrast, offering programmatic content in a group format also aids in maximizing the number of clients reached given the available program resources. Here also, a balance must be established in program design among (a) maximum number of clients that the program aims to reach, (b) the duration and intensity of the program activities offered (i.e., the "program dose," such as number of sessions), and (c) the quality of the program content. The best-designed health promotion programs seek to maximize coverage in all three areas while balancing this with the limitations of staff size, the staff expertise and experience, and the number of hours of face-to-face contact that the staff can offer clients.

DESIGN

Outlining Program Goals and Objectives

The design of health promotion programs for Latino populations can benefit from the use of a sequential analysis involving clear programmatic steps. Winett, King, and Altman (1994) present such a framework consisting of three *conceptual steps* (problem definition, explication of theories and values, and multilevel analysis) and *four strategic steps* (specification of goals, design of the intervention, implementation of the intervention, and assessment of impact).

Regarding the conceptual steps in planning a health promotion program for disadvantaged Latinos, it is important to define the targeted group explicitly and to use public health and health psychology knowledge to identify a viable prevention intervention. For these clients, a disease-specific intervention (e.g., diabetes prevention) might set a goal of reducing the prevalence of obesity within a targeted group of disadvantaged (Group 1) Latinos, ages 25 to 40 years. However, to do so, the proposed program also must consider the complex of multiple health risk factors that covary with obesity among these disadvantaged Latinos (Marks, Garcia, & Solis, 1990). Such co-related factors might include limited access to health care, an exposure to impoverished living conditions that prompts high levels of stress, and comorbidity with other health problems (e.g., tuberculosis) (Carter-Pokras, 1994; Giachello, 1994).

For example, in planning a program for diabetes risk reduction among disadvantaged Latinos (Group 1), the apparent "individual" problem of being overweight must be conceptualized and defined within the broader context of a family system, both core and extended, in which members consume and are reinforced for consuming high-fat foods on a daily basis and often attend various cultural family activities and celebrations such as baptisms, *quinceñeras,* weddings, and birthday parties where high-fat foods often are served.

As a sequential framework for program planning and design, Windsor et al. (1994) present a 10-step framework for guiding the development of a health program (pp. 66-97). These steps are (1) analyzing the health problem among the population at risk; (2) delineating behaviors to resolve the problem; (3) delineating needed information; (4) identifying needed resources; (5) identifying related resources; (6) enumerating expected changes and how to measure them; (7) selecting behaviors to change and outcomes to measure; (8) designing educational and behavioral interventions; (9) developing organizational arrangements, logistics, and personnel training; and (10) developing a budget and an administrative plan.

This detailed outline clarifies the major activities that *ideally* precede the development of a sound health promotion program. In the experience of the present authors in their work with Latino organizations and populations, this stepwise outline offers a useful tool for program planning. However, program planners often do not or cannot follow each of these steps in sequence, and program planners sometimes inherit certain starting conditions, as described previously, that disallow the conducting of several of these steps while prompting the need to act on other steps. Indeed, some of the starting conditions identified previously as origins of health promotion require adjustment in a program planner's progression through an idealized sequence of steps for program planning as recommended by Windsor and colleagues (1994).

Relating Population Need to Program Goals

Several major challenges complicate program design for Latino populations. First, as noted previously, within most Latino communities nationwide, limited local data exist on incidence and prevalence rates for various diseases and disorders, particularly as these might be associated with key sociocultural factors relevant to Latinos. At best, public health departments within some communities collect surveillance data that include an ethnicity/race variable, thus allowing a link between rates of disease and a broad, nonspecific ethnic/racial category such as "Hispanic." In some instances, data on a more specific ethnic/racial category such as "Mexican American/Chicano" are collected and are available. However, more specific and refined analyses, such as by level of acculturation or by more specific moderators of the Latino subpopulation as mentioned earlier in this chapter, seldom are possible because data with such variables seldom are collected. Unfortunately, this situation involving inadequate databases on Latino characteristics limits the extent to which a proposed intervention can be tailored to the specific needs of a subpopulation of Latinos and other minorities when using existing institutional databases (Anderson, 1995). One notable exception to this problem has been the Hispanic Health and Nutrition Examination Study (HHANES) during the period 1982 to 1984, which surveyed the Latino population while giving special attention to Latino/Hispanic health issues. However, this data set is now becoming old.

A second major problem that limits the ability to design a tailored health promotion program for Latinos based on empirical data is that few Latino-specific theoretical frameworks exist that clarify the potential relationship between cultural identity as a Latino and the factors involved in disease risk development or in risk avoidance. For example, the appearance of a high age-adjusted prevalence rate of disease for a Latino group will indicate that a problem exists, but such data do not offer a viable and culturally relevant explanatory mechanism on the underlying process that governs the development of a given health problem.

A few theoretical frameworks currently are available that provide an initial cultural framework that, with some extrapolation, offers sociocultural perspectives on precursors of disorder and disease among Latinos. These works include studies on the role of the family and acculturative process in drug abuse and adolescent problem behaviors (Szapocznik & Kurtines, 1989), the development of ethnic identity (Bernal & Knight, 1993), the role of traditionalism-modernism and cultural mismatch in the development of psychological disorders in Latinos and other minorities (Ramirez, 1991), the effects of social migration and social affiliation on urban survival (Rogler, 1994; Rogler et al., 1991), and the influence of living in the U.S.-Mexico border environment (Martinez, 1994). Moreover, although mainstream psychology has offered several important theoretical perspectives that relate to health and behavior such as Bandura's (1977, 1986) Social Learning Theory and has offered several health-oriented theories (Glanz, Lewis, & Rimer, 1990), little empirical data exist on the applicability and limits of effect for each of these theoretical approaches as related to health promotion with various Latino populations.

Thus, in program design, when progressing to Step 2 (explication of theories and values) in Winett et al.'s (1994) conceptual steps, developers of health promotion programs for Latinos, if using theory at all, in the past have simply applied extant theory (e.g., Social Learning Theory) to Latinos while ignoring or minimizing the role of Latino cultural and gender issues. Unfortunately, as applied to Latinos, ignoring the factors of ethnicity, gender, and local community characteristics can compromise a program's capacity to implement and attain its goals effectively with Latinos from the local community. Currently, more work is needed on the development of Latino health theory and on the analysis of the process of health problem etiology and development as this is mediated by various Latino sociocultural factors.

Proposing Ideal and Achievable Program Outcomes

In working with minority populations, many dedicated program planners tend to propose lofty programmatic goals and objectives. Doing so is easy when seeking to improve the health status of disadvantaged (Group 1) Latino populations (the least acculturated, least educated, and poorest Latinos). Yet, in working with this subpopulation, given its members' difficult life situation, setting modest but attainable goals and designing a program that addresses barriers to full participation are key approaches to successful health promotion.

As one issue among this subpopulation of disadvantaged Latinos, the learning of program content does not always progress in a cumulative and linear fashion. For example, in a 10-session cancer prevention program that covers issues of prevention through screening, self-examinations, and healthy diet and lifestyles, a typical Latino program participant from the disadvantaged group (Group 1) might miss 3 to 6 of the 10 sessions because of transportation problems, unexpected family emergencies, personal illness, competing family priorities, and/or waning interest. Thus, a 10-session program might succeed in imparting only half of its program content, that is, a 50% acquisition of "program dose."

This situation prompts the need for the program planner to incorporate *repetition and review* into the design of a health promotion program curriculum and to set modest program goals. A rule of thumb is to anticipate that disadvantaged group clients will exhibit a 50% acquisition of program content relative to expected learning and/or skills development if learning had occurred efficiently in a linear and cumulative fashion. This situation should prompt the program planner to set achievable goals and learning objectives at a level of 50% of the ideal or total program content.

By contrast, in working with the more advantaged Latinos, those with higher education and high acculturation (Group 4) and perhaps those of high education and low acculturation (Group 2) (see Figure 7.4), goals and learning objectives set at 80% of the ideal might be realistic. For example, among these more advantaged Latinos, an 80% attendance rate (8 of the 10 sessions), 80% correct learning on a knowledge test, skills acquisition at 80% of maximum, and course passage by 80% of the group of participants would be realistic goals, whereas these goals set at 50% would be more realistic for Latinos from the disadvantaged group (Group 1).

These experiences prompt the emerging view that health education learning among disadvantaged Latinos progresses in a "spiral" rather than in a cumulative "linear" fashion. Revisiting and reviewing prior health education messages or skills, emphasizing process in learning as well as content, and flexibility in working with varying combinations of participants within the group constitute culturally responsive strategies in program design that respond to the health education needs of disadvantaged Latino clients.

Developing the Intervention

A series of key questions must be raised in developing a sound health promotion intervention for Latinos, especially for those who are most economically disadvantaged. These questions include the following:

1. How can the health promotion program command clients' attention, interest, and initial participation?
2. How will the program feature cultural aspects that will attract and motivate clients' commitment to participate and clients' sustained adherence to program activities?
3. How will the program maximize its delivery of health-related outcomes in light of the multiple barriers to full client participation that affect the most disadvantaged Latinos?
4. How will the program effectively measure or document the impact on Latino clients' health that occurs as a direct consequence of clients' involvement in this health promotion program?

In working with the most disadvantaged Latinos, their complex and barrier-laden living conditions prompt the need for innovation yet feasibility in the design and implementation of effective health promotion programs.

As an initial strategy, to establish contact with targeted disadvantaged Latinos, *community outreach* is essential, whether solely to invite their participation or to export actual program and service delivery to their community. Outreach is facilitated through a partnership with local community leaders and with community-based organizations, local clinics, churches, and other community agencies. However, such partnerships develop only after many months of relationship building with community leaders and agencies. This relationship building must be characterized by commitment, trust, action, and demonstrated accomplishment (Castro et al., 1995).

Also, this process of outreach is facilitated by the recruitment and training of *peer health leaders* (*Promotoras* or *Promotores*), members of the targeted community who, in consultation with established community leaders and organizations, are identified, recruited, screened, and trained as health promotion aides. Being residents of the targeted community, these peer health leaders have frequent contact with members of their community and can serve both as active role models of healthy activity and as purveyors of health education messages. Peer health leaders also can serve as community consultants and/or advisers on the cultural relevance and cultural effectiveness of the intervention.

Strategies for Strengthening the Intervention

A major but elusive goal in the design of effective health promotion programs is to design a *potent* intervention, one that has the capacity to produce significant changes in health-related behavior, that is, an intervention that has a significant and perhaps large *effect size* (Castro, Coe, Gutierres, & Saenz, 1996). Unfortunately, most community-based intervention programs exhibit, at best, a moderate effect size and often exhibit a small effect size. This means that these programs produce only a limited change in a targeted behavior among members of the targeted community group or population. Clearly, changing the specific behaviors of a group of individuals as they live their daily lives within a community setting is a most challenging task.

A few strategies have been offered to strengthen a proposed health promotion intervention. One strategy, *maintaining intervention fidelity,* focuses on delivering the planned intervention consistently and in the manner in which it was designed (Hansen & Collins, 1994). This quality control activity seeks to ensure that all clients receive a "complete dose" of the intervention protocol and that they receive it in the same manner. Clearly, a complementary strategy that aims to ensure that all clients receive the maximum intervention dose is to promote *full client participation and adherence* with the intervention's activities. However, for Latinos, the effectiveness of these two strategies for promoting healthy behavior change is contingent on the availability of a well-designed intervention protocol that is matched culturally to the needs of the targeted group.

Accordingly, another strategy for enhancing program effect is to *develop a culturally relevant intervention,* one that appeals to members of the targeted audience. An appealing intervention will capture clients' interest and motivate their participation. Such interventions can be developed only under conditions of *cultural competence,* that is, when the program planner fully understands the beliefs, values, preferences, and norms that govern the health behaviors of members of the targeted ethnic/racial group. Having such *cultural insights* into the nuances and dynamics of client behavior is a hallmark of cultural competence.

A related strategy for enhancing program effect that is based on cultural competence with a targeted group or subpopulation is to *target appropriate mediators* of relevant behavior change (Hansen & Collins, 1994). Here also, identifying and targeting such mediators is possible only when the program planner understands well the culture of the targeted group and has a working or an established model of the relationship between the cognitive mediators and the behavior change that is prompted by these mediators.

Mediators of behavior change are cognitive and behavioral factors that, if changed in the healthy direction, will introduce subsequent change in a targeted behavior. For example, increasing a client's *knowledge* about the benefits of aerobic exercise, building *commitment* to exercise, and teaching the client *skills* in how to exercise would prompt and reward exercise behavior. Here, eight important mediators of healthy behavior change observed in community prevention intervention programs are (a) increasing *knowledge* about a health behavior, (b) modifying *normative beliefs* about a health behavior, (c) changing *values* related to the health behavior, (d) building *commitments* toward a health behavior, (e) changing the client's *life orientation* toward one that is compatible with a health behavior, (f) changing the client's *self-concept* as related to a health behavior, (g) increasing the client's sense of *self-efficacy* in relation to accomplishing the health behavior, and (h) building *personal skills* for enacting the health behavior (Hansen, 1992).

Another strategy to enhance intervention effect is to *establish environmental contingencies that will prompt or reward healthy behavior change* (Kazdin, 1994). For a given cultural group, this also requires in-depth knowledge of the cultural and environmental contexts that govern the occurrence of a targeted behavior and of the reinforcing consequences that can maintain that health-related behavior. Here again, cultural competence on the part of the program planner will offer insights into the *naturally occurring cultural conditions* that prompt or reward unhealthy behavior and into the changes in the cultural environment that must be made to prompt and reward healthy behavior.

Finally, another key strategy is to *develop a system of social support,* a system that will prompt and maintain healthy behavior change within a given community setting. Given the central role of *la familia Latina* (family) in Latino cultures, a culturally effective health promotion program for Latinos should include a family support module. This module should offer educational information on *what constitutes healthy behavior* for the targeted client and on how family members can and should provide *social reinforcement* to help their family member. Appeals such as *"Ayudale, por que es tu hermano(a)"* ("Help him because he is your brother" or

"Help her because she is your sister") emphasize the Latino value of family unity and mutual support.

Next, the concept of social reinforcement can be conveyed by illustrating the family member's role in offering the client differential reinforcement for healthy behaviors. The client's family members can learn culturally appropriate skills to discourage or communicate disapproval of an unhealthy behavior (e.g., smoking is discouraged, and disapproval is expressed when it occurs) while also learning culturally appropriate skills on how healthy behavior can be encouraged and approved (e.g., walking for exercise can be encouraged, and social reward or approval can be offered when it occurs). How to organize members of Latino family systems to offer guidance and support to a family member for healthy behavior change is an area in need of future research and program evaluation. Similarly, a health promotion program's use of *Promotoras* or *Promotores* (peer health leaders) serves as another source of social reinforcement for guiding and maintaining healthy behavior change.

Considerations in Program Evaluation

A program's evaluation plan should not be an afterthought; instead, it should serve as an integral component of the total health promotion program as it is being designed. In formal program evaluation research, an experimentally sound evaluation design features an *intervention group,* a *control group,* and the randomization of clients or schools to each of these groups, depending on the unit of analysis. However, for many health promotion programs, such design elegance seldom is possible. Typical in such programs is the absence of a control group and of randomization; by contrast, the opportunity to obtain multiple measures of client progress often is available. These conditions yield naturally a *one-group repeated-measures design.* This design does have weaknesses relevant to the evaluation goal of drawing absolute conclusions that the intervention is the sole source of effect as measured by specified behavior change outcomes; that is, the design demonstrates high *internal validity.*

Nonetheless, this one-group repeated-measures design does allow program evaluators to draw reasonable conclusions on program effects based on observed changes from pretest to posttest on targeted health behavior outcome measures. Here, it should be emphasized that internal validity is *not* an "all or nothing" condition but rather a matter of degree. Accordingly, a well-developed single-group repeated-measures design can yield useful and reasonably valid data on program effects. If well implemented, this design can yield a sound conclusion that observed changes in behavior are *likely* the result of the intervention, although other factors such as history and maturation also might have contributed to the observed outcomes. For many community service programs, such evidence of program effect, whether or not it is *solely* attributable to the program itself, is useful information that suggests program effectiveness and offers evidence that the program merits serious consideration for continued funding.

In addition, under this single-group design, much valuable *process data* on the way in which the program operates can be gathered using structured or unstructured qualitative data collection methods. Gathering such data using an "open systems" approach aims to document the chronological series of events that "tell the story" of the program's development and possible effectiveness. The well-planned and reliable collection of *narrative data* that are collected on a weekly basis from key program participants (e.g., clients, health educators, administrators) generates a stream of storytelling data that reflects the temporal growth of the program and its possible effects, as seen by various members of the health promotion team and their clients.

Then, using inductive (data-integrative) methods, program evaluators can begin building a process-related program description by piecing together these various accounts. Thematic extraction methods, such as those described from grounded theory (e.g., open coding, axial coding, selective coding, process analysis, case analysis, model building), can be used to build a rich and reliable account of program process (Miles & Huberman, 1994; Strauss & Corbin, 1990). Here, descriptive narrative files can be analyzed by the old-fashioned "cut and paste" method or by creating computer narrative data files and using a computerized narrative data analysis program such as QSR NUD-IST (Qualitative Solutions, 1995) to aid in narrative analysis, discovery of new ideas, and inductive model building.

IMPLEMENTATION

Allowing Flexibility in Program Development

Once a program operates effectively by developing "programmatic momentum," the program will develop "a life of its own." Although programmatic guidelines give a program its direction, the program also is likely to develop in a few unique and unexpected ways. Alert program managers will make an effort to evaluate the usefulness of unexpected developments in relation to initial program goals and objectives. Some of these unique developments can then be expanded and considered in the development of a new cycle of the program.

Staff Development and Administrative Leadership

Three important programmatic aspects of an effective health promotion program involve (a) preparing clients by advising them on guidelines for their participation, (b) enhancing the cultural competence of program staff, and (c) enhancing the cultural competence of the program's administrative staff and infrastructure. At the point of program delivery, the client-provider working relationship is enhanced by *client education* (clearly advising clients as to what is expected in their participation) and *provider education* (enhancing the cultural competence skills of the provider or health educator). By suggestion, increasing the cultural competence of program staff will increase their effectiveness in delivering the health promotion intervention to the targeted audience. At the program level, increasing cultural competence in program design aims to strengthen the impact of the intervention.

One factor that seldom is discussed regarding health promotion program design and implementation, but one that is critical to program effectiveness, is administrative leadership. The best administrators of health promotion programs with Latino populations are those who (a) have knowledge of the local community and an organized vision of the program's purpose and direction and can communicate this to the staff on a regular basis; (b) build commitment and morale among program staff; (c) give all staff an appropriate voice regarding program policies and procedures; (d) plan meetings, as needed, to speak personally with community leaders and other community stakeholders so as to build and maintain *personalismo* (personalized relations) and *confianza* (trust) and to demonstrate a "commitment from the top" in giving an ear and a voice to the community in relation to program goals and objectives; (e) maintain a balance between scientific agendas and cultural competence agendas in the ongoing evolution of the program; (f) are *proactive* in anticipating problems and in searching for solutions that optimize program effectiveness given the available resources; (g) inspire staff and community confidence in their abilities as dedicated workers whose agendas are driven by the goal of enhancing the health and welfare of the local community; and (h) exhibit strength and integrity in responding forcefully on behalf of the program if and when the program is accosted by sources that harbor political or social opposition.

An administrator's attention to these issues, in consultation with staff and/or the program's advisory board, will prompt effective decision making on behalf of the project. Effective administrative leadership also involves making programmatic decisions that enhance the project by (a) garnering support for the program from the local community and from the funding agency, (b) strengthening staff morale and commitment to project goals, (c) maintaining fidelity in program implementation, (d) identifying serendipitous developments that can be added to the program to enhance its effectiveness, (e) ensuring effective gathering and processing of program evaluation data that aid in documenting program development and effectiveness, and (f) meeting regularly with staff to assess program activities, engaging in problem solving, and planning for future activities and program growth. Effective program administration and management may be a hidden factor not examined closely in the past, a factor that may contribute significantly to a health promotion program's overall effectiveness in enhancing the health of members of the local community.

EVALUATION

Relating Evaluation Design to Programmatic Realities

In parallel with program design and implementation, cultural competence in the evaluation of community-based health promotion programs for Latino populations also requires in-depth knowledge and appreciation of issues that affect program effectiveness with various Latino populations. Clearly, a program that fails to elicit and sustain client participation will suffer from a limited program effect (Castro et al., 1995), thus yielding limited or null health outcomes that could otherwise be attributable to the health promotion program's activities and interventions (Windsor et al., 1994).

The evaluation program itself should include culturally relevant measures that aptly evaluate the impact of program outcomes and the implementation process as specifically relevant for members of the targeted group of Latinos. Accordingly, the assessment protocol must consist of survey or interview items or questions that are tailored to the linguistic and educational aptitudes of members of the targeted population. In working with various Latino populations, developing conceptually parallel assessment forms in both Spanish and English often is necessary (see Appendixes A and B). The availability of simple, easily administered, clinically useful measures that are reliable and valid for use with various Latino populations (i.e., available in both English and Spanish) remains an important area for research and development that can aid in the design and implementation of health promotion programs for Latinos (Marin & Marin, 1991).

Process and outcome information that aids in program evaluation includes the systemic collection of well-planned program information on client adherence, on sources of disruption to program participation, and on programmatic health outcomes. In turn, these results aid in the improvement of the health program's content, structure, and operations when this information is fed back in a timely fashion. Moreover, three types of client *baseline information* (collected at intake) will aid in describing and understanding the characteristics of the participating clientele. These major types of data—that is, data on sociocultural resources, on subjective health culture, and on access to health services—will aid in describing and understanding the characteristics of the participating clientele. This information also is of considerable value in program monitoring and future planning. In particular, simple descriptive data on the acculturative and sociocultural characteristics of clients who participated in the program, as compared to those who dropped out, yield valuable programmatic information on which clients the program has reached effectively and which clients the program has failed to engage and benefit.

A similar strategy in the use of baseline and ongoing monitoring data can be implemented, perhaps more effectively, in the clinical setting. As a client completes a treatment or follow-up session, the administration of a simple and brief form or card can generate significant process data for monitoring the client's progress and for evaluating program effects. The goal is to administer a simple form on a regular basis such that it becomes a routine and standard aspect of a client's visit. Unfortunately, many clinical settings do not plan and fail to implement such an evaluation system at the beginning of a program. As a result, when it is introduced "after the fact," staff might become resistant to the implementation of a "new" procedure, or a client's progress evaluation might need to be conducted retrospectively, thus yielding less reliable data.

By contrast, using the principle of participation, involving program or clinic staff in the planning, design, and implementation of the program evaluation plan builds their ownership and participation. This can be a particularly useful strategy during the present era of accountability, when program funding and program survival often are contingent on documenting program effectiveness. Moreover, and beyond the issue of funding, program staff who are committed to the provision of effective services to their clientele can be encouraged to participate in the evaluation effort by advising them that their effectiveness as interventionists and their contributions toward enhancing the health of their community can be documented via their active participation in the overall evaluation effort.

RECOMMENDATIONS FOR HEALTH PROMOTION PROGRAMS SERVING LATINOS

1. Health promotion programs that serve minority populations should take a *cultural relativist* orientation toward the design and delivery of a health promotion program that meets the needs of the local minority population. Here, mainstream conceptual frameworks such as Social Learning Theory can be used as primary frameworks for program design. However, more must be done to identify and incorporate *culturally specific* factors (e.g., ethnicity, level of acculturation, gender identification, location of residence in the local community) that must be considered in tailoring the program to the unique needs of the local targeted group.

2. Health promotion programs that serve minority populations must establish strong relations with the communities that they serve. This includes outreach to these communities. Consistent with this effort, program leaders (e.g., administrators, project directors, health educators) must personally go into the community, at least periodically, to communicate and demonstrate commitment and support "from the top" for the health promotion partnership.

3. Health promotion programs, including research studies, should involve selected community leaders or representatives in the decision-making process that governs program operations. Some social scientists would argue that community people are not trained to offer scientific advice and counsel on scientific matters. Although this is generally true, selected community leaders can offer culturally relevant contextual information such as information on need or on what community residents like. Such commentary or advice can help fortify a health promotion program, in part by "grounding" it in the true needs of the local community. Such community input should be seen *not* as *encroachment* but rather as *enrichment* for the scientific and programmatic agendas that govern the health promotion program. Moreover, such actions contribute significantly toward making the program culturally competent as related specifically to the needs of the local targeted population.

4. Health promotion program delivery personnel, such as health educators, should engage in simple but regular monitoring of health promotion experiences and discovery. Such simple but consistent feedback will serve as *ongoing documentation* of programmatic events and of observations or discoveries obtained from "frontline workers," those who are involved in program delivery on a daily basis. Who is in a better position to comment on programmatic observation problems, discoveries, and solutions?

APPENDIX A
General Acculturation Index (English Version)

Please circle the choice that is true for you. Then, add the circled scores to obtain the SUM below. Then, divide the SUM by 5 to obtain the General Acculturation Index value.

1. I speak:
    1. Only Spanish
    2. Spanish better than English
    3. Both English and Spanish equally well
    4. English better than Spanish
    5. Only English

2. I read:
    1. Only Spanish
    2. Spanish better than English
    3. Both English and Spanish equally well
    4. English better than Spanish
    5. Only English

3. My early life from childhood to 21 years of age was spent:
    1. Only in Latin America (Mexico, Central America, South America) or the Caribbean (e.g., Cuba, Puerto Rico)
    2. Mostly in Latin America or the Caribbean
    3. Equally in Latin America or the Caribbean and in the United States
    4. Mainly in the United States and some time in Latin America or the Caribbean
    5. Only in the United States

4. Currently, my circle of friends includes:
    1. Almost exclusively Hispanics/Latinos (e.g., Chicanos/Mexican Americans, Puerto Ricans, Cubans, Colombians, Dominicans)
    2. Mainly Hispanics/Latinos
    3. Equally Hispanics/Latinos and Americans from the United States (e.g., Anglo-Americans, African Americans, Asians/Pacific Islanders)

4. Mainly Americans from the United States
5. Almost entirely Americans from the United States

5. In relation to having a Latino/Hispanic background, I feel:
   1. Very proud
   2. Proud
   3. Somewhat proud
   4. Little pride
   5. No pride (or circle 5 if you are *not* of Latino/Hispanic background)

____ = SUM

Acculturation Index = SUM / 5 = ____

APPENDIX B
Indice General de Aculturación (Spanish version)

Por favor, circule el número de la selección que sea más correcta para usted. Luego calcule la SUMA. Divida la SUMA entre cinco para obtener su Indice General de Aculturación.

1. Yo hablo:
   1. Solamente español (castellano)
   2. El español mejor que el inglés
   3. El inglés y el español por igual
   4. El inglés mejor que el español
   5. Solamente inglés

2. Yo leo:
   1. Solamente español (castellano)
   2. El español mejor que el inglés
   3. El inglés y el español por igual
   4. El inglés mejor que el español
   5. Solamente inglés

3. Mi juventud desde la infacia hasta los 21 años de edad la vivi:
   1. Solamente en Latinoamérica (México, Centroamerica, Sudamerica) o en el Caribe (e.g., Cuba, Puerto Rico)
   2. Principalmente Latinoamérica o el Caribe
   3. En Latinoamérica/el Caribe y en los Estados Unidos por igual
   4. Principalmente en los Estados Unidos y un tiempo en Latinoamérica/el Caribe
   5. Solamente en los Estados Unidos

4. Actualmente mi círculo de amigos está formado de:
    1. Casi exclusivamente hispanos/latinos (e.g., chicanos, mexicoamericanos, puertorriqueños, cubanos, colombianos, dominicanos)
    2. Principalmente hispanos/latinos
    3. Mexicanos/hispanos y angloamericanos (e.g., norteamericanos, africoamericanos (negros), asiaticoamericanos)
    4. Principalmente angloamericanos
    5. Casi exclusivamente angloamericanos

5. En relación con mis raíces latinas/hispanas me siento:
    1. Muy orgulloso(a)
    2. Orgulloso(a)
    3. Algo orgulloso(a)
    4. Un poco orgulloso(a)
    5. Nada orgulloso(a), o no tengo raíces latinas/hispanas

_____ = SUMA

Indice de Aculturación = SUMA / 5 = _____

NOTE

1. The literature on Latino health has no consensus regarding the preferred term to use when referring to persons of Latin American heritage who live in the United States. Both *Hispanic* and *Latino* are used extensively, although U.S. government documents, including the census, use the term *Hispanic*. Given this mixed usage in the literature, the present chapter uses the terms *Latino* and *Hispanic* interchangeably.

REFERENCES

Ajzen, I., & Fishbein, M. (1980). *Understanding attitudes and predicting social behavior.* Englewood Cliffs, NJ: Prentice Hall.

Anderson, N. B. (1995). Summary of task group research recommendations. *Health Psychology, 14,* 649-653.

Balcazar, H., Castro, F. G., & Krull, J. L. (1995). Cancer risk reduction in Mexican American women: The role of acculturation, education, and health risk factors. *Health Education Quarterly, 22,* 61-84.

Bandura, A. (1977). *Social learning theory.* Englewood Cliffs, NJ: Prentice Hall.

Bandura, A. (1986). *Social foundations of thought and action: A social cognitive theory.* Englewood Cliffs, NJ: Prentice Hall.

Barona, A., & Miller, J. A. (1994). Short Acculturation Scale for Hispanic Youth (SASH-Y): A preliminary report. *Hispanic Journal of Behavioral Sciences, 16,* 155-162.

Becker, M. H. (1974). The health belief model and personal health behavior. *Health Education Monographs, 2,* 324-473.

Bernal, M. E., & Knight, G. P. (1993). *Ethnic identity: Formation and transmission among Hispanics and other minorities.* Albany: State University of New York Press.

Carter-Pokras, O. (1994). Health profile. In C. W. Molina & M. Aguirre-Molina (Eds.), *Latino health in the U.S.: A growing challenge.* Washington, DC: American Public Health Association.

Castro, F. G. (1988). *Southern California Social Survey.* Unpublished manuscript, University of California, Los Angeles.

Castro, F. G. (1998). Cultural competence training in clinical psychology: Assessment, clinical intervention, and research. In C. D. Belar (Ed.). *Comprehensive clinical psychology: Sociocultural and individual differences.* (Vol. 10, pp. 127-140). New York: Pergamon.

Castro, F. G., Coe, K., Gutierres, S., & Saenz, D. (1996). Designing health promotion programs for Latinos. In P. M. Kato & T. Mann (Eds.), *Handbook of diversity issues in health psychology: Issues of age, gender and orientation, and ethnicity.* New York: Plenum.

Castro, F. G., Elder, J., Coe, K., Tafoya-Barraza, H. M., Moratto, S., Campbell, N., & Talavera, G. (1995). Mobilizing churches for health promotion in Latino communities: *Compañeros en la Salud. Journal of the National Cancer Institute Monographs, 18,* 127-135.

Castro, F. G., & Gutierres, S. E. (1997). Drug and alcohol use among rural Mexican Americans. In E. B. Robertson, Z. Sloboda, G. M. Boyd, L. Beatty, & N. J. Kozel (Eds.), *Rural substance abuse: State of knowledge and issues.* NIDA Research Monograph No. 168, pp. 498-533. Rockville, MD: National Institute on Drug Abuse.

Council on Scientific Affairs. (1991). Hispanic health in the United States. *Journal of the American Medical Association, 265,* 248-252.

Cross, T. L., Bazron, B. J., Dennis, K. W., & Isaacs, M. R. (1989). *Toward a culturally competent system of care.* Washington, DC: Georgetown University Child Development Center.

Cuellar, I., Arnold, B., & Maldonado, R. (1995). Acculturation Rating Scale for Mexican-Americans. II: A revision of the original ARMSA Scale. *Hispanic Journal of Behavioral Sciences, 17,* 275-304.

Cuellar, I., Harris, L. C., & Jasso, R. (1980). An acculturation rating scale for Mexican American normal and clinical populations. *Hispanic Journal of Behavioral Sciences, 2,* 199-217.

Fishbein, M. (1967). Attitude and the prediction of behavior: Results of a survey sample. In M. Fishbein (Ed.), *Readings in attitude theory and measurement.* New York: John Wiley.

Giachello, A. L. (1994). Issues of access and use. In C. W. Molina & M. Aguirre-Molina (Eds.), *Latino health in the U.S.: A growing challenge.* Washington, DC: American Public Health Association.

Glanz, K., Lewis, F. M., & Rimer, B. K. (1990). *Health behavior and health education.* San Francisco: Jossey-Bass.

Green, L. W., Kreuter, M. W., Deeds, S. G., & Partridge, K. D. (1980). *Health education planning: A diagnostic approach.* Mountain View, CA: Mayfield.

Hale, C. B. (1992). Demographic profile of African Americans. In R. L. Braithwaite & S. E. Taylor (Eds.), *Health issues in the black community.* San Francisco: Jossey-Bass.

Hansen, W. B. (1992). School-based substance abuse prevention: A review of the state of the art in curriculum, 1980-1990. *Health Education Research, 7,* 403-430.

Hansen, W. B., & Collins, L. M. (1994). Seven ways to increase power without increasing N. In L. M. Collins & L. A. Seitz (Eds.), *Advances in data analysis for prevention intervention research* (NIDA Research Monograph No. 142). Rockville, MD: National Institute on Drug Abuse.

Hochbaum, G. M. (1958). *Public participation in medical screening programs: A sociopsychological study* (PHS Publication No. 572). Washington, DC: Public Health Service.

Kazdin, A. (1994). *Behavior modification in applied settings* (5th ed.). Pacific Grove, CA: Brooks/Cole.

Kim, S., McLeod, J. H., & Shantzis, C. (1992). Cultural competence for evaluators working with Asian American communities: Some practical considerations. In M. A. Orlandi, R. Weston, & L. G. Epstein (Eds.), *Cultural competence for evaluators.* Rockville, MD: Office of Substance Abuse Prevention.

Marin, G., & Marin, B. V. (1991). *Research with Hispanic populations.* Newbury Park, CA: Sage.

Marin, G., Sabogal, F., Marin, B. V., Otero-Sabogal, R., & Perez-Stable, E. J. (1987). Development of a short acculturation scale for Hispanics. *Hispanic Journal of Behavioral Sciences, 9,* 183-205.

Marks, G., Garcia, M., & Solis, J. M. (1990). Health risk behaviors of Hispanics in the United States: Findings from HHANES, 1982-84. *American Journal of Public Health, 80*(Suppl.), 20-26.

Martinez, O. J. (1994). *Border people: Life and society in the U.S.-Mexico borderlands.* Tucson: University of Arizona Press.

Miles, M. B., & Huberman, A. M. (1994). *Qualitative data analysis: An expanded sourcebook* (2nd ed.). Thousand Oaks, CA: Sage.

Minkler, M. (1990). Improving health through community organization. In K. Glanz, F. M. Lewis, & B. K. Rimer (Eds.), *Health behavior and health education: Theory, research, and practice.* San Francisco: Jossey-Bass.

Orlandi, M. A., Landers, C., Weston, R., & Haley, N. (1990). Diffusion of health promotion innovations. In K. Glanz, F. M. Lewis, & B. K. Rimer (Eds.), *Health behavior and health education.* San Francisco: Jossey-Bass.

Orlandi, M. A., Weston, R., & Epstein, L. G. (1992). *Cultural competence for evaluators.* Rockville, MD: Office of Substance Abuse Prevention.

Perry, C. L., Baranowski, T., & Parcel, G. (1990). How individuals, environments, and health behavior interact: Social learning theory. In K. Glanz, F. M. Lewis, & B. K. Rimer (Eds.), *Health behavior and health education.* San Francisco: Jossey-Bass.

Qualitative Solutions. (1995). *User's guide for QSR NUD-IST.* Thousand Oaks, CA: Sage.

Ramirez, M. (1991). *Psychotherapy and counseling with minorities: A cognitive approach to individual and cultural differences.* Elmsford, NY: Pergamon.

Rogers, E. M. (1983). *Diffusion of innovation* (3rd ed.). New York: Free Press.

Rogler, L. H. (1994). International migrations: A framework for directing research. *American Psychologist, 49,* 701-708.

Rogler, L. H., Cortes, D. E., & Malgady, R. G. (1991). Acculturation and mental health status among Hispanics. *American Psychologist, 46,* 585-597.

Rosenstock, I. M. (1990) The health belief model: Explaining health behavior through expectancies. In K. Glanz, F. M. Lewis, & B. K. Rimer (Eds.), *Health behavior and health education.* San Francisco: Jossey-Bass.

Rossi, P. H., & Freeman, H. E. (1989). *Evaluation: A systematic approach* (4th ed.). Newbury Park, CA: Sage.

Strauss, A., & Corbin, J. (1990). *Basics of qualitative research: Grounded theory procedures and techniques.* Newbury Park, CA: Sage.

Szapocznik, J., & Kurtines, W. M. (1989). *Breakthroughs in family therapy with drug abusing and problem youth.* New York: Springer.

Tobler, N. S. (1986). Meta-analysis of 143 adolescent drug prevention programs: Quantitative outcome results of program participants compared to a control or comparison group. *Journal of Drug Issues, 16,* 537-567.

U.S. Department of Commerce. (1993). *We the American Hispanics.* Washington, DC: Government Printing Office.

Watson, D. L., & Tharp, R. G. (1989). *Self-directed behavior: Self-modification for personal adjustment* (5th ed.). Pacific Grove, CA: Brooks/Cole.

Windsor, R., Baranowski, T., Clark, N., & Cutter, G. (1994). *Evaluation of health promotion, health education, and disease prevention programs* (2nd ed.). Mountain View, CA: Mayfield.

Winett, R. A., King, A. C., & Altman, D. G. (1994). *Health psychology and public health: An integrative approach.* Boston: Allyn & Bacon.

8

Community-Level Diabetes Control in a Texas Barrio

A Case Study

AMELIE G. RAMIREZ
ROBERTO VILLARREAL
PATRICIA CHALELA

The overall prevalence rate in the United States for non-insulin-dependent diabetes mellitus (NIDDM), also called Type II diabetes, is approximately 12 million people or 6% of the population (Davidson, 1991). NIDDM, which is generally found in men and women over 30 years of age, accounts for about 90% of all diabetes cases. The other major form of diabetes, insulin-dependent diabetes mellitus (IDDM), generally strikes people under 30 years of age and accounts for nearly all of the remaining 10% of diabetes cases. Baxter et al. (1993) report that NIDDM is two to five times more prevalent among Hispanics than among the general U.S. population. Diabetes prevalence among Mexican Americans is between 10% and 12%, with 95% of cases classified as NIDDM (Baxter et al., 1993). This estimate is very close to findings of a 14.1% prevalence for NIDDM in Mexico City (Llanos & Libman, 1994). Among Mexican Americans, low-income men and women experience diabetes at a higher rate than do their more affluent counterparts, a pattern that apparently is linked to obesity prevalence in the lower income population.

AUTHORS' NOTE: The authors thank Rick Marshall for his assistance in preparing this case study. The authors also recognize the contributions of Karen Stamm, Virginia Ramirez, Irene Garza, Jesus de la Torre, and Sarah Harding in the implementation of the *A Su Salud En Acción* program for diabetes prevention. Finally, the authors thank the survey research firm, the Office of Survey Research at the University of Texas at Austin, the outreach staff, and community volunteers whose assistance was vital to this project's success. In addition, the financial support of the Texas Diabetes Council and the Texas Diabetes Institute made this program possible.

The catastrophic effects of NIDDM at an early age among Mexican Americans require the study of diabetes and its risk factors to develop culturally sensitive and appropriate prevention programs. This case study describes a theory-based community intervention that focuses on encouraging positive lifestyle-related behaviors (proper diet, exercise, and screening) in a predominantly Mexican American community, with the purpose of delaying the onset of the disease in this population.

Prevalence. Mexican American predisposition to NIDDM, central obesity, and other medical disorders have been associated with Native American genes, which typically comprise about one third of Mexican Americans' genetic heritage (Dietschy, 1991). Not surprisingly, other groups, particularly Native Americans, have high rates of diabetes mellitus. Pima Indians of Arizona have the highest incidence and prevalence of diabetes in the world (40% to 50% incidence for those over 35 years of age, adjusted prevalence 26.5 per 1,000 persons over 35 years of age) (Knowler, Bennett, Hammon, & Miller, 1978). Daniel and Gamble (1995) report similar increased risk among Canadian Indian groups. In Mexican Americans, evidence indicates that diabetes primarily results from greater resistance to insulin rather than from decreased blood levels of insulin, according to the San Antonio Heart Study (Haffner, Miettinen, & Stern, 1996).

Mortality outcomes. Diabetes is recognized as an underlying cause of excess premature death. A recent World Health Organization (WHO) study of 10 cohort sites worldwide found that both NIDDM and IDDM were responsible for excess mortality in every site (Wang, Heady, Stevens, & Fuller, 1996). Excess mortality was greater for IDDM subjects than for NIDDM subjects, yet NIDDM also was responsible for higher age standardized mortality ratios (1.92 for men, 2.36 for women, with 1 = normal mortality ratio), even when subjects with hypertension and proteinuria were excluded. The WHO study also found that time since onset of diabetes was a strong risk factor for early mortality and that hypertension and proteinuria accounted for most of the excess mortality among diabetics. Many other studies have confirmed the link between diabetes and deaths due to hypertension and proteinuria (Balkau et al., 1993; Jarrett, 1989; Moss, Klein, & Klein, 1991). Often, diabetes is the underlying cause of death but is not recorded as such. Hanis et al. (1993) found that 33% of premature deaths among Mexican Americans in Starr County, Texas, were among diabetics and that retinopathy was a strong predictor of early mortality. Fully 60% of diabetic premature deaths were attributed to heart disease in Starr County. U.S. standardized mortality ratios for Starr County diabetics were 3.6 and 4.2 for men and women, respectively.

Morbidity outcomes. The typical diabetic experiences considerable disease complications including increased risk of hypertension and obesity (Connolly & Kesson, 1996). Complications that affect vision (retinopathy), kidney function (nephropathy), and nerve and muscle function (neuropathy) also are common (Chalela-Alvarez, 1995). One U.S. study indicated that diabetics were 10 times more likely to require hospitalization for cardiovascular disorders, 15 times more likely to need treatment for peripheral vascular disorders, and 22 times more likely to be treated for skin ulcers and gangrene than the general U.S. population (Jacobs, Sena, & Fox, 1991). Lavery et al. (1996) reported that California Hispanics who suffer from diabetes had the highest proportion of amputations (82.7%) among three ethnic groups (African Americans 61.6%, Anglos 56.8%).

Financial outcomes. All of these factors combine to place significant economic burdens on diabetes patients and society. Data on costs to Mexican Americans with diabetes are lacking; however, national studies in the United States and Finland help give some idea of this economic burden. In 1987, $5.1 billion was spent on late-stage diabetic complications in U.S. hospitals. Cardiovascular complications accounted for 74% of the cost, and renal disease accounted for 10% (Jacobs et al., 1991). A Finnish study indicated that drug-treated diabetes patients consumed 5.8% of total direct health care costs (Kangas et al., 1996). On average, diabetics expended three times the amount of resources of non-diabetic patients. Inpatient care accounted for 81% of the direct costs for diabetic patients.

Outreach potential. Unlike many diseases, diabetes is not laden with gender-specific disease notions. Fitzgerald, Anderson, and Davis (1995) found that attitudes and practices concerning diabetes (both IDDM and NIDDM) between males and females were similar, with only minor differences noted. Health care providers also tended to give the same recommendations to men and women. Hampson, Glascow, and Foster (1995) found that diabetic patients' coping strategies mirrored their perceptions of self-efficacy and treatment effectiveness. Other researchers (Pham, Fortin, & Thibaudeau, 1996) found that in spite of perception, many NIDDM patients seemed ignorant of the vital role exercise plays in diabetes control and that less than half followed diet guidelines 80% of the time. They also found that social support, particularly from family members, was a key factor in exercise compliance, suggesting that family education is an important tool in diabetes prevention.

Because screening aids in early detection and treatment of diabetes, this represents an encouraging area in which to focus health promotion intervention. Glucose screening is inexpensive and underused in Mexican American communities. For early-stage diabetes, often all that is prescribed is a good diet and exercise program. With early diabetes detection, onset of hypertension, neuropathy, nephropathy, and retinopathy can be delayed, lessened in impact, or prevented altogether (National Coalition of Hispanic Health and Human Services Organization, 1989; Tuomilehto, Tuomilehto-Wolf, Zimmet, Alberti, & Keen, 1992). Although several studies do not recommend diabetes screening for low-risk populations (Newman, Nelson, & Scheer, 1994; Paterson, 1993; Worrall, 1991), Mexican Americans represent a high-risk population that could greatly benefit from increased screening compliance (Chalela-Alvarez, 1995).

Purpose

This case study presents program methods, implementation evaluation results, and preliminary outcomes for a study called *A Su Salud En Acción* (To Your Health in Action), demonstrating the application of the A Su Salud En Acción health promotion model to diabetes (NIDDM). The objective of this study was to conduct a community education demonstration project in a Hispanic community to (a) learn about the community's knowledge, attitudes, and practices regarding diabetes; (b) develop an educational community intervention based on the A Su Salud En Acción model; (c) enhance the community's knowledge, attitudes, and protective behaviors about diabetes; and (d) promote screening for diabetes.

METHODS

Target Population

Program activities were concentrated in, but not limited to, an 11-census tract area on the west side of San Antonio, Texas, with a population of 65,758. Mexican Americans comprised 90% of this community. According to a 1993 U.S. census report, more than 42,000 (64%) of these individuals were age 18 years or over (U.S. Bureau of the Census, 1993). Of these, 10,144 majes and 13,071 females were in the critical age range for NIDDM (30 years or over). Only 12% of the population spoke English exclusively, and nearly 19% said they either spoke Spanish only or spoke English very poorly. Although all but 10% of the population consisted of U.S. citizens, 17% were foreign born. Among persons over 24 years of age, 48% had less than a ninth-grade education and 69% had not graduated from high school. Census figures indicated that 48% of the target population lived below the poverty line, and the unemployment rate was 16%. Of those who were employed, 57% made less than $15,000 per year.

Initial Research

A research firm conducted a telephone baseline survey using a questionnaire prepared by A Su Salud En Acción staff. A project director supervised 27 interviewers. Within the data collection team, 85% of the interviewers were bilingual (the interview instrument was available in both English and Spanish). Prior to conducting the survey, a pilot test was performed in selected census tracts among San Antonio residents with the same demographic characteristics as the target population.

Although the at-home personal interview is the standard method for collecting information among this population, telephone survey methods were used because of feasibility factors, time constraints, and economic factors. A phone list purchased for the project target area was compiled from three separate record sources: telephone system, voter registration, and driver's license records. Interviewers, who conducted telephone inquiries until the specified number of surveys were completed, reached respondents in 98% of the homes. To be eligible, respondents had to be Hispanics age 35 years or over. The refusal rate was based on the number of refusals per total phone numbers called, whereas the response rate was calculated as the number of completed interviews divided by the combined number of completed interviews and refusals. The study used computer-assisted telephone interview methodology because it considerably reduces the element of human error and facilitates data handling after survey completion.

Survey questions included background variables (demographics, access to health care, quality of care, acculturation, social contacts, and media exposure) and outcome variables (knowledge, attitudes, behaviors, screening prevalence, and diabetes care-related issues). The survey instrument, which consisted of 78 questions, took approximately 20 minutes to administer in English or Spanish. To ensure correct translation and cultural sensitivity, the back-translation method was employed. This means that after a document is translated, it is translated back into the original language by another person, and then the original version is compared against the two translations so that errors can be revised.

A total of 3,123 calls yielded 800 completed interviews. This reflected an 84% response rate among eligible homes and a 5% refusal rate among all homes called. The average age of respondents was 59 years, and men and women were nearly equally represented. One quarter of the respondents were diabetics.

Program Design:
Efficacy of the A Su Salud En Acción Model

One effective way in which to reach Mexican Americans is through media-based public health campaigns (Ramirez, Cousins, & Santos, 1986). However, such programs must be culturally meaningful and sensitive to the heterogeneous needs of the Mexican American community. The A Su Salud En Acción model is a theory-based approach to behavior change that has proven effective in other cross-cultural settings. This approach combines two communication techniques: (a) role modeling in which individuals who demonstrate positive behaviors are promoted in broadcast and print media and (b) mobilizing a natural community social network to prompt and reinforce the imitation of the media role models (McAlister, 1991). Prime examples of this two-pronged approach are the North Karelia Project in Finland and *A Su Salud* (To Your Health) in Eagle Pass, Texas (Puska et al., 1985, 1986, 1987; Neittaanmaki, Koskela, Puska, & McAlister, 1980; Ramirez & McAlister, 1988; Ramirez et al., 1995). A Su Salud, which was developed to encourage smoking prevention and cessation among Mexican Americans, achieved positive results (McAlister, Ramirez, & Amezcua, 1992). Although this model was later applied to diet and cancer screening in San Antonio (McAlister et al., 1995), it had not been applied to diabetes prevention. The following sections describe its adaptation to this area of health promotion and disease prevention.

TABLE 8.1 Theoretical Sources for Message Content Areas

Cognitive Influences on Behavior	Theoretical Sources
Self-efficacy (skill)	Social cognitive learning theory (Bandura, 1986)
Response efficacy (benefits)	Health belief model (Becker, Maiman, Kirscht, Haefner, & Drachmann, 1977)
Attitudes (evaluation)	Theory of reasoned action (Fishbein & Ajzen, 1975)
Perceived risk	Health belief model (Becker et al., 1977)
Barriers	Health belief model (Becker et al., 1977)
Perceived norms/social support	Theory of reasoned action (Fishbein & Ajzen, 1975)
Perceived incentives/consequences	Social cognitive learning theory (Bandura, 1986)

Media Development

Behavioral journalism. A Su Salud En Acción used several forms of mass media including radio, print, and television in both English and Spanish. Stories in the media focused on role models who were recruited from the community and reflected the same ethnic and cultural characteristics as the target audience. These were men and women who had demonstrated some degree of success in a given behavior change (e.g., cutting down on high-fat food consumption). Through social modeling, the program promoted healthy behaviors and motivated people to action. It also focused on modifying preferences and perceptions within the target population. In particular, awareness of self-efficacy issues, barriers to service and action, and the role of social pressure in shaping outcomes were explored (Table 8.1). The benefits of good health practices also were highlighted.

Community participation. Focus groups in the community yielded information on the target population's media preferences. Based on this information, local television and radio stations were contacted, and partnerships were spawned. These partnerships were formalized in writing, with information covering the project's genesis, examples of role modeling, tentative quarterly media schedules, and content outlines included in the negotiations. Each party contributed a clear statement of its responsibilities and interests. The various media channels agreed to provide regular air time or column space. For its part, the A Su Salud En Acción staff provided role models, interview questions, background material, and expert commentary on topics of discussion.

Specific criteria were established for role models. To be selected, an individual had to be Hispanic, 18 to 65 years of age, and of low income and had to have made a behavior change that reduced the risk of diabetes. Role models were identified through numerous community organizations (churches, social and civic organizations, community health clinics, small businesses, and schools) and through community outreach by program staff and volunteers.

The concepts for the media health segments were drawn from a variety of theories to maximize the effectiveness of education, skills training, persuasion, and stages of change (McAlister, Orlandi, Puska, Zbylot, & Bye, 1991; Prochaska & DiClemente, 1994) (Table 8.1). Based on this analysis and guided by a quarterly topic schedule, the program's staff produced media messages in the form of news articles, scripts, and flyers. This method simplified interview analysis, clarified behavioral messages, and eased content classification. It also enhanced campaign monitoring using process evaluation tools.

Mass media. A chief goal of the intervention was to provide a steady stream of messages across as many different media channels as possible. From May 1994 to December 1995, this was in large part achieved through regular television and newspaper coverage and through two intensive campaigns aimed at promoting diabetes awareness and screening. Quarterly newscasts on the most widely watched local Spanish-language television station (KNMX) were aired on diabetes-related topics. In addition, major newspapers in English (*San Antonio Express-News*) and Spanish (*La Prensa*) carried stories on a monthly basis. The *San Antonio Express-News* had a daily circulation of 220,000, whereas *La Prensa,* a weekly newspaper, reported a circulation of 50,000.

Billboards. From April to October 1995, 20 billboards strategically placed throughout the target area focused on increased awareness of diabetes risk, benefits of exercise in fighting the disease, and the impact of healthy dietary habits (e.g., adding more vegetables to soups) on diabetes control. Billboards also advertised the availability of a free diabetes booklet and free screening examinations.

Radio. In July and August 1995, three Spanish-language radio stations (KXTN, KCOR, and KROM) aired 60-second health promotion commercials during drive-time, mid-day, and evening hours. These commercials emphasized diabetes awareness and low-cost screenings available through the county health clinic. The stations also provided free public service announcements to supplement the paid spots.

Narrowcast media. Project print materials were developed to promote and re-inforce the mass media messages and to present modeling stories in a small media format. The print products included newsletters with calendars, a 32-page diabetes booklet, and recipe flyers. These facilitated interpersonal contact by volunteers with their peers within the community. Other project-generated materials, which were specifically designed to aid the volunteer network mainte-nance, included quarterly bilingual volunteer bulletins and a 162-page cookbook.

The monthly newsletters, which contained a calendar of events, role model stories, and specific health tips (e.g., diabetes screening locations, times, and phone numbers), were distributed by outreach staff and volunteers (see "Community Organization" subsection). The 32-page bilingual booklet, titled *Diabetes,* incorporated photographs and quotes from role models, all describing what they were doing to prevent diabetes. Their stories and photos accompanied the basic information about diabetes and "how to" suggestions and tips for risk behavior modification that comprised the booklet's copy. The booklets were distributed in the community through volunteers, who gave them to family and friends, and through various area organizations (e.g., churches, clinics, businesses, schools). In addition, about 600 were mailed directly to participants in the baseline survey. Both the booklets and the newsletters were written for an audience with a reading level of fifth grade or lower. Graphic elements of relevance to the target audience were incorporated into the design whenever possible.

To encourage additional interpersonal contact with the community, a bilingual mid-month recipe flyer was produced. The flyer typically provided directions for preparing a traditional Mexican menu item (low fat, high nutrient, and high fiber) and a brief role model message. The recipes, provided by volunteers or other community members, were reprinted from the cookbook, which contained 47 dishes, preparation guidelines, a simple explanation of the different food groups and daily nutritional requirements, fat and fiber facts, and photos of the contributors. Dietitians, who provided helpful cooking tips, tested each recipe to quantify and standardize ingredient measures.

Community Organization

A full-time community coordinator supervised community outreach activities, networker recruitment, and the efforts of two part-time community outreach workers. The role of outreach workers was to help identify, recruit, train, and maintain peer networkers. This was achieved through contact with neighbors, either in person or over the telephone. Once recruited, volunteer networkers distributed small media materials each month and reinforced mass media messages promoting diabetes risk reduction behaviors. In addition to their formal social reinforcement role, the networkers also were instrumental in identifying role models within the community for use in the media campaign. Recruitment of volunteers required networking among opinion leaders, institutions, and community groups. Organizations, agencies, small retailers, and churches within the study area provided names of potential networkers.

Initial networker training focused on (a) describing the content of the monthly bulletin, (b) explaining the importance of interpersonal communication during distribution, and (c) emphasizing respect for the sociocultural environment. Particular attention was paid to observing cultural traditions such as respecting the schedules of others, maintaining confidentiality, and never approaching a person of the opposite sex who might be alone in the house. Basic training techniques were offered in the proper use of positive social reinforcement and the avoidance of prejudice, criticism, and conflict. Training also reinforced project benefits, goals, and personal self-efficacy.

Quarterly refresher sessions for volunteers offered practical information, reported on network activities, and encouraged leadership development. Training sessions also served to familiarize the peer networkers with health care technologies and to alleviate fears and alienation associated with medical care and procedures. These sessions included tours of health care sites and presentations by speakers with expertise in diabetes detection, treatment, and research. By seating participants in a circle and mixing staff and networkers, interaction increased and reticence to express real needs and experiences decreased.

Peer Network

Keeping volunteers motivated is as much art as it is social science. As incentives, networkers were given identification buttons with their photos, certificates to mark completion of training, canvas bags with educational materials, T-shirts with the project logo, refrigerator magnets, and (after 6 months of participation) a cookbook. Volunteers also were recognized in the quarterly networker newsletter. Personal events, such as birthdays and anniversaries, were acknowledged with cards in the mail. In addition, a summer picnic and a Christmas party each year provided opportunities for group celebrations and team building.

After the first year of program activity, organizational sites were recruited to augment distribution of small media materials. Organizations included small businesses, churches, senior nutrition centers, and community health centers. The quantity of materials disseminated was based on the number of customers or members that regularly attended each site and the interest displayed by the particular organization's leadership personnel.

Implementation and Process Evaluation

Several forms were designed to facilitate process data collection and to monitor the conceptual and applied development of A Su Salud En Acción. The data collected from these forms were coded and entered using FoxPro data management software and then were analyzed by the project evaluation staff. In addition to these project-generated measures, the information on telephone calls from the public requesting screening information and diabetes booklets was recorded.

Data analysis was performed using SPSS for Macintosh, a statistical analysis program, and focused on calculations of frequencies. Forms contributing to this database were (a) Organization Contact Forms to record information such as type of group contact, contact person, and number of potential volunteers; (b) Volunteer Recruitment Forms to register potential volunteers who wished to enroll in the project; (c) Training Evaluation Forms to evaluate each training session so that adjustments could be made to improve effectiveness; (d) Volunteer Profile Forms (updated weekly) to provide an inventory of the volunteers with the basic data needed for further evaluation; (e) Media Production Forms (updated monthly) to record all mass media activities; (f) Small Media Distribution Forms (updated monthly) to record distribution of materials by volunteers and sites; (g) Volunteer Survey Forms (distributed quarterly) to evaluate project activities and volunteer interests, needs, and attrition; and (h) Role Model Inventory Forms (updated periodically) to provide an inventory of the role models participating in the project.

Regular staff meetings were conducted to review community and media target activities and to aid in problem solving. These meetings also helped in gathering and confirming field data not collected by other means.

RESULTS

The results focus on baseline survey findings, media and community outreach outcomes, and process data gathered on diabetes screening. Comprehensive results of the intervention were not available at the time of this report.

Preliminary Telephone Survey Results

In the initial research phase, the telephone survey found that diabetic respondents tended to be more economically disadvantaged and less educated than their nondiabetic counterparts. A significantly larger number of diabetic men than nondiabetic men were unemployed $(p < .01)$ and had incomes of less than $10,000 per year $(p < .05)$. In addition, a larger (but nonsignificant) number of men and women with diabetes had not completed high school. Despite the higher unemployment rate among diabetic men, this group was significantly more likely to be insured $(p < .05)$. The overall proportion of respondents who spoke Spanish only was approximately 20%. The number who reported Spanish as their primary language was about the same for diabetic and nondiabetic men, as was the case for women (see Table 8.2). Approximately 1 out of 4 respondents was diabetic. Moreover, 4 out of 5 persons in the sample had at least one family member who had suffered from diabetes (Table 8.2). Despite the high incidence of NIDDM in the target population, as reflected in this survey sample, researchers found that general and specific knowledge of the disease was alarmingly low. Most notable were the gaps in knowledge with regard to diabetes causes, symptoms, and complications among both the diabetic and nondiabetic groups. Table 8.3 reflects that 1 out of 3 respondents could not define diabetes, 39% lacked knowledge about the complications, nearly half were unable to list symptoms, and a large majority failed to articulate the causes of diabetes or even to realize that age is a risk factor for the disease. Respondents who did not believe themselves to be diabetic were understandably less informed than were diabetics surveyed. Diabetic respondents had significantly better knowledge than did nondiabetics with regard to symptoms (66% vs. 49%, $p < .01$) and complications (68% vs. 59%, $p < .05$). However, their understanding of the cause of diabetes was not significantly better than that of nondiabetics. Knowledge of risk factors—vital to prevention—was even lower. However, most respondents in the sample (65%)

TABLE 8.2 Demographics of "A Su Salud En Acción" Study: Telephone Survey Respondents, San Antonio, Texas, 1994 (percentages)

	Diabetics			*Nondiabetics*			*Total Sample*
	Male (n = 87)	*Female (n = 97)*	*Total (n = 184)*	*Male (n = 312)*	*Female (n = 303)*	*Total (n = 615)*	*(n = 799)*
Less than a high school education	48.2	61.9	55.4	43.6	56.4	49.9	51.2
Income under $10,000	43.7*	77.3	61.4*	34.3	71.0	52.4	54.4
Spanish primary language	16.1	23.7	20.1	17.3	26.5	21.8	21.4
No insurance	21.8*	33.0	27.7	33.3	28.7	31.1	30.3
Employed	31.0**	17.5	23.9**	51.0	20.5	35.9	33.2
Family history of diabetes	82.8	87.6	85.3	78.5	79.5	79.0	80.5

$*p < .05, **p < .01.$

TABLE 8.3 Knowledge of Diabetes Among "A Su Salud En Acción" Program: Telephone Survey Respondents, San Antonio, Texas, 1994 (percentages)

	Diabetics			*Nondiabetics*			*Total Sample*
	Male (n = 87)	*Female (n = 97)*	*Total (n = 184)*	*Male (n = 312)*	*Female (n = 303)*	*Total (n = 615)*	*(n = 799)*
Don't know what diabetes is	17.2**	30.9	24.5*	38.5	30.0	34.3	32.0
Don't know its causes	81.6	80.4	81.0	82.1	87.8	84.9	84.0
Don't know its symptoms	32.2**	35.1*	33.7**	55.4	47.2	51.4	47.3
Don't know its complications	28.7*	35.1	32.1	43.6	38.9	41.3	39.2
Don't perceive age as risk	100.0	100.0	100.0**	77.9	82.8	80.3	84.9
Don't perceive ethnicity as risk	33.3	29.9	31.5	33.7	39.9	36.7	35.5

$*p < .05, **p < .01.$

were aware that being Mexican American increased one's risk of experiencing diabetes.

Reported behaviors related to diabetes demonstrated several critical areas of need (Table 8.4), particularly among nondiabetics, the population that should be concerned about delaying disease onset or preventing it altogether. Only about half of respondents in this group reported maintaining proper diets, and 4 out of 10 said they did not exercise regularly. More than one quarter of nondiabetics surveyed never had been screened for diabetes. Compliance of diabetics questioned was significantly better than that of nondiabetics in the critical areas of screening and diet ($p < .01$) but not with regard to exercise.

TABLE 8.4 Behaviors Among "A Su Salud En Acción" Program: Telephone Survey
Respondents, San Antonio Texas, 1994 (percentages)

	Diabetics			Nondiabetics			Total Sample
	Male (n = 87)	Female (n = 97)	Total (n = 184)	Male (n = 312)	Female (n = 303)	Total (n = 615)	(n = 799)
Have ever been screened	97.7**	96.9**	97.3**	60.9	72.9	66.8	73.8
Screened in past 6 months	87.4**	87.6**	87.5**	33.3	41.9	37.6	50.9
Watch diet	62.1**	79.4**	71.2**	41.7	50.2	45.9	51.7
Exercise	64.4	60.8	62.5	60.6	55.8	58.2	59.2

$*p < .05$, $**p < .01$.

TABLE 8.5 Sample of Media Content by Theoretical Concept

Theoretical Concept	Number of Times Concept Used	Explanation
Self-efficacy	11	"But you can arm yourself against diabetes."
Response efficacy	10	Thanks to his walking and healthy diet, Role Model A is fit and active. He controls his diabetes with insulin.
Attitudes	10	"I took it more seriously after a cousin died from diabetes."
Perceived risk	14	"For many Mexican Americans living in the United States, diabetes is like a time bomb ready to go off."
Barriers	7	Deciding to make healthier meals is a great step forward. But sometimes the rest of the family does not go along.
Social support	20	"I like the company of the ladies here. I have been able to lose weight, which is really good."
Incentives and conse-quences	17	Uncontrolled diabetes is known to cause blindness, kidney failure, and loss of feeling in legs and feet.
Perceived norms	10	Do not wait until you are overweight.

NOTE: Total number of media presentations = 26 (billboard = 3, radio = 8, television = 5, newspaper = 10).

Media Outcomes

During 1994 and 1995, 73 stories about diabetes appeared in San Antonio's
mass media outlets (18 television stories, 42 newspaper articles, and 13 radio
segments). These stories featured 79 role models from the community. The radio
campaign during July and August 1995 aired 11 different commercials for a total
of 168 exposures. Whereas all television and radio segments were in Spanish, 18
newspaper articles focused on the English-speaking community. Analysis performed on a sample of media presentations revealed that social support (in the

TABLE 8.6 "A Su Salud En Acción" Narrowcast Media Diabetes Topics, 1994 to 1995

Diabetes screening: Free, fast, easy	Nutrition fights diabetes
Recommend diabetes screening to a friend	Diabetes risk factors
Stand up to diabetes (foot care)	Signs of diabetes
You might not need insulin all your life	Tests for diabetes
Young people must fight diabetes, too	Exercise helps control diabetes
Fight diabetes with exercise	Weight loss wins "new life" (for diabetics)
Control diabetes now, avoid problems later	Make this the year of getting thinner: Healthy eating in the real world
You can learn how to avoid diabetes	Exercise combats both cancer and diabetes
Diabetes will not fence him in	Taking care of eyes and feet
Diabetes: Prevention is the key	A shot of truth about insulin
Healthy choices when eating out	Self-defense against diabetes
Cactus cools diabetes (high fiber benefits)	Obesity factor in diabetes
Team up for good health (family exercise)	Gene factor in diabetes
One step cuts two killers	A heart-to-heart talk about diabetes
Jose will not step back (don't fear diabetes)	Dad and son work together against diabetes
Fighting diabetes step by step	

form of free or low-cost screening), perceptions of incentives, consequences of diabetes-related behavior, and perceptions of risk were the major focal points of the media campaign (Table 8.5).

Diabetes risk reduction behaviors were the emphasis of 34 newsletters produced in 1994 and 1995. Table 8.6 lists the titles of those articles dedicated specifically to diabetes. Nearly 400,000 narrowcast media (print materials) related to diabetes were distributed. In addition, 10,000 copies of the booklet *Diabetes* initially were printed and distributed. However, due to demand in the community and elsewhere, since that 1994 first printing, 55,000 more copies have been printed for dissemination.

Community Outreach

During the course of the intervention, 610 community networkers were recruited and trained. These consisted of three types of networkers: individual networkers ($n = 328$) who distributed newsletters to groups or community organizations, site networkers ($n = 268$) who distributed newsletters in retail sites and other businesses, and church networkers ($n = 14$) who distributed newsletters in churches. Volunteer recruitment was conducted primarily at health fairs and during special presentations to organizations. Also effective was recruitment through referrals made by active networkers.

The majority of volunteers were women ($n = 311$ or 94%), predominantly housewives (60%). Approximately 48% of networkers had high school diplomas or higher degrees, with only 15% having full-time employment outside the home. Although the ages ranged from 21 to 84 years, most were between 35 and 60 years, and the median age was 48 years.

With regard to language proficiency, 92% were bilingual to some degree, with 78% able to speak, read, and write in Spanish and 48% possessing similar skills in English. The large majority of the volunteers were married (69%), and a number of volunteers also were widowed (14%).

A total of 37 community organizations had working partnerships with A Su Salud En Acción, enabling the program to maximize its outreach in the target community. Of these organizations, 14 were nutrition centers. A total of 261,716 calendars were distributed to networkers and their constituents during the 18 months of the study. The top four channels of dissemination were schools, businesses, individual volunteers, and clinics (Table 8.7).

At the end of 1995, 530 (87%) individual and organizational networkers still were active. This represented an attrition rate among individuals, businesses, and churches of 18%, 8%, and 8%, respectively. For individual networkers, the primary reason for leaving the program was mobility. Business closings accounted for most of the attrition among sites.

Screening Outcomes

Diabetes screenings were offered free to the public and were administered by a trained registered nurse. The services, which were available for an entire year, were well publicized by A Su Salud En Acción. From June 1994 to September 1995, A Su Salud En Acción media and community outreach efforts were responsible for 575 first-time screening referrals at the county clinic. That is, nearly 65% of all first-time referrals during this period were attributable to A Su Salud En Acción activities (Figure 8.1). Analysis showed that more than half of the program's referrals were due to print media exposure. Combined with volunteer contacts, this amounted to three fourths of A Su Salud En Acción-related screenings. The average age of the program's referrals was 55.7 years. Because the mean age of those referrals testing positive was 57.9 years and of those testing negative was 47.6 years, this would indicate that A Su Salud En Acción referrals tended to be at greater risk for diabetes compared to other first-time referrals.

CONCLUSIONS

The preliminary results from the baseline telephone survey found that many persons from the target community were in need of diabetes information to help

TABLE 8.7 Small Media Distribution, May 1994 to December 1995 (numbers of newsletters or recipe flyers distributed)

Sites	1994 Quarter				1995 Quarter					Total
	2nd	3rd	4th	Subtotal	1st	2nd	3rd	4th	Subtotal	
Schools (n = 14)	0	6,546	13,318	19,864	18,772	17,068	11,170	14,850	61,860	81,724
Businesses[a] (n = 169)	4,120	9,196	6,475	19,791	8,325	8,675	9,637	7,550	34,187	53,978
Individuals (n = 269)	5,985	9,742	6,504	22,231	9,805	6,412	9,226	3,331	28,774	51,005
Clinics (n = 30)	800	4,120	2,175	7,095	3,925	3,925	4,400	3,065	15,315	22,410
Local organizations (n = 13)	2,800	1,800	2,000	6,600	5,225	2,500	2,675	1,140	11,540	18,140
Nutrition sites (n = 14)	2,285	3,280	1,100	6,665	1,925	2,505	2,345	1,610	8,385	15,050
Churches (n = 13)	0	1,775	4,480	6,255	2,200	2,385	1,675	1,759	8,019	14,274
Other (n = 8)	280	750	580	1,610	840	890	1,095	700	3,525	5,135
Totals	16,270	37,209	36,632	90,111	51,017	44,360	42,223	34,005	171,605	261,716

a. Includes restaurants, grocery stores, pharmacies, beauty salons, flower shops. Participation of businesses increased over time. Also in January 1995, a monthly recipe flyer was added to the distribution network.

183

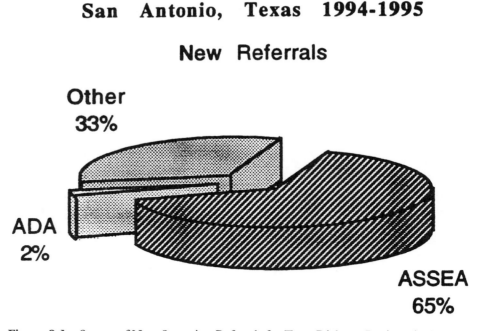

Figure 8.1   Source of New Screening Referrals for Texas Diabetes Institute in San Antonio, 1994 to 1995

them understand the nature of the disease, its cause, and its early warning signs. Far too few nondiabetic respondents in this high-risk population could define diabetes, its cause, or its symptoms. Respondents also were less knowledgeable than expected about risk factors attributing to this devastating disease. Those who were diabetic were somewhat more knowledgeable about symptoms; however, they had a poor understanding of what causes diabetes, the complications associated with the disease, and what measures can be taken to control their diabetes.

Preliminary data from the reported screening outcomes showed a positive impact of A Su Salud En Acción intervention efforts. Anecdotal evidence of the program's impact was encouraging as well. For example, response to the booklet *Diabetes* was excellent, as reflected by the numerous letters from health care providers seeking additional copies for their patients. One nurse practitioner described the publication as "the most popular diabetes literature we have ever stocked" and said that health care providers in her office "prefer to use this literature over others that we have [available]." Another nurse reported that a previously noncompliant diabetic patient carried the booklet to her doctor's appointment and, subsequently, took her insulin dosage daily and switched to a healthier diet.

Evaluation of A Su Salud En Acción's strategies and outcomes revealed several implementation components that proved either more or less effective than others. Lessons learned through this study included the following:

- Maintaining community input is important to ensure that health messages are on target and reflect the real-life struggles of underserved populations in trying to access health services.

- Use of print media is more effective than other mass media (radio and television) in promoting screening and educational classes. This finding was surprising given the literacy level of the target community.

- Using behavioral theories to develop the content for the media helps to keep a clear focus on the message for each diabetes segment.

- Community outreach and participation is a must. This process was critical in reaching a large number of persons and encouraging them to be proactive about their health.

- Community self-esteem is enhanced by focusing on positive health changes instead of on negative consequences.

An example of a less successful measure follows:

- Selective mass media (e.g., radio, billboards) avenues were not effective in encouraging community residents to participate in diabetes screening, even when services were offered free of charge.

The Mexican American population records a lower incidence of heart disease and certain cancers but not of diabetes. Although extensive controversy over the ability to prevent diabetes exists, action must be taken to reach high-risk populations, such as Mexican Americans, to reduce the devastating effect of this disease on individuals, their family members, and the public. Therefore, more targeted education programs directed at all age levels are needed to promote proper nutrition, increased exercise, and regular medical examinations. We must intervene before the risk factors escalate beyond control. Health promotion programs, such as the one described in this chapter, need to be conducted over long periods of time, and all staff involved in program implementation must be highly dedicated to promoting and maintaining positive lifestyle behaviors in the community.

REFERENCES

Balkau, B., Eschwege, E., Papoz, L., Richard, J. L., Claude, J. R., Warnet, J. M., & Ducimetiere, P. (1993). Risk factors of early death in non-insulin-dependent diabetes and men with known glucose tolerance status. *British Medical Journal, 307,* 295-299.

Bandura, A. (1986). *Social foundations of thought and action: A social cognitive theory.* Englewood Cliffs, NJ: Prentice Hall.

Baxter, J., Hamman, R. F., Lopez, T. K., Marshall, J. A., Hoag, S., & Swenson, C. J. (1993). Excess incidence of known non-insulin-dependent diabetes mellitus (NIDDM) in Hispanics compared with non-Hispanic whites in the San Luis Valley, Colorado. *Ethnicity and Disease, 3*(1), 11-21.

Becker, M., Maiman, L. A., Kirscht, J. P., Haefner, D. P., & Drachmann, R. H. (1977). The health belief model and prediction of dietary compliance: A field experiment. *Journal of Health and Social Behavior, 18,* 348-366.

Chalela-Alvarez, P. (1995). *Measuring the effectiveness of specialized training for volunteers on diabetes screening behaviors among Mexican Americans.* Unpublished thesis, University of Texas Health Science Center.

Connolly, V. M., & Kesson, C. M. (1996). Socioeconomic status and clustering of cardiovascular disease risk factors in diabetic patients. *Diabetes Care, 19,* 419-422.

Daniel, M., & Gamble, D. (1995). Diabetes and Canada's aboriginal peoples: The need for primary prevention. *International Journal of Nursing Studies, 32,* 243-259.

Davidson, M. B. (1991). *Diabetes mellitus: Diagnosis and treatment* (3rd ed.). New York: Churchill Livingstone.

Dietschy, J. M. (1991). *Medical grand rounds: The origins, genetics and diseases of Mexican-Americans.* Unpublished manuscript, University of Texas Southwestern Medical Center, San Antonio.

Fishbein, M., & Ajzen, I. (1975). *Belief, attitude, and behavior: An introduction to theory and research.* Reading, MA: Addison-Wesley.

Fitzgerald, J. T., Anderson, R. M., & Davis, W. K. (1995). Gender differences in diabetes attitudes and adherence. *Diabetes Education, 21,* 523-529.

Haffner, S. M., Miettinen, H., & Stern, M. P. (1996). Non-diabetic Mexican-Americans do not have reduced insulin responses relative to non-diabetic non-Hispanic whites. *Diabetes Care, 19,* 67-69.

Hampson, S. E., Glasgow, R. E., & Foster, L. S. (1995). Personal models of diabetes among older adults: Relationship to self-management and other variables. *The Diabetes Educator, 21,* 300-397.

Hanis, C. L., Chu, H. H., Lawson, K., Hewett-Emmett, D., Barton, S. A., Schull, W. J., & Garcia, S. A. (1993). Mortality of Mexican Americans with NIDDM: Retinopathy and other predictors in Starr County, Texas. *Diabetes Care, 16,* 82-89.

Jacobs, J., Sena, M., & Fox, N. (1991). The cost of hospitalization for the late complications of diabetes in the United States. *Diabetic Medicine, 8*(Suppl.), S23-S29.

Jarrett, R. J. (1989). Epidemiology and public health aspects of non-insulin-dependent diabetes mellitus. *Epidemiologic Reviews, 11,* 151-171.

Kangas, T., Aro, S., Koivisto, V. A., Salinto, M., Laakso, M., & Reunanen, A. (1996). Structure and costs of health care of diabetic patients in Finland. *Diabetes Care, 19,* 494-497.

Knowler, W. C., Bennett, P. H., Hammon, R. F., & Miller, M. (1978). Diabetes incidence and prevalence in Pima Indians: A 19-fold greater incidence than in Rochester, Minnesota. *American Journal of Public Health, 108,* 497-505.

Lavery, L. A., Ashry, H. R., Van Houtum, W., Pugh, J. A., Harkless, L. B., & Basu, S. (1996). Variation in the incidence and proportion of diabetes-related amputations in minorities. *Diabetes Care, 19,* 48-52.

Llanos, G., & Libman, I. (1994). Diabetes in the Americas. *Bulletin of the Pan American Health Organization, 28,* 285-301.

McAlister, A. (1991). Population behavior change: A theory-based approach. *Journal of Public Health Policy, 12,* 345-361.

McAlister, A., Fernandez-Esquer, M., Ramirez, A. G., Trevino, F., Gallion, K. J., Villarreal, R., Pulley, L., Hu, S., Torres, I., & Zhang, Q. (1995). Community level cancer control in a Texas barrio. II: Base-line and preliminary outcome findings. *Journal of the National Cancer Institute Monographs, 18,* 123-126.

McAlister, A., Orlandi, M., Puska, P., Zbylot, P., & Bye, L. L. (1991). Behavior modification in public health: Principles and illustrations. In W. W. Holland, R. Detels, & E. G. Knox (Eds.), *Oxford textbook of public health.* London: Oxford Medical Publications.

McAlister, A., Ramirez, A., & Amezcua, C. (1992). Smoking cessation in Texas-Mexico border communities: A quasi-experimental panel study. *American Journal of Health Promotion, 6,* 274-279.

Moss, S. E., Klein, R., & Klein, B. E. (1991). Cause-specific mortality in a population based study of diabetes. *American Journal of Public Health, 81,* 1158-1162.

National Coalition of Hispanic Health and Human Services Organization. (1989). *Diabetes and Hispanics: A resource for providers.* Washington, DC: Author.

Neittaanmaki, L., Koskela, K., Puska, P., & McAlister. A. (1980). The role of lay workers in community health equation: Experiences of the North Karalia project. *Scandinavian Journal of Social Medicine, 8*(1), 1-7.

Newman, W. P., Nelson, R., & Scheer, K. (1994). Community screening for diabetes: Low detection rate in a low-risk population. *Diabetes Care, 17,* 363-365.

Paterson, K. R. (1993). Population screening for diabetes mellitus: Professional advisory committee of the British Diabetic Association. *Diabetes Medicine, 10,* 777-781.

Pham, D., Fortin, F., & Thibaudeau, M. F. (1996). The role of the health belief model in amputees' self-evaluation of adherence to diabetes self-care behaviors. *The Diabetes Educator, 22*(2), 126-132.

Prochaska, J. O., & DiClemente, C. C. (1994). *The transtheoretical approach: Crossing traditional boundaries of therapy.* Malabar, FL: Krieger.

Puska, P., Koskela, K., McAlister, A., Mayranen, H., Smolander, A., Moiso, S., Viri, L., Korpelainen, V., & Rogers, E. M. (1986). Use of lay opinion leaders to promote diffusion of health innovations in a community program: Lessons learned from the North Karelia project. *Bulletin of the World Health Organization, 64,* 437-446.

Puska, P., McAlister, A., Niemensivu, H., Piha, T., Wiio, J., & Koskela, K. (1987). A television format for national health promotion: Finland's "Keys to Health." *Public Health Reports, 102,* 263-269.

Puska, P., Wiio, J., McAlister, A., Koskela, K., Mayranen, H., Smolander, A., Pekkola, J., & Maccoby, N. (1985). Planned use of mass media in national health promotion: The Keys to Health TV program in 1982 in Finland. *Canadian Journal of Public Health, 76,* 336-342.

Ramirez, A. G., Cousins, J. H., & Santos, Y. (1986). A media-based acculturation scale for Mexican Americans: Application to public health education programs. *Family and Community Health, 12,* 345-361.

Ramirez, A. G., & McAlister, A. (1988). A mass media campaign: A Su Salud. *Preventive Medicine, 17,* 608-621.

Ramirez, A. G., McAlister, A., Gallion, K. J., Ramirez, V., Garza, I. R., Stamm, K., de la Torres, J., & Chalela, P. (1995). Community level cancer control in a Texas barrio. I: Theoretical basis, implementation, and process evaluation. *Journal of the National Cancer Institute Monographs, 18,* 117-122.

Tuomilehto, J., Tuomilehto-Wolf, E., Zimmet, P., Alberti, K. G. M. M., & Keen, H. (1992). Primary prevention of diabetes mellitus. In K. G. M. M. Alberti, R. A. DeFronzo, H. Keen, & P. Zimmet (Eds.), *International textbook of diabetes mellitus.* New York: John Wiley.

U.S. Bureau of the Census. (1993). *1990 census of population and housing: Population and housing characteristics for census tracts and block numbering areas, San Antonio, TX MSA* (CPH-3-292). Washington, DC: Government Printing Office.

Wang, S., Heady, J., Stevens, L., & Fuller, J. H. (1996). Excess mortality and its relation to hypertension and proteinuria in diabetic patients. *Diabetes Care, 19,* 305-312.

Worral, G. (1991). Screening healthy people for diabetes: Is it worthwhile? *Journal of Family Practice, 33*(2), 155-160.

9

Tips for Working With Hispanic Populations

ROBERT M. HUFF
MICHAEL V. KLINE

There are many terms used to describe persons who trace their ancestry back to Spain, the most common of which are *Hispanic* and *Latino*. Suarez and Ramirez, in Chapter 6 of this volume, commented that it is more appropriate to use terms that actually identify the country of origin of the individual or population group (e.g., Mexican American, Guatemalan American) because this recognizes that these diverse ethnic groups have customs and behaviors that are unique to them despite the fact that they might share a common ancestral language and other more general cultural characteristics. Thus, the health promoter is urged to consider this suggested approach not only because it is a more accurate way in which to describe Hispanic population groups and individuals but also because it can serve as the first step in becoming more culturally competent and sensitive to the diversity of peoples who have been labeled as having Hispanic or Latino origins.

This brief "tips" chapter seeks to provide comments, suggestions, and recommendations for working with these different ethnic groups in health promotion or disease prevention (HPDP) activities. These tips are taken from Chapters 6, 7, and 8 as well as from other sources (Huff, Chapter 2, this volume; Huff & Kline, Chapter 1, this volume; Minkler, 1990) and are meant to be only general starting points when thinking about designing HPDP programs for Hispanic population groups.

CULTURAL COMPETENCE

As noted in Chapter 1, health promoters need to develop cultural competency skills for working across multicultural population groups. This is an especially important issue when working with Hispanic populations because there is a great diversity of ethnic differences that must be considered if one hopes to be successful in one's HPDP efforts. The following tips for the health promoter can help facilitate that process:

▶ Seek to learn the history and immigration patterns of the specific ethnic group you will be targeting for HPDP interventions or services.

▶ Become familiar with the group's specific cultural values, beliefs, and ways of life including forms of address and other verbal and nonverbal communication patterns, food preferences, attitudes toward health and disease, and related cultural characteristics that differentiate this group from other Hispanic populations.

▶ Seek to incorporate these cultural values, beliefs, and ways of life into the HPDP programs or services where appropriate and possible.

▶ Be aware that the degree to which Spanish is used as the primary language of the specific ethnic group will depend on a variety of factors including generational level, age, and gender. Assessment is the key to understanding.

▶ Be aware that acculturation is a critical factor in explaining risk behavior and health status. The more traditional the individual or group, the less likely the individual or group is to know about, understand, or practice Western approaches to HPDP.

▶ Understand that the measurement of acculturation is an important activity for understanding how traditional, acculturated, and assimilated a specific ethnic group may be. There are a variety of scales that can be used, and you are urged to read Chapters 1, 6, 7, and 8 for a more detailed discussion of this process.

▶ Understand that family and family support are extremely important core values among Hispanic population groups.

▶ Be aware that avoiding conflict and achieving harmony in interpersonal relationships is a strong cultural value.

▶ Be aware that respect is an extremely important factor in all relationships and especially in HPDP encounters.

▶ Examine your own perceptions, stereotypes, and prejudices toward the target group and be willing to suspend judgments (where they exist) in favor of learning who these people really are rather than who or what you might think they are. This is a critical first step in developing cultural competence and sensitivity.

▶ Take the time to make multiple visits to the community in which the target group lives. Talk with community leaders and residents, visit important cultural sites within the community, eat at local restaurants, attend local events, and otherwise become familiar with the community's ways of life.

▶ Seek to establish early and continuing support from the community for any HPDP programs and services that are to be offered.

HEALTH BELIEFS AND PRACTICES

There are a variety of health beliefs and practices that characterize the many different Hispanic population groups residing in the United States. An understanding of these can help the health promoter to develop an increased understanding of and sensitivity to the differences he or she is likely to encounter and also can provide for opportunities to incorporate these differences into his or her HPDP programs and services. Thus, the health promoter should keep the following in mind:

▶ Recognize that belief in folk illnesses still is a strong cultural characteristic among many traditional Hispanic population groups. Developing an understanding of some of these illnesses and their traditional treatments can help you to be more effective in the design of specific HPDP intervention and treatment services.

▶ Recognize that *fatalism,* the belief that one has no control over one's health outcomes, is a common attitude among many traditional Hispanic population groups.

▶ Understand that there are a number of explanatory models used to make sense of health and disease and that these are generally associated with the social, psychological, and physical domains.

▶ Where differences exist between the explanatory models of the target group and yourself, you will need to make efforts to ameliorate or otherwise find ways in which to work within these different frames of reference.

▶ Consider becoming more familiar with traditional healing practices where these exist in the community because this may provide opportunities to bring beneficial practices into the biomedical framework while also modifying those practices that might be potentially harmful.

▶ Remember that *curanderismo* is a traditional health care system that still is used today and often is the first system used when an illness or other disorder is detected in a family member. Those who use this system are generally not inclined to discuss this with a Western health care practitioner.

▶ Remember that decisions associated with seeking medical care and/or participating actively in a prescribed treatment or health program might involve the head of the household (or other family members), whose decisions will be based on what this individual feels is best for the family.

▶ Be aware that beliefs and expectations about health care treatment may enhance or impede the group's participation in the health program or service. Thus, there is a need to explore these beliefs and expectations in the needs assessment or initial health care encounter.

▶ Recognize that traditional folk healers often are the first health practitioners consulted because they are culturally acceptable, willing to make house calls, and far less expensive than the Western health care system.

PROGRAM PLANNING CONSIDERATIONS

Preparing to design and carry out an HPDP program for a Hispanic population group requires that the planner be culturally competent and sensitive to the differences in how its members view and operate in the world and how the target group sees this same process. Thus, the health promoter should consider the following comments and suggestions as he or she begins the program planning process:

▶ Involve the community in every aspect of the program planning process from needs assessment to evaluation of final outcomes.

▶ Seek to develop positive alliances with the leadership of the community as you begin considerations about the programs and services that might be needed by the community.

▶ Review all previous HPDP program efforts in the community to identify potential community resources and assets, interventions that have worked, and any other factors that have played or might play a role in the new program or service to be offered.

▶ Ask yourself whether the program or service being developed will be culturally acceptable to the target group. That is, will the program or service come into conflict with the target group's values, beliefs, attitudes, and knowledge about the problem?

▶ Ask yourself: Where there is a potential or real conflict, how can the program or service be tailored to better fit the needs and interests of the target group to be served?

▶ Ask yourself: What are the potential barriers that might be encountered that would hinder participation in the HPDP program or service? How might you overcome these?

▶ Wherever possible, seek to eliminate obstacles to participation in the HPDP program or service. This may involve simplifying how the target group enrolls in or accesses the service or program, bringing the program or service to the target group, making sure that the program or service is offered in the language of the target group, making sure that any follow-up activities that might be required of participants are simplified, relevant, easily understood, and so on.

▶ Consider employing the principles of *relevance* and *participation* when designing the program or service, that is, starting your program or service where the target group is and involving its members' active participation throughout the entire process from design through evaluation.

▶ Be sure that the goals, objectives, and interventions of the evolving HPDP program or service reflect the felt needs of the community wherever possible. Where there is a lack of perception from the community about the value or need for the evolving program, consider developing strategies to increase awareness of the need before launching the full-blown program.

▶ Remember that the employment of local community members in the planning, implementation, and evaluation of HPDP programs and services has been found to be very effective for delivering high-quality programs to the community.

▶ Make sure that the organization or agency involved in designing the program or service has a mission, policy, procedures, organizational structure, and staff that reflect a sense of cultural competence and sensitivity to the target group on which the program or service is being focused.

NEEDS ASSESSMENT

In general, all successful HPDP programs and services have as their foundation extensive data to help them better understand and address the specific health needs and interests of their target populations. It is critical that the health promoter take the time to adequately determine the characteristics of the target group he or she will be serving including factors such as morbidity and mortality, historic and immigration patterns, specific cultural characteristics, demographics, health care access and use patterns, and related variables. Huff and Kline, in Chapter 26 of this volume, present a cultural assessment framework that can help provide guidelines for the assessment areas that should be considered when preparing to develop the needs assessment component of their program planning process. In addition, the following suggestions may be useful in the needs assessment process:

▶ Be aware that no matter what planning model may be employed, it is essential that a cultural assessment be included in the other data gathered in the baseline study of the target group.

▶ Make sure that needs assessment instruments reflect the linguistic, literacy, and cultural symbols and values of the community.

▶ Be aware that standardized needs assessment instruments designed for the mainstream culture might have little meaning in Latino communities. Thus, instruments will need to be shaped to reflect the community in which they are administered.

▶ Where possible, train and use community members to assist in the data collection process because this can help facilitate community ownership of the program or service being developed and can provide perspectives that might have otherwise been missed by a non-community member.

▶ Be sure to include key community members (both formal and informal) in the community needs assessment process because they might be able to speak to both the real and felt needs of the community.

▶ Be aware that key informants might not always be in touch with the community's needs and that they might be operating with their own agendas in mind. Thus, always seek to triangulate the data that are gathered from those who are used as key informants using focus group data and other data gathered as a part of the baseline assessment of the community.

▶ Consider including acculturation measures in the needs assessment instrument.

▶ Focus groups can be a useful and effective approach to determining the knowledge, attitudes, behaviors, and felt needs of the community.

▶ Be sure to assess the types of media used within the community because this might be a critical factor when the program or service is ready to go on-line and marketing activities are being planned. It also relates to acculturation levels in the community.

▶ When designing questions for survey instruments or interviews, be sure to employ a *back translation* process if the questions are to be administered in a language other than English.

▶ Be sure that assessment and evaluation efforts reflect the needs, interests, and values of the stakeholders within the community.

INTERVENTION CONSIDERATIONS

Well-planned and culturally appropriate interventions are critical to the successful implementation of HPDP programs and services for Latino population groups. Pasick, D'Onofrio, and Otero-Sabogal (1996) describe a process of cultural tailoring that may be useful to the health promoter because it encourages the recognition of the need to design interventions that are specific to the cultural characteristics of the target group. The health promoter also may wish to consider the following comments and suggestions as he or she begins the design phase of the program planning process:

▶ Recognize that the development of culturally appropriate interventions requires consideration of available community resources and inclusion of important cultural themes of the target group. For example, *family* is one of the strongest core values of traditional Hispanic culture, so interventions that have a family focus might prove more effective than those that focus on the individual.

▶ Be aware that "one size fits all" is not a useful approach to intervention design. Programs and services need to be tailored to the target groups they will serve.

▶ Linguistic, literacy, gender relevance, and other cultural factors must be considered in the design of the intervention to be carried out in the community.

▶ Remember that using captive audiences and unconventional sites for the delivery of HPDP programs and services can be a highly effective approach to reaching and involving the community. This may involve home parties, parks and other recreation areas, social groups, and other locations where community members might gather.

▶ Be aware that interventions such as role modeling and use of community social networks can be useful approaches for demonstrating and reinforcing individual behavior change.

▶ Be aware that developing partnerships with local media (e.g., radio, television, newspapers) for the dissemination of health education and health promotion information can be a valuable and effective approach for both marketing the program or service and reinforcing the successes of program participants who may be recruited as role models for the community in which the program or service has been targeted.

▶ Recognize that the use of behavioral theory to guide development of intervention approaches is central to well-conceived and appropriately designed intervention strategies (Frankish, Lovato, & Shannon, Chapter 3, this volume).

▶ Recognize that the recruitment and training of a group of community peer networkers who can distribute program materials and reinforce messages can be an extremely effective method for maintaining community involvement and support for the HPDP program or service.

▶ Seek to develop interventions that focus on positive health changes rather than on negative or fear-arousing consequences.

▶ Remember that development of educational materials must reflect relevant cultural values, themes, and learning styles of the target group for which they are designed.

▶ All materials used in the HPDP program that are written in a language other than English must be *back translated* and pilot tested to ensure that they say what was meant and that the messages are clear and understandable to the target group.

▶ Always assess the cultural appropriateness of any pictures, models, dolls, or other educational materials prior to their inclusion in the program because some materials might make the target group uncomfortable.

▶ Remember that employing and training community members to facilitate educational programs in the community is a valuable and effective approach for implementing an HPDP program or service.

EVALUATION CONSIDERATIONS

Evaluation is central to understanding how well a program or service is doing in meeting the needs of the clientele it is serving. For this reason, the health promoter is urged to consider the following recommendations:

▶ Seek to develop evaluation strategies, methods, and instruments that reflect an understanding of current theory and practice in the evaluation and research literature.

▶ Evaluation of HPDP programs and services should include culturally relevant measures for evaluating the impact of the program or service on the target group.

▶ Assessment and evaluation items must be tailored to the educational and linguistic capabilities of the target group for which they are intended. Here again, back translation of items will be an important consideration in the development of the assessment and evaluation instruments.

▶ Recognize that evaluation and assessment are processes for which it frequently is difficult to gain support, even from the most sophisticated of groups. Efforts to explain underlying assumptions governing these processes, as well as the methods and anticipated outcomes from these activities, can help make explicit what often is unclear to those inexperienced in evaluation and can motivate increased interest and support for evaluation and assessment methods and procedures.

▶ Recognize that providing evaluation and assessment training for community members who will be involved in the provision of the HPDP program or service can help promote increased input and support for evaluation efforts. This also can extend the number of staff and community supporters who can be involved in data collection activities related to assessment and evaluation activities.

▶ Evaluation efforts need to consider the needs and interests of the stakeholders both in the community and in the agency providing the HPDP program or service.

▶ Evaluation criteria should be elicited from the community in which the program or service is being offered because its members are the ones who know what is important to them.

▶ Evaluators should recognize that HPDP participants from the community might have limited test-taking skills or abilities. Thus, efforts to design evaluation methods should reflect these potentialities by seeking approaches that are within the relevant experiences and skills of the target group.

▶ Be sure to design evaluation and assessment reporting and feedback mechanisms to ensure that the target community is regularly informed about how well the program or service is functioning to improve the health issue or problem for which it was designed.

REFERENCES

Minkler, M. (1990). Improving health through community organization. In K. Glanz, F. M. Lewis, & B. K. Rimer (Eds.), *Health behavior and health education: Theory, research, and practice*. San Francisco: Jossey-Bass.

Pasick, R. J., D'Onofrio, C. N., & Otero-Sabogal, R. (1996). Similarities and differences across cultures: Questions to inform a third generation for health promotion research. *Health Education Quarterly, 23*(Suppl.), S142-S161.

PART **3**

*African American
Populations*

10

Promoting Health Among Black American Populations

An Overview

JOYCE W. HOPP
PATTI HERRING

Black Americans, who constituted 12.5% of the U.S. population in 1990, will constitute 15% by the year 2020, as predicted by the U.S. Bureau of the Census (1992). Blacks, however, suffer disproportionately from preventable diseases and premature deaths. This chapter explores the extent of this disparity and the historical and current factors that may contribute to it. It also alerts the health professional to the health beliefs, behaviors, and cultural context in which black Americans function as a basis for understanding their health promotion and health care needs.

In the year 2020, nearly one out of five children of school age and one out of six adults of prime working age (25 to 54 years) will be black. Thomas (1992) points out that although rising numbers of blacks will be represented in both influential occupations and positions, they also will be among the poorest, the least educated, and the jobless. Throughout the 20th century, blacks have lagged behind whites in terms of life expectancy; whereas life expectancy has risen to 76 years for the overall population, it has fallen to 69 years for blacks (U.S. Bureau of the Census, 1992).

The extent of the disparity between black and white populations was first documented in 1980. The *Report of the Secretary's Task Force on Black and Minority Health* (Heckler, 1985) documented that blacks suffered nearly 60,000 excess deaths per year. Although the prevalences of cardiovascular disease and stroke are similar in both populations, the mortality rates are higher for black Americans (Magnus, 1991). Black men, in particular, are twice as likely as white men to die from strokes or heart attacks (Caplan, 1991). Hypertension is more prevalent among black Americans than among whites. Black American men under 45 years of age have a 10 times greater chance of dying from high blood pressure than do white men (Magnus, 1991).

Maternal mortality rates for black women are three times higher than those for white women (Aday, 1993). Black neonates born in the United States have an increased risk of low birthweight and perinatal mortality (Cabral, Fried, Levenson, Amaro, & Zuckerman, 1990).

More black Americans than whites smoke, although black Americans smoke an average of 20% fewer cigarettes; however, they have a higher incidence of lung cancer (Magnus, 1991). More than 44% of black women over 20 years of age are overweight, compared to 27% of women in general (U.S. Department of Health and Human Services [U.S. DHHS], 1990b).

Black Americans come from a wide variety of backgrounds and cultural experiences, which in turn influence their health behaviors. But they share traditional health beliefs and practices, which can affect many aspects of their interactions with the health care delivery system and public health.

BLACK SUBCULTURAL DIVERSITY

Although all blacks in the United States often are labeled as *African Americans,* foreign-born and immigrant blacks who have not become acculturated into the American culture might not identify with American-born blacks and, therefore, might not classify themselves as African Americans. Many blacks who emigrated to the United States from Africa, Great Britain, and the islands of the Caribbean, even though their ancestors may have been enslaved prior to emigration, might not identify with the descendants of slaves in the United States. Some blacks are Spanish speaking, emigrating from Central American countries. Thus, blacks in the United States represent a wide range of backgrounds with a variety of beliefs and customs, so that a single label does not fit all blacks. Following are definitions used in the literature:

African Americans: This term usually refers to American-born blacks only, excluding foreign-born blacks.

Afrocentricity: This is a way of interpreting the history, culture, and behavior of blacks around the world. From this perspective, African history is seen as a diaspora, and the history of black Americans is understood as part of the story of that dispersion (Coughlin, 1987).

Blacks: This term is used by the U.S. Bureau of the Census to denote the race of individuals. The authors use this label to refer to both foreign- and American-born blacks.

Ethnicity: This is a social concept designating a people group as opposed to race, which is a biological term. Ethnic groups are distinguished by characteristics such as names, language, accents, and religion (Adams, 1995).

Minority: Vander Zanden (1972) describes this as "a sociological term that refers to a culturally or physically distinctive social group whose members experience various disadvantages at the hands of another social group" (quoted in Adams, 1995, p. 6).

HISTORICAL PERSPECTIVE: A BRIEF OVERVIEW OF BLACK AMERICAN HISTORY IN THE UNITED STATES

Slavery Within the United States

No discussion of black culture would be complete without mentioning the effect of slavery on this group of Americans. Black Americans' cultural personality and breeding are strongly shaped by the slavery experiences of their ancestors. Slavery has significantly shaped black culture more than has any other factor.

Slavery, according to Sowell (1994), "is one of the oldest and most widespread institutions on Earth" (p. 186). The practice affected the lives of countless people of various ethnic groups around the world for generations. Slavery existed in the Western Hemisphere before Columbus's ships appeared on the horizon, and it existed in Europe, Asia, Africa, and the Middle East for thousands of years.

What, then, distinguishes the black American slavery experience? Blacks did not consensually come to America seeking a land of freedom, as did other migrants. During their more than two centuries of bondage, however, their many ancestral languages and cultures faded away and their genetic differences were combined to produce the American blacks. Thus, American blacks were a cultural and biological product of the New World rather than direct descendants of any given African nation or culture (Sowell, 1994).

American blacks also have different histories according to the time of acquiring freedom. Although most American blacks were freed by the Emancipation Proclamation of 1863, about a half million were free before then. These "free persons of color" had a history, a culture, and a set of values that continue to distinguish their descendants from other blacks well into the 20th century. A third small, but important, segment of the black population consists of emigrants from the West Indies. They, too, have had an economic and social history very different from that of other blacks (Sowell, 1981).

A variety of ceremonial or ritual behaviors accompanied the slaves from Africa. Most African religions were tribal; however, Islam and voodoo were practiced by some tribes. Voodoo is a blend of Christian, African, and other beliefs related to both religion and health practices. Researchers have reported that medical care for ill slaves was, at best, inconsistent (Guillory, 1987). Most slave owners insisted that slaves immediately inform them of any illness. Many blacks, however, preferred self-treatment or treatment by black herb/root doctors or influential conjurers. Slave owners always watched for malingerers; one way of dealing with the potential of faked illness was to make the medicine worse than the complaint (Guillory, 1987).

Because of slavery, the level of trust that blacks had for white physicians was either very low or nonexistent. This mistrust survives, to a certain extent, even today. Individuals who survived the experience of slavery formed a society that had little resemblance to the proud and independent stance of their ancestors (Guillory, 1987).

Social and psychological means of control by slave owners, in addition to armed guards, were not sufficient to control the potential for rebellion or runaways. An additional means was the maintenance of ignorance among the slaves. This ignorance included not only the absence of formal education but also the lack of knowledge of the geographical area. Unfamiliarity with the area reduced the risk of successful escapes (Sowell, 1994).

Urban slaves, often domestic servants, were different from rural field hands. Urban slaves were much more likely to be able to read and write because of their wider access to resources. They also were more likely to have social contact with free blacks in the cities. Frederick Douglas observed that urban slaves were almost free citizens. He knew this from personal experience as an urban slave before he escaped to the North to become a leader of his people (Sowell, 1994).

Following the abolition of slavery, many blacks continued to live on farms. Families depended on extended family members for health care. Many older family members served as midwives and root doctors. Health care rarely was sought outside the community because of lack of trust, money, knowledge of available health care, and transportation. Reliance on ethnomedicine flourished.

Slavery as an institution is gone from the United States, but its effects are being felt into the 21st century.

Post-1950s Health Care Reform and Black America

Important events that led to more equal access to medical care and improved health status for black Americans were (a) the Civil Rights Act of 1964, (b) Medicaid-Medicare legislation of 1965, and (c) Title VI of the Civil Rights Act, which prohibited racial discrimination in any institution receiving federal funds, thus giving hospitals a powerful incentive to alter their practices. In spite of increased access to medical care services, however, black Americans continue to have disproportionately large numbers of premature and excess deaths compared to the white majority (Thomas, 1992).

McCord and Freeman's (1990) study of excess mortality in Harlem, New York, shows that, due largely to high levels of homicide, drug- and alcohol-related deaths, and cardiovascular disease, the men of this inner-city community were less likely to reach their 65th birthdays than were men in Bangladesh, a resource-poor nation. Blacks are more often the victims of crime; Page, Kitchin-Becker, Solovan, Golec, and Hebert (1992) found that black city residents were four times as likely to die from homicide than were white city residents and that blacks represented two thirds of all known murder suspects.

McBride (1993) postulates that the history of black health care has occurred in three main phases: *engagement* (mid-1960s to mid-1970s), *submersion* (late 1970s to mid-1980s), and *crisis recognition* (late 1980s to present). During the engagement phase, a community health policy orientation prevailed as the national government targeted resources to health care programs for needy blacks and other poor Americans. Neighborhood health centers were replaced by community health centers, which included a variety of ambulatory multispecialty services. In the submersion phase, health professionals and political leaders experienced a newfound inclusion in health policy, but the government reduced medical resources for the inner-city poor. By the time of the crisis recognition phase, leaders of the black community were able to make the point that the specific disease problems and access needs of the black poor were intertwined with the many general sources of stress in the black community, namely high unemployment, overburdened community services and public hospitals, drug abuse, fear and violence in the neighborhood, and the overburdening of single mothers.

URBANIZATION

Just as the urban and rural blacks had different experiences during slavery, so too do the urban and rural blacks of today. In the early part of the 20th century, many blacks migrated to the northern cities from rural areas in the South. This migration increased after World War II. In 1910, 73% of all black Americans lived in rural areas; by 1960, 73% lived in urban environments (Guillory, 1987).

Health care was more available to blacks in the cities but still was inferior to that available to whites. Cancer incidence is higher among blacks living in urban areas as opposed to rural areas. Although the reasons for this difference are unclear, it appears that urban blacks are exposed to more environmental hazards and other risk factors. Urban blacks seek health care more frequently and practice more preventive measures, whereas rural blacks, especially those who are poor, do not seek medical care until the problems are serious. Often, the black client's response to the history of poor health care and inhumane treatment in the past is to stay away from health care facilities (Guillory, 1987).

TRADITIONAL HEALTH BELIEFS AND PRACTICES

Just as there is diversity among blacks in terms of heritage, background, and culture, so too are there individual variations in beliefs. Congress and Lyons (1992) attribute these variations to the duration of stay in the United States, age, and economic status. New immigrants tend to share beliefs directly related to their cultural backgrounds, whereas those who have lived in America longer tend to possess a greater belief in the scientific medical model. Few studies differentiate among subgroups of black Americans, although recent usage of the term *non-Hispanic black* indicates that researchers are recognizing that difference.

Congress and Lyons (1992) also point out that socioeconomic status is a significant factor in diverse cultural beliefs on health and treatment. The economically deprived are more likely to retain the beliefs and values of their countries of origin than are their middle-class counterparts from the same culture. It is important that the practitioner understand the effect of socioeconomic factors on his or her clients' health beliefs and their ability to use health care services. Many health care practitioners tend to treat the poor in a paternalistic fashion.

American-born blacks share many traditional beliefs with foreign-born blacks, but the reasons why they continue to use traditional healing methods and self-treatment regimens are somewhat different. Traditional health was perhaps the only health system accessible to everyone in Africa. Some 80% of Africans used traditional healing methods, which have been sustained over the years partly because they are acceptable, available, and affordable (Airhihenbuwa & Harrison, 1993). The use of traditional remedies to prevent, treat, and cure illness dates back to the dawn of time. The reliance on informal folk healers by the American black population has roots in the fact that their access to more formalized American health care was denied, first by slavery and then by segregation. Second- and third-generation blacks raised in northern urban areas since civil rights legislation may be less influenced by these traditional southern black beliefs (Congress & Lyons, 1992).

Caribbean blacks may be especially influenced by their native countries, particularly if they are undocumented immigrants, because of their recent arrival in the United States, with limited access to the formal health care system. The beliefs of some Haitians regarding the causes, treatment, and prevention of illness differ significantly from U.S. health practices. Many attribute diseases to supernatural causes.

Snow (1983), in her extensive research of traditional health beliefs among blacks, reports that individuals who come into contact with orthodox medicine contrary to their traditional health beliefs often will react by ignoring the prescribed treatment, misusing the treatment, complaining about the quality of care they are receiving, or seeking treatment from a folk healer. Folk healers often become the only health care providers for low-income blacks.

Some folk healers are considered to be sorcerers with magical powers either to cause or to cure illness. They acquire this special gift when they are "born with the veil," the veil being the amniotic sac that surrounds and protects the baby during pregnancy. It is believed that a child born with the veil will have power to see and hear ghosts and to foretell the future (Rich, 1976).

Folk healers often offer themselves to the blacks in urban ghettos by advertising their services (Snow, 1978). Although some provide useful services, others use their acclaimed power to manipulate and swindle money from the gullible. Sometimes, their treatment works, and when it fails, believers are convinced that it failed because the victim was beyond hope. Webb (1971) reports that folk medicine is grounded on belief, not knowledge; thus, it requires only occasional successes for it to maintain its power and control over believers.

Good health is considered harmony with nature; illness and bad health, on the other hand, are viewed as disharmony with nature that may be caused by a variety of factors (Jacques, 1976). Therefore, blacks tend to classify illness into two categories: natural and unnatural (Congress & Lyons, 1992). This categorization affects the methods that traditional health practitioners use to treat or cure an illness. The majority of practitioners and followers believe that illness can be cured if only special care is taken to follow the prescribed plan of the master (God). Thus, causes of illness generally fall into three domains: divine punishment, environmental hazards, and impaired social relationships (Snow, 1974).

Natural illnesses can result from stress; cold; impurities in the water, air, or food; improper eating habits or diet; weakness; or lack of moderation in daily activities. They are considered nature's calling card as punishment for sin; natural illnesses can be visited on sinners directly or on their children. Hence, disorders such as mental retardation, seizures, and deformities demonstrate that innocent children suffer the consequences of their parents' misdeeds or sins. It is believed that illness is predictable and according to God's plan (Gregg & Curry, 1994).

Rotter's (1966) external locus of control construct explains the traditional black belief that evil influences may be blamed for illnesses or mishaps. This is matched by the belief that magical means are needed to bring about the desired behavior. Snow (1974) maintains that sympathetic magic is believed to link the body with forces in nature, whereas external forces are thrust on individuals who must learn to manipulate them for their own well being. Natural illness can occur at any time; individuals are susceptible at various times, depending on factors such as drinking too much, staying out too late, eating the wrong types of foods, fighting with neighbors, failing to pay, failing to wear protective charms during certain periods of life, and lunar or planetary cycles (Flaskerud & Rush, 1989).

The cause of an illness is more important than its manifestation in the body. For example, stroke is variously believed to be caused by taking a bath during the menstrual period, eating red meat, or punishment by God. An illness such as this is considered to be a test of faith that might not be explained in the lifetime of those afflicted; they might only learn the reason when they reach heaven. Because the illness is regarded as God's punishment, it cannot be treated or cured by human medicine. Gregg and Curry (1994) quote the philosophy expressed thusly: "You got to die with something; one day you got to leave here. . . . When it's time to go, it's time to go" (p. 522). The only prescription to follow to obtain a cure is to admit the sin, be sorry for having committed it, and vow to improve in the future.

Unnatural illnesses are caused by the evil influences of the devil, and many times they are induced by witchcraft or caused by demons or bad spirits (Jacques, 1976). Unnatural illness can be terrifying to individuals because they usually do not respond to self-treatment or remedies administered by friends, relatives, or practitioners (Snow, 1978). In such cases, the use of conjurers or voodoo doctors is needed to manipulate the spirits or demons (Guillory, 1987). As Snow (1978) explains, magic gives people the illusion that they have a measure of control over events.

Specific aids, such as soap, incense, lotions, aerosol sprays, candles, and oils, have been sold in lower-class black neighborhoods for the purposes of keeping away evil spirits, bringing luck at Bingo games or the races, and keeping spouses at home. Webb (1971) reports that some of these seemingly primitive remedies are successful because of the psychotherapeutic quality of such medicine to heal or destroy, as in voodoo deaths.

Worry, according to traditional beliefs of many blacks, is the main component in the course of unnatural illness. When worry is prolonged, the individual cannot sleep, eat, or perform everyday activities. According to folk healers, too much worry causes someone to "go crazy" (Snow, 1978).

The remedies for treating calamities caused by evil influences include food, medicine, antidotes, healing, and prayer proposed to God by a medium with unusual powers (Snow, 1974). Other cures and treatments include external aids such as magic and visible protection in the form of prayer, cards, charms, and asafetida bags (Snow, 1983). Guillory (1987) reports that other folk remedies include eating garlic for hypertension, drinking teas made from herbs for colds, applying tallow to the chest and covering it with a cloth for colds, pouring kerosene into cuts as a disinfectant, and wearing garlic around the neck to keep from catching disease. Use of vinegar, Epsom salts, Ben-Gay, and copper wire or bracelets for arthritis; horehound tea or buttermilk for diabetes; and tea made of rabbit tobacco and pine top for asthma is common.

The health practitioner should acquaint himself or herself with the cultural beliefs and practices of the black Americans the practitioner treats and determine which may be beneficial or potentially hazardous. Replacing dangerous practices with alternatives is possible if done sensitively. For example, the use of marijuana teas for respiratory conditions can be discouraged by explaining the reason for concern and then recommending an alternate herb tea acceptable to the patient and family.

How does a health practitioner learn the specific cultural beliefs and practices of individuals? The best sources are patients themselves. Another source is office staff members who reside in the community or who are of the same ethnocultural background as the patients. Probing into nonbiomedical illness customs may initially be met with apprehension, but if the topic is approached in a sincere and nonjudgmental style, it is surprising how much information can be obtained from patients themselves.

Williams (1996) points out that Black American churches have been the most important social institution in the black community. Churches frequently offered the only respite from the continuous repression of slavery and afforded the only places where members could exercise leadership. Black churches today function as centers for health screening, promotion, and counseling. Clergy deal with marital and family problems, drug and alcohol problems, financial problems, and HIV/AIDS, all of which directly affect the health of their parishioners.

The health practitioner needs to be sensitive to the religious beliefs of his or her patients and be alert for opportunities to learn of potential treatment or prevention. The health practitioner does not need to hold the same religious beliefs but needs to recognize their effect on patients' lives and prognoses. Open-ended questions such as "What does your belief in God mean to you now?" and "How does your belief in God's direction in your life make a difference?" may be used to elicit the patient's beliefs in relation to a health problem.

SOCIODEMOGRAPHIC CHARACTERISTICS OF BLACK AMERICAN POPULATIONS

Black Americans live in all regions of the country and are represented in every socioeconomic group. One third live in poverty, a rate three times that of the white population. More than half live in central cities, areas often typified by poverty, poor schools, crowded housing, and unemployment and exposed to a pervasive drug culture and periodic street violence and high levels of stress (U.S. DHHS, 1990b).

Population growth. The black population in the United States increased an average of 1.4% per year between 1980 and 1992, compared to 0.6% for the white population and 0.9% for the total population. Fully 84% of the growth in the black population was from natural increase, or the excess of births over deaths. Immigration, which increased substantially since 1980 for the black population, accounted for the remaining 16% (U.S. Bureau of the Census, 1992).

Sex and age distribution. Both black and white populations have aged since 1980. The black population had a median age of 28.2 years in 1992, compared to 24.8 years in 1980. The corresponding median ages for whites were 34.3 and 30.8 years, respectively. Compared to the white population, a larger proportion of the black population was under 18 years of age, and a smaller proportion was age 65 years or over. Only 15% of the black population was age 55 years or over, compared to 22% of the white population. Among both blacks and whites, there were more females in this older age group (U.S. Bureau of the Census, 1992).

Marital status and households. Since 1980, the number of black households has risen at a faster pace (29%) than the number of white households (15%). This differential growth can be attributed in part to greater increases in black householders than white householders who are separated, divorced, or never married as well as the higher growth rate of the adult black population. Black families maintained by women with no spouses present rose from 40% to 46%, and those maintained by men with no spouses present from 4% to 7%; this increase in black families maintained by women was slower than the sharp rise of the 1970s, during which the rate jumped from 28% to 40%. The proportion of children living with two parents has declined since 1980 for both blacks and whites; in 1992, 36% of black children under 18 years of age lived with both parents, compared to 42% in 1980, a 16% decline. In the same time period, white families had a 6% decline, going from 83% in 1980 to 77% in 1992 (U.S. Bureau of the Census, 1992).

Economic characteristics. In 1992, blacks made up 11% of the total labor force in the United States and 21% of the unemployed. They comprised twice the proportion of the unemployed as they did of the employed, a condition unchanged from 1980 to 1992. The per capita income of the black population in

1992 ($9,170) was about 60% that of the white population ($15,510), with a similar ratio (.59) in both 1979 and 1989. Black median family income in 1991 ($21,550) was 57% that for whites ($37,780).

A person's earning power is positively correlated to educational attainment. A substantial difference is evident in comparing workers with high school diplomas to those with bachelor's degrees. Blacks with bachelor's degrees or more had earnings 66% higher than those possessing only high school diplomas. In 1992, black males earned 80% of what white males earned. When education was taken into consideration, however, black males with college educations attained earnings parity with comparably educated white males in several occupations but not in executive, administrative, or managerial positions (U.S. Bureau of the Census, 1992).

Educational attainment. Black adults made notable progress in attaining high school diplomas during the 1980s. In 1980, 51% of blacks age 25 years or over had attained high school diplomas; by 1992, 68% had done so. The corresponding rates for whites were 71% and 81%, respectively. In 1980, 8% of black adults had bachelor's degrees or more; by 1992, this proportion had increased to 12% (U.S. Bureau of the Census, 1992).

Poverty rates. The proportion of black persons in poverty has fluctuated little since the mid-1960s. The 1991 poverty rate for blacks (33%) was three times that for whites (11%), compared to the corresponding 1979 rates of 31% and 9%, respectively. Approximately 4.5 million (46%) of all black-related children under 18 years of age were in poor families, compared to 8.3 million (16%) of white-related children. Three times as many black persons (29%) as white persons (9%) age 55 years or over were poor in 1991. Approximately 34% of all poor black persons lived in the South, whereas white persons age 55 years or over who were below the poverty level were more likely to reside in the North or West region (62%) (U.S. Bureau of the Census, 1992).

The homeless. Black Americans are disproportionately represented among the homeless. In New York City, about 25% of the population is black, but black Americans comprise 73% of the city's homeless people (Institute of Medicine, 1988). Similarly, blacks make up 7.5% of Ohio's population but 11% of the state's homeless (Braithwaite & Taylor, 1992).

HEALTH AND DISEASE PATTERNS AMONG BLACK AMERICANS

Differences in health status of blacks and whites have been documented in the United States as long as health data have been collected. These differences persist in spite of large increases in life expectancy and improvements in the health status of the general population (Thomas, 1992).

Diabetes. Diabetes is 33% more common among blacks than among whites. More than 2.1 million black Americans have diabetes. The rates of diabetes prevalence are 160% higher in black Americans than in the general population (Gavin, 1995). The highest rates are among black women, especially those who are overweight. The complications of diabetes—heart attack, stroke, kidney failure, blindness, and limb amputation—are more prevalent among blacks with diabetes than among whites with diabetes. Black women with diabetes are nearly seven times more likely to die from ischemic heart disease than are black women without diabetes (Will & Casper, 1996). Among blacks 65 to 74 years of age, one in four has diabetes.

Cardiovascular disease and stroke. Cardiovascular diseases are the leading cause of death for black Americans, as they are for the entire U.S. population. Between 1972 and 1992, the coronary heart disease death rate declined about 49%, and stroke death rate declined about 58% (U.S. DHHS, 1996). Despite these gains, for black Americans the death rates for coronary heart disease and stroke were 155 and 45 per 100,000, respectively, compared to 113 and 26 per 100,000 for the total population. End-stage renal disease actually increased from 13.9 to 14.4 per 100,000 for the total population and 34 to 43 per 100,000 for blacks (U.S. DHHS, 1995).

Hypertension. Hypertension is defined as sustained blood pressure of 140/90 mm Hg in individuals age 18 years or over. Hypertension is a significant component of the relative risk for heart disease, stroke, and end-stage renal disease. The single most powerful determinant for hypertension is ethnicity. High blood pressure is much more common among blacks of both genders than among the total population. Severe hypertension is present four times as often among black men as among white men (U.S. DHHS, 1990b). Hypertension kills 15 times as many black males as white males in the age 15- to 40-year age group and 7 times as many black females as white females in any age group.

Genetic and physiological differences alone are unlikely to explain race differences in blood pressure. There are cultural variations in the relationship between age and blood pressure levels (Williams, 1992). Cross-cultural studies indicate that blood pressure within racial groups varies by geographical or social context. Williams (1992) points out that blood pressure levels in West Africans are generally lower than those in U.S. and Caribbean blacks. When black populations in Africa move from their original communities to large urban centers, their blood pressure increases.

Livingston and colleagues report that church affiliation was inversely related to blood pressure among black residents sampled in Maryland (Livingstone, Levine, & Moore, 1991). A study of blacks and whites in North Carolina provides direct evidence that social support is related to blood pressure among blacks (Williams, 1992). Health behaviors, such as excessive intake of alcohol, sodium, and dietary fat as well as inadequate physical activity, also are determinants of high blood pressure (Williams, 1990b). Many of the preferred foods among black Americans, including pork products, fried foods, and baked goods, are high in saturated fat, total fat, and sodium content (Magnus, 1991). Changing the types of foods and the methods of food preparation, as well as an increased level of physical activity, could potentially control hypertension without medication.

Stroke. Black men die from stroke at almost twice the rate of men in the total population, and black men's risk of nonfatal stroke also is higher (U.S. DHHS, 1990b). The incidence of stroke among southern blacks is nearly double that of southern whites, especially among the rural poor. The so-called "Stroke Belt," encompassing the southeastern United States, largely owes its higher stroke mortality to the black population living there.

Sickle cell anemia. This genetic blood disease, in which abnormal hemoglobin molecules fail to release sufficient oxygen to the tissues, affects more than 80,000 black Americans. The sickle cell trait, although more common in blacks, appears to result not from race but rather from geographic origin (Williams, Lavisso-Mourey, & Warren, 1994). Approximately 1 in 12 black babies in the United States is born with a genetic tendency to transmit the trait to offspring. It can result in severe pain, stroke, organ failure, and a life span shortened by 30 years. Health care providers need to screen individuals for this trait and support ongoing research into effective treatment. Although bone marrow transplants have successfully cured young patients with symptomatic sickle cell disease, there is risk of a fatal outcome (Walters et al., 1996).

Cancer. The incidence of cancer and the mortality rate for cancer have increased at an unprecedented rate in the black community over the past 30 years. The overall cancer incidence rate for blacks went up 27%, compared to an increase of 12% for whites. The cancer mortality rate is 27% higher for blacks than for other racial groups and has increased by nearly 50% over the past 30 years. This figure represents a 10% increase among black women and a 77% increase among black men (American Cancer Society, 1989).

Cancer sites in which blacks have significantly higher increases in incidence and mortality rates include the lung, colon-rectum, prostate, and esophagus. The number one site of cancer among black men is the digestive system, with an incidence rate of 123.5 per 100,000 (U.S. DHHS, 1989). Black patients are less likely than white patients to undergo surgical resection (68% vs. 78%), even after controlling for age, comorbidity, and location and extent of tumor. Black patients also are more like to die (2-year mortality rate of 40% vs. 33.5% in white patients) (Cooper, Yuan, Landefeld, & Rimm, 1996). Cancer of the prostate is more prevalent in black men, and black women have cervical cancer more than twice as often as do white women. When adjusted for social class, the black-white differential falls by 60% but does not disappear (Millon-Underwood & Sander, 1990).

Cigarette smoking prevalence is higher among black Americans, although whites tend to smoke more cigarettes per day than do blacks. Prevalence of smoking among white (38.3%) and Hispanic high school students (34%) is higher than among non-Hispanic black students (19.2%). Male black students are more than twice as likely (27.8%) as females (12.2%) to be current smokers (Office of Smoking and Health, 1996). Despite the fact that blacks smoke 20% fewer cigarettes, they have a higher incidence of lung cancer (Magnus, 1991).

Whether a person gets cancer depends on exposure to cancer-causing substances, a family history of cancer, and other factors. Whether a person dies from cancer depends on the availability of screening, the point at which the cancer is detected, and the type of treatment received. The latter are telltale markers of the quality and accessibility of health care, all of which reveal that black Americans come up short.

Infant mortality. Black babies are twice as likely as white babies to die before their first birthday (U.S. DHHS, 1990b). High rates of low birthweight among black babies account for many of these deaths, but even normal weight black babies have a greater risk of death. Black infant mortality rates are higher not only for babies in the first month of life but also for those between 1 month and 1 year of age. The gap between black and white rates of neonatal, postneonatal, and infant mortality continues to widen. In 1980, the total black infant mortality rate for live births (22.2%) was twice that for white babies (10.9%). By 1989, the black rate (18.6%) was 2.3 times the white rate (8.1%). Infant mortality rates, according to several studies, were higher for mothers with less than 12 years of schooling and lower for those with 16 or more years of schooling (Kleinman, Fingerhut, & Prager, 1990).

Only 61% of black women receive prenatal care in the first trimester of pregnancy (U.S. DHHS, 1990b). Each $1 spent on prenatal care saves between $3 and $20 in medical expenses in the infant's first year of life (Gorman, 1991).

Teenage pregnancy. Adolescent pregnancy is a major concern, according to *Healthy People 2000* (U.S. DHHS, 1990b), because of its social and economic consequences as much as its health effects. There are higher risks of infant mortality and low birthweight, especially for very young pregnant girls. But even greater risks indirectly threaten the health of both mothers and babies because of the patterns of poverty and low educational attainment that often become entrenched as a result of early childbearing. Actual rates of childbirth among black teenagers have dropped since the 1960s; however, because the number of girls in this population has risen by 20%, the total number of births has increased. Birthrates for black girls younger than 15 years of age were nearly five times higher than those for white girls in 1987 (U.S. DHHS, 1990b).

Obesity. Black women have a higher prevalence of obesity than do either white women or black men. In every age group above 20 years, 20% to 50% of black women are overweight compared to 10% to 20% of white women (Magnus, 1991). The rate of obesity increases with age; among black women in the 45- to

67-year age group, 60% are more than 20% above their ideal weights (Bowen, Tomoyasu, & Cause, 1991).

Bowen et al. (1991) attribute the weight problem of the population to three major risk factors, which they term the "triple threat": gender, race, and poverty. They contend that race and class play powerful but often neglected roles in women's weight and in the perceptions and attitudes that accompany it. Magnus (1991) reports that studies have found that obesity is six times more common among poor women than among affluent women.

Ethnic differences probably are not due to anthropometric differences, genetic differences, or differences in caloric intake between black and white females. Williams (1992) postulates that differences in physical exercise may be an important contributor to obesity in black females. Black women are more likely to be poor, to be single parents, and to reside in poor neighborhoods, making it difficult to find the facilities and opportunities to obtain physical exercise.

Bowen et al. (1991) suggests that obesity among poor blacks may be due to an external locus of control. Poor people often perceive that they cannot control their lives or the events in their environments. This sense of powerlessness reflects the limited choices imposed by economics; money creates choices, and without it you have none.

The dietary contribution to obesity also must be considered. Although "soul food" is thought to be for blacks only, this is a misconception. It is difficult to say who eats more of the so-called soul food—urban blacks, rural blacks, or their white counterparts. Bloch (1983) points out that the scraps of food and leftovers from the slavemasters' tables were the origin of much of the soul food. It was not the native food of the black community; rather, it had its roots in slavery, not in Africa. The diet of West Africa consists of mainly cereals, green vegetables, peas, beans, cassava, yams, and sweet potatoes. Slavemasters in the United States, however, fed their slaves as little as possible of the cheapest food available, which most often was pork and dried corn. Slaves contrived to make edible meals from pigs' trotters, knuckles, tails, ears, snouts, necks, stomachs (hog maw), and intestines (chitterlings). They marinated and smothered these and other scraps with seasonings such as Louisiana hot sauce and served them with turnips and collard greens, black-eyed peas, and hot cornbread, dishes that today are known as soul food (Mutumbi, 1981).

In recent years, pigs feet and chitterlings have been replaced in many black households by smoked sugared ham, pork chops, and barbecued ribs. Diets have expanded to include larger quantities of highly refined convenience foods. Frying and the frequent use of pork and pork fat continue to contribute a high content of saturated fats to the diet, a factor associated with increased risk of cancer and heart disease (Guillory, 1987).

Lactose intolerance. Fully 70% to 80% of adult blacks are estimated to be lactose intolerant, compared to 5% to 19% of whites (Kiple, 1981). Lactose intolerance, due to sufficient levels of the lactase enzyme, often is unrecognized in infants and leads to nausea, bloating, and diarrhea from drinking milk and using milk products. The condition worsens with age and may have adverse effects on the health of individuals unless it is recognized and appropriate dietary accommodations are made.

Mental health. Although blacks more often are exposed to social conditions considered to be important antecedents of psychiatric disorders, they do not have higher rates of mental illness than do whites (Williams, 1990a). According to the National Institute of Mental Health's Epidemiologic Catchment Area Program studies, 14% of black males had psychiatric disorders, compared to 13% of white males (Williams, 1992). In addition, 27% of black males in institutions had psychiatric disorders, compared to 26% of white males. Recently, there has been an increase in suicide rates among black males that peak in the 25- to 34-year age group, whereas white male rates peak for those age 65 years or over.

Williams (1990a) comments, "The overall evidence on black mental health clearly indicates that there are important resources and strengths in the black community that [are] protecting the community from the onslaught of pathogenic stressors" (p. 26). One of these important and neglected resources probably is black churches. Renewed research attention should be given to the possible health-promoting functions of religious involvement.

Historically, the major diagnostic category of mentally ill blacks was tertiary syphilis. The infamous Tuskegee study[1] corroborates this.

Chemical dependency. Chemical dependence, particularly the use of illegal drugs such as crack, marijuana, and PCP, is a major threat to the black community. Its dramatic impact is evidenced by increased crime, wanton violence, mental disorders, family disruptions, and social problems in school and on the job.

The impact of cocaine abuse results in an unprecedented number of children being abused, neglected, or mistreated. Many parents seeking the next crack fix abandon their young children in the streets and hospitals. They sell food stamps and their children's clothes for drug money. Some have even sold their children as prostitutes. The neglected children eat what they can find and spend hours— sometimes days—alone. Some 6-year-olds have been found taking care of their younger brothers and sisters.

More so than with any other drug, crack addicts are found among young mothers with small children, few child-rearing skills, and no spouses to share the load. In the extended family, even some of the grandparents are addicted. The rates of infant mortality, sudden infant death syndrome, child abuse, and HIV infection are significantly linked to maternal substance abuse, most often caused by crack/cocaine but also by other illegal drugs and alcohol.

Violence, homicide, and intentional injuries. Violence is a public health issue with an impact on quality of life. Violent behavior is committed disproportionately by young males (late teens to early 30s) situated in the lowest levels of socioeconomic status. They are more likely to be not only the perpetrators but also the victims of violence. Although there is an overrepresentation of blacks (44% of all homicide victims are black) and other nonwhites in U.S. violence statistics, Page et al. (1992) point out that socioeconomic status is a better predictor of violence than is racial status.

Many black children and adolescents grow up in poverty, which increases their exposure to and experience with violence. Thus, they are at risk for using or experiencing violence in their interpersonal relationships. In some neighborhoods, close to 25% of elementary and high school students have seen someone killed (Bell & Jenkins, 1990).

Bell and Jenkins (1990) state that when women kill their partners, the women often have been physically abused and are acting in self-defense. Black men are more likely than white men to be killed by spouses who are acting in self-defense. Approximately 1 in 29 black males becomes a murder victim. By comparison, 1 in 124 black females, 1 in 186 white males, and 1 in 606 white females become murder victims (Page et al., 1992).

Violence prevention should include family and school interventions designed to teach children and parents problem-solving skills for conflict resolution, anger control, communication skills, and substance abuse prevention (Page et al., 1992).

HIV/AIDS. AIDS, a communicable disease first identified in 1981, is caused by the human immunodeficiency virus primarily transmitted through semen, vaginal fluid, blood, or breast milk of infected people. Individuals often are infected and are infectious without knowledge of their HIV status, although there are various blood tests widely available to determine that status. The virus may lie dormant within the body, producing no symptoms, for up to 10 years, yet HIV-infected persons can be transmitting the virus to other individuals, usually through sexual intercourse (oral, vaginal, or anal) or through needle sharing among intravenous drug users.

At present, there is no vaccine available to prevent the infection by the virus. Early treatment may delay progression to AIDS. The use of antiviral agents also may prevent the transmission of the virus from mothers to their unborn infants. Treatment with a combination of protease inhibitors has been shown to clear HIV from the blood of infected individuals for up to 1 year.

Of the reported cases of AIDS in the United States, 53% are among whites and 30% are among black Americans, although only 12% of the U.S. population is black. The rate of AIDS among blacks is more than triple that among whites. Among women and children, the gap is even wider. Black women's risk of contracting AIDS is 10 to 15 times higher than that of white women. Black children account for more than 50% of all children with AIDS (U.S. DHHS, 1990b).

Intravenous drug-related HIV infection has been the primary mode of transmission for blacks. Most blacks with AIDS are either homosexual/bisexual men (35% to 38%) or heterosexual men and women who use intravenous drugs (38%) (Chng & Fridinger, 1994).

Barriers to preventive efforts include poverty, inadequate health care, mistrust, lack of knowledge, and low educational levels. The daily struggle for survival may make it difficult to consider preventive measures for a disease that can take a decade to develop. The risk is compounded for those who must resort to prostitution to ensure a ready supply of crack/cocaine or other drugs. Individuals who drink heavily or take drugs are more likely to engage in unprotected sex (U.S. DHHS, 1990a).

Fewer sources of health care, support for home care, and hospices have been available to members of minority communities. Blacks with AIDS might delay seeking help, leading to a shorter survival period after diagnosis than that for whites.

Black churches are beginning to be more accepting of persons with AIDS, although the belief that HIV is a divine indictment for a sinful life persists. Black churches, like many white fundamentalist churches, preach sexual fidelity and a drug-free life as the only solution to the HIV problem.

NATIONAL GOALS: IMPLICATIONS FOR HEALTH PROMOTION AND DISEASE PREVENTION AMONG BLACK AMERICANS

Since 1980, the United States has been setting national goals by decades, the most recent being published in *Healthy People 2000* (U.S. DHHS, 1990b). In 1990, the federal government established the Office of Minority Health to coordinate departmental efforts to reduce excess mortality and morbidity among blacks and other minorities. This office publishes regular updates on progress toward the national goals. In addition, it established a nationwide hotline (800-444-6472) to sources of information, maintaining a database of organizations and volunteers to assist in local minority health programs.

Healthy People 2000 lists nearly 50 objectives targeting black Americans. They range from reducing risk factors such as cigarette smoking, obesity, and teenage pregnancies to increasing the span of healthy life to at least 60 years. The goals are a recognition that medical care alone will not eliminate the devastating impact of chronic disease, the rate of infant mortality, and the burden of homicide and violence. Most of the goals are based on the assumption that individuals can control their own destinies in significant ways. This assumption means that the black community as a whole might not get to the promised land of *Healthy People 2000* because there exists a correlation between poor health and socioeconomic status.

Availability and Accessibility of Health Care and Resources

According to *Healthy People 2000* (U.S. DHHS, 1990b), "Statistics demonstrate with sharp clarity that blacks do not receive enough early, routine, and preventive care" (p. 33). Early prenatal care can reduce low birthweight and prevent infant deaths. Early detection of cancer can increase survival rates. Appropriate medical care can reduce the frequency and severity of the complications of diabetes. Information about actual use of health services confirms the lack of use among blacks. They make fewer annual visits to physicians than do whites, and black mothers are twice as likely as white mothers to receive no health care or care only in the final trimester of their pregnancies. Hospital emergency rooms and clinics are a more common source of medical care for blacks than for whites. In addition, 20% of blacks report no usual source of medical care, compared to 13% of whites. In 1986, 23% of blacks had no private or public medical insurance, compared to 14% of whites (U.S. DHHS, 1990b).

Studies have revealed that blacks are half as likely as whites to receive bypass operations for coronary artery disease. Of those undergoing dialysis for kidney disease, whites were 33% more likely to get kidney transplants. Blacks who were hospitalized for pneumonia received less intensive treatment than did whites (Gorman, 1991).

Correcting the inequities in health care alone will not solve the health problems of black Americans. Even those studies that find a positive impact for physician services note that the effect of medical care is small when compared to that of nonmedical variables (Williams & Collins, 1995). A reduction in cigarette smoking would do more to improve health than would an increase in medical expenditures. Goldman and Cook (1984) analyzed the decline in ischemic heart disease between 1968 and 1976. They found that changes in lifestyle saved more lives than did all medical interventions combined. Louis Sullivan, former Secretary of Health and Human Services, stated, "Stopping smoking, losing weight, and cutting down on alcohol consumption could eliminate up to 45% of deaths from cardiovascular disease, 23% of the deaths from cancer, and more than 50% of the disabling complications of diabetes" (quoted in Gorman, 1991, p. 52).

Caveats When Generalizing About Health and Black Americans

Stereotypes may be commonplace and convenient for conservation of thought, but they have no place in a health worker's practice. As this chapter has shown, black Americans have been shaped by 400 years of history, the forces of slavery, migration, and socioeconomic status. There are as great a number of differences within the black American population group as among it and other population groups in the United States. Health professionals should remember the following caveats when working with individuals who consider themselves black Americans:

- Not all black Americans share the same history or culture; many are immigrants who may or may not identify with the term *African American*.
- Health beliefs and practices will vary between urban and rural blacks and between countries of origin.
- Socioeconomic status has a greater impact on health status than does ethnicity.
- Lifestyle risk factors are more important predictors of diseases than is ethnicity (e.g., intravenous drug use and HIV infection).
- Health promotion and health care programs need to be tailored to the identified needs of individuals wherever possible; health beliefs and concerns can be elicited by asking individuals in a manner that demonstrates genuine care and concern.

CHAPTER SUMMARY AND RECOMMENDATIONS

Black Americans, through their 400-year history in the United States, have a legacy that results in their suffering a disproportionate rate of disease, less access to and use of curative and preventive health care, and a mistrust of the health care system. Many continue to rely on self-care and ethnomedicine and on the extended family primarily or in parallel with scientific medical care.

Health beliefs and practices vary according to the degree of acculturation, country of origin, education level, socioeconomic level, and time of acquiring freedom historically. The health care practitioner should avail himself or herself of the information available from the literature and directly from patients and community members with whom the practitioner works in planning appropriate programs of health care and health promotion. The health practitioner should use community resources, such as black churches, that are respected as an integral part of black communities. The practitioner also should respond positively to the challenge to add to the body of knowledge about differences among subgroups by reporting, through case studies or other qualitative methods, the results of his or her observations and interactions with these members of American society.

NOTE

1. Jones's (1981) publication, *Bad Blood: The Tuskegee Syphilis Experiment—A Tragedy of Race and Medicine,* records the 40-year government-sponsored study of rural black men with syphilis to monitor the venereal disease's long-term effects. Although 399 men were examined, they never were treated. Even after the discovery of penicillin during the 1940s, their symptoms were left unchecked. Although they received free physical examinations, free rides to and from the clinics, and burial stipends, they were deceived into thinking that they were receiving treatment. Nearly 100 of the men died from direct complications of the disease. The study was discontinued after public outcry in 1972.

REFERENCES

Adams, D. L. (1995). Cultural diversity and institutional inequity. In D. L. Adams (Ed.), *Health issues for women of color.* Thousand Oaks, CA: Sage.

Aday, L. A. (1993). *At risk in America: The health and health care needs of vulnerable populations in the United States.* San Francisco: Jossey-Bass.

Airhihenbuwa, C. O., & Harrison, I. E. (1993). Traditional medicine in Africa: Past, present and future. In P. Conrad & E. Gallagher (Eds.), *Healing and health care in developing countries.* Philadelphia: Temple University Press.

American Cancer Society. (1989). *Cancer facts and figures.* New York: Author.

Bell, C., & Jenkins, E. (1990). Preventing black homocide. In J. Dewart (Ed.), *The state of Black America, 1990.* New York: National Urban League.

Bloch, B. (1983). Nursing care of black patients. In M. S. Orgue, B. Bloch, & L. S. Monrroy (Eds.), *Ethnic nursing care: A multi-cultural approach.* St. Louis, MO: C. V. Mosby.

Bowen, D. J., Tomoyasu, N., & Cause, A. M. (1991). The triple threat: A discussion of gender, class and race differences in weight. *Women and Health, 17,* 123-143.

Braithwaite, R. L., & Taylor, S. E. (Eds.). (1992). *Health issues in the black community.* San Francisco: Jossey-Bass.

Cabral, H., Fried, L. E., Levenson, S., Amaro, H., & Zuckerman, B. (1990). Foreign-born and U.S. born black women: Differences in health behaviors and birth outcomes. *American Journal of Public Health, 80,* 70-72.

Caplan, L. R. (1991). Cardiovascular disease and stroke in African-Americans and other racial minorities in the United States: Strokes in African-Americans. *American Health Association Scientific Statement: Special Report, 83,* 1469-1470.

Chng, C. L., & Fridinger, F. W. (1994). The African American community and HIV: Personal reflections. *Journal of Health Education, 25,* 51-55.

Congress, E. P., & Lyons, B. P. (1992). Cultural differences in health beliefs: Implications for social work practice in health care settings. *Social Work in Health Care, 17*(3), 81-96.

Cooper, G. S., Yuan, Z., Landefeld, C. S., & Rimm, A. A. (1996). Surgery for colorectal cancer: Race-related differences in rates and survival among Medicare beneficiaries. *American Journal of Public Health, 86,* 582-586.

Coughlin, E. K. (1987, October 28). Scholars work to refine Africa-centered view of the life and history of black Americans. *Chronicle of Higher Education,* p. 32.

Flaskerud, J. H., & Rush, C. E. (1989). AIDS and traditional health beliefs and practices of black women. *Nursing Research, 38,* 210-215.

Gavin, J. R. (1995, February). Testimony to the Congressional Black Caucus Health Brain Trust. *Diabetes Dispatch: News from the American Diabetes Association,* pp. 53-55.

Goldman, L., & Cook, E. F. (1984). The decline in ischemic heart disease: An analysis of the comparative effects of medical interventions and changes in lifestyles. *Annals of Internal Medicine, 101,* 825-836.

Gorman, C. (1991, September 16). Why blacks die young. *Time,* p. 52.

Gregg, J., & Curry, R. H. (1994). Explanatory models for cancer among African-American women at two Atlanta neighborhood health centers: The implications for a cancer screening program. *Social Science Medicine, 39,* 519-526.

Guillory, J. (1987). Ethnic perspectives of cancer nursing: The black American. *Oncology Nursing Forum, 14*(3), 66-69.

Heckler, M. M. (1985). *Report of the Secretary's Task Force on Black and Minority Health,* Vol. 1: *Executive summary.* Washington, DC: Government Printing Office.

Institute of Medicine. (1988). *Homelessness, health and human needs.* Washington, DC: National Academy Press.

Jacques, G. (1976). Cultural health traditions: A black perspective. In M. F. Blanck & P. P. Paxton (Eds.), *Providing safe nursing care for ethnic people of color.* Norwalk, CT: Appleton-Century-Crofts.

Jones, J. H. (1981). *Bad blood: The Tuskegee Syphilis Experiment—A tragedy of race and medicine.* New York: Free Press.

Kiple, K. (1981). *Another dimension to the black diaspora: Diet, disease and racism.* New York: Cambridge University Press.

Kleinman, J. C., Fingerhut, L. A., & Prager, K. (1990). Differences in infant mortality by race, nativity status, and other maternal characteristics. *American Journal of Diseases of Children, 145,* 194-199.

Livingstone, L. R., Levine, D. M., & Moore, R. D. (1991). Social integration and black intraracial variation in blood pressure. Cited in Williams, D. R. (1992). Black-white differences in blood pressure: The role of social factors. *Ethnicity and Disease, 2,* 125-141.

Magnus, M. H. (1991). Cardiovascular health among African-Americans: A review of the health status, risk reduction and intervention strategies. *American Journal of Health Promotion, 5,* 282-290.

McBride, D. (1993). Black America: From community health care to crisis medicine. *Journal of Health Politics, Policy and Law, 18,* 319-334.

McCord, C., & Freeman, H. P. (1990, January 18). Excess mortality in Harlem. *New England Journal of Medicine,* pp. 173-177.

Millon-Underwood, S., & Sander, E. (1990). Factors contributing to health promotion behaviors among African American men. *Nursing Oncology Forum, 17,* 707-712.

Mutumbi, D. (1981, July). African homeland. *East West Journal,* pp. 38-41.

Office of Smoking and Health, Division of Adolescent and School Health, National Center for Chronic Disease Prevention and Health Promotion. (1996). Tobacco use and usual source of cigarettes among high school students: United States, 1995. *Journal of School Health, 66*(6), 222-224.

Page, R. M., Kitchin-Becker, S., Solovan, D., Golec, T. L., & Hebert, D. L. (1992). Interpersonal violence: A priority issue for health education. *Journal of Health Education, 23,* 286-292.

Rich, C. (1976). Born with the veil: Black folklore in Louisiana. *Journal of American Folklore, 89,* 328-335.

Rotter, J. B. (1966). Generalized expectancies for internal versus external control of reinforcement. *Psychological Monographs, 80* (No. 609).

Snow, L. F. (1974). Folk medical beliefs and their implications for care of patients. *Annals of Internal Medicine 81,* 82-96.

Snow, L. F. (1978). Sorcerers, saints and charlatans: Black folk healers in urban America. *Culture, Medicine and Psychiatry, 2,* 69-106.

Snow, L. F. (1983). Traditional health beliefs and practices among lower class black Americans. *Western Journal of Medicine, 139,* 820-828.

Sowell, T. (1981). *Ethnic America: A history.* New York: HarperCollins.

Sowell, T. (1994). *Race and culture: A world view.* New York: HarperCollins.

Thomas, S. B. (1992). Health status of the black community in the 21st century: A futuristic perspective for health education. *Journal of Health Education, 23,* 7-13.

U.S. Bureau of the Census. (1992). *The black population in the United States: March 1992.* Washington, DC: Government Printing Office.

U.S. Department of Health and Human Services. (1989). *Cancer statistics review 1973-1985.* Washington, DC: National Cancer Institute.

U.S. Department of Health and Human Services. (1990a). *Closing the gap: AIDS/HIV infection and minorities.* Washington, DC: Government Printing Office.

U.S. Department of Health and Human Services. (1990b). *Healthy People 2000.* Washington, DC: Government Printing Office.

U.S. Department of Health and Human Services. (1996, May 3). Healthy People 2000 progress report for heart disease and stroke. *Morbidity and Mortality Weekly Report,* p. 17.

U.S. Department of Health and Human Services. (1995). *Progress report for heart disease and stroke.* Washington, DC: Government Printing Office.

Vander Zanden, J. (1972). *American minority relations* (3rd ed.). New York: Rondal.

Walters, M. C., Patience, M., Leisenring, W., Eckman, J. W., Scott, J. P., Mentzer, W. C., Davies, S. E., Ohene-Frempong, K., Bernaudin, F., Matthews, D. C., Storm, R., & Sullivan, K. M. (1996, August 8). Bone marrow transplantation for sickle cell disease. *New England Journal of Medicine,* pp. 369-376.

Webb, J. Y. (1971). Louisiana voodoo and superstitions related to health. *HSMHA Health Reports, 86,* 291-301.

Will, J. C., & Casper, M. (1996). The contribution of diabetes to early deaths from ischemic heart disease: U.S. gender and racial comparisons. *American Journal of Public Health, 86,* 576-579.

Williams, D. R. (1990a). Social structure and the health status of black males. *Challenge: A Journal of Research on Black Men, 1,* 25-46.

Williams, D. R. (1990b). Socioeconomic differentials in health: A review and redirection. *Social Psychology Quarterly, 53,* 81-99.

Williams, D. R. (1992). Black-white differences in blood pressure: The role of social factors. *Ethnicity and Disease, 2,* 125-141.

Williams, D. R. (1996). The health of the African American population. In S. Petrosa & R. Rhomboid (Eds.), *Origins and destinies: Immigration, race and ethnicity in America.* Belmont, CA: Wadsworth.

Williams, D. R., & Collins, C. (1995). U.S. socioeconomic and racial differences in health: Patterns and explanations. *Annual Review of Sociology, 21,* 349-386.

Williams, D. R., Lavisso-Mourey, R., & Warren, R. C. (1994). The concept of race and health status in America. *Public Health Reports, 109,* 28-41.

11

Health Promotion Planning in African American Communities

MARY ASHLEY

In developing health promotion and disease prevention (HPDP) programs for Americans of African ancestry, health promoters providing such programs must research, understand, and appreciate the history of African Americans in this country. Through this process, the health promoter and planning team will have an opportunity to address their own prejudices and stereotypes while learning about the community targeted for intervention. Special attention should be focused on the history of institutionalized racism and discrimination experienced by African Americans with respect to health care, educational opportunities, housing, and employment.

The early 20th century found most blacks living in the southern United States without any formalized system of health care. In addition, many were living in substandard housing under poor sanitary conditions and with less than adequate nutritional resources. Those blacks who migrated to the urban North found their living conditions to be somewhat better, although poverty, substandard living conditions, and inadequate health care continued to be problematic (Quinn, 1996). Such conditions greatly affected the health status of black Americans, and the vestige of these conditions still is apparent in many black communities today. Racism continues to be a major contributor to disparate health outcomes between black and white Americans, with structural inequities and institutional racism in the health care system and health education infrastructures (Byrd, 1990; Byrd & Clayton, 1993; Hirsch, 1991). This disparity in health status has been widely discussed by a number of writers since early in this century. Many of these agree that factors related to lifestyle, reduced access to health care resources, a lack of health insurance, limited knowledge of HPDP behaviors and practices increased exposure to environmental hazards and toxins, and certain genetic variables have been major contributors to this problem (DuBois, 1903; Haynes, 1975). They also have noted that many of the health problems experienced by this population are preventable.

The purpose of this chapter is to provide a framework in which to inform the health promoter's approach to strategies that can be employed in the assessment, planning, implementation, and evaluation of HPDP programs and activities targeting African American communities. For clarity, it should be noted that the terms *black* and *African American* are used interchangeably because many researchers continue to use them in this manner. Because the factors inherent in the health status of African Americans.are complex and long-standing, the task of achieving parity also is complex and multifaceted. HPDP programs play a major role in addressing the existing disparities between whites and African Americans.

BRIEF OVERVIEW OF AFRICAN AMERICAN CULTURAL AND HEALTH ISSUES

African Americans are not a homogeneous group. There is great diversity within populations in general, and there is much variation in attitudes, behaviors, and values regarding health, health promotion, and disease prevention (Herring & Montgomery, 1996). Contrary to what some may believe, slavery was not the genesis of differences in African Americans as a group. Because slaves were brought from different regions, they came with different languages, values, health beliefs and practices, and religious orientations. Within the slave culture, they were differentiated by skin color, class, social status, religious beliefs, physical health and physique, and job assignments (Byrd, 1990). These variations in cultural attributes significantly influence the patterns of access and use of health promotion activities within the African American community. However, because of the American experience, most African Americans have developed cultural values that are similar.

African Americans lag behind many other U.S. populations on virtually all health status indicators. In fact, six of these account for most of this disparity: cancer, heart disease and stroke, homicide and unintentional injuries, infant mortality, diabetes, and substance abuse (Quinn, 1996; U.S. Department of Health and Human Services, 1995). As can be seen, all of these indicators can be prevented or controlled. That these disparities continue unabated was the topic of a report by McGinnis and Lee (1995) in which they observed that the 7-year gap in life expectancy between blacks and whites continues to be a problem and has, in fact, widened since 1980. The inability to narrow this gap suggests that social factors such as education, employment, public access, and other factors outside the traditional health arenas might have a significant impact on health outcomes. Sociocultural and behavioral lifestyle issues are highly correlated with these disparities (Zelasko, 1995). Health education as a primary tool for HPDP is potentially an efficient and effective strategy for improving the health status of all Americans. This is especially true in poor minority communities in which the most elementary information about disease and disease prevention very often is absent. Because the primary focus of prevention is on knowledge, attitudes, and behaviors that are amenable to change, the range of prevention strategies in these communities should span early childhood to the most senior members of the community (Haynes & Ashley, 1993).

Where and how to develop the needed strategies to improve the health of African American and other minority communities is an important issue. Penn and his colleagues suggest that whatever health problems exist in a community can be effectively resolved if they are addressed within the social context of each ethnocultural group (Penn, Kar, Kramer, Skinner, & Zambrana, 1995). This would seem to reflect the concept of starting where the people are when designing HPDP strategies and interventions. Of necessity, all HPDP programs should be grounded in scientific theory that has been tested in the populations to be affected by the project. The elements for achieving successful programs in the African American community are no different in their basic tenets from those in any other community. The application of these elements may differ, but there must be adherence to the basic constructs common to all HPDP program planning efforts—needs assessment, program plan development, implementation, and evaluation. The following sections focus on how each of these elements may be successfully applied to programs developed for African American communities where the target group may be welfare recipients or upper-middle-class individuals and families.

NEEDS ASSESSMENT

The health promoter's first task in program development is to conduct a needs assessment to determine the wants, needs, and perceptions of the community regarding HPDP programs and services. A major hurdle in this process is in gaining access to the community. African Americans have a healthy suspicion about programs that have their roots in traditional Western health institutions. This is because many of these communities have seen programs and services come and go at the seeming whim of the institutions and granting agencies that have brought them into the community. Entrée to the community many times is another delicate matter. Even individuals of the same ethnic background are suspect because they often are educated and trained by institutions outside of the community and might be seen as sharing the values and attitudes of these institutions rather than those of the community in which they will be working. The health promoter will find it necessary to prove that he or she is sincere in his or her concerns about the community regardless of the health promoter's ethnic origin. Forging relationships and involvement of community members from the beginning and throughout the entire life of the program will be a critical ingredient. This includes developing positive alliances with both the formal and informal leadership of the community, joining with trusted members of the community, and identifying and working with an individual or community organization that can assist the health promoter in gaining access to other individuals, groups, and organizations in the targeted population to be served by the HPDP program or service. A failure to connect with key persons in the community can undermine even the most sincere efforts of the health promoter. Finding these key leaders is not always an easy matter. There may be different leaders for different health issues. For example, in one urban community in which the author was involved, the leadership was divided among three powerful black women. In this case, a failure to involve any one of them was tantamount to disaster. Thus, identifying those people who are the major players in the community, including what their perceived and real roles are with respect to health issues, is an absolutely critical activity to undertake.

So, how does the health promoter find and meet these important people? The health promoter might begin by being seen in the community, attending community events, going to church in the community, and engaging in other similar activities where the health promoter may be approached by someone who can assist him or her or even champion the cause of the program. In addition, compiling a list of key individuals and organizations such as religious and civic leaders, local citizens groups, community coalitions with a health focus, non-health organizations (e.g., 100 Black Men, 100 Black Women, the Links, Eastern Star, the Masons), sororities, fraternities, and historically black colleges and universities within the community can be most helpful. Fully engaging a community in HPDP planning efforts and processes might be more difficult in rural settings. Local ministers and other religious leaders have been successfully enlisted for health program support in rural areas, and the use of lay health advisers has been found to be very effective in delivering HPDP programs and services (Eng & Hatch, 1991). Once these people and organizations have been identified, the health promoter must realize that they might have different purposes and agendas that may or may not include health. A case in point is churches, which frequently are mentioned in the literature as ideal sites for health programs. Churches are not easy targets for such involvement. Ministers are busy people, and they frequently are approached to assist with many causes of which health programs are but one of many different issues. Church size and the educational level of the minister have been identified as the strongest predictors of participation, with larger churches and better educated ministers more likely to participate in HPDP programs (Quinn, Billingsley, & Caldwell, 1994).

Once the health promoter has made and cultivated the necessary contacts, the next step is to develop a planning committee of appropriate people including individuals to be served by the HPDP program or service. A group of 15 to 20 individuals is a good working size, and keeping the group together is of utmost importance to ensure continuity and representative involvement of the community in the planning process. The health promoter will find that regular contact with group members from the community is one strategy that works especially well in fostering trust, friendship, and motivation to stay involved in the working relationship. Although conventional wisdom dictates that the health promoter maintain a strictly professional relationship, personal experience has demonstrated that interacting in the real-life events of individuals within the community is enriching for those involved and provides a glimpse, at a deeper level, into the barriers and incentives that motivate action within the community.

Depending on the population to be served and the behaviors being targeted for change, the health promoter will need to have at his or her disposal a "bag" of possible strategies for involving community residents in the needs assessment process. Different behavioral issues might call for different data collection approaches. For instance, open discussions within a community forum setting might be appropriate for exploring issues and behaviors relating to hypertension. However, the more private issues such as sexuality might best lend themselves to personal interviews. Regardless of the strategy selected, any procedures or instruments used to collect the needed data must be pretested with the group that will be the focus of the assessment process. Criteria for the design and use of an instrument should include appropriate literacy level and appropriate language and cultural symbols for the target population, and it should be culturally relevant. Frequently, standardized questionnaires are developed for the majority culture and contain questions that have little or no meaning in the lives of the target population. This became evident to the author when she was reviewing a telephone survey instrument for breast health. Many of the questions needed restructuring for use in the African American community. Unfortunately, many surveys being developed in the university setting have little input from those in the minority communities who are to be targeted for assessment using these instruments. Occasionally, these types of instruments are pilot tested by having African American students or clerical staff critique the instrument. But this does not constitute an adequate pretest because it does not represent a sufficient review by a cross section of the community in which the instrument will be employed. Cottrell et al. (1995) describe tasks that community groups can help facilitate in the needs assessment process. These include identification of community needs, identification of issues that should be considered and included in the needs assessment instrument, and priorities of the community in which the needs assessment and subsequent HPDP program or service will occur. A variety of strategies should be used to collect data for the needs assessment. Cottrell et al. suggest four major domains to explore when conducting assessments in inner-city communities:

- *Historical information:* This includes historical events, major conflicts and concerns of the community such as civil unrest and the manner in which the community has related to police and other public agencies, demographic changes such as the influx of other ethnic groups, and the reputation and perceptions of health care providers and health institutions in the community.

- *Economic and political information:* This includes the socioeconomic levels within the community such as the percentages of families classified as lower, middle, and upper-middle income; the percentage of families receiving public assistance; educational levels; ownership of local businesses; identification of the primary providers of health services to the community; the structure and involvement of local political representatives in helping to resolve perceived problems in the community; and the organizations that successfully serve the community.

- *Traditional or culture-specific issues:* This includes how the target group defines health and illness; common beliefs and health practices that carry over from previous generations such as the use of herbs and faith healers; the predominant family structures in the community; the role of women as formal and informal leaders; the channels of communication that are used in the community to convey health and other types of information; what various age and gender groups perceive as the major health problems of the community; general beliefs about disease causation, prevention, and treatment; the use of nontraditional medicine; experience with the existing health delivery system; and the community's usual sources for health information.

- *Religious issues:* This includes identification of the religious leaders in the community and the level and types of involvement religious organizations in the community have with health issues and problems. There are several predominant religious groups found in African American communities including Baptist, Methodist, and members of the charismatic or Holiness Faith. The author has noted that it often is very difficult to motivate a church to deal with certain issues such as teen pregnancy, safer sex, and issues regarding AIDS. In one case with which the author was involved, even cancer education and prevention was an unacceptable area for one church to be involved in until the minister's wife was diagnosed with this disease. Religion plays a major role in illness and quality-of-life issues in the African American community, and although this has many positive benefits, it also can serve to foster fatalistic attitudes and feelings of hopelessness in some members of the community.

Strategies for collecting needs assessment data will vary with the community and the health issues to be addressed. Some suggested strategies that have been successfully used include community surveys (both self-administered and assisted questionnaires), focus groups, direct interviews, community forums, and the collection of health services data. A brief description of each of these might prove useful to those who are less familiar with these approaches.

Community Surveys

Community surveys can be used for any target group and nearly any target behavior. The most critical factor to be considered in the use of this approach is that of the literacy level of the instrument. Because of the African American experience in the educational system, the reading skills within the community might be low. This is especially true for older individuals in both rural and urban settings. The health promoter should be watchful for older citizens who say that they left their glasses at home and adolescents who clown around when asked to complete a questionnaire or other form. This might be an indication of an inability to read. They also might make marks on the questionnaire or form without being able to read, which might give a false impression of the literacy level of the individual or of the true needs of the community. For example, in one study with which the author was involved, a project instrument was being tested for a program to assist senior citizens with taking multiple medications. During the pretesting of the instrument, it became apparent that a number of participants were not completing the form, and their most common reason was that they did not have their glasses. The health educator in the setting decided to read each question and record responses from participants, which resulted in being able to conduct a successful pilot test of the instrument. This approach must, however, be done with sensitivity and respect so as not to embarrass participants.

Several venues have been successfully used in collecting needs assessment data in African American communities. The first of these is the convenience sample approach taken at locations throughout the community. Although this is not a randomized sample, it can help to provide valuable information from community residents. For example, community grocery stores are an ideal location in which to conduct this type of data collection. Store managers usually are cooperative, especially if the health promoter uses incentives from their stores. Because shoppers often are primarily female, the use of other unconventional sites to capture a sufficient sample of males should be explored. These might include the local recreation center, pool halls, asphalt basketball courts, and barber shops. Other sites for women might include laundromats, nail shops, and beauty salons.

Focus Groups

The use of the focus group is a qualitative needs assessment strategy that has been identified as an efficient way in which to collect data about existing knowledge, attitudes, and beliefs that may be supporting or maintaining health-damaging behaviors in any given target community (Morgan, 1993). This method requires the selection of a diverse group of 8 to 12 people from the target group for which interventions are to be planned. The objective is to provide the group members with the opportunity to discuss their perceptions and experiences regarding the HPDP needs within their community. The information generated from the analysis of the group's responses can assist in establishing priorities and clarifying issues and problems that might not be considered in more traditional designs for health education and health promotion intervention (Lorig et al., 1996).

Direct Interviews

Direct face-to-face interviews can be another effective way in which to generate information about the needs and interests of the community for HPDP programs and services. This approach requires skill and a knowledge of the community including the "turfs," factions, and agendas of the organizations and recognized leaders (both formal and informal) in the community. This was brought home to the author very clearly in a program targeted to senior citizens in an inner-city community. A committee was organized to discuss and plan the program, but one individual who was a major influence on senior issues in the community was left out of the planning group. The result of this error in not recognizing and including this important community person was that it delayed implementation of the program by several months. The lesson learned was that it is critical to involve all individuals and organizations, at least initially, in the planning efforts, even though they might actually oppose a particular HPDP project. Obviously, this can present challenges, but it also presents opportunities for education and compromise that might be needed to ensure the success of the program.

It is important to include a diverse cross section of the community if the health promoter is doing direct interviews, and it is especially important to include members of the target group on whom the program will be focused. Service providers also should be interviewed because they might be able to provide in-depth information and perspectives on current services and use patterns of the target group that might provide insight to the planning team. They also might be able to provide additional suggestions for HPDP content, format, and logistics of potential interventions. This interaction also may serve to facilitate their buy-in and support for the proposed intervention (Jemmatt & Jemmatt, 1992).

Community Forums

The community forum approach allows for the involvement of significantly greater numbers of individuals from the community to voice their issues and concerns about the needs of the community. It is especially useful when broad community issues are to be discussed. Generally, a community forum might involve 50 or more people and organizations from the community, all coming together under one roof to talk. This approach frequently is used by represen-tatives of local government to gather input on specific program activities and resource distribution allocations. Using the community forum method requires that the meeting be carefully thought out and planned to ensure that the discussion that occurs is not monopolized by a few individuals and especially by those who might represent a dissenting point of view.

Community forums often surface issues that the health promoter has no immediate ability to address. For instance, a forum might be called to address a health-related issue, but the participants want to discuss issues that have greater relevance for them at that moment such as crime, violence in the community, jobs, street lighting, and other community concerns. In this case, it is important to recognize that the health promoter can work with other individuals and agencies within the community to begin addressing these issues while at the same time working to resolve the health issues or problems that were the reason for the forum to be held. When planning a forum on a specific health issue, be sure that you have presenters who can speak to the level of the audience while at the same time being attentive to the issues raised by the participants. Regardless of what might be discussed in the meeting, the forum should be closed with a reminder of why it was called (the health promoter's issues) and some suggestions about where to go from that point with respect to all the issues that were raised. Remember that any community forum will be shaped within the context of what may be happening in the community at the time of the event. The climate on the day of the forum may be different from what was expected, and this may result in outcomes other than those intended. So, be prepared.

Health Services Data

Throughout the country in both small and large communities, there are agencies that collect information about their citizens. Both vital statistics and other health data are published on a regular basis by county health departments, and many private and federal agencies also publish information on health issues of the general public. Of concern here is that although these data identify the problems that are of the most concern to public health officials and health care providers, these issues might not be perceived as major concerns within local communities. In a study conducted at Drew University in Los Angeles, it was observed that African Americans did not perceive themselves to be at risk for cancer at the same level as did whites. In this unpublished study, it also was noted that gangs and violence were cited most often by adults as major problems for the community. By contrast, there was not a single instance in which infant mortality was identified by the community as a major health issue. In this case, it appears that the community's responses were a reflection of age and personal experience rather than of any sense of there being a widespread health problem in the community. Thus, it might be necessary to increase the community's perceptions and understanding of a particular health issue or problem before any major intervention work can be carried out.

The needs assessment process also should seek to gather data about the communication and information sources the community uses to stay informed or to find out what may be happening. This would include local newspaper, television, and radio resources used by the community because these can help to give insight into community functioning and also can serve as major communication channels for promoting the HPDP program or service to be offered in the community. The list of strategies discussed here is by no means exhaustive. The planner will need to be creative and flexible in deciding what approaches will work best in his or her targeted community, and the best approach is generally a combination of all of these. Whenever possible, community members should be included in helping to carry out the assessment activities, and training components to prepare these community members will need to be built into the needs assessment process. This also carries over into the analysis of the data that are gathered. Be sure to build in a reporting process to inform the community of the results of the assessment process using plain language rather than professional jargon, which can serve to confuse community residents. The better the community members understand the health promoter, the easier it is for them to believe the health promoter is really interested in them.

PROGRAM PLANNING

Fueled by the findings in the assessment phase, the planning process begins. The health promoter must consider a theoretical model or framework for the program to be developed. Because there are a number of possible theoretical models and frameworks available to the planner, selecting an appropriate one can be a frustrating process. Few HPDP programs use the strict models identified in the health promotion and education literature. Hochbaum, Sorenson, and Lorig (1992) observe that it might be difficult to apply some of the theories currently available but comment that they still can be useful guides for selecting or developing the most promising approaches to a given situation. Frequently, the choice is to use a combination of theories that may focus on both predicting change and measuring actual behavioral outcomes (Clark & McLeroy, 1995). Ryan and Heaney (1993) suggest a process for selecting a workable theory that begins by first knowing the specific target population, the behaviors that are to be targeted, and the goals and objectives the program will try to reach. They also identify criteria for selecting a useful theory using questions such as the following:

- Does the theory complement and flow with the worldview of the target group?
- Has the theory been tested on a population similar to the one to be served in the developing program?
- Has the theory been used in a program similar to the one being developed?
- Has the theory been successfully used in other programs with the target population?
- Does the theory make sense to the health promoter?

Two theories that are similar in their approach and that have usefulness in addressing HPDP programs in African American communities are social learning theory and the theory of planned change. Social learning theory, which was renamed social cognitive theory by Bandura (1986), is concerned with the cognitive, environmental, and behavioral variables that help describe human behavior and learning. The application of this theory is discussed extensively by Ryan and Heaney (1993), who note three factors involved in the behavior change process that must be modified for a new behavior to be acquired, performed, and sustained over time. These include having the necessary skills to perform the desired behavior, believing that one is capable of carrying out the new behavior, and believing that performing the desired behavior will result in a desired outcome. These three variables are especially important when addressing issues in the black community. The theory of planned behavior (Ajzen, 1991; Ajzen & Driver, 1991; Ajzen & Madden, 1986), which is an extension of the theory of reasoned action (Fishbein, 1967), is discussed by Gielen and colleagues as a plausible theory for use in HPDP efforts (Gielen, Wilson, Faden, Wilson, & Harvilchuck, 1995). They note that the theory seeks to predict behavioral intention to actually carry out any given behavior on the basis of personal beliefs about performing the behavior including evaluation of possible outcomes of the behavior, attitudes toward the behavior, the influence of normative and subjective beliefs, motivations to comply with normative pressures, and perceived behavioral control including barriers and resources necessary to perform the behavior (Gielen et al., 1995). These models are valuable frameworks, not only for thinking about health behavior change in the African American community but also because they suggest areas for inclusion in the needs assessment process that can provide data on current knowledge, attitudes, and beliefs held by the target group. With this information, interventions can be structured that take into account the areas where deficits may exist and where work needs to be done to facilitate new health-promoting behaviors within the target group.

Once decisions have been reached about a theoretical approach to the health issue or problem, the health promoter will need to turn his or her attention to the more practical issues of planning the program. This includes consideration of the planning team, that is, the need to maintain and perhaps expand the team's membership to ensure that all parties that have a stake in the outcome of the proposed program or service are involved in the process. It is important to cultivate and care for the planning team to help facilitate its members' ongoing commitment and motivation in the planning, implementation, and evaluation process. Thus, periodic reassessment of the quality of the core group with respect to whether it represents the diversity of the target group the health promoter is trying to reach will be necessary; where indicated, new members might need to be added. It is important that planning sessions be made public and held in an easily accessible and safe location such as a church, school, or library in the community. An agenda should be included with every meeting, and some discussion of what it will take to plan and carry out a program should be included so that the planning team members have some sense of the magnitude of the work that may be required of them. Blacks have a healthy learned skepticism about new programs and projects starting in the community. Historical events and personal experiences have fostered a negative attitude about being used as "guinea pigs" by local agencies and outside organizations such as state and federal agencies, colleges, and universities where projects have been initiated and then abandoned because of loss of funding, leaving no lasting benefits to the community and its residents.

Following assessment of needs in the community and organization of the planning team, goals and measurable objectives need to be determined, based on the resources and limitations of the planning agency and community. Boundaries must be set, priorities must be listed and agreed on, and compromise must be reached where this is necessary. An honest discussion of all these issues can help foster respect for the program staff who have the responsibility of seeing that the program is developed and carried out. The health promoter will need to be sensitive to the needs of planning team members because some will have their own vested interests that they will hope to promote through their involvement in the planning efforts. Identifying these interests early on in the process can help to minimize and/or bring into focus what these interests might be and how they might be addressed to benefit all parties to the planning process and the community in general. During the actual planning process, the health promoter should not forget relevant behavioral and environmental precursors, especially those that can be controlled by changes in behavior such as smoking, substance abuse, stress, uncontrolled high blood pressure, diet and nutrition, exercise, use of prenatal and other health services, easy access to weapons of violence, and related factors.

Accessibility to appropriate health services is an important consideration, and the planner needs to pay attention to the real and perceived barriers that may be preventing the target group from participation in or use of these, particularly as these same issues may carry over to participation or lack thereof in the program being planned. Often, it is a matter of competing priorities in the African American community, that is, basic survival needs such as food, shelter, safety, child care, and employment. There also may be cultural issues such as obesity, a condition that has an impact on cardiovascular disease and cancer and is more socially acceptable for many older black women. Environmental factors such as lack of transportation and unsafe neighborhoods may affect the willingness of community members to participate in affordable HPDP programs such as walking and bicycling.

Lack of knowledge about health issues and prevention practices within the target group is a major consideration for those working in low-income African American communities. This often is manifested in a general belief in the community that residents are not at risk for unfavorable outcomes as a result of their lifestyle practices. A major part of developing and improving a culture of health promotion in African American communities will be instilling a sense of awareness about individual health risks. For example, in a series of focus groups conducted with involvement of the author in Southern California that focused on breast and prostrate cancer, participants expressed a lack of knowledge about their risks for acquiring these diseases. This suggests that a major emphasis should be placed on awareness and risks before or in conjunction with efforts to teach and promote screening and periodic checkups for specific health conditions.

IMPLEMENTATION

Marin and his colleagues (1995) describe a set of criteria that should be considered when planning interventions for underserved population groups. They note that the intervention must be based on the cultural values of the target group, that it should reflect the subjective cultural characteristics of the members of the group to be served by the intervention, and that the intervention should reflect the behavioral preferences and expectations of the target group. This speaks to the need for including a cultural assessment as part of the overall needs assessment process carried out by the health promoter and planning team.

As intervention design begins, it will be important that all activities necessary to carry out the stated objectives of the program are thoroughly explored by planning team members, especially by those who represent the community being served. This can help to identify issues that may have been missed or overlooked in the assessment phase and to identify potential strategies that might be unrealistic for the community and target group to be served by the program. Program interventions and the activities associated with them must be carefully written out to include what is to be done, by whom, when, and where. As interventions are developed, they should be pilot tested with members of the community using focus group processes or other procedures to ensure that the interventions are acceptable, understandable, and relevant to the target group. This is especially important with respect to the use of educational materials developed by the mainstream culture because these might not be culturally sensitive and appropriate to the literacy levels of the community in which they are to be used. This might require developing materials locally to ensure that they are culturally relevant and meaningful to the intervention group.

The use of traditional HPDP strategies for implementing interventions has not met with great success in African American communities. Thus, the planner should consider nontraditional sites and captive audiences, that is, planning to implement interventions at churches, laundromats, nail shops, beauty salons, barber shops, family and class reunions, social clubs and organizations, and home health parties cultivated by the planning team and organized by interested community members. It should be noted that the author has observed the difficulty of getting intervention participants to attend multiple sessions of an intervention, so the health promoter might want to explore other avenues where more than one intervention may be needed to deal with a health issue or problem. Because African Americans do depend a great deal on what their doctors tell them, education sessions should be integrated into the clinical encounter whenever possible. This also may help to overcome the multiple education session problem if sessions are scheduled to coincide with follow-up clinical visits.

In an effort to highlight some of the suggestions that have been made thus far, the following example is offered to illuminate some strategies that were successfully used for working with African American and other minority populations in the inner-city areas of Los Angeles. Beginning in the mid-1970s at the Martin Luther King Jr. General Hospital/Drew Medical Center in Los Angeles, the author and one of the editors of this book were involved in planning, implementing, and evaluating a program to reduce the numbers of community residents who had uncontrolled hypertension. The program began as a result of information gathered at a local health fair that revealed a significantly low level of knowledge about hypertension in the community. Participants in blood pressure screening offered at the health fair were unaware of their blood pressure levels and of the impact of elevated blood pressure on health outcomes.

The program began by offering blood pressure screenings to captive audiences at every opportunity including community health fairs, churches, senior citizen programs, community group meetings, schools and the local community college, and the lobby of the hospital itself. On these occasions, individuals were offered screening and a simple questionnaire to further assess the knowledge level of the community with respect to hypertension. The results confirmed that knowledge levels were low and needed to be addressed. A three-pronged program using community residents as major partners in the development and implementation of a hypertension control program was begun. To address the knowledge issues in the community, a preventive health education team was organized that included two community workers, health educators, allied health personnel, and a physician. The team had as its primary goal to provide innovative educational experiences about hypertension throughout the community and developed educational materials, songs, dance routines, lectures, and individual educational sessions to get the high blood pressure message out.

The second component of the program focused on training and certification of a cadre of community residents to conduct screening and educational sessions throughout the community. These community workers were able to provide screening and individual/group education to hundreds of individuals living in the community. In addition, they were responsible for identifying, referring, and following up on individuals with elevated blood pressure using hospital and community clinical services.

Providing effective, accessible care was the third prong of the program. To accomplish this goal, the team focused on the clinical setting including staff attitudes and the actual physical environment of the hypertension clinic, which was established specifically to diagnose, treat, and follow patients with hypertension. Trained community workers were assigned to conduct education in the clinic, which was transformed to create an atmosphere conducive to education; that is, the walls of the clinic were painted with scenes that depicted behaviors associated with control of hypertension including proper meal planning with low-salt/low-fat diets, smoking cessation, exercise, stress management, medication adherence, and making regular doctor visits at the clinic. Small group discussion proved to be the most effective method of education in this setting. It allowed for participants to discuss their issues and to receive suggestions for how to take better care of themselves from both the community workers and their peers. There always was a trained community worker or health educator on hand to correct misconceptions and misinformation and to suggest workable alternatives to control problems the patient might have. The scenes on the walls provided a complete visual outline of the concepts for controlling high blood pressure and were a reinforcement reminder to patients at each visit of their responsibility in the treatment process.

This brief example suggests that the health promotion planner will need to consider multiple intervention strategies and especially those that have been found to be successful in African American communities. Once intervention strategies have been determined, it is time to consider how these will be evaluated for effectiveness.

EVALUATION

Evaluation of programs is a very important task. It provides a basis for program planning and improvement as well as information needed to make funding decisions. Evaluation can be viewed as a process of inquiry and comparison in which issues such as how well the program functioned to meet its stated objectives, how well the staff performed in their program tasks, how much learning and behavior change might have occurred from pre- to postprogram, and how much money was spent to achieve desired outcomes (Dignan & Carr, 1987; Green & Kreuter, 1991).

It is important for traditionally trained evaluators, who place a great deal of emphasis on objective, logical, and rational aspects of behavior and who may distrust factors that reflect the specific physical and emotional features of a particular disease or condition, to recognize and understand that there are nonquantifiable features that are important in determining what is measured, what methods are used, and how the results are interpreted (Gay, 1985). A first step in any evaluation process is to determine the purpose of the evaluation, the questions that need to be addressed, who the stakeholders are and what their specific interests and needs might be, how decisions will be made based on evaluation data, and what resources will be needed to carry out evaluation activities. Priorities will need to be set to address each of these questions to ensure that an adequate and appropriate evaluation strategy is designed.

In general, one can view evaluation as having several major levels including process, impact, and outcome. Another level known as formative evaluation is concerned with the collection of data at the beginning of program development, that is, the process of designing and conducting a needs assessment at the outset of a program to target the HPDP program or service appropriately. Process evaluation provides an assessment of the program as it is being developed and during the time it is actually up and running. This is a very important aspect of the evaluation of a program, particularly for communities with little history of successful health promotion programming. This helps to provide an opportunity to carefully monitor how well the program is functioning at all levels and to make changes throughout implementation when problems are detected rather than waiting until the program is over.

Process evaluation strategies can take a number of forms including the use of direct interviews of clients and staff participating in the program; focus groups; monitoring attendance records; pre- and posttesting for changes in knowledge, attitudes, and behaviors; and similar types of activities. Using the earlier example of the three-pronged hypertension program, evaluation centered on pre- and posttesting for changes in knowledge, attitudes, and behaviors; attendance at educational sessions; satisfaction with program services; the keeping of scheduled clinic appointments; follow-through with referrals from community screening activities; staff performance with respect to screening services in the community and education sessions for which they had responsibility; and improvements in the control of blood pressure levels, based on chart reviews and follow-up screenings of community members and hypertension clinic patients. It is critical to regularly report findings to the planning team and the community using language that is clear, understandable, and jargon free to ensure that all constituencies associated with the program are aware of how the program is functioning, what changes may be needed, and what they can do to assist in the process of program monitoring and improvement.

Summative evaluation is concerned with two major levels of assessment: *impact evaluation* and *outcome evaluation*. Impact evaluation is concerned with measuring and summarizing short-term changes in knowledge, attitudes, and behaviors over the duration of the project, based on all the data that were collected at the process level. One also would expect to summarize data related to staff performance, budget, marketing, and other items related to program functioning. The value in doing this type of evaluation is to present findings to all constituencies involved in the program and to be able to ascertain how well the program did in the short run. It also provides new baseline data (formative evaluation) for the next iteration of the program.

Outcome evaluation measures the long-term effects of a program on morbidity and mortality. This is an area that often is difficult to evaluate by the health promoter because many community programs are short-lived and funds to continue long-term monitoring frequently are not available. Nevertheless, where one does have the capacity to follow a cohort of program participants over time, this can be a very valuable opportunity to identify changes or variations in the knowledge, attitudes, and behaviors of the group and to provide opportunities to reengage program participants by offering update sessions to help them become current with changes and to reinforce the knowledge, attitudes, and skills that were a part of the program's original implementation. Evaluation is the cornerstone of all HPDP program efforts. The health promoter should make a special effort to include all levels of evaluation possible in every program he or she plans. Without the data available through this process, there is no way of knowing what effects the program is having on the population participating in its interventions.

CHAPTER SUMMARY AND RECOMMENDATIONS

This chapter has sought to describe program planning, implementation, and evaluation strategies that can be helpful when working with African American communities. There is an urgent need to make HPDP programs and services more accessible to all segments of this population group. There are and have been initiatives at all levels of government, universities, and the private sector to address and enhance HPDP efforts. Some of these have been quite successful, although major gaps still remain to be addressed in others. A starting point for HPDP program planning in African American communities would be to give consideration to the following key issues:

- Research should be conducted by the health promoter to identify the values, beliefs, practices, and barriers one might encounter within the different segments of the population targeted for intervention.
- There must be a willingness to understand the important aspects of black culture such as language, music, religion, and social life within the context of social history and racism in America. This also means assessing one's own values and beliefs as these relate to the target population.
- Health promoters must be willing to invest time and energy to make certain that there is a partnership with the community that ensures that community members are involved in every step of the planning, implementation, and evaluation process.
- The health promoter should have an in-depth knowledge of the perceived needs of the community to be served. This includes an understanding of the community's health beliefs and practices and how these affect the traditional biomedical model of health care delivery.

- The health promoter must be equipped with a variety of strategies for working in the African American community and be able to employ these effectively in all phases of program plan development. In addition, intervention strategies must be comprehensive, multifaceted, and culturally relevant to the community.

- HPDP programs and services, including the messages sent to the community about these, must be developed within the context of the lives of individuals and norms of the community in which they live.

- The health promoter must be able to garner the necessary support from local organizations, local and national politicians, and influential individuals within the community.

This list of recommendations is by no means exhaustive. It represents a few salient points that have been covered in the body of this chapter. In spite of what seem like insurmountable barriers, there are many audiences in the black community that are eager to learn and assist in improving the health outcomes for themselves, their families, and their neighbors.

REFERENCES

Ajzen, I. (1991). The theory of planned behavior. *Organizational Behavior and Human Decision Processes, 50,* 179-211.

Ajzen, I., & Driver, B. L. (1991). Prediction of leisure participation from behavioral, normative, and control beliefs: An application of the theory of planned behavior. *Leisure Sciences, 13,* 185-204.

Ajzen, I., & Madden, T. J. (1986). Prediction of goal-directed behavior: Attitudes, intentions, and perceived behavioral control. *Journal of Experimental Social Psychology, 22,* 453-474.

Bandura, A. (1986). *Social foundations of thought and action: A social cognitive theory.* Englewood Cliffs, NJ: Prentice Hall.

Byrd, W. M. (1990). Race biology and health care: Reassessing a relationship. *Journal of Health Care for the Poor and Underserved, 1,* 278-292.

Byrd, W. M., & Clayton, L. A. (1993). The African American cancer crisis. Part 2: A prescription. *Journal of Health Care for the Poor and Underserved, 4,* 102-116.

Clark, N. M., & McLeroy, K. R. (1995). Creating capacity through health education: What we know and what we don't. *Health Education Quarterly, 22,* 273-289.

Cottrell, M. A., Davis, W., Schlaff, A., Liburd, L., Orenstein, D., & Presley, C. L. (1996). *Promoting healthy lifestyles in inner-city minority communities.* Washington, DC: U.S. Department of Health and Human Services.

Dignan, M. B., & Carr, P. A. (1987). *Program planning for health education and health promotion.* Philadelphia: Lea & Febiger.

DuBois, W. E. B. (1903). *The souls of black folk: Essays and sketches.* Bend, OR: A. C. McClurg.

Eng, E., & Hatch, J. W. (1991). Networking between agencies: The lay health advisor model. *Human Services, 10,* 123-146.

Fishbein, M. (Ed.). (1967). *Readings in attitude theory and measurement.* New York: John Wiley.

Gay, G. (1985). *Expressively black: The cultural basis of ethnic identity.* New York: Praeger.

Gielen, A. C., Wilson, M. E. H., Faden, R. R., Wilson, L., & Harvilchuck, J. D. (1995). In home injury prevention practices for infants and toddlers: The role of parental beliefs, barriers and housing quality. *Health Education Quarterly, 22,* 85-95.

Green, L. W., & Kreuter, M. W. (1991). *Health promotion planning: An educational and environmental approach.* Mountain View, CA: Mayfield.

Haynes, M., & Ashley, M. (1993). Making cancer prevention available for black Americans. In V. Devita, S. Humezn, & S. Rosenberg (Eds.), *Cancer prevention.* Philadelphia: J. B. Lippincott.

Haynes, M. A. (1975). The gap in health status between black and white Americans. In R. A. Williams (Ed.), *Textbook of black related diseases.* New York: McGraw-Hill.

Herring, P., & Montgomery, S. (1996). Health beliefs, health values and prevention, health promotion activities of black and white women: A comparative study. *Journal of Wellness Perspectives, 12,* 188-197.

Hirsch, J. (1991). Race, genetics and scientific integrity. *Journal of Health Care for the Poor and Underserved, 2,* 331-334.

Hochbaum, G. M., Sorenson, J. R., & Lorig, K. (1992). Theories in health education practice. *Health Education Quarterly, 19,* 295-313.

Jemmatt, L. S., & Jemmatt, J. B. (1992). Increasing condom use interventions among sexually active black adolescent women. *Nursing Research, 41,* 273-278.

Lorig, K., Stewart, A., Ritter, P., Gonzales, V., Laurent, D., & Lynch, J. (1996). *Outcome measures for health education and other health care interventions.* Thousand Oaks, CA: Sage.

Marin, G., Burhansstipanov, L., Connell, C. M., Gielen, A. C., Helitzer, A. D., Lorig, K., Morisky, D. E., Tenney, M., & Thomas, S. (1995). A research agenda for health education among underserved populations. *Health Education Quarterly, 22,* 346-363.

McGinnis, J. M., & Lee, P. R. (1995). Healthy People 2000 at mid decade. *Journal of the American Medical Association, 273,* 1123-1140.

Morgan, D. (1993). *Successful focus groups: Advancing the state of the art.* Newbury Park, CA: Sage.

Penn, N. E., Kar, S., Kramer, J., Skinner, J., & Zambrana, R. E. (1995). Ethnic minorities, health care systems and behavior. *Health Psychology, 14,* 641-646.

Quinn, S. C., Billingsley, A., & Caldwell, C. (1994). The characteristics of northern black churches and community outreach programs. *American Journal of Public Health, 84,* 575-579.

Quinn, T. S. (1996). The National Negro Health Week, 1991 to 1995: A descriptive account. *Journal of Wellness, 12*(4), 172-179.

Ryan, M. V., & Heaney, C. (1993). What's the use of theory? *Health Education Quarterly, 19,* 315-330.

U.S. Department of Health and Human Services. (1995). *Report of the Secretaries Task Force on Black and Minority Health, Vol. 1: Executive Summary.* Washington, DC: Government Printing Office.

Zelasko, C. (1995). Wellness programming: A paradigm for a Medicaid population. *Journal of Wellness Perspectives, 2*(3), 16-27.

12

Promoting Health in African American Populations

A Case Study

GINA M. WINGOOD

AIDS has rapidly emerged as a serious public health threat for women. In the United States, the fastest growing sector of people with AIDS are women between the ages of 18 and 44 years (Centers for Disease Control and Prevention [CDC], 1990). Unfortunately, AIDS and HIV infection disproportionately affect ethnic minority women in the United States. In 1993, AIDS incidence rates were 73 per 100,000 among African American women, 32 per 100,000 among Hispanic women, and only 5 per 100,000 among white women (CDC, 1994b). The death rate from AIDS for African American women is 10 times that for white women, and AIDS is the leading cause of death among African American women between the ages of 25 and 44 years (CDC, 1994a). Since the epidemic was first recognized in 1981, women have outnumbered men in the heterosexual contact transmission category in the United States (Guinan & Hardy, 1987). Among individuals with heterosexually contracted HIV infection, 61% are women (CDC, 1994c, p. 5). Sexual acquisition of HIV infection is most prevalent among young adult women between the ages of 20 to 24 years of age with 49% of these females who have been infected acquiring HIV through heterosexual contact. From 1988 through 1992, AIDS cases among women 20 to 24 years of age increased markedly, with the greatest increase observed among African American women who reported heterosexual contact as their primary risk exposure category ("AIDS Among Racial/Ethnic Minorities," 1994).

AUTHOR'S NOTE: In this chapter, the pronoun *we* refers to the investigators who conducted the research of which the author was a part.

BACKGROUND OF THE CASE STUDY

The development of an effective therapeutic treatment or prophylactic vaccine might not become a reality in the foreseeable future. Thus, reducing the risk of HIV infection among sexually active women requires the adoption of preventive strategies that effectively inhibit viral transmission (Bandura, 1994; DiClemente & Peterson, 1994). Behavioral interventions, based on theories of health behavior and designed to reduce HIV-related sexual risk practices, are critical for preventing further acceleration of HIV among women. Although behavioral interventions have been developed for a number of at-risk populations (Choi & Coates, 1994), programs developed specifically for women have lagged behind those developed for other populations (Wingood & DiClemente, 1996). A paucity of published empirical literature exists describing interventions targeted specifically toward women. Of these studies, there are even fewer published reports evaluating their effectiveness in modifying risk behaviors. Indeed, most of the available literature addressing the threat of HIV for women consists of recommendations for the content of interventions (Wingood & DiClemente, 1996). Thus, there is an urgent need to develop and evaluate HIV prevention programs designed to promote the adoption and maintenance of HIV prevention strategies, especially condom use, among women.

ISSUES ADDRESSED BY THE CASE STUDY

A primary HIV prevention strategy for women who are sexually active is to use condoms consistently and correctly during sexual intercourse (Roper, Peterson, & Curran, 1993). Although condoms are an efficacious method for prohibiting transmission of sexually transmitted disease (STD) pathogens including HIV, their effectiveness as a risk reduction strategy is dependent on consistent and proper use (Cates & Stone, 1992; De Vincenzi, 1994; Laurian, Peynet, & Verroust, 1989; Saracco, Musicco, Nicolosi, et al., 1993). Unfortunately, many economically disadvantaged African American women encounter numerous socioeconomic, behavioral, cultural, and gender-related obstacles that make practicing consistent condom use a formidable challenge (Auerbach, Wypijewska, Keith, & Brodie, 1994; Fullilove, Fullilove, Bowser, Haynes, & Gross, 1990; Moore, Harrison, & Doll, 1994; Wingood & DiClemente, 1992).

The case study presented in this chapter addresses the question of how to design a culturally and gender-sensitive, community-based, HIV sexual risk reduction program for African American women.

THE USE OF PSYCHOLOGICAL THEORIES
FOR DESIGNING INTERVENTIONS

Theoretical models provide guidance in the design and implementation phases of HIV prevention programs, assisting in the selection of key constructs to be targeted for intervention and the identification of appropriate intervention strategies designed to modify those targeted constructs (DiClemente & Peterson, 1994). One model that is particularly useful as a foundation for developing sexual risk reduction behavior change interventions, especially for women and ethnic minority populations, is social cognitive theory (Bandura, 1994). Social cognitive theory is a social psychological model that examines social, environmental, behavioral, and personal influences on an individual's behavior. According to social cognitive theory, providing information alone to individuals might not be sufficient to influence their adoption or maintenance of HIV-preventive behavior (e.g., condom use during sexual intercourse). Changing an individual's behavior requires developing and refining their skills in self-motivation, their ability to use these skills effectively and consistently under difficult circumstances, and their ability to receive the appropriate resources and social supports. Successful behavior change, therefore, requires a strong belief in one's self-efficacy to perform a specific behavior. Neglecting the use of psychosocial models in HIV prevention research makes it difficult to understand how and why individuals change their behavior.

The distinguishing feature of HIV prevention interventions based on social cognitive theory is their inclusion of skills training and strategies to modify perceived peer or partner normative beliefs about risk-taking behavior. Skills training usually emphasizes developing and refining condom use and social competency skills. Social competency skills include talking with a partner about sex and condom use (sexual communication), negotiating condom use with a sex partner, assertively asking a partner to use condoms, and refusing to have unsafe sex. Developing and refining these skills entails using a variety of interactive learning techniques such as observing others demonstrating these skills (social modeling) and actively participating in interactive role-playing to facilitate acquisition and mastery of sexual risk reduction skills. Many of the effective interventions for women are based on this model. However, prevention interventions that emphasize only individual behavior change efforts is shortsighted. To design a maximally effective HIV prevention intervention for women, we also must address the social factors underlying the condition.

The Utility of Social Theories for Designing Interventions

Many of the issues that must be addressed when designing and implementing HIV prevention interventions for women are social factors. Therefore, to design maximally effective HIV prevention interventions for women, psychological theories of behavior change should not be used in isolation from social theories. The limitations of many psychological theories is that they fail to address the social aspects of the HIV epidemic, particularly among ethnic minority women (Wingood & DiClemente, 1992, 1995).

To date, the majority of HIV risk reduction interventions for women are gender neutral (Wingood & DiClemente, 1995). Gender-neutral interventions, or interventions that do not differ between the sexes, implicitly assume static "sex roles" while obscuring potentially modifiable social processes that influence women's risk of HIV infection. This approach to risk reduction fails to recognize the importance of social sexual relationships between women and men and how these relationships may adversely affect a women's ability to adopt and maintain HIV-preventive behavior. HIV prevention researchers should use both social theories and psychological theories to understand how a specific health condition is socially produced and maintained.

This case study illustrates how use of a social theory, the theory of gender and power, increased understanding of the social factors that increase women's vulnerability to HIV. It then applies the theory of gender and power and social cognitive theory as guides in designing an effective HIV prevention intervention for young adult African American women.

CONCEPTUAL SOCIAL FRAMEWORK FOR ADDRESSING THE ISSUES IN THE CASE STUDY

When researchers consider women's issues by looking at women's families and primary relationships, the factors that affect sexual decision making, and economic concerns, they often fail to apply a theoretical framework for understanding gender differences or the social factors that may be uniquely important for promoting risk reduction among women (Wingood & DiClemente, 1995). One theory that may be particularly applicable for understanding women's sexual behavior and developing appropriate risk reduction intervention programs is the theory of gender and power.

The theory of gender and power incorporates three overlapping but distinct structures that serve to explain the culturally bound roles between men and women (Connell, 1987). Because women's vulnerability to HIV infection is closely intertwined with their gendered roles, a theory that examines gender relations is crucial for understanding women's risk behaviors and HIV risk reduction practices in a gendered manner. According to the theory of gender and power, the division of labor, the structure of power, and the structure of cathexis are the three major tenets that characterize relationships between men and women.

The sexual division of labor is an allocation of particular types of work to certain categories of people (Connell, 1987). This allocation becomes a constraint on human behavior. The sexual division of labor is manifested in the segregation of unpaid work—namely housework and child care to women—and inequalities in wages and educational attainment between the sexes. The sexual division of labor highlights women's socioeconomic vulnerability to HIV. The markedly higher HIV seroprevalence among African American women in inner-city environments should be considered within the context of occupational sex segregation, that is, the assignment of more women than men to part-time, casual, and marginal jobs, forcing women into positions that do not have a significant earning potential and excluding women from acquiring marketable skills (Sorenson &

Verbrugge, 1987). This unequal positioning may influence women to engage in prostitution or to exchange sex for money or drugs to survive, further placing them at risk for HIV.

The division of labor also is evident in the limited availability of affordable drug treatment programs for women. Women who use drugs or whose partners use drugs often are poorly educated, unemployed, or underemployed and struggle to meet daily survival needs of their families (Hankins, 1990). Economic and insurance constraints represent formidable barriers to accessing drug treatment services (Quinn, 1991). Moreover, drug treatment programs often either refuse admission to pregnant women or fail to provide child care. The lack of accessible and affordable drug treatment programs for women may further exacerbate their risk of HIV. Similarly, this structure is evident in the lack of affordable STD services for many economically disenfranchised women. As STDs facilitate the transmission of HIV (Wasserheit, 1992), the higher incidence of STDs among African American women may contribute to the higher incidence of HIV in this ethnic population (Rolfs & Nakashima, 1990).

Women's vulnerability to HIV also can be viewed as a reflection of the distribution of social and economic power. The association of power with the demarcation between men and women's work also serves to constrain gender relations (Connell, 1987). Inequalities in power between the sexes form the basis for the sexual division of power. This structure deals with issues such as control, authority, and coercion within heterosexual relationships. The physical assault of women by male partners, now estimated to affect 2 million women every year, is at the heart of the structure of power (Straus & Gelles, 1990). A recent study conducted among a community-based sample of African American women reported that women who had physically abusive partners were less likely to use condoms, less likely to negotiate safer sex, and more worried about acquiring HIV compared with women who were not in abusive relationships (Wingood & DiClemente, 1997a). This structure is manifested by the fact that approximately 20% of adult women, 15% of college women, and 12% of adolescent girls have experienced sexual abuse and assault during their lifetimes (Koss, 1988). Estimates for the prevalence of rape among African American women are even higher (Wyatt, 1990a). Several studies have documented the acquisition of STDs (Irwin, Edlin, Wong, et al., 1995) including HIV transmission among women who have been raped (Claydon et al., 1991). In addition, compared to women without such histories, female survivors of childhood sexual abuse are more likely to engage in prostitution than are women without such histories (Zierler et al., 1991), initiate sexual intercourse earlier (Wyatt, 1990b), report higher STD rates (Wingood & DiClemente, 1998), and less likely to use condoms, further exacerbating their risk for HIV (Wingood & DiClemente, 1997b). The constraints of power in heterosexual relationships are evident in norms supporting male control over condom use and the difficulty women have in negotiating safer sex (Wingood & DiClemente, 1997b, 1998; Worth, 1990). A recent study conducted among African Americans reported that women whose partners never used condoms were three time more likely to have partners who were resistant to using condoms and twice as likely to feel uncomfortable negotiating safer sex (Wingood & DiClemente, 1997b, 1998).

In addition to the medical establishment, social rules about sexual behavior often are enforced by other social institutions such as the media and churches. The caricature of women in the mass media is rooted in an unequal exchange and an imbalance of social power. These popular cultural prescriptions foster the norm of fulfilling sexual obligations to men that, in turn, may further increase women's vulnerability to HIV by reducing the likelihood that women will assertively deny sexual intercourse or demand the use of condoms (D'Emilio & Freedman, 1988). The Baptist and Catholic churches have internal systems of morality that equate sexuality with procreation, further placing many African American women at risk for HIV (D'Emilio & Freedman, 1988).

Decisions women make about engaging in safer sex also are influenced in various ways by normative and emotional factors. The structure of cathexis localizes the social norms that govern appropriate sexual behavior for women and characterizes the erotic and affective influences in relationships (Connell, 1987). This structure creates the norms for women's passiveness in sexual relationships and normalizes men having multiple female sexual partners, placing women at further risk for HIV (D'Emilio & Freedman, 1988). This structure rationalizes that women fail to negotiate safer sex because doing so would undermine the trust and intimacy in relationships. This structure of cathexis is evident in the attraction of older men to younger women, and vice versa, as sexual relationships often are erotically characterized by women's submission and men's dominance, making women more vulnerable to HIV (Finkelhor & Associates, 1986).

The structure of cathexis is further evident in the emotional ties that mothers have with their children. Women's concern for securing food, shelter, and money for their children may take priority over purchasing condoms and practicing safer sex. This may be a particularly strong barrier to risk reduction among African American women given the strong cultural value placed on child rearing (Amaro, 1995).

This structure also explains why the sex ratio imbalance in the African American community makes it difficult for African American women to exert control over their partners by asking them use condoms. Among African Americans, there are far more available women than available men. This sex ratio imbalance may hinder women's ability to form meaningful emotional and sexual attachments with men. When this situation is coupled with women's desire to feel connected to men, women might find it difficult to exert any restrictions, and particularly constraints for safer sex, on their partners. Further intensifying the situation, the underrepresented gender, men, may view their options as limitless, resulting in less pressure to develop commitments and greater power within relationships, and may perceive that it is unnecessary for them to practice safer sex, placing themselves and their sex partners at risk for HIV (Mays & Cochran, 1988).

Examining the gender-based economic, power, cultural, and relational aspects of sexuality may assist us in understanding African American women's risk of sexually acquired HIV infection.

PROGRAM SETTING FROM WHICH THE CASE STUDY EMERGED

The most effective interventions build on the strengths and resources found within a community. This process fosters positive collaborations between researchers and the community, roots an intervention within the community, and allows researchers the opportunity to identify motivated individuals within the neighborhood to assist in developing and implementing the intervention (Freudenberg et al., 1995). Adopting these guiding principles, we established a partnership with the local African American community-based organization, the Bayview-Hunter's Point Foundation, the second largest African American, community-based organization in San Francisco. The foundation provides legal, mental health, medical, and social services to the residents of the Bayview-Hunter's Point neighborhood. The Bayview-Hunter's Point neighborhood is 84% African American. In addition, 24% of the total households are below the poverty line, and the median family income is 34% lower than the median family income for San Francisco in general (Bowser, 1988). The long-standing relationship between the foundation and the community lent credibility to our program as being sensitive to the needs of the residents.

The tripartite partnership among the foundation, the community residents, and ourselves undoubtedly influenced the adoption of our HIV prevention program by African American women in the community. This partnership facilitated our ability to conduct qualitative research, which led to our gaining a better understanding of the social context of sexual decision making among young adult African American women in the community. This partnership also allowed us to work with women from the community to design the HIV sexual risk reduction intervention manual. Having young adult African American women from the community assist in developing the manual made the vignettes more realistic, tailored the manual to the linguistic and cultural influences pervasive in the community, created a more developmentally appropriate intervention, and captured the essence of being a sexually active, young adult African American woman in the community. Finally, the partnership allowed us to identify motivated African American female peers to implement the intervention.

THE CASE STUDY PROGRAM

Objectives of the Program

The study had three main objectives: (a) to design a gender-sensitive, community-based HIV sexual risk reduction intervention for young adult African American women; (b) to use indigenous peers to implement the HIV sexual risk reduction program for young adult women; and (c) to evaluate the efficacy of this community-based HIV sexual risk reduction intervention to enhance the adoption and maintenance of consistent condom use among young adult African American women (DiClemente & Wingood, 1995).

Design

Women were recruited from the Bayview-Hunter's Point community of San Francisco. Women were recruited over an 11-month period from February 1993 through December 1993 using street outreach and media advertisements placed throughout the community. Indigenous African American women field recruiters, who were familiar with the Bayview-Hunter's Point neighborhood, approached and screened women for eligibility at the local unemployment office, the social security office, public laundry facilities, beauty salons, grocery stores, health clinics, and the local Aid to Families with Dependent Children office. Inclusion criteria consisted of being a sexually active, heterosexual African American woman, 18 to 29 years of age, residing in the Bayview-Hunter's Point neighborhood. Exclusion criteria included use of crack/cocaine in the previous 3 months or a history of injection drug use. Interviews were conducted at the Bayview-Hunter's Point Foundation, an African American community-based organization with a long history of providing social and medical services in this community. Prior to the interview, each participant completed a tracking form that included her name, address, and telephone number as well as the address and phone number of a close confidant. After each participant was informed of the purpose of the investigation, was informed of procedures to protect confidentiality, and provided written informed consent, a trained African American woman interviewer administered a face-to-face, 45-minute private interview. On completing the baseline interview, each woman was compensated $10 for her time.

The project director, using a random numbers table, generated a listing that identified the treatment assignment for each participant who completed a baseline assessment and entered her treatment allocation into the log book. Then, 1 week prior to implementation of the treatment conditions, the project director telephoned each participant to inform her of the start date for her treatment condition. On completing the baseline interview, each woman was randomly assigned to one of three study conditions: a five-session social skills intervention condition ($n = 53$), a one-session HIV education condition ($n = 35$), or a delayed HIV education control condition ($n = 40$). The study design was a randomized, single-blind controlled trial. To encourage compliance, the project director telephoned each participant the day prior to implementation of her treatment condition.

At 3 months postintervention, the project director contacted and scheduled each participant to return for a follow-up interview using a modified version of the baseline interview to assess changes in consistent condom use and theoretically important constructs thought to mediate condom use. Each participant completed a follow-up interview administered by an interviewer who was blinded to the participant's treatment assignment. A reimbursement of $20 was provided to each participant on completion of the 3-month follow-up interview.

Implementation Issues and Scheme

Because this intervention was designed for African American women, the topic of HIV prevention should be contextualized within a framework that addresses African American cultural pride, gender awareness, and values prioritized by African American women. Women in the HIV social skills intervention received five 2-hour weekly group sessions implemented by two African American women peer health educators. The five-session HIV sexual risk reduction program is known as SISTA (Sisters Informing Sisters about Topics on AIDS). The acronym SISTA was chosen because this name represents the sisterhood that African American women share with one another.

The project motto also was designed to be culturally appropriate for young African American women: "SISTA love is strong. SISTA love is safe. SISTA love is surviving." The statement "SISTA love is strong" is reflective of the strong pride and dignity that African American women possess. The statement "SISTA love is safe" refers to our desire to create a norm of safer sex and the establishment of safer relationships. The statement "SISTA love is surviving" refers to the legacy of African American women surviving through hardship. Woven throughout the entire intervention are issues that personally address African American young women when attempting to protect themselves from HIV infection. The intervention addresses barriers faced by African American women when practicing or attempting to practice safer sex. Furthermore, the intervention discusses those aspects of the African American culture that act as facilitators and that may make practicing safer sex more of a norm for this population. HIV prevention activities and structural factors were incorporated into the intervention to enhance its appropriateness for young African American women. As discussed earlier, financial constraints are prevalent with this population; therefore, we provided bus tokens to all participants, and child care was available on-site for all women needing this service. In addition, before each session, participants read and discussed a poem by an African American female artist that related to the particular session. Furthermore, each session was tailored to be culturally relevant for young African American women.

The first session emphasized gender and ethnic pride. Prior to imparting risk reduction knowledge, skills, and norms to women, we wanted to listen to the women talk about their lives, goals, and dreams and to have them assert their self-worth. We felt that it was essential for the participants to build their self-esteem and personal self-confidence before discussing issues related to sexuality and HIV. This process allowed us to embed the values of young African American women within the HIV prevention messages and vignettes. During this session, the women discussed the positive attributes of being African American women, identified personal African American women role models, and engaged in values clarification exercises. At the end of this session, the participants framed postcards designed by African American female artists, and the peer and health educators discussed how these artists served as positive role models for African American women.

The second session emphasized HIV risk reduction information by increasing participants' knowledge about HIV-associated risk behaviors and preventive strategies. To enhance the participants' perceived risk of HIV, the session also discussed how the HIV epidemic disproportionately affects African American women compared to white women. Participants viewed and discussed an HIV educational video, *AIDS: Me and My Baby,* which encouraged women to take responsibility for sexual decision making. This session focused on staying safe not only for themselves but also for their children and families, as unity and the family are values that are highly prioritized by many African Americans. This session also discussed the social relations that places African American women at greater risk for acquiring HIV. During this activity, the women discussed the consequences of having sexual partners who injected drugs or who had been in jail and may have had sex with other men.

The third session emphasized sexual assertiveness and communication training. Participants were first taught the differences among, and the consequences of, being assertive, passive, and aggressive in a relationship. The women were taught to distinguish among these communication styles in nonsexual vignettes using scenarios common to African American women. For example, one non-sexual scenario modeled how a young African American woman assertively communicated to her beautician the need to restyle her braids prior to leaving the salon such that they would appear more attractive. Women were then taught an assertiveness model to assist them in managing risky sexual situations. The assertiveness model, known as the SISTAS assertiveness model, had six steps: thinking of oneself first, using the information the woman gained to practice safer sex, assessing the situation, stating the trouble the woman had with her partner, informing the partner of the woman's concern in an assertive manner, and suggesting alternatives that both partners can be comfortable with if safer sex is not an option. Subsequent to learning the SISTAS assertiveness model, the women applied the model to assist them in negotiating the safer sex vignettes. All exercises modeled by the peer health educators were role-played by participants in several practice situations, with the peer health educators providing corrective feedback.

The fourth session emphasized enhancing proper condom use skills and fostering positive norms toward consistent condom use. The health educator first sought to dispel many of the myths and misconceptions that many African American women have regarding condoms and their use. Then, the peer educators conducted condom use demonstrations with African American phallic replicas. The condom application skills subsequently were role-played by participants. Norm-setting exercises focused on establishing the perception of consistent condom use as becoming more normative with young adult African American males and females.

The fifth session emphasized coping skills. During this session, the health educator defined *coping* and discussed adaptive and maladaptive coping styles.

The vignettes focused on refining women's assertiveness skills to avoid sex when under the influence of alcohol, if a condom was not accessible, or if her sexual partner was abusive. At the end of this session, the participants read a poem or story that illustrated how they had grown as African American women from the SISTA project. At the end of the fifth session, the women received certificates of empowerment, signed by the project director, congratulating the women on their achievements.

Evaluation Issues and Scheme

Analyses were performed only on prespecified hypotheses using an "intention to treat" protocol in which participants were analyzed in their original randomized conditions, regardless of number of sessions attended (Pocock, 1993). Baseline differences among the three treatment conditions for continuous variables were assessed using analysis of variance, and differences for categorical variables were assessed using contingency table analyses (Fleiss, 1973). Intervention effects were evaluated using logistic regression models, adjusting for corresponding baseline outcome variables (Hosmer & Lemeshow, 1989). Logistic regression was employed because of the binomial nature of several outcome variables and the markedly skewed distribution underlying scale scores. Consistent condom use was the primary outcome variable. Secondary outcome variables included HIV knowledge, sexual self-control, sexual assertiveness and communication, partner norms, and condom use skills. The primary predictor variable was treatment condition. Variables identified at baseline that approached statistical significance $(p \leq .10)$ among treatment conditions and were theoretically important potential confounders were included in logistic regression models as covariates (Hosmer & Lemeshow, 1989). Model statistics computed included adjusted odds ratios and corresponding 95% confidence intervals to assess the significance and magnitude of the associations between the treatment conditions and outcome variables.

Results of the Case Study Program

A total of 128 African American women 18 to 29 years of age $(M = 23.2, SD = 3.8)$ completed baseline interviews. The equivalence of sociodemographic sexual behavior in the past 3 months and outcome variables (HIV knowledge, sexual self-control, condom use skills, communication skills, assertiveness skills, partner norms supportive of safer sex, and consistent condom use in the past 3 months) across the three treatment conditions was assessed at baseline and follow-up. At follow-up, length of relationship and income remained different across treatment conditions. Therefore, length of relationship and income level were entered as covariates in logistic regression analyses.

Of the 128 participants completing baseline interviews, 100 (78.1%) completed 3-month follow-up interviews. Follow-up rates differed by treatment condition, with 48 (90.6%) participants in the social skills intervention, 29 (82.9%) participants in the HIV education condition, and 23 (57.5%) partici-

TABLE 12.1 Evaluation of Program Effects on HIV Knowledge, Coping Skills, Interpersonal Skills, Partner Norms, and Consistent Condom Use at 3-Month Follow-Up: Social Skills Intervention Condition and Delayed HIV Education Control Condition

Variable	Social Skills Intervention Condition		Delayed HIV Education Condition		Adjusted Odds Ratio	95% Confidence Interval	p
	Baseline (%)	3-Month Follow-Up (%)	Baseline (%)	3-Month Follow-Up (%)			
HIV knowledge							
High HIV knowledge	41.7	56.6	26.1	40.0	1.4	0.82-2.36	.22
Cognitive coping skills							
High sexual self-control	60.4	61.2	52.2	41.7	1.9	1.00-3.60	.05
Interpersonal skills							
High communication skills	80.4	89.4	86.4	65.2	4.1	1.67-10.00	.002
High assertiveness skills	56.3	61.2	39.1	37.5	1.8	1.01-3.27	.05
High condom use skills	47.9	51.2	43.5	35.0	1.3	0.63-2.51	.52
Partner norms							
Perceive partner norms supportive of safer sex	33.3	53.1	38.1	25.0	2.1	1.08-3.87	.03
Condom use behavior							
Consistent condom use	35.4	46.9	21.7	29.2	2.1	1.03-4.15	.04

NOTE: Delayed HIV education control condition is the referent for calculation of odds ratios. Baseline and follow-up percentages are unadjusted by covariates. Odds ratios are adjusted by corresponding baseline variable, length of current relationship, and income level.

pants in the delayed HIV education control condition completing 3-month follow-up interviews.

Table 12.1 summarizes the results of logistic regression analyses examining changes in outcome variables for the social skills intervention compared to the delayed HIV education control condition. Participants in the social skills intervention, compared to those in the delayed HIV education control condition, were twice as likely to practice consistent condom use, nearly twice as likely to have greater sexual self-control, four times as likely to engage in sexual communication, nearly twice as likely to be sexually assertive, and twice as likely to have sex partners whose norms were supportive of consistent condom use.

No statistically significant differences in outcome variables were observed between the HIV education condition relative to the delayed HIV education control condition (Table 12.2).

Discussion of the Case Study Program

This study is the first randomized controlled trial of a community-based sexual risk reduction intervention for economically disenfranchised young adult African

TABLE 12.2 Evaluation of Program Effects on HIV Knowledge, Coping Skills, Interpersonal Skills, Partner Norms, and Consistent Condom Use at 3-Month Follow-Up: HIV Education-Only Treatment Condition and Delayed HIV Education Control Condition

Variable	HIV Education-Only Condition		Delayed HIV Education Condition		Adjusted Odds Ratio	95% Confidence Interval	p
	Baseline (%)	3-Month Follow-Up (%)	Baseline (%)	Month Follow-Up (%)			
HIV knowledge							
High HIV knowledge	48.3	48.6	26.1	40.0	0.9	0.54-1.76	.94
Cognitive coping skills							
High sexual self-control	55.2	48.3	52.2	41.7	0.9	0.42-1.74	.67
Interpersonal skills							
High communication skills	75.0	62.1	86.4	65.2	0.5	0.25-1.13	.10
High assertiveness skills	51.7	44.8	39.1	37.5	0.8	0.43-1.61	.58
High condom use skills	55.2	46.2	43.5	35.0	1.5	0.66-3.52	.28
Partner norms							
Perceive partner norms supportive of safer sex	39.3	48.3	38.1	25.0	1.1	0.56-2.28	.73
Condom use behavior							
Consistent condom use	20.7	37.9	21.7	29.2	1.1	0.55-2.40	.71

NOTE: Delayed HIV education control condition is the referent for calculation of odds ratios. Baseline and follow-up percentages are unadjusted by covariates. Odds ratios are adjusted by corresponding baseline variable, length of current relationship, and income level.

American women. Women's self-reports indicate that significant changes were made in theoretically important areas of HIV prevention, interpersonal skills, cognitive coping skills such as sexual self-control, partner norms, and (most important) consistent condom use. The inference that the increase in consistent condom use is attributable to the social skills intervention is strengthened by concomitant favorable changes in theoretically important HIV preventive skills and norms.

One methodological characteristic of the present study that differentiates it from other randomized controlled behavior change interventions designed to enhance condom use is the classification of the outcome variable. Consistent condom use was selected as the primary outcome measure, based on findings from prospective studies indicating that condoms, when used consistently, can provide a 70% to 100% reduction in the risk of HIV transmission (Fineberg, 1988). In particular, the most recent findings, from the European Study Group on Heterosexual Transmission of HIV (De Vincenzi, 1994), observed no seroconversions among couples who used condoms consistently, whereas among inconsistent condom users the seroconversion rate was significantly higher, 4.8 per 100 person-years. Moreover, predictions based on mathematical modeling suggest that, irrespective of the number of sexual partners and the prevalence of HIV among potential sex partners, consistent condom use can substantially reduce the risk of sexually transmitted HIV infection relative to never or half-time condom use (Cates & Stone, 1992; Roper et al., 1993). Thus, because empirical evidence supports the clinical and public health significance of consistent condom use for preventing HIV infection, future behavior change interventions should assess consistent condom use as a primary outcome measure for evaluating program efficacy.

ANALYSIS OF THE CASE STUDY

What Worked?

The effectiveness of this intervention may be attributed, in large part, to the focus on gender relations in which HIV sexual risk behaviors occur. In managing safer sex, women have to exercise influence over both themselves and their sexual partners (Bandura, 1994). However, few HIV prevention interventions have been based on theoretical models that address gender relations (Wingood & DiClemente, 1995, 1996). The theory of gender and power (Connell, 1987), a gender-appropriate model useful for understanding relationship dynamics, provided a framework for developing and implementing the social skills intervention. In particular, the social skills intervention addressed how to successfully negotiate safer sex and foster favorable partner norms supportive of consistent condom use within the context of a heterosexual relationship in which women often are in unequal positions of power relative to men.

This intervention's effectiveness also might have been the result of using African American women peer health educators to implement the HIV social skills intervention. Peer educators are more effective at facilitating the acquisition of social skills through modeling exercises that emphasize skills mastery, such as sexual communication and assertiveness, and dispelling perceptions of high-risk behavior as normative.

What Did Not Work?

Although this study demonstrated that young adult women can be taught skills to encourage their sex partners' consistent use of condoms and that several theoretically important mediators associated with the adoption of this HIV prevention strategy can be enhanced, no differences were observed for two other important mediators: condom use skills and HIV risk reduction knowledge. Condom use skills may take longer for women to acquire and to feel confident in using these skills. With respect to HIV risk reduction knowledge, both the social skills intervention and the delayed HIV education control condition demonstrated high baseline HIV knowledge scores, suggesting that efforts to disseminate HIV information have been effective. Although differences were observed between the social skills intervention and the delayed HIV education control condition, achieving statistical significance was difficult because of a ceiling effect.

A subsidiary analysis evaluating the efficacy of the HIV education condition relative to the delayed HIV education control condition identified no statistically significant differences in consistent condom use or theoretically important mediators of HIV preventive behavior. These findings corroborate previous research that suggests that providing HIV risk reduction information, in and of itself, is not sufficient to motivate the adoption of preventive behavior (DiClemente & Peterson, 1994). In general, interventions that are theory driven, emphasize intrapersonal and interpersonal factors, provide skills training, and attempt to modify social norms have been more effective at promoting the use of HIV preventive behaviors (Coates, 1990; Fisher & Fisher, 1992).

VALUE OF THE STUDY TO THE FIELD

There are several key programmatic features that appear to be associated with changing African American women's high-risk sexual behaviors. Foremost is that programs need to be tailored to meet the specific needs of the target population. "Tailoring" would include ensuring that the intervention was culturally sensitive and gender relevant (Wingood & DiClemente, 1992). Simply having African American peers implementing the HIV intervention curricula or using HIV education brochures illustrating African American women on the cover is not enough. The intervention should contextualize the topic of HIV prevention within the framework of sessions that address African American cultural pride, gender awareness, and values prioritized by African American women.

Second, HIV prevention interventions for women that are guided by psychological theories, in particular social cognitive theory, provide skills training in condom use and sexual communication, emphasize social support for behavior change, and are more effective at promoting the adoption and maintenance of condom use (DiClemente & Peterson, 1994; Wingood & DiClemente, 1996). Furthermore, most effective HIV prevention interventions for women also apply a social structural framework or emphasize gender-related influences such as stressors facing women, gender-based power imbalances within the relationship, and sexual assertiveness (Wingood & DiClemente, 1996). Although HIV preventive skills clearly are important, unsafe sexual behavior often not only is the result of a deficit of knowledge, motivation, or skills but also has meaning within a woman's personal relationships and sociocultural context.

Third, effective HIV prevention interventions for women often are multiple-session programs. Interventions in which women receive 8 to 10 hours of HIV prevention education and skills training are more effective at enhancing and maintaining condom use than are single-session interventions (Wingood & DiClemente, 1996).

Another key objective is to maintain a narrow focus on reducing sexual risk-taking behaviors. Thus, each sexual risk behavior targeted for change, whether it is enhancing condom use, reducing the number of sexual partners, or even postponing sexual intercourse, should be clearly specified with appropriate strategies designed to address the behavior directly. This is of critical importance because too often prevention programs have targeted a broad spectrum of risk behaviors for change without including behavior-specific strategies in the programs.

Finally, most effective HIV prevention interventions for women are peer led (Wingood & DiClemente, 1996). Theoretically, peer involvement offers a number of advantages over traditional didactic HIV prevention interventions. Derived from social cognitive theory and based on developmental theory, peer-facilitated interventions recruit and train peers indigenous to a large target population to serve as leaders, educators, and counselors. When working with young adults, peer-led interventions offer a number of advantages relative to professional or adult-led programs. Peers may be more effective teachers of social skills, may be more influential models of health-promoting behavior, and can serve as credible role models because they are members of the young adults' social milieu. Peers also can help to change normative expectations about the frequency of the targeted behavior in the peer group. Finally, peers can offer social support for performance of desired behaviors and for avoidance of health-damaging behaviors. These advantages are particularly important when educating young adult women in inner-city environments where social networks are limited and social norms, which may encourage and support risk-taking behavior, are highly influential (DiClemente & Houston-Hamilton, 1989). Several studies have successfully used peer-based models for reducing high-risk sexual behavior in women (Wingood & DiClemente, 1996). Clearly, peer involvement in the implementation of HIV prevention interventions warrants further consideration as one strategy for enhancing programmatic efficacy.

The present study represents the first evaluation of an intervention designed to increase consistent condom use among a community-recruited sample of women. The findings suggest that a culturally appropriate, gender-tailored intervention that emphasizes social skills training and attempts to modify partner norms may be effective at enhancing consistent condom use and psychosocial mediators associated with this HIV preventive behavior.

In the absence of an effective prophylactic vaccine or cure, interventions designed to enhance the use of HIV preventive behaviors are urgently needed to avert further escalation of new infections, particularly among African American women at high risk for sexually acquired HIV infection. Given the epidemiological significance of consistent condom use as an effective strategy in preventing HIV infection relative to any other use of condoms during sexual intercourse (Roper et al., 1993), interventions that emphasize and assess the adoption of consistent condom use may have a greater public health impact on reducing HIV incidence. Ultimately, however, controlling the HIV epidemic among inner-city women is dependent not only on the development and evaluation of gender-tailored prevention interventions but also on how effectively these interventions can be translated into existing community prevention activities and how rapidly they can be disseminated to high-risk urban centers.

REFERENCES

AIDS among racial/ethnic minorities: U.S., 1993. (1994). *Morbidity and Mortality Weekly Reports, 43,* 653-655.

Amaro, H. (1995). Love, sex, and power: Considering women's realities in HIV prevention. *American Psychologist, 50,* 437-447.

Auerbach, J. D., Wypijewska, C., Keith, H., & Brodie, H. (1994). *AIDS and behavior: An integrated approach.* Washington, DC: National Academy Press.

Bandura, A. (1994). Social cognitive theory and exercise of control over HIV infection. In R. J. DiClemente & J. Peterson (Eds.), *Preventing AIDS: Theories and methods of behavioral interventions.* New York: Plenum.

Bowser, B. P. (1988). Bayview-Hunter's Point: San Francisco's black ghetto revisited. *Urban Anthropology, 17,* 383-400.

Cates, W., & Stone, K. M. (1992). Family planning, sexually transmitted diseases and contraceptive choice: A literature update—Part 1. *Family Planning Perspectives, 24,* 75-84.

Centers for Disease Control and Prevention. (1990). AIDS among women—United States. *Mortality and Morbidity Weekly Report, 39,* 845-846.

Centers for Disease Control and Prevention. (1994a). AIDS among racial/ethnic minorities: United States, 1993. *Morbidity & Mortality Weekly Report, 43,* 644-647.

Centers for Disease Control and Prevention. (1994b). Heterosexually acquired AIDS: United States 1993. *Morbidity & Mortality Weekly Report, 43,* 155-160.

Centers for Disease Control and Prevention. (1994c). Mid-year edition. *HIV/AIDS Surveillance Report, 6,* 5-10.

Choi, K. H., & Coates, T. J. (1994). Prevention of HIV infection. *AIDS, 8,* 1371-1389.

Claydon, E., Murphy, S., Osborne, E. M., Kitchen, V., Smith, J. R., & Harris, J. R. (1991). Rape and HIV. *International Journal of STDs and AIDS, 2,* 200-201.

Coates, T. J. (1990). Strategies for modifying sexual behavior for primary and secondary prevention of HIV disease. *Journal of Consulting Clinical Psychology, 58,* 57-69.

Connell, R. W. (1987). *Gender and power.* Stanford, CA: Stanford University Press.

D'Emilio, J., & Freedman, E. B. (1988). *Intimate matters: A history of sexuality in America.* New York: Harper & Row.

De Vincenzi, I. (1994). A longitudinal study of human immunodeficiency virus transmission by heterosexual partners. *New England Journal of Medicine, 331,* 341-346.

DiClemente, R. J., Houston-Hamilton, A. (1989). Strategies for prevention of human immunodeficiency virus infection among minority adolescents. *Health Education, 20,* 39-43.

DiClemente, R. J., & Peterson, J. (1994). Changing HIV/AIDS risk behaviors: The role of behavioral interventions. In R. J. DiClemente & J. Peterson (Eds.), *Preventing AIDS: Theories and methods of behavioral interventions.* New York: Plenum.

DiClemente, R. J., & Wingood, G. M. (1995). A randomized controlled trial of an HIV sexual risk-reduction intervention for young African-American women. *Journal of the American Medical Association, 274,* 1271-1276.

Fineberg, H. V. (1988). Education to prevent AIDS: Prospects and obstacles. *Science, 239,* 592-596.

Finkelhor, D., & Associates. (1986). *A sourcebook on child sexual abuse.* Beverly Hills, CA: Sage.

Fisher, J. D., & Fisher, W. A. (1992). Changing AIDS-risk behavior. *Psychology Bulletin, 111,* 455-474.

Fleiss, J. L. (1973). *Statistical methods for rates and proportions.* New York: John Wiley.

Freudenberg, N., Eng, E., Flay, B., Parcel, G., Rogers, T., & Wallerstein, N. (1995). Strengthening individual and community capacity to prevent disease and promote health: In search of relevant theories and principles. *Health Education Quarterly, 22,* 290-306.

Fullilove, M. T., Fullilove, R., Bowser, B. P., Haynes, K., & Gross, S. A. (1990). Black women and AIDS: Gender rules. *Journal of Sexual Research, 27,* 47-64.

Guinan, M., & Hardy, A. (1987). Epidemiology of AIDS in women in the United States. *Journal of the American Medical Association, 257,* 2039-2042.

Hankins, C. (1990). Issues involving women, children and AIDS primarily in the developed world. *AIDS, 3,* 443-448.

Hosmer, D. W., & Lemeshow, S. (1989). *Applied logistic regression.* New York: John Wiley.

Irwin, K. L., Edlin, B. R., Wong, L., et al. (1995). Urban rape survivors: Characteristics and prevalence of human immunodeficiency virus and other sexually transmitted infections—Multicenter Crack Cocaine and HIV Infection Study Team. *Obstetrics & Gynecology, 85,* 330-336.

Koss, M. P. (1988). Hidden rape: Sexual aggression and victimization in a national sample of students in higher education. In A. W. Burgess (Ed.), *Rape and sexual assault.* New York: Garland.

Laurian, Y., Peynet, J., & Verroust, F. (1989). HIV infection in sexual partners of HIV seropositive patients with hemophilia. *New England Journal of Medicine, 320,* 183.

Mays, V. M., & Cochran, S. D. (1988). Issues in the perception of AIDS risk and risk reduction activities by black and Hispanic/Latina women. *American Psychologist, 43,* 949-957.

Moore, J. S., Harrison, J. S.., & Doll, L. S. (1994). Interventions for sexually active, heterosexual women in the United States. In R. J. DiClemente & J. Peterson (Eds.), *Preventing AIDS: Theories and methods of behavioral interventions.* New York: Plenum.

Pocock, S. J. (1993). *Clinical trials: A practical approach.* New York: John Wiley.

Quinn, S. C. (1991). AIDS and the African-American woman: The triple burden of race, class and gender. *Health Education Quarterly, 20,* 305-320.

Rolfs, R. T., & Nakashima, A. K. (1990). Epidemiology of primary and secondary syphilis in the United States, 1981 through 1989. *Journal of the American Medical Association, 264,* 1432-1437.

Roper, W. L., Peterson, H. B., & Curran, J. W. (1993). Commentary: Condoms and HIV/STD prevention—Clarifying the message. *American Journal of Public Health, 83,* 501-503.

Saracco, A., Musicco, M., Nicolosi, A., et al. (1993). Man-to-woman sexual transmission of HIV: Longitudinal study of 343 steady partners of infected men. *Journal of Acquired Immune Deficiency Syndrome, 6,* 497-502.

Sorenson, G., & Verbrugge, L. M. (1987). Women, work and health. *Annual Review of Public Health, 8,* 235-251.

Straus, M. A., & Gelles, R. J. (1990). *Physical violence in American families: Risk factors and adaptations to violence in 8,145 families.* New Brunswick, NJ: Transaction Publishers.

Wasserheit, J. (1992). Epidemiological synergy: Interrelationships between human immunodeficiency virus infection and other sexually transmitted diseases. *Sexually Transmitted Diseases, 9,* 61-77.

Wingood, G. M., & DiClemente, R. J. (1992). Cultural, gender and psychosocial influences on HIV-related behavior of African-American female adolescents: Implications for the development of tailored prevention programs. *Ethnicity and Disease, 2,* 381-388.

Wingood, G. M., & DiClemente, R. J. (1995). Understanding the role of gender relations in HIV prevention research. *American Journal of Public Health, 85,* 592.

Wingood, G. M., DiClemente, R. J. (1996). HIV sexual risk reduction interventions for women: A review. *American Journal of Preventive Medicine, 12,* 209-217.

Wingood, G. M., & DiClemente, R. J. (1997a). Child sexual abuse, HIV sexual risk and gender relations of African-American women. *American Journal of Preventive Medicine, 13,* 380-384.

Wingood, G. M., & DiClemente, R. J. (1997b). Effects of having a physically abusive partner on the condom use and sexual negotiation practices of young adult African-American women. *American Journal of Public Health, 87,* 1016-1018.

Wingood, G. M., & DiClemente, R. J. (1998). Partner influences and gender-related factors associated with noncondom use among young adult African-American women. *American Journal of Community Psychology, 26,* 29-53.

Worth, D. (1990). Sexual decision making and AIDS: Why condom promotion among vulnerable women is likely to fail. *Studies in Family Planning, 20,* 297-307.

Wyatt, G. E. (1990a). *Hearings before the Select Committee on Children, Youth, and Families of the House of Representatives* (101st Congress, 2nd session, testimony of Gail E. Wyatt). Washington, DC: Government Printing Office.

Wyatt, G. E. (1990b). The relationship between child sexual abuse and adolescent sexual functioning in Afro-American and white American women. *Annals of the New York Academy of the Sciences, pp.* 111-121.

Zierler, S., Feingold, L., Laufer, D., Velentgas, P., Kantrowitz-Gordon, I., & Mayer, K. (1991). Adult survivors of childhood sexual abuse and subsequent risk of HIV infection. *American Journal of Public Health, 81,* 572-575.

13

Tips for Working With African American Populations

ROBERT M. HUFF
MICHAEL V. KLINE

The term *African American* often is used to label black populations that represent a wide diversity of ethnic and cultural backgrounds. Many of these peoples do not perceive or identify themselves as African American. That is, they may identify with Haitian, British, Brazilian, or any number of other cultural or ethnic groups (Hopp & Herring, Chapter 10, this volume). As Hopp and Herring observed in Chapter 10, new immigrants who have not acculturated into the mainstream culture of the United States might not identify with American-born blacks, nor will they necessarily identify with those who are descended from the slaves who were brought into the United States early in its history. Thus, it is important to recognize that, like other cultural groups described in this book, one cannot conveniently place everyone into the one broad category of "African American" without first noting that this is being done with the knowledge that the term is not necessarily an accurate representation of the group being discussed. The caveat to the reader is to determine the particular term(s) the target group uses to describe itself and how that group's cultural characteristics, including its history, immigration patterns, acculturation and assimilation levels, socio-economic status, and generational and other related factors, are similar to or different from those of the mainstream culture before launching into major needs assessment and other planning activities.

This brief "tips" chapter draws from the three preceding chapters (Hopp & Herring, Chapter 10; Ashley, Chapter 11; and Wingood, Chapter 12) as well as from a number of other sources (Huff, Chapter 2, this volume; Huff & Kline, Chapter 1, this volume; Locks & Boateng, 1996; Willis, 1992) and is only a beginning list of suggestions and recommendations for working with this large and very diverse group of people.

CULTURAL COMPETENCE

Anyone involved in the delivery of health promotion and disease prevention (HPDP) programs and services needs to develop cultural competence and sensitivity to the differences between themselves and the multicultural group with which they will be working. This is no less true for those working with groups broadly classified as "African American," "black," or another term reflecting this particular population grouping. Thus, the health promoter is encouraged to consider the following suggestions related to cultural competence:

▶ Research the history of the target group to be involved in the HPDP program or service and seek to become familiar with its members' cultural values, beliefs, and ways of life as a people living in the United States.

▶ Remember that there is a great diversity of backgrounds and countries of origin for this population group and that this also means there is likely to be a significant diversity of beliefs and practices different from those of the individuals planning the HPDP intervention or service.

▶ Examine your own perceptions, stereotypes, and prejudices toward the target group and be willing to suspend judgments, where they exist, in favor of learning who these people really are instead of who you might think they are. This is one of the most important steps you can take toward cultural competence and sensitivity.

▶ Take the time to make multiple visits to the community where the target group lives. Talk with community leaders and members, visit important sites within the community, eat at local restaurants, attend local events, and otherwise become familiar with the community's ways of life.

▶ Seek to establish early and continuing support from the community for any HPDP programs and services that are to be offered.

▶ Recognize that there is a healthy suspicion in some black communities about programs and services coming from existing health institutions both inside and outside the community. This might be a result of having a history with institutions that sought to offer intervention programs and services, research projects, or other types of programs or services that did not continue after the funding ran out and everyone left.

▶ Be aware that just because an individual from an institution or agency might be of the same ethnic group as the community, this will not necessarily guarantee that person entry into or trust from the community. Having been trained outside the community might place that person in an "outsider" frame, and the individual will need to demonstrate his or her sincerity and true interest in helping the community to deal with its particular needs and concerns.

HEALTH BELIEFS AND PRACTICES

There is a wide variety of health beliefs and practices that characterize this broad multicultural population group, and the need to assess what these beliefs and practices are early in the intervention planning process cannot be stressed enough. The health promoter is encouraged once again to review the history of the target group, speak to the formal and informal leaders in the community about their perceptions of the health beliefs and practices of the community, and work to suspend their judgments about these. Not doing so might lead to conflict and to a failure of the program or service to achieve the goals and objectives it has set for and with the community. Thus, the health promoter should consider the following tips:

▶ Identify and seek to understand the explanatory models that the individuals within the community use to make sense of and deal with threats to their personal health and well-being.

▶ Expect that there will be a range of explanatory models that are employed across this broad multicultural population group, ranging from very traditional folk health beliefs and practices to those reflective of the current biomedical model.

▶ Where differences exist between the explanatory models of the target group and your explanatory models, make efforts to ameliorate or otherwise find ways in which to work within these different frames of reference and perception.

▶ Consider becoming more familiar with traditional healing practices where these are prevalent in the community because this may provide opportunities to bring beneficial practices into the biomedical framework while also modifying those practices that can potentially be harmful.

▶ Be aware that variations in health beliefs and practices can be attributed to a variety of variables including socioeconomic status, education, area of residence, access to health care services, health insurance, and other related factors.

▶ Recognize that the use of traditional folk healing practices can be linked to a number of factors including the ease of access to traditional healers and medicines within the community, their cultural acceptability, and their expense (which often is far less than what is charged in the Western biomedical system).

▶ Remember that traditional folk healers sometimes are the first and only health practitioners used by low-income blacks for all the reasons cited earlier in this discussion.

▶ Remember that traditional explanations for illness and disease often fall into two general categories: *natural causes* (including cold, stress, and improper eating or lack of moderation in one's daily life) and *unnatural causes* (resulting from witchcraft practices including voodoo, hoodoo, bad spirits, and other works of the devil).

▶ Be aware that, in general, the Western biomedical system is highly respected and used for serious medical problems, although folk healing traditions also may be employed.

PROGRAM PLANNING CONSIDERATIONS

Program planning for HPDP is a systematic, all-encompassing process whose aim is to create highly effective, well-structured and -implemented interventions for promoting change of health-damaging behaviors to more positive health-promoting behaviors within individuals, small groups, communities, and the larger society (Kline, Chapter 4, this volume). Keeping in mind the basic program planning considerations espoused by the many contributors to this book, the following suggestions and recommendations also should be considered by the health promoter:

▶ The community must be involved in every aspect of the program planning process, from needs assessment through evaluation.

▶ It is very important to begin developing positive alliances with the leadership of the community as you consider developing HPDP programs and services for the community.

▶ Be sure that HPDP programs and services reflect the values, beliefs, and interests of the community in which they are targeted.

▶ Review all previous HPDP program efforts in the community to identify potential community resources and assets, interventions that have been found to enhance or impede the successful adaptation of programs in the community, and any other factors that might play a role in the new program or service to be developed.

▶ Be sure that the goals, objectives, and interventions of the HPDP program or service reflect the felt needs of the target group. Where community needs and interests do not meet this criterion, consider developing strategies to increase awareness of those less well-known issues that might exist prior to launching a full-blown program or service that is not considered important by the community.

▶ Be aware that the employment of an indigenous model for planning and carrying out an HPDP program or service in the community has been found to be an extremely effective approach for delivering high-quality programs to the community.

NEEDS ASSESSMENT CONSIDERATIONS

Well designed and conducted needs assessment processes can provide a strong baseline for understanding the health and other social needs of a community. The process should be rigorous and should consider not only the usual targets of assessment (e.g., morbidity and mortality rates, demographics) but also the cultural factors that can affect the successful implementation of an HPDP program or service. The reader is encouraged to review the cultural assessment framework presented in Chapter 26 (Huff & Kline, this volume) as well as the following suggestions as he or she prepares assessment instruments and methodologies:

▶ Be aware that no matter what planning model may be employed, it will be essential that a cultural assessment be included in the other data gathered in the baseline study of the target group.

▶ Needs assessment instruments need to reflect the linguistic, literacy, and cultural symbols and values of the community.

▶ Standardized needs assessment instruments designed for the mainstream culture often have little meaning in black communities. Thus, instruments will need to be shaped to reflect the community in which they are to be administered.

▶ Consider including acculturation measures in the community assessment process.

▶ Where possible, seek to involve community members in identifying key informants who can speak to the real and felt needs of the community including the resources that might be available in the community to support HPDP activities.

▶ Be aware that key informants might not always know what the issues are in the community or might be operating with their own agendas in mind. Thus, always seek to triangulate the data that are gathered from those who are involved as key informants, using focus group data and other data gathered as a part of the baseline assessment of the community.

▶ Be sure to include assessment of the media resources and channels that are used by members of the community because these might play an important role in the marketing of the program or service developed by community representatives and yourself.

▶ Recognize that the PRECEDE model can be a useful framework for identifying and describing health behaviors with respect to their predisposing, enabling, and reinforcing factors and can help point the way toward the design of interventions that accurately target the factors most amenable to change.

▶ Seek to involve community members in the actual conduct of needs assessment activities because this can help foster involvement and ownership of the program or service to be developed.

▶ Be sure that assessment and evaluation efforts reflect the needs, interests, and values of the stakeholders within the community.

INTERVENTION CONSIDERATIONS

The design of well-planned and culturally appropriate interventions is critical to the success of any HPDP program or service offered in a community. *Cultural tailoring* encourages the planner to design intervention strategies, methods, and materials to the specific cultural characteristics of the target group and should be an integral component of the design process (Pasick, D'Onofrio, & Otero-Sabogal, 1996). With these ideas in mind, the health promoter also might wish to consider the following additional comments and suggestions as the individual begins the intervention phase of his or her work:

▶ Recognize that "one size fits all" is not a useful approach to intervention design. A program needs to be tailored to the target group for which it is intended.

▶ Be aware that the most effective HPDP interventions are built on the community's strengths, resources, and assets, all of which serve to foster community ownership and involvement with the HPDP program or service being developed.

▶ Be aware that intervention design needs to include significant involvement from the target group whose members will be the recipients of the program or service.

▶ Linguistic, literacy, gender relevance, and other cultural factors must be considered in the design of the intervention to be carried out in the community.

▶ Recognize that using captive audiences and unconventional sites for an HPDP program or service can be a highly effective approach to reaching the community. These might include laundromats, social clubs, hair and nail salons, home parties, family reunions, and other locations and events likely to draw community members.

▶ Churches often have been used as sites for conducting HPDP programs, but you should be aware that these sites are not always the easiest to involve in HPDP efforts because many of them have their own causes, which may or may not have a health focus.

▶ If you are designing educational sessions for the community, then be aware that it often is difficult to get community members to attend such sessions, especially if they are multiple sessions. Taking the intervention to the community rather than having the community come to the intervention might be much more effective.

► Be aware that the use of peer educators from the community has been found to be a very effective method for delivering HPDP programs or services to the community.

► Intervention design should be theory based because these types of intervention designs have been found to be much more effective than those without that type of foundation.

► Consider the learning styles of the target group when designing interventions and seek to incorporate educational approaches that reflect these ways of learning within the target population.

► Development of educational materials must reflect relevant cultural values, themes, and literacy levels of the target group for which they are intended.

► Recognize that developing partnerships with local media can be an effective way in which to disseminate information about the HPDP program or service being planned and offered to the community.

► Seek to develop interventions that focus on positive health changes rather than those with negative or fear-arousing consequences.

EVALUATION CONSIDERATIONS

Evaluation is at the heart of all well-conceived HPDP programs and must be among the first considerations when planning an HPDP program or service. It begins with formative assessment to establish baseline information for building a program and continues through process, impact, and outcome evaluation to measure the success of the program or service in achieving its identified objectives. For this reason, the health promoter is encouraged to consider the following recommendations:

► Seek to develop evaluation strategies, methods, and instruments that reflect an understanding of current theory and practice in the evaluation and research literature.

► Recognize that evaluation and assessment are processes that frequently are difficult to gain support for, even in the most sophisticated of groups. Thus, an effort to explain underlying assumptions governing these processes and the methods and anticipated outcomes of assessment and evaluation activities can serve to strengthen support and involvement of the community and planning group in these most important activities.

► Be aware that providing evaluation and assessment training for the community can help foster support for and empower the community to become more actively involved in data collection efforts related to assessment and evaluation activities.

▶ Evaluation and assessment measures should be culturally relevant and tailored to the linguistic and educational capabilities of the target group.

▶ Evaluation must consider the needs and interests of the stakeholders within both the community and the agency providing the HPDP program or service.

▶ Evaluation processes must include the participation of the community, and the criteria for evaluation should be sought from the community because its members are the ones who know what is important to them.

▶ Recognize that HPDP program participants might have limited test-taking skills or abilities. Thus, efforts to design evaluation methods should reflect these potentialities by seeking approaches that are within the relevant experiences of the target group whenever possible.

▶ Be sure to design evaluation and assessment reporting and feedback mechanisms to ensure that the target community is regularly made aware of how well the program is functioning to improve the health issues or problems for which it was designed.

REFERENCES

Locks, S., & Boateng, L. (1996). Black/African Americans. In J. G. Lipson, S. L. Dibble, & P. A. Minarik (Eds.), *Culture and nursing care: A pocket guide*. San Francisco: UCSF Nursing Press.

Pasick, R. J., D'Onofrio, C. N., & Otero-Sabogal, R. (1996). Similarities and differences across cultures: Questions to inform a third generation for health promotion research. *Health Education Quarterly, 23*(Suppl.), S142-S161.

Willis, W. (1992). Families with African American roots. In E. W. Lynch & M. J. Hanson (Eds.), *Developing cross-cultural competence: A guide to working with young children and their families*. Baltimore, MD: Paul H. Brookes.

PART 4

American Indian and Alaska Native Populations

14

American Indian and Alaska Native Populations in the United States

An Overview

FELICIA SCHANCHE HODGE
LARRI FREDERICKS

A variety of terms are used interchangeably for Native North Americans such as *Indian, American Indian, Native, aborigine, indigenous people, First Nation, First People,* and *First American.* The search for a single name, however, has not been successful. In the United States, the term *Native American* has been used but has fallen out of favor recently because anyone born in North or South America may claim to be a Native American. The term *American Indian* currently is in favor despite its misnomer; *Indian* still carries the stigma of being bestowed on tribal groups by European explorers in search of the Indian subcontinent of Asia. As such, the term fails to define the originary status of pre-Columbian American peoples. That the Inuit, Yupik, and Aleut peoples of Alaska consider themselves distinct from other indigenous North American peoples compromises the term *American Indian* even further, as these groups of Alaskan peoples do not wish to be called *Indian.* Thus, when generalizations of the entire group are necessary, it is preferred to use the terms *American Indians* and *Alaska Natives.*

Native peoples in the United States do not form a single ethnic group, and they always have resisted a homogeneous definition. They are better understood as thousands of distinct communities and cultures. Many American Indian and Alaska Native peoples have distinct languages, religious beliefs, ceremonies, and sociopolitical organizations. Characterizing this diverse array of cultures and peoples with one inclusive name undercuts any effort to assess cultural development specific to time and place, encouraging common misunderstandings based on preconceived assumptions. In recognizing them by their specific tribal or community identities such as Apache, Hopi, or Cherokee, we distinguish these peoples from others in ways that they themselves always have preferred. These tribal names usually mean "the people" or "the real people," in reference to themselves as set apart from the rest of the world. Such identifications more accurately capture the unique and varied tribal and cultural distinctions found among American Indian and Alaska Native peoples.

Culture areas, such as the sub-Arctic and the Southwest, are used to describe geographical areas in which several American Indian nations lived and shared a similar ecological environment and, hence, similar methods of food production such as hunting and gathering or horticulture. Nevertheless, within a specific culture area, there may be several very different cultures and a multiplicity of languages and dialects, such as in the Southwest, where the Navajo speak an Athabascan language, whereas the Zuni speak a Penntian language. Culture areas have been used by anthropologists primarily to reconstruct how Indians lived prior to Western contact after the year 1500. However, the manner in which American Indians and Alaska Natives live today is more determined by political and economic relations with the United States than by the ecological environments of the precontact period. For example, Alaska and California are listed as separate cultural areas rather than as part of the sub-Arctic and West Coast because of their unique histories and relations with non-Indians. The following list of culture areas draws on the basic anthropological culture areas but also takes into account the people who live in the culture area; their cultural, social, and political histories; and major contemporary issues.

DIVERSITY OF SUBGROUPS

Northeastern Indians

The culture area defined as Northeast is noted for its "relative degree of cultural cohesiveness" despite its wide variety of environmental and ecological conditions (Champagne, 1994). The demographic settlement of contemporary Indian tribes in the Northeast is the result of intensified struggles for land brought about by the arrival of European settlers. Tribal displacement resulting from such struggle during the 16th and 17th centuries contributed to an unending cycle of dislocation and Indian population decline resulting from infectious diseases contracted from European immigrants. Continual contact with European explorers and settlers from 1497 onward had made it increasingly difficult for the Iroquois and Algonkian tribes to maintain land holdings and traditional means of support, that is, horticulture and hunting.

The culture area in the Northeast, then, is determined not only by Indian subjection to colonial law but also to changing economic "environments" such as the decline of the fur trade in the mid-19th century. Having had to abandon a subsistence economy for one based on trade, northeastern tribes had no alternative but to sell lands to meet their need for manufactured goods once those markets failed. Whereas coastal Indians such as the Algonkians found themselves subject to English colonial law in the 17th century, tribes such as the Iroquois were emulated by late 18th-century white Americans for their spirit of democracy and liberty. American Indian political custom, as such, played a constructive role in the very formation of early American government as the colonies sought their independence from Britain.

Despite the peaceful assimilation of the Algonkian Indians into colonial coastal communities and the subsequent role the Iroquois fulfilled in forging the early American nation, American Indians suffered from both the loss of tribal lands and their vulnerability to European diseases throughout the 19th century. The reservation became the final refuge for those who had survived the processes of social and economic isolation well into the 20th century (Grinde, 1994).

Southeastern Indians

The major tribes of the American Southeast are the Catawba, the Cherokee, the Creek, the Chickasaw, the Choctaw, and the Seminole. Their common territory is bounded by the Atlantic Ocean, the Gulf of Mexico, the Trinity River in present-day Texas, and the Ohio River. Southeastern Indian tribes share a widespread traditional culture known as Mississippian, a term referring to practices associated with the construction of ceremonial mounds central to the village and its cultivated fields of corn, beans, and squash.

Southeastern peoples shared a balanced economy centering on agriculture and supported by hunting wildlife. Such a subsistence-level economy had been kept in balance by spiritual beliefs and ritual practice. For example, hunting never exceeded actual food requirements, and killing itself was preceded by prayer to animal spirits. Excessive slaughter was commonly forbidden among tribal groups.

The spiritual values common to the southeastern tribes center on the spirit of balance and harmony with other humans, the natural world, and the spirit world. All things had spirits, either good or evil, and success in life depended on the careful cultivation of these spirits. Just as European settlement uprooted the balance of American Indians in the Northeast, tribal cultures of the Southeast suffered widespread disruption of traditional life over the course of three centuries beginning in the years 1540 and 1541. A new economy, based on trade for profit, usurped and replaced a traditional subsistence economy, sending tribal life into disarray. American Indians were ill prepared to incorporate commercialism based on product and profit into a spiritual tradition that had evolved on need-based hunting and self-sufficient agriculture.

Despite the upheaval caused by such foreign intervention, subsequent loss of tribal lands, widespread migrations westward, the emergence of mixed-blood families, and the collapse of traditional village life, the tribes of the Southeast have been remarkably resilient in surviving four centuries of change. For many of the Native peoples living in the Southeast today, the past 20 years have been a period of marked population growth for both urban- and rural-dwelling Indians (O'Donnell, 1994).

Southwestern Indians

Southwestern Indian culture is the product of a coherent cultural network dating back to the Aztecs. Early Indian settlements centered around agricultural communities defined by an architecture of multistory buildings and large ceremonial centers. The major peoples of this area include the Hopi, the Pueblo, and the Athabascan-speaking Navajo and Apache, who migrated south from the sub-Arctic region sometime around the 13th century. The nomadic Apache people mixed with agriculture-based village peoples such as the Navajo. Interchange or cultural heritage engendered new ceremonial and performance forms such as ritual dance. New and complex themes emerged, underlying traditional creation myths previously held sacred in the region.

The Spanish intervention in the early 16th century brought tight control of village peoples and widespread suppression of traditional cultural practices. American Indians faced hardships such as forced labor, military conscription, and compulsory religious conversion. Southwestern tribes such as the Navajo, the Apache, and the Ute, a hunting and gathering people, resisted intervention, defending themselves with the military power at their disposal. The emigration of the Comanche people into New Mexico from their Shoshoni homeland complicated the cultural dynamics of the region. By the mid-18th century, they were the dominant bison-hunting people of the southern Plains and the Southwest. Their trade dominance grew in influence as they soon controlled the horse and gun trade, selling to the Spanish themselves. Intertribal warfare was on the rise during this period, with the Comanche often allied with the Spanish in battles against the Apache and the Navajo. By the mid-1800s, the U.S. military entered the region, meeting strong opposition from Indian tribes collectively, particularly the Apache.

The modern southwestern Indian region, then, brings together the Apache, the Hopi, the Navajo, and the Pueblo people of New Mexico. Each culture offers distinct contributions to the area. The Navajo nation, as the largest group within the area (as well as within the entire United States), possesses the potential for significant consolidation of political power given its size. The Hopi and the Pueblo peoples have been known throughout the centuries for their talents in the narrative and visual arts. The Pueblo have produced many well-known artists, novelists, poets, scholars, and painters among their people. The southwestern culture area remains a vital center for the transmission of American Indian culture (Ortiz, 1994).

Northern Plains Indians

Despite a long history of economic and political forces amassed to destroy Plains culture, tribal communities have maintained their integrity and have endured into the late 20th century. The tribes we now associate with the High Plains had in fact migrated to the area from points farther east. Migration took place during the colonial period after 1650 as European settlement expansion forced many Indians westward.

Tribes such as the Cheyenne were among those forced westward into the Northern Plains as Iroquois expansion after 1650 pushed southern Canadian peoples and tribes in the Great Lakes region out of their lands. By the 1700s, the Cheyenne had occupied North Dakota and were subsisting on the cultivation of corn, the use of horses, and the hunting of buffalo.

Although the common non-Indian perception of Indian culture evokes an image of the nomadic Indian hunter/warrior, such a stereotype is at odds with American Indian history in the centuries preceding the rapid expansion of colonial settlements. Before the 1700s, most Indians in the East were farmers, living without horses. Nevertheless, Plains culture survived and advanced for two centuries until U.S. military forces "pacified" the Plains Indians, confining survivors to reservations. By the late 1870s, U.S. hunters had virtually slaughtered the large herds of buffalo, and without adequate buffalo supplies as a major food source, the Plains Indian culture no longer was possible.

Contemporary reservation life is the product of flexibility and endurance. The Plains Indians have absorbed western settlement without abandoning their cultural practice. Traditional practices such as powwows, tribal fairs, sun dances, sweat ceremonies, and naming rituals have survived the historical process of colonization and expansion into Indian lands. Tribes such as the Crow, the Sioux, and the Cheyenne remain alive and well, despite the widespread poverty and isolation that characterizes life on the Northern Plains reservations (Clow, 1994).

Northwest Coast Indians

The Northwest Coast is bounded by southeastern Alaska, western portions of British Columbia, and the states of Washington and Oregon. The cultures of the area have remained defiantly unique, despite the forces of demographic change beginning in the late 18th century. Tribal economies depended heavily on salmon and cedar as Indians worked both the Pacific Ocean and the forests of the Pacific Northwest.

Scholars reconstructing these early cultures see evidence that tribes worked both as traders and as farmers. Tribes such as the Tlingit were fishermen, whereas the Haida of southeast Alaska are better known for their woodworking skills and the craft of totemic art. A third group, the Tsimshian, sometimes are collectively known as the *northern matrilineal tribes* because of their distinctive form of social organization. Scattered among these major groups are dozens of distinct tribes and bands residing in southwest mainland British Columbia, southeast Vancouver Island, and much of western Washington. Linguistic diversity typifies the area, with several bands of such diverse tribes residing along the Oregon Coast and inland in the Willamette River Valley.

It is perhaps this combination of linguistic and cultural diversity that has enabled tribes of this area to participate in American and Canadian society without having lost their unique traditional roots. As Native communities in Alaska, British Columbia, Washington, and Oregon begin to assert their sovereignty as a means to develop economically and politically, they will continue to bring about positive change in a culturally sensitive manner (Boxberger, 1994).

Alaska Natives

There are four major indigenous groups in Alaska: the Aleut, the Eskimo (Yupik and Inuit), the coastal Tlingit and Haida, and the Athabascan. The Aleut people occupied small villages scattered throughout the Aleutian Islands, whereas the Eskimo peoples resided in an environment that spans mountain ranges, deep fjords, tundra, and flat coastal lowlands of the Arctic province. Yupik and Inuit peoples are "central-based wanderers" who spent part of the year moving from place to place while spending the other months as stationary settlers. The Tlingit, Haida, and Tsimshian occupied southeastern Alaska. The northern Athabascan people occupied a vast territory that extended through most of interior Alaska, bordered by the Arctic to the north and the temperate forests to the south.

Alaska Native culture has survived the adverse impact of competing colonial forces vying for Native lands. Whereas the Russians' hostile colonial enterprise occupied much of the 18th century, American colonialists seeking economic reward sought to legislate laws in favor of white settlements through most of the 19th century. As in other North American indigenous cultures, a subsistence economy was central to the lives of most Alaska Natives. Unlike their European American counterparts, these peoples have managed to retain subsistence economic models well into the 20th century. Many Natives consider themselves first and foremost hunters and fishermen. There also is evidence that subsistence economies are not only resilient but even growing in certain villages.

Tribal sovereignty is at the core of Alaska Native tribal government. Villages often maintain a right to self-rule, forming their own governments. Alaska Natives believe in exercising their local power to provide for self-sufficient village economies throughout the area (Maas, 1994).

Oklahoma Indians

Today, as in the past, Oklahoma is the home of the largest number of Indian tribes and peoples within the United States. A total of 38 federally recognized Indian nations continue to exercise their sovereign tribal status within Oklahoma. The great majority of these tribes are not indigenous to Oklahoma; rather, they were "resettled" in the state, most involuntarily, under the 19th-century federal Indian removal policy. Driven out of the South on what historians call "The Trail of Tears," tens of thousands of Indians from the Five Civilized Tribes—the Choctaw, the Chickasaw, the Creek, the Cherokee, and the Seminole—perished on forced marches that often were conducted in the dead of winter. Prior to the American Civil War, other tribes, including the Quapaw, the Seneca, and the Shawnee, also were removed to what is now Oklahoma.

Indian tribes in Oklahoma have worked to maintain their own sovereign governments from precontact times through forced removal and the bitter betrayal of statehood up to the present. The Five Civilized Tribes achieved a level of literacy and economic prosperity exceeding that of many other states by the mid-19th century.

Today, Oklahoma's Indian population reflects a demographics with great diversity in its large numbers. The current generation of Oklahoma's Indians are producing children who are combinations such as Choctaw-Ponca-Cheyenne-Delaware and Cherokee-Osage-Omaha-Creek-Apache. Contemporary Oklahoma tribes seem to be undergoing a revived interest in old ways and an increased pride in Indian identity (Strickland, 1994).

Indians of the Plateau, Great Basin, and Rocky Mountains

The Indian peoples of this area continue to live in their ancestral homes. The boundaries of this region span a distance between the states of Washington and Utah and from California to Wyoming. Given such a wide expanse of geographical distance, there is great variety in the cultural and economic systems of the region's tribes. Given that some cultures have remained intact over the past three centuries, all of the tribes enjoy a rich oral tradition about their origins, and tribal elders consider the stories to be both literature and history.

Today, tribes such as the Shoshoni and the Bannock have made the transition to the realities of a modern American economy. They often are employed in ranching, farming, and small business. They own their own agricultural enterprise and a construction business. Most important is the 20,000-acre irrigation project that the tribe operates, providing water to Indians and non-Indians alike. Other tribes have made strides in educational and economic self-determination. The Warm Springs of Oregon and the Yakima people of Washington are active in both of these areas, with major investments in the local lumber and utility industries. The Yakima have been successful in maintaining their own spiritual beliefs and promoting their own economic self-determination.

The Indians of this region are a diverse group of cultures. Although they have suffered tremendous losses to the forces of European colonial expansion, they, like so many other tribal groups from other geographical areas, have survived. Since the 1960s, the tribes have asserted themselves with greater force, offering tribally managed educational, health, and economic development programs. This type of innovative spirit, which has served them so well in the past, will be a source of strength in the coming century, as the Indians of this culture area continue on the road toward reclamation and reconstruction of traditional tribal sovereignty (Trafzer, 1994).

California Indians

The Native peoples of California, like almost all American Indian and Native Alaskan tribes, believe that they originated in North America. Traditional origin stories tell of a creator or creators whose awesome powers brought forth the physical universe and all plant and animal life. This cultural centrism created the precedent that tribal territories were sacred and intimately connected to the divine intentions of the Creator. Consequently, land, place, and sacred sites all had a tie to the Creation and to traditional events that were the major events and symbols in Indian history.

The Native Californian worldview centered around seeking a balance between physical and spiritual well-being at the extended family and tribal levels. Such a balance is based on the idea of reciprocity. Just as the individual or village would bring forth an offering to the spirit world, humans would in turn expect a favorable relationship with the spirit engaged. In addition, reciprocity formed the basis of economic relationships among individuals, extended families, and neighboring villages.

Such a worldview was brutally tested during the Spanish colonization of California. The Spanish Empire's plan was to reduce the numerous free and independent Native hunting and collecting villages and societies into a mass of peon laborers. Survival for California Indians remained difficult well into the late 19th century. Mission life was unbearable, and death through the transmission of European diseases took a much heavier toll on the Indian population. Some tribes and village populations had virtually disappeared from the face of the Earth. Those Indians who had survived the ravaging effects of infectious disease were confronted with violence from white settlers and the U.S. military throughout the 19th century.

Faced with the reality of complete extinction, California Indians have fought through the numerous legal channels made sparingly available to them since the early 1900s. Since that time, the California Indian population has grown to more than 200,000. Although it will take far longer than a century to reclaim what had been lost to a relentless series of policies designed specifically to destroy Indian culture and tribal life, much is now in the process of changing. Although issues such as poverty and health still threaten California Indians going into the next century, many tribes are reclaiming the strength found in original identity, as they look through the specter of their recent past, to reclaim that spirit of reciprocity governing the world of their ancestors (Castillo, 1994).

HISTORICAL PERSPECTIVES: A BRIEF OVERVIEW OF AMERICAN INDIAN AND ALASKA NATIVE HISTORY IN NORTH AMERICA

When European explorers first stepped ashore on North American soil, they encountered a wide variety of American Indian cultures that had existed in every region of the continent for thousands of years. North America was not a "vacant" continent as early European explorers had believed. To the contrary, some of the regions first touched by Europeans were in fact the homelands of the continent's most complex cultures. In the southeastern United States, tribal societies developed hereditary leadership, long-distance trading networks, and elaborate systems for obtaining and displaying wealth. With the arrival of Europeans in North America, many fully developed Indian cultures suffered catastrophic collapse. European diseases, warfare, and the social disruptions caused by loss of resources forever changed the people of this continent, but it did not destroy them. American Indians found many ways of adapting to change.

By the 1450s, many American Indian civilizations had risen and disappeared. During the years before Columbus's arrival, Indians were developing rich and diverse cultures and were engaging in agricultural development, cultivating uniquely American crops such as corn, tomatoes, potatoes, green beans, squash, pumpkins, and tobacco. They were living in teepees, Quonsets, longhouses, A-frames, pueblos, hogans, sod huts, or other types of dwellings. During this time, American Indians also were gaining considerable knowledge about medicine and astronomy and were developing a wide variety of music, art, and literature. Historians estimate that the American Indian population numbered between 1 and 2 million when Columbus landed in 1492. In a letter to the Queen of Spain, Columbus called these Natives a race of hardy people (Brown, 1970, p. 1). Early physicians, traders, and explorers remarked about the extraordinarily good health of the Natives, noting that Native peoples were clean, good looking, without apparent illness, and peaceful (Brown, 1970). With the arrival of the Europeans came the epidemic of diseases that killed hundreds of thousands of Indians. At the turn of this century, Native Indians were reduced to a paltry 200,000. More than 200 (out of an estimated 700) tribes became extinct. American Indians were ill prepared to fight off the diseases and illnesses brought over with the early settlers. Unlike the Europeans, who had built up a natural immunity through prior exposure, Indians had no natural immunity to smallpox, measles, tuberculosis, or typhoid. Indian people lived in small communities with clean water, sanitation, and healthy food that were free from the diseases that were so widespread in the European countries.

Today, the American Indians have increased to the numbers reported 500 years ago and have organized themselves into social and political groups concerned over the health and social welfare of their members. Meanwhile, the U.S. federal policy toward Indians has had a significant impact on the development of the Indian social and political groups. The history of American Indian federal policies can be roughly divided into four major periods since 1880:

1880–1932, assimilation and incorporation: During this period, the policy of the federal government was to "civilize" Indians and incorporate them into mainstream society. Boarding schools were built as a means to educate Indian youths in the ways of whites.

1933–1945, indirect rule: The federal government had a major role in reorganizing Indian social and political groups. Traditional Indian leadership was reorganized into counsels that adopted Western rules and structures.

1946–1960, termination: A serious termination policy proved to be significantly damaging to tribes as wholesale "termination" of tribes took effect. This resulted in loss of services, Indian "status," and Indian land. The intent was to end the "Indian problem" by terminating tribes.

1961–1990s, economic development and self-determination: This period marks tribal re-emergence as American Indians and Alaska Natives develop new models for economic sufficiency. This process provides the financial means for reclaiming a level of self-determination widespread among pre-Columbian American peoples. Tribes begin to take over major aspects of federal programs and services. (Young & Kim, 1993, p. 7)

The 1960s marked a major turning point in U.S. Indian policy. By the mid-1960s, the threat of termination of Indian reservations had subsided, and new government programs were introduced aimed at eliminating poverty in the United States. Many Indian reservations and tribal governments benefited from the new programs, and government policy became redirected, allowing reservation-based tribal governments more control over local administration of government programs. Local management of community reservations, largely managed by the Bureau of Indian Affairs since the 1880s, became the theme of the new U.S. Indian policy. This policy, called "self-determination," characterized most of the period from 1965 to 1996 and became the policy for Indian affairs for the foreseeable future. Through the 1960s and 1970s, reservation-based tribal governments received considerable federal funding to service reservation needs such as housing, health, community action, and education. During the 1980s, federal funding available to Indians declined, and inflation made the smaller level of funding worth even less.

The 1980s, however, increasingly saw Indian communities work to gain more control over reservation governments, over reservation industry and mineral resources, and over education and other reservation institutions that were generally managed through the Bureau of Indian Affairs. With the passage of Public Laws 93-638 and 94-437, as well as more recent administrative processes providing for "self-governance" and "self-determination," the funding base for the power of the Indian health care delivery system has shifted to the wants and needs of tribal entities. This has resulted in the disbursement of "tribal shares," which has contributed to the reduction of the Indian Health Service (IHS) staff and program offices. In the future, it is anticipated that most Indian reservation communities will work toward furthering the goals of cultural and political self-determination.

SOCIODEMOGRAPHIC CHARACTERISTICS OF AMERICAN INDIAN AND ALASKA NATIVE POPULATIONS

The U.S. census reports 2.3 million American Indians, Eskimo, and Aleut residing in the United States, representing .09% of the U.S. population (Russell, 1996), the smallest racial minority in the United States. There are more than 500 federally recognized tribes and more than 100 state and non-federally recognized tribes and bands. The federal government recognizes 310 reservations, 217 Alaska Native villages, 12 Alaska Native regional corporations, 50 American Indian trust lands, and 17 tribal jurisdiction statistical areas. Most reservations are clustered in 35 states, primarily in the western half of the United States. Approximately one half of the American Indian population lives in the West, with the remainder residing primarily in the South (27%), Midwest (18%), and East (6%) (U.S. Bureau of the Census, 1990).

The American Indian of today can be described as the poorest, least educated, and most neglected minority group in the United States. Identified problems include a pattern of poverty, social problems, and diseases unparalleled among major ethnic groups.

Nationally, American Indians have one of the youngest populations comparatively. According to the 1990 census, 34% of the general population was younger than 15 years, and 6% was older than 65 years (U.S. Department of Health and Human Services [U.S. DHHS], 1994). The median age for Indians was 24.2 years, compared to 32.9 years for all U.S. races (U.S. DHHS, 1994). Accounting for the younger population characteristics of the Indian community may be the high Indian birthrate. The American Indian live birthrate of 27.3 per 1,000 for the period 1990 to 1992 was 67% higher than the rate for all U.S. races of 16.3 per 1,000 during that period (U.S. DHHS, 1995b).

The social and economic profile of American Indians indicates that the Indian population differs substantially from U.S. residents in general. The Indian population is younger, with larger families that are more likely to be maintained by adult females. American Indians are less likely to have a higher education and more likely to be unemployed. Median income is lower, and Indian families have higher rates of poverty. Data from the 1990 census report the following statistics: Approximately 15% of Indian households are headed by females; 65.3% of American Indians age 25 years or older completed high school degrees or higher, compared to 75.2% of all U.S. races; less than one half reported earning bachelor's degrees (8.9% vs. 20.3%); 16.2% of Indian males were unemployed, compared to 6.4% for all U.S. races; the median income for Native households in 1989 was $19,897, which was two thirds the national median income of $30,056; and in all age categories except those over 75 years, American Indians ranked higher in reported percentage below poverty level than did any other ethnic group (U.S. Bureau of the Census, 1992).

One of the most difficult problems affecting the American Indian community is the school dropout rate. Data from the 1990 census report that among persons age 25 years or over, approximately 20% had not finished high school and that, of these, 32% had less than a ninth-grade education (U.S. Bureau of the Census, 1992). In the Indian foster care system, 45% of the school-age children are in special education or individual education programs (Division of General Pediatrics and Adolescent Health, 1992).

ACCULTURATION, INTEGRATION, AND GROWTH OF AMERICAN INDIAN AND ALASKA NATIVE POPULATIONS IN THE UNITED STATES

The multiplicity of tribes within the United States is further complicated by the increasing migration of American Indians and Alaska Natives to urban areas. More than 50% of American Indians and Alaska Natives reside in large metropolitan areas. This migration pattern has brought about new concerns for Native people. Migration to the city brings isolation because the urban environment lacks the network of family and community support found in the rural reservation/rancheria/village areas. Urban Indians tend to live dispersed within the larger population in the city, thus losing important support systems. Life in large metropolitan areas often can be more bleak and stressful. More than half of urban Indians sampled in a recent study (Hodge, Fredericks, & Kipnis, 1996) did not have enough money for food, clothing, housing, and other necessities of life. They also reported more fears about the safety of their neighborhoods and having been the victims of theft more frequently than did Indians living in rural areas. Furthermore, urban Indians were more likely to be unemployed, with 54% having been out of work for 1 month or more in the previous 3 months. Overall, urban Indians reported being more mobile and reported higher smoking rates, higher unemployment, less social support systems, and more "hassles" than did American Indians in the rural sites or reservations sampled. For more than 500 years, Indians have been forced to assimilate into mainstream society, resulting in deterioration of culture and ethnic identity. Long-term isolation from reservations and traditional homelands may contribute to the breakdown of social support systems among urban Indians.

The early reports on Indians in the city tended to create a generalized composite view of urban life for Indians. Today, it is counterproductive to talk about "the urban Indian" in the singular because the adjustment patterns, recreational behavior, and employment and educational expectations vary as much as the people classified as Indian and Alaska Native. The urban Indian, like the rural or reservation-based Indian, does not fit neatly into one unified category. Rather, any effort to construct a composite American Indian is undercut by the multiple levels of adjustment experienced by numerous and differing groups of American Indians within a variety of urban environments.

Most of the past research has been done on the first generation of Bureau of Indian Affairs relocatees into the cities during the 1950s and 1960s. Today, there is a generation of urban-dwelling Indians who never have seen their reservations, spoken their native tongues, or listened to their tribal elders. They are the urban Indians born in San Francisco, Los Angeles, Denver, or Anchorage—reared away from their traditional roots.

In the city, being Indian is tied to participating in the life of the Indian community. This aspect of life, more than anything else, identifies someone as Indian because it is a public statement of belonging, commitment, and pride. Even though the urban Indian has a community—a social network of other Indians—this sense of community differs dramatically from prescriptive cultural formation. Urban life has undone traditional tribal identity for some American Indians, posing a new set of challenges for the reclamation and nurturing of Indian tradition within the postmodern world.

HEALTH AND DISEASE AMONG AMERICAN INDIANS AND ALASKA NATIVES

An Overview of the Issues

The health status of American Indians currently is at a critical stage. Whereas Indians once died of acute infections such as smallpox, measles, and diphtheria, today they die of chronic diseases such as alcoholism, heart disease, cancer, and diabetes. The federal IHS reports that American Indians continue to present with extremely high disease rates for common, easily treatable illness and health problems. The five leading causes of death—diseases of the circulatory system; accidents, violence, and poisoning; diseases of the digestive system; neoplasm; and diseases of the respiratory system—accounted for nearly 80% of the total Indian deaths in 1992 and have changed little in order of importance over the years (U.S. DHHS, 1992).

The IHS reports that during the period 1989 to 1991, the Indian age-adjusted mortality rates for the following causes were considerably higher than those for all U.S. races:

Tuberculosis: 440% greater

Alcoholism: 430% higher

Accidents: 165% higher

Diabetes mellitus: 154% higher

Homicide: 50% higher

Pneumonia and influenza: 46% higher

Suicide: 43% higher (U.S. DHHS, 1994)

The high rates of sexually transmitted disease and teen pregnancy among American Indians indicate a high potential for heterosexual transmission of AIDS. The incidence of syphilis among Indians is three times greater for Indians than for non-Indians (U.S. Congress, Office of Technology Assessment, 1986).

American Indians are more likely to die in accidents than are those in the general U.S. population. The American Indian accident rate for the period 1990 to 1991 was higher for all ages relative to the general population. For Indian youths (ages 1 to 14 years), the rate was twice as high (23.5 vs. 12.4 per 100,000). For Indians between the ages of 15 and 41 years, the accident death rate was more than twice as high (99.4 vs. 42.5 per 100,000). For Indian adults (ages 25 to 44 years), the death rate from accidents was 3.3 times higher (107.4 vs. 32.6 per 100,000). And for older Indians (ages 45 to 64 years), the rate was 232.3 per 100,000 (vs. 226.2 per 100,000) (U.S. Bureau of the Census, 1992).

Diabetes is one of the leading causes of outpatient visits for the adult age group at IHS facilities. Indian deaths due to renal failure alone were reported to be 290% higher than the national average (U.S. DHHS, 1993).

In 1995, alcohol mortality was 5.5 times the rate for all other U.S. races combined (37.2 vs. 6.8 per 100,000) (U.S. DHHS, 1995a). Fetal alcohol syndrome was 33 times higher among Indians than among non-Indians.

Suicide is the second leading cause of death for Indian adolescents. In 1992, 21% of females and 12% of males reported ever having attempted suicide. Suicidal attempts and ideation were strongly associated with emotional stress, history of abuse, chemical use, and family problems, particularly violence and suicide by other family members. Nearly half (44.6%) of emotionally distressed adolescents have attempted suicide, compared to 16.9% of youths in general (Division of General Pediatrics and Adolescent Health, 1992).

A study of American Indian adults in northern California found a depressive symptomology (case rate using the Center for Epidemiologic Studies–Depression scale) of 41%, which is more than triple the U.S. general population rate of 16%. Women scored higher than men, unemployed scored higher than employed, and age exhibited a curvilinear effect, with higher rates found in late adolescence and early adulthood (Hodge & Kipnis, 1996).

Cancer is the second leading cause of death among Indian women over 45 years of age. The 5-year survival rate for easily treated cancers such as cervical cancer is poorer than that for any other ethnic group (U.S. DHHS, 1991).

Behavioral Impact on Health Status

Today, American Indians are dying from chronic diseases that are largely attributed to environmental conditions and behavioral patterns. Acculturation and assimilation have contributed to the adoption of unhealthy behavioral patterns and habits such as smoking, drinking alcohol, and injuries and accidents. Behavioral influences have resulted in poverty, illness, and increased social disruption.

The prevalence of smoking among American Indians is twice the rate of that reported for the general population (Hodge et al., 1995). The rates of smoking among Indian women of childbearing age (18 to 44 years) are very high (43%). In some western states, more than 50% of adult Indians smoke cigarettes. Two out of five Indian deaths are attributable to smoking (Hodge et al., 1991). Smoking increases rates of cardiovascular disease, cancer (including cervical, lung, oral cavity, esophageal, bladder, kidney, and pancreas), low birthweight, birth defects, and sudden infant death syndrome. American Indians experience increased rates of premature death due to cardiovascular disease and cancer, two of the leading causes of death in this population. The American Indian 5-year survival rate for all cancers is the poorest recorded for all ethnic groups.

The historical importance of tobacco to American Indian culture is multidimensional. The role of tobacco in religious and ceremonial practices has been complicated by its economic importance for the American Indian population. As a cash crop, tobacco has provided economic security for American Indians for generations. In the traditional usage, tobacco is a gift of the Earth. It is used as a spiritual communicator and as a cleansing agent. Tobacco is given as a gift to healers and often is used in healing ceremonies. Tobacco also has become one of the few sources of economic stability on otherwise poor rural reservation areas. Small vendors (e.g., smoke shops) are able to make a living by selling tax-free tobacco products on Indian lands. This economic incentive in areas where unemployment is high presents a barrier to smoking cessation and control now that it is clear that smoking presents an undeniable health hazard for Indians and non-Indians alike.

Alcoholism among American Indians has reached epidemic proportions and has been described as the number one health problem among Indians. The federal government reports that the Indian alcoholism death rate is more than five times greater than that reported for all U.S. races (U.S. DHHS, 1995a). Of the 10 leading causes of death for American Indians and Alaska Natives, four are alcohol related. The death rate from cirrhosis is five times higher among American Indians and Alaska Natives ages 25 to 44 years than for the general population. At least 80% of homicides, suicides, and motor vehicle accidents in the American Indian population are alcohol related. Cigarette smoking combined with alcohol usage place American Indians at risk for throat cancer and neoplasms of the pharynx. They also contribute to accidents, home fires, and violence.

Accidents and violence, often a consequence of alcohol or substance abuse, accounted for 21% of all Indian deaths during the period 1990 to 1992, almost three times the national figure. Accidents and violence also are a leading cause of inpatient and outpatient care for Indians (U.S. DHHS, 1992). The IHS has determined that 75% of all accidental deaths to American Indians are alcohol related.

Impact of Environmental Contamination on Health Status

Health status is a function of a variety of factors such as behavior, environment, heredity, and health services. Of these, the poisoning of the environment is an irreversible harm that will threaten generations of American Indians.

In the late 19th and early 20th centuries, gold, timber, minerals, and water were mined, harvested, and harnessed in the West. Many Indian reservations were found to be rich in minerals sought by non-Indians. Little thought was given to environmental consequences, which resulted in extensive damage to land, posing a new threat to Indian health. For instance, arsenic used in mining camps contaminated the water. Logging disrupted the game supply and damaged the land; dams erected on rivers for electrical power changed the course of water to downstream sites and halted the annual migration of salmon. Newer riches were sought from the land. Uranium mining on the Navajo reservation left many Indians with a new disease—cancer and radiation poisoning.

Development of reservation resources has brought environmental concerns that mirror those of the United States as a whole. For instance, trace metal content in teeth of postindustrial Hopis is similar to that found in California suburban residents showing contamination from heavy metals. Indian reservations are on federal land and, as such, often are near toxic waste dumps. Contaminated water supplies, contaminated soil, and even air quality are now more commonplace on reservation sites. It is not too surprising that we are seeing an increase of cancers and other health problems related to the environmental contamination of Indian lands.

Four of the five leading causes of hospitalization at IHS facilities (respiratory illness, digestive system diseases, injuries and poisoning, and circulatory ailments) have potential environmental causes, and three of the five leading causes of outpatient visits (respiratory diseases, nervous system and sense organ ailments, and endocrine, nutrition, and metabolic disorders) might have environmental linkages.

Many of these elevated disease risks are due to poverty, excessive use of alcohol and tobacco, lack of health care services, and high risk-taking behavior (Valway,

Kileen, Paisano, & Ortiz, 1991). In addition, individuals engaged in occupations such as uranium mining have elevated risks of chronic lung diseases, silicosis, lung cancer, and other radiation-related malignancies (U.S. DHHS, 1992). Because of the lack of disposal facilities, hazardous wastes from mining, agriculture, and petroleum extraction have contaminated many Indian lands in the western states of Utah, Arizona, New Mexico, California, and Washington, where Indian lands carry high burdens of industrial toxins. This has led to contamination of air, water, and soil and to despoliation of sacred grounds. In addition, this contamination has affected agriculture such as berries and the reeds and willows used in traditional basket weaving. Forest trails and rural roadsides often are sprayed with weed-retarding chemicals and other highly toxic pesticides, thus affecting potential agriculture used for food or crafts.

Urban Indian residents share with poor inner-city communities high exposure to lead-based paints, air pollution, noise, unsanitary plumbing, and exposure to urban toxic and industrial wastes. These environmental impacts are not the only changes affecting Indian health. Stress caused from unemployment and relocation to large cities created new problems. Indians found themselves moved to large metropolitan areas where they were unaccustomed to "city living." They no longer could hunt, fish, or grow their food; a self-sufficient subsistence lifestyle had become a way of the past. Their family members were too far away to visit. Bad habits acquired in their new neighborhoods contributed to poor health. Cigarette smoking, poor eating habits, alcoholism, and dysfunctional families added to the stress.

Overview of the Indian Health Service

American Indians and Alaska Natives have a special relationship with the federal government in regard to their medical care. Indians living on or near their reservations are eligible for medical services at IHS facilities. Although IHS services are not limited to reservation-based Indians, IHS clinical facilities usually are found on or near reservations and receive most of the federal funds allocated for Indian health.

The U.S. DHHS, primarily through the IHS of the Public Health Service, is responsible for providing health and medical services to American Indians and Alaska Natives. The Indian Self-Determination and Education Assistance Act of 1975 (amended in 1988, 1990, and 1994) gave Indian tribes the capability of contracting directly with the IHS for the management and control of their own health programs. These contracted programs are commonly referred to as "638 contracts." Thus, the Self-Determination and Education Assistance Act enabled Indians to become more actively involved in determining their health care for the first time.

Currently, the IHS program consists of both IHS and tribally operated hospitals, clinics, and health centers as well as its Contract Health Services component. Services are coordinated through its regional administrative units called IHS area offices. IHS facilities and Indian-operated clinics are able to enter into contracts with outside facilities and physicians to provide services needed.

The operation of the IHS health service delivery system is managed through local administrative units called *service units*. A service unit is the basic health organization for a geographical area served by the IHS program. These are defined areas, usually centered around a single federal reservation in the continental United States or a population concentrated in Alaska. The service units are grouped into larger cultural-demographic-geographic management jurisdictions that are administered by IHS area offices (U.S. DHHS, 1994).

Healthy People 2000 Objectives: Implications for Health Promotion and Disease Prevention Among American Indians and Alaska Natives

The *Healthy People 2000: National Health Promotion and Disease Prevention Objectives* provide a standard goal toward which all Americans can strive—equitable health status for all racial/ethnic groups by the year 2000. For American Indians, these objectives require close consideration because there is a dearth of data on American Indians to monitor progress. Most cancer registries do not record data specific to American Indians. Most statistical reports do not isolate and report on American Indian morbidity and mortality because the Indian population is a fraction (.08%) of the total U.S. population.

To reach the goal of equitable health status for all racial/ethnic groups by the year 2000, appropriate health care services are required. American Indians and Alaska Natives have little chance of reaching the *Healthy People 2000* objectives, given current levels of resources and services, because there is a significant lack of services and resources with which to support targeted culturally appropriate community-based programs and services. Currently, the IHS provides health care services to one half or less of the total Indian population. This federal agency provides both primary care and inpatient care to American Indians living on or near reservations or approved areas. Migration to large metropolitan areas has resulted in loss of health care services to a significant number of Indians. It also has resulted in increased health problems due to poverty, stress, and violence. The health needs of the American Indian population have changed, and the health care delivery system must change as well to meet these needs.

The American Indian experience with regard to risk factors is both alarming and disgraceful. Serious behavioral and social problems, leading to injuries and early death, are well known. Suicide rates are rising, and deaths due to homicide, accidents, and injuries are one of the leading causes of Indian mortality. Newer threats to Indian health such as cancer, diabetes, nutritional diseases, and other illnesses due to changing behavioral and to environmental contaminants are on the rise. These behavioral problems have become epidemic and contribute heavily to death and disease. They must become the priority areas to control if we are to reach the *Healthy People 2000* objectives.

HEALTH BELIEFS AND PRACTICES AMONG AMERICAN INDIAN AND ALASKA NATIVE POPULATIONS: A GENERAL OVERVIEW

There are numerous health beliefs and practices within the various American Indian and Alaska Native tribes. Many tribes continue to practice traditional ceremonies that are tied to maintaining balance and well-being. The use of medicine men, traditional healers, and herbal remedies and medicines is a continued practice in many rural and urban areas. The extent of these and other culturally influenced health beliefs and practices vary from one tribe to another.

Differences in culturally based beliefs about risk factors for illness in general are characteristics that need to be better understood because these factors affect the acceptance and use of medical care services. Modesty, taboos, and use of traditional healing practices are important elements of a cultural belief system maintained among American Indians and Alaska Natives.

In all American Indian and Alaska Native cultures, interactions on all levels contain the fundamental element of *respect*. Respect is how one presents himself or herself to the world and how one acts. Respect is tied to being Indian and Native. Elders will state that respect means not talking about oneself, not bragging about what one has done or will do; it means not talking back, and treating everyone as equal and good. It also means giving back and sharing what is given to one. How one is treated and how one treats others are very important. Respect is valued as the core of being Indian and Native.

In addition, Indian and Native people place a very high value on cultural sensitivity, and "the most important features sought [by] health care staff are treatment with respect and kindliness and understanding of American Indian and Alaska Native ways" (Bennett, 1992, p. 2). Culturally sensitive care is not traditional medicine, nor is it care provided by only those from within that culture or ethnic group; rather, it is care that is open and accepting of other worldviews and styles of interactions. It is care that is "comfortable" for both the provider and the patient and that embodies a primary philosophy that is firmly rooted in the concepts of "caring" and "healing."

BARRIERS TO HEALTH PROMOTION AND DISEASE PREVENTION IN AMERICAN INDIAN AND ALASKA NATIVE POPULATIONS

There are several significant barriers to Indian health care. These can be identified as (a) cultural barriers, (b) system barriers, and (c) financial barriers. Over the years, American Indians have been forced to assimilate rapidly into mainstream society with consequent deterioration of culture and ethnic identity. American Indian youths, in particular, are strongly affected by the adverse conditions affecting their family units. High mobility of long-standing urban residents and reservation-based new arrivals to urban areas, disintegration of the family unit, high unemployment rates, and serious behavioral and emotional problems of adults add to the problems.

A significant portion of the American Indian population receives health care services from the IHS, a part of the federal Public Health Service. Health services to Indians actually began in the Department of War as an attempt to control the spread of epidemics to military post personnel and their families. The IHS was designed primarily for Indians residing on reservation lands. Today, however, more than 50% of Indians reside in large metropolitan areas, where access to health services is limited. The health care delivery system has developed into a dual system in which a "cradle-to-grave" system is operating in rural reservation sites and a limited piecemeal system is operating in several urban sites.

Although the health services components of rural and urban Indian clinics are similar to mainstream health clinics, they are unique because of their attention to cultural sensitivity and their ability to communicate effectively with their service population. The IHS provides most, if not all, of the rural Indian clinic funding resources. For urban Indian clinics, the IHS provides less than 50% of their total funding base. Urban Indian programs always have been viewed as separate programs from the IHS's reservation-oriented direct services system.

CHAPTER SUMMARY

Some 500 years ago, the Native peoples of North America roamed the vast continent of North America. Their subsistence economy, which depended on nature and the land, was physically and spiritually healthy. Some tribes became farmers and grew corn and squash; others were hunters and gatherers following the seasons. Game animals were stalked, and physical exercise was a way of life. Diseases caused by poor nutrition, such as heart disease, diabetes, high blood pressure, and obesity, were unknown.

American Indian culture has lost its measure of self-sufficiency to the relentless processes of acculturation and assimilation brought about by the economic forces of urbanization and industrialization. Today, many Indians no longer fish and stalk game animals; they cannot hunt buffalo because the buffalo are gone—exterminated by the settlers. Salmon fishing in the Northwest has been restricted due to the barriers placed by the dams. Cities have been erected over traditional sites. Herbs and healing medicines have been plowed under the ground or paved over for highways. Nuclear plants, toxic waste dumps, and contaminated waste have infected reservation lands with pollutants.

Since the arrival of European settlers, the American Indian population has survived policies of genocide, cultural assimilation, and social disruption. None of these destructive forces, however, has carried the potential threat to land, livelihood, and future generations as has the current contamination and toxic damage to Indian lands. The answer to controlling or eliminating this contamination might lie in educating Indians to the extent and enormity of the threat to tribal lands.

The magnitude of health problems confronting American Indians, ranging from the emotional and psychological to the physiological, presents a formidable challenge to health educators. The key to responding to these health problems is understanding the cultural context under which they present themselves. Also, health providers must understand that the unique historical context of our First Americans as an indigenous people sheds light on the ability and desire of American Indians and Alaska Natives to survive.

REFERENCES

Bennet, T. (1992). *American Indians in California: Status and access to health care* (monograph series). San Francisco: University of California, San Francisco, Institute for Health Policy Studies.

Boxberger, D. (1994). Northwest Coast Indians. In D. Champagne (Ed.), *The Native North American almanac.* Detroit, MI: Gale Research.

Brown, D. (1970). *Bury my heart at Wounded Knee: An Indian history of the American West.* New York: Holt, Rinehart & Winston.

Castillo, E. (1994). California Indians. In D. Champagne (Ed.), *The Native North American almanac.* Detroit, MI: Gale Research.

Champagne, D. (Ed.). (1994). *The Native North American almanac.* Detroit, MI: Gale Research.

Clow, R. (1994). Northern Plains Indians. In D. Champagne (Ed.), *The Native North American almanac.* Detroit, MI: Gale Research.

Division of General Pediatrics and Adolescent Health. (1992). *The state of Native American youth health.* Minneapolis: University of Minnesota.

Grinde, D., Jr. (1994). Northeastern Indians. In D. Champagne (Ed.), *The Native North American almanac.* Detroit, MI: Gale Research.

Hodge, F. S. (1991). *Tribal tobacco policy workbook.* Unpublished manuscript, Northwest Portland Area Indian Health Board.

Hodge, F. S., Cummings, S. R., Fredericks, L., Kipnis, P., Williams, M., & Teehee, K. (1995). Prevalence of smoking among adult American Indian clinic users in northern California. *Preventive Medicine, 24,* 441-446.

Hodge, F., Fredericks, L., & Kipnis, P. (1996). Urban-rural contrasts, patient and smoking patterns in northern California American Indian clinics. *Cancer, 78,* 1623-1628.

Hodge, F. S., & Kipnis, P. (1996). Demoralization: A useful concept for case management with Native Americans. In P. Manoleas (Ed.), *The cross-cultural practice of clinical case management in mental health.* New York: Hawthorn.

Maas, D. (1994). Alaska Natives. In D. Champagne (Ed.), *The Native North American almanac.* Detroit, MI: Gale Research.

O'Donnell, J. (1994). Southeastern Indians. In D. Champagne (Ed.), *The Native North American almanac.* Detroit, MI: Gale Research.

Ortiz, R. D. (1994). Southwestern Indians. In D. Champagne (Ed.), *The Native North American almanac.* Detroit, MI: Gale Research.

Russell, C. (1996). *The official guide to racial and ethnic diversity.* Ithaca, NY: New Strategist Publications.

Strickland, R. (1994). Oklahoma Indians. In D. Champagne (Ed.), *The Native North American almanac.* Detroit, MI: Gale Research.

Trafzer, C. E. (1994). Indians of the Plateau, Great Basin, and Rocky Mountains. In D. Champagne (Ed.), *The Native North American almanac.* Detroit, MI: Gale Research.

U.S. Bureau of the Census. (1990). *Census of the population: Characteristics of the population.* Washington, DC: Government Printing Office.

U.S. Bureau of the Census. (1992). *Minority economic profiles* (Tables CPH-L-92, 93, 94, and 95). Washington, DC: Government Printing Office.

U.S. Department of Health and Human Services.(1991). *American Indian task force report on the year 2000 health promotion objectives and recommendations for California.* Rockville, MD: Indian Health Service.

U.S. Department of Health and Human Services. (1992). *Trends in Indian health.* Rockville, MD: Indian Health Service.

U.S. Department of Health and Human Services. (1993). *Regional differences in Indian health.* Rockville, MD: Indian Health Service.

U.S. Department of Health and Human Services. (1994). *Trends in Indian health.* Rockville, MD: Indian Health Service.

U.S. Department of Health and Human Services. (1995a). *Regional differences in Indian health* (charts). Rockville, MD: Indian Health Service.

U.S. Department of Health and Human Services. (1995b). *Trends in Indian health* (tables). Rockville, MD: Indian Health Service.

Valway, S., Kileen, M., Paisano, T., & Ortiz, E. (1991). *Cancer mortality among Native Americans in the United States: Regional differences in Indian health, 1984-1987.* Rockville, MD: Indian Health Service.

Young, I. S., & Kim, E. C. (1993). *American mosaic: Selected readings on American multicultural heritage.* Englewood Cliffs, NJ: Prentice Hall.

15

Assessment, Program Planning, and Evaluation in Indian Country

Toward a Postcolonial Practice

BONNIE M. DURAN
EDUARDO F. DURAN

This chapter discusses the pleasures and challenges of conducting public health needs assessment, program planning and implementation, and evaluation in "Indian Country."[1] It begins with a discussion of potentially unconscious elements of the practitioner's conceptual framework and the multiple functions and outcomes of health promotion and disease prevention (HPDP) efforts. It then outlines standard public health approaches to needs assessment, planning and implementation, and evaluation and specific nuances of that work in Indian Country.

So long as Native American and Alaska Native communities suffer disproportionately from disease, trauma, and other social problems, HPDP efforts will be indispensable. Conducting these efforts affords multiple pleasures and challenges for Native American groups and public health professionals, and it achieves multiple outcomes.

The authors support a postcolonial approach to work in Native communities (Duran & Duran, 1995). This approach is inherently hybrid. It uses the latest that public health and other social science disciplines have to offer in assessment, planning, and evaluation while anchoring HPDP efforts within Native American control and in Native American social, cultural, and spiritual knowledge. In addition to improving health status, an inherent aim of many Native American-controlled HPDP efforts is to empower people and transform ethnocentric social structures and social science. In this sense, they are founded on the public health principle of social justice.

Constructing a Workable Conceptual Framework

Conceptual frameworks typically include the theory of etiology and theory of change for the health issues or problems for which interventions are planned. More fundamentally, conceptual frameworks include, among other things, our assumptions about target populations, motivations for wanting to work with specific groups, and ideas about the roles professionals and community representatives assume in that work. It is useful to make conceptual frameworks explicit (an exercise in self-reflection) when working in environments that might be organized by worldviews, historical experiences, and principles that are different from our own (Marcus & Fischer, 1986).

Successful working relationships between Native American communities and health professionals are dependent on overcoming misconceptions and clarifying assumptions about both Native peoples[2] and public health practice. For example, popular culture beliefs about Native people's homogeneity are misguided. A crucial step in liberating Native subjectivities from the straitjacket of binary oppositions (white/Indian) is gaining an understanding of the diversity of Native communities and perspectives (Fleming, 1992; Prakash, 1995). In 1492, more cultural and linguistic diversity existed on this continent than could be found in all of Europe. The differences among tribes still account for 50% of American cultural diversity (Berkhofer, 1979; Hodgkenson, 1990). Native heterogeneity is marked by differences in language, normative beliefs and behavior, gender roles, spiritual practices, migration, social class, economic opportunity, openness to other cultures, religion, and history, among other differences.

In addition to differences among tribes, differences among tribal members and groups are significant. It is inaccurate to assume that all members of one tribe share opinions about matters such as the role of government, tradition, spirituality, and economic development. Like all communities in the postmodern social context, tribal groups can be highly factionalized. For example, individuals in impoverished communities where social service funds are an important source of revenue often are stratified by access to federal and other public resources (Ong, 1987).

Attitudes toward outsiders vary among Native American groups. Social research and interventions in Indian Country have left many participants feeling exploited and mistrustful (Beauvais & Trimble, 1992). The issue of European Americans and other non-Indians working in communities of color, therefore, is a common concern of Natives and others. The subject is overly simplified once again by the unvoiced assumption of a binary opposition (Euro-American perspective/Native perspective). There are numerous perspectives, characterized as ranging from conservative to radical, in all ethnic groups. A decision to match ideological positions may alleviate tensions among individuals and groups trying to work together.

Understanding the motivation for wanting to work in ethnic communities different from one's own is an important focus of professional reflection. A research assistant, for example, recently told the authors that she wanted to work with Native Americans to voice their concerns to people in power. The authors' response was to ask her whether her anthropology education included a course in ventriloquism. Can any research or researcher hope to speak authentically of the experience of the "other"? This thorny problem is partially addressed through participatory and collaborative public health practice and through efforts of historically marginalized groups to increase public health practice capacities of their own.

The ideal situation for the public health practitioner wanting to work with Native peoples is to be contracted by, or to work directly under the supervision of, the tribe or Native community agency itself. Because this is *not* how most public health projects are initiated, many tribes have established policies that give their communities more control over outside research and evaluation. The tribal or agency institutional review board is gaining popularity as a way in which to control the amount and type of research and programs conducted on reservations or in Indian agencies. Tribal council or board approval is, at the very least, commonly required to begin any intervention work.

Many tribes and Native organizations have developed their own planning, research, and development divisions to respond to knowledge and intervention needs more directly. Sovereignty, always a paramount tribal concern, is furthered by the widespread American political trend toward state and local control of social service funds (block granting). Toward this end, tribes are taking over federal programs and funding (Public Law 93-638) from federal government entities such as the Indian Health Service (IHS) and the Bureau of Indian Affairs, and many professionally trained Native Americans are moving from federal jobs to tribal agencies and other Native-controlled enterprises.

MULTIPLE FUNCTIONS OF HEALTH PROMOTION AND DISEASE PREVENTION PROJECTS IN INDIAN COUNTRY

The recognition that politics and science are inextricably linked and, therefore, significant aspects of program planning, implementation, and evaluation is infusing social service fields (Greene, 1994; Habermas, 1988; Institute of Medicine, 1988; Keller, 1992; Lincoln & Denzin, 1994; Tesh, 1988). Fundamental to this position is the acknowledgment that science and HPDP efforts are enacted by people, embodied as we all are by multiple subject positions—ethnicity, gender, class, sexual orientation, region, and so on. The recipients or audiences of HPDP efforts are likewise situated and may desire projects for different reasons— cultural, spiritual, political, economic, medical, bureaucratic, and so on.

Tribal leaders often see HPDP funds as economic and employment opportunities as well as opportunities to raise the health consciousness and status of their communities. A common positive, but not well-documented, outcome of intervention efforts is employment development. The authors recently documented a trend toward upward employment mobility by staff of a primary prevention project among tribes in eastern California. This upward mobility was accomplished, in part, by the training, experience, and self-confidence provided by the HPDP intervention.

Cultural integration and community building are other important outcomes of HPDP projects (Minkler & Wallerstein, 1997). Social and cultural activities and relationships constitute Native American communities as such and inscribe meaning to identity. Implementing efforts that are rooted in cultural and spiritual tradition helps to reestablish tribal and family social networks as well as forms of social control that were lost largely through government efforts to eradicate Indian culture (O'Brien, 1989). Community building is accomplished through the opportunity for Native people to come together and affirm their commitment to each other and healthful lifestyles. Many of these outcomes are captured through attention to changes in the number and type of, as well as participation in, community activities and concomitant tribal or agency policies regarding community events.

CLASSIC NEEDS ASSESSMENT AND ISSUES PARTICULAR TO NATIVE COMMUNITIES

Classic needs assessment describes health and social service requirements in a geographic or social area and then estimates the relative importance of those needs in the context of available resources (Siegel, Attkisson, & Carson, 1987). Needs assessment is an integral component of a cyclical public health core functions framework in which assessment informs policy that guides assurance activities.

Needs Assessment Process Issues

Within Native communities, increasing local capacity to conduct assessments and assuaging historical mistrust are important goals. Developing an inclusive and empowering process, therefore, requires attention to and planning of the *procedures* of assessment. The public health practitioner who has trained and worked within formal organizations often is oriented toward outcomes rather than process and, therefore, is less attuned to issues of process.

Empowering processes include oversight power by community leaders and an opportunity for community members to voice their satisfaction, concerns, and complaints about health assessment and subsequent services. Within the IHS, for example, some service units are beginning to work closely with tribal health boards in defining and addressing health needs and projects in their regions. In this case, tribal health boards have an informal approval authority on IHS yearly strategic plans. Reservation-based town hall meetings provide an opportunity for the dissemination of epidemiological data on health status and the space for dialogue about the needs and quality of services from a community perspective. A space for community input must be designed into the system, regardless of whether or not people immediately take advantage of the opportunity to speak. Patience is the real mark of commitment in Native communities.

Although processes can be designed to improve community control and participation, the practitioner should not be discouraged or surprised if he or she encounters resistance to his or her efforts. Regarding the degree to which colonial structures share similarities, Scott (1990) asserts, "They will, other things equal, elicit reactions and patterns of resistance that are also broadly comparable" (p. xi). He identifies four types of political discourse produced by historically marginalized groups:

1. *Public discourse:* official ideology of relations between oppressed and oppressor that takes as its basis the flattering self-image of elites
2. *Hidden transcript:* subordinates gathering outside the gaze of power and constructing a sharply critical political and cultural discourse
3. *Coded counter hegemonic discourse:* subordinate groups making use of disguise and anonymity to find an avenue for the veiled expression of hidden transcripts within public discourse
4. *Open defiance:* a public refusal to comply with words, gestures, or other signs of normative compliance; a public announcement of the intention to engage in conflict

A public unveiling of "hidden transcripts" resulting in community conflict is a sign that disenfranchised groups are realizing and exercising their inherent power. Building an allied base from within the community, developing cross-cultural communication skills, and cultivating sensitivity to the historical bases of conflict and mistrust are ways to prevent or lessen conflicts. If the HPDP practitioner is confident of his or her cross-cultural competence (which is ideally based on successful experience with a multitude of ethnic groups different from the practitioner's own rather than on classroom success), then not taking the conflict personally is an important attitudinal approach. Time, commitment, knowledge, and sensitivity will be recognized by tribal leaders and will be rewarded with trust.

If serious conflicts do arise, then appealing to either informal or formal processes of mediation, based on tribal adjudication methods, may clear up misunderstandings. Some tribal governments have established programs for conflict resolution based on traditional Native forms of social control. In areas where formal programs have not been developed, there may be tribal members or groups known for mediation. Postcolonial practice requires the commitment to build communication and mediation skills and to work through conflict.

Compiling Existing Data

A standard element of needs assessment includes the compilation and synthesis of existing social indicator, epidemiological, and health service data. Although health service utilization data have their limitations in capturing population health status, the national office of the IHS compiles and synthesizes data on morbidity and mortality yearly. Two annual publications, *Trends in Indian Health* (U.S. Department of Health and Human Services [DHHS], 1995b) and *Regional Differences in Indian Health* (U.S. DHHS, 1995a), are excellent starting points for understanding the distribution of disease and trauma in Indian Country. The

IHS national office and some area offices[3] also are monitoring the progress of objectives from *Healthy People 2000* (U.S. DHHS, 1991). Other entities with responsibility for Native specific research and evaluation are useful sources of data. The national IHS Office of Research and Evaluation in Rockville, Maryland, the Native American and Alaska Native Center for Mental Health Research at the University of Colorado, and the Center on Alcohol and Substance Abuse at the University of New Mexico have produced or compiled excellent reports about Native health status, health problems, health services, and their correlates.

On a regional level, IHS area offices are starting to compile and synthesize data for smaller geographic locations. In New Mexico, for example, health service utilization data are available for small tribal areas and, in some cases, for reservation towns (R. Gollub, IHS office in Albuquerque, New Mexico, personal communication, September 1996). Unfortunately, the IHS is not yet collecting widespread health service outcome data. Fairly accurate denominators (i.e., total population numbers needed to calculate rates) are available from the national census or tribal census. Federal regulations allow the IHS to conduct population health surveys, but probability sample surveys involve a more complex approval process. The 1991-1992 Navajo Health and Nutrition Examination Survey (NHANES) is an example of the type of health and behavioral survey that may be available by IHS area office or tribe (C. Percy, Navaho area IHS office, personal communication, September 1996).

Regional business associations are useful sources of data on urban Indian communities. These entities often compile census and market data by ethnicity. Information about education and poverty levels, household makeup, and other social indicators is available for free or for a small fee. The Bureau of Indian Affairs regional offices and tribal economic development offices have comparable data for rural or reservation residents.

Some states, working alone or with the IHS, are beginning to oversample Native population in their Behavioral Risk Factor Surveys. State vital statistics offices also provide Native birth and death records including demographics and community of residence. Tribal health departments have conducted or sponsored community health surveys and needs assessments. Tribal health departments are crucial sources of survey data, needs assessment data, and (most important) collaboration.

Primary Data Collection

In comprehensive needs assessments, population-based community surveys are important sources of information about the community's perceptions of capacities and needs. Client utilization data capture information about a specific segment of the community, whereas population surveys provide access to sections of the population that might not, for a variety of reasons, use existing public resources. Community surveys are best undertaken either under the direction of or in conjunction with tribal health departments, tribal councils, or urban health or social service agencies. As stated earlier, many tribes and Indian organizations have an internal institutional review board process that governs all research activities.

Developing a realistic sampling frame requires collaboration with individuals very knowledgeable about Native residence and social network patterns. Although random or probability sampling is the most rigorous approach, this type of sampling for Native communities is problematic in both rural and urban areas. In most urban areas, the cost of probability sampling is prohibitive. Native researchers and others, however, have uncovered important patterns and insights about health-related needs, behavior, and attitudes by using purposive, convenience, and quota sampling.[4]

Key Informants in Indian Country

Key informants are important sources of information about community health status, community concerns, and health-related behavioral patterns, attitudes, and beliefs (Siegel et al., 1987). In the standard approach, key informants include personnel from social and health service agencies, schools, economic development endeavors, police and fire departments, and the like. Long-term community residents not in an official capacity also are a meaningful source of community knowledge. In Native communities, it is important to include information from cultural, spiritual, and political leaders. Each reservation town may have a person or family teaching cultural arts such as singing, drumming, dancing, and regalia design. Spiritual people and their helpers, medicine women and men, sweat lodge leaders, "road men," sobriety group leaders, and other religious or spiritual workers not only provide insight into assessment efforts but also support and provide legitimacy for the health practitioner's work. Often, there are advocacy groups working on salient community issues such as environmental, educational, and economic development concerns. These individuals illuminate the current political climate and help identify "natural helpers," people who, because of some characteristic highly valued in the culture, are influential and respected. Youths are another important source of information, particularly about the way in which they are influenced and affected by the variety of adolescent subcultural trends. For example, the authors' research in eastern California found that many Native adolescents identified highly with the vibrant Latino culture in the area and claimed Latino ethnicity on school-based surveys.

Talking to many types of individuals provides insight into community capacities and needs. If the forums or interviews are thorough, then the health practitioner probably will uncover differences of opinion about key community issues; he or she should be prepared to hear some venting. It is important not to be seen as taking sides or as supporting any position on these issues until the assessment is complete. Although it is impossible to be "disembodied" or totally neutral in any assessment, it is possible to minimize perceptions of working for any particular community political group or contingent.

Accessing Existing Community Capacity

The work of John McKnight and his colleagues at Northwestern University has increased awareness of the inherent capacity of communities to define and solve problems (Kretzmann & McKnight, 1993; McKnight & Kretzmann, 1990). His social problem analysis assumes a decline in "social integration" brought about by huge economic shifts and social service intrusion into the natural helping process and capabilities at the local level. His amelioration strategies, then, work to revive or improve local capacities by focusing on their strengths. Even before the groundbreaking work of McKnight and his colleagues, using existing talent and capacity had been a common practice in Indian Country. McKnight's work, however, reminds us that everyone in the community has something to offer. His "skills-capturing instrument" (McKnight & Kretzmann, 1990) provides a good template for similar efforts in Native communities. Community natural helpers can assist in distinguishing those skills specific to Native communities (e.g., community organizing, public speaking, powwow and other events organizing, facilitating, training, emceeing).

Building on community capacity is an ongoing approach in Native communities. Native-specific projects already employed include traditional, social, cultural, and spiritual practices (Beauvais & LaBoueff, 1985; Duran, 1996; Duran & Duran, 1995; May, 1986; Parker, 1990; Schinke, Gilchrist, Schilling, & Walker, 1986; Slagle & Weibel-Orlando, 1986; U.S. DHHS, 1990; Weibel-Orlando, 1989).

Accessing existing community capacity is institutionalized in the federal Indian Preference Hiring Act of 1975. Indian hiring preference accomplishes the agenda of community capacity building in numerous ways. It might, however, increase the need for training and supervision in Western bureaucratic modes of implementation, program maintenance, and organizing and documenting labor. In this situation, optimal project functioning is dependent on adequate mechanisms for oversight, training, and technical assistance.

Tying It All Together: Postcolonial Convergent Analysis

In a rational policy model, the distribution of resources is dependent on the relative importance, costs, and benefits of addressing any particular health problem compared to all others (Siegel et al., 1987). The postcolonial, self-determined, or empowerment approach that is adopted by many tribes and Native communities, however, also determines value from the perspective of community stakeholders and traditional values. An important principle of this approach is that Native community values, beliefs, and knowledge are valid and integral to the process of valuing (Duran & Duran, 1995). Standard cost-benefit analysis is a necessary but not a sufficient method for determining community needs or program priorities.

Once community needs are documented and prioritized, program planning directs action toward the amelioration of health problems and the promotion of healthful practices.

PROGRAM PLANNING IN NATIVE COMMUNITIES

Without adequate planning, many HPDP efforts in Indian Country fall into "activity traps." Compelled by the dual desires for visibility in the community and the provision of multiple recreation or social activities, activity traps occur when staff conduct health-related activities or events without linking them to causal and change theories or to specific health outcomes. These activity traps often rest on an unarticulated rational model; increased knowledge produces better attitudes that change behavior. This approach assumes that human action is primarily voluntary and conscious, that all ill health is a result of lack of knowledge, and that knowledge alone will produce the environmental and behavior change needed to protect and improve health status. Systematic problem analysis, program planning, and applied theory overcome this simplistic model. A well-informed and systematic planning process serves to define resource needs and increases performance and morale of prevention staff who understand their roles and can observe the concrete effects of their work.

The ecological perspective (McLeroy, Bibeau, Steckler, & Glanz, 1988) is a very useful framework for defining etiological factors. This approach, emphasizing determinants in the intrapersonal, interpersonal, institutional, community, and public policy spheres, seeks to define contributing factors at multiple levels of analysis. Epidemiological, social, and medical research findings and field experience are used to determine the extent to which certain factors contribute to or protect against disease, trauma, and other social problems. Using the ecological perspective enables one to recognize that Native peoples are not always the appropriate target of change, although the aim is improved Native American health status. Institutional practices, mainstream attitudes and beliefs, and economic policies are emphasized as having a direct impact on Native health status. Krieger (1994) reminds us that certain factors contribute more to poor health status than do others. She supports an "ecosocial" approach rather than an individualistic biomedical conception of disease, which does not adequately reflect the unequal contribution of factors. This warning is important for workers in Native communities where "commonsense" etiological understanding often includes the effects of historical processes, colonization, racism, cultural hegemony, poverty, and other outcomes of unequal power relations.

The contemporary HPDP field is rich with theories of change that include not only educational activities but also advocacy, organizational change efforts, policy development, economic supports, environmental change, and multimethod programs (Glanz, Lewis, & Rimer, 1990). Articulating the theories of change also is a prerequisite for good evaluation (Connell, Kubisch, Schoor, & Weiss, 1995).

Having identified and prioritized those problems most affecting a particular community (and subpopulations of that community), and having chosen appropriate etiological theories and thus targets of change, program planning proceeds toward devising interventions with a specific goal, a specific target, and measurable outcome objectives in mind. As with assessment efforts, program planning in Native communities is a collaborative effort that actively involves key leaders and members of the target population.

The logic model (U.S. DHHS, 1993), a five-step process, provides a simple and sensible approach to planning. Promoted by the Center for Substance Abuse Prevention, which has funded numerous community-based interventions in Indian Country since 1987, the logic model delineates core variables in HPDP planning. Logic model categories have been successfully adapted to employ Native community values (Edwards, Seaman, Drews, & Edwards, 1995).

The Logic Model

In Step 1, *problem identification,* the planner makes succinct statements about measurable intervention aims across ecological domains—reduce alcohol and drug use, decrease obesity rates, reduce unprotected sexual activity, increase screening behavior, and so on. The factors most alterable and most significant are targeted for change. This information is garnered from existing epidemiological and other research about the correlates of problems and from experience at the local level about the antecedents to problems. In Step 2, the *assumptions and literature* that support the problem identification are delineated. For each of the problems or risk factors, there is an assumption that the factor is related to the current or subsequent problem. In Step 3, *program objectives* are selected. The planner takes the problem statement and turns it into an action statement indicating what needs to be done to alleviate the problem or condition or to promote the protective factor. Each objective should specify a single measurable quantifiable result and should be accomplishable with existing resources and within the program time frame. In Step 4, *program strategies* for achieving the objectives should always be based on culturally appropriate theories of change. For example, in Table 15.1, the sobriety, coping, and bicultural skills curriculum is based on principles of social learning theory. In Step 5, *anticipated outcomes* assist the evaluation process by clearly delineating the results of the program. This step identifies the outcome indexes that the planner needs to determine whether his or her intervention was effective in fulfilling its objectives.

Operationalizing Theory

Subsequent to developing a causal theory, change theories help explain and delineate how those factors identified in disease and illness causality are best manipulated. Change theory is "operationalized" in the context of the practitioner's health problem and target population (Stanton, Black, Engle, & Pelto, 1992). Operationalization involves four steps: (a) defining components of the theory or model, (b) translating the component for the targeted behavior within the culture, (c) determining options for intervention design, and (d) determining content of intervention. Table 15.2 illustrates the first steps in this task using social cognitive theory for an alcohol, tobacco, and other drugs (ATOD) prevention program with high-risk youths in one reservation population. This type of joint activity with a variety of interested people (e.g., parents, youths, teachers,

TABLE 15.1 Logic Model for Alcohol, Tobacco, and Other Drug Prevention for a Specific Subpopulation of American Indian Youths

Level	Problem Identification	Assumptions and Literature	Project Objectives	Program Strategies	Anticipated Outcomes
Individual	Lack of sobriety skills; poor positive Native ethnic group identification	Experience of prevention workers (Trimble, Padilla, & Bell, 1987)	Reduce ATOD use; increase sobriety and coping skills; increase positive cultural identification	12-week sobriety skills curriculum; 12-week Native cultural education curriculum	Increased coping and sobriety skills; increased bicultural competency
Peer	Lack of peer support for nonuse	Experience of prevention workers (Trimble et al., 1987)	Create ATOD nonusing support/peer groups	Peer-managed self-control; Native American youth groups	Nonusing peer groups; perceptions of peer use decreased
School	Lack of commitment to school; low teacher expectations of Native youths; hostile environment	Parents and community leaders unhappy with what they perceive as racism in the schools	Reduce school-based racism; increase teacher cultural competency	Community organizing; school staff competency training; enforced school policy against racist activities	School mission includes honoring diversity; increased cultural competency; higher teacher expectations of Native youths
Community	Lack of clear-cut sanctions against use	Experience of prevention workers (Trimble et al., 1987)	Increase community sanctions against use by youths	Community organizing to change tribal council policies	Tribal policy concerning ATOD at community events, buildings

NOTE: ATOD = alcohol, tobacco, and other drugs.

health board members, prevention staff) brings many people experience and wisdom to bear on the problem and encourages communities and agencies to support the intervention.

Implementation

Green and Kreuter (1991) assert that textbooks can offer little implementation advice to improve on a "good plan, an adequate budget, good organizational and policy support, good training and supervision of staff, and good monitoring in the process evaluation stage" (p. 205). Program policies and procedures, however, also are key implementation tools for program design, program management, and staff accountability. For example, program policy and procedure manuals might include brief statements about the intervention target population, participant disqualification and reinstatement, rules for staff reimbursement for

TABLE 15.2 Operationalization of Social Cognitive Theory to Alcohol, Tobacco, and Other Drug Prevention Among Indian Youths

Define Theory Components	Cultural Interpretation	Determine Options for Intervention	Determine Content of Intervention
Behavioral capacity	Drinking alleviates stress or anger Fun involves drinking	Increase level of sobriety and coping skills Increase ATOD-free recreational activities	Adopt 12-week curriculum in intervention in youth groups Sponsor six community events during year
Expectations	Drinking is part of Indian social life Nonusing will isolate youths from Indian peer group No role for Indians in mainstream culture Success in school means acting "white"	Cultural education about history of ATOD in Indian Country Parental and teacher training to increase expectations of youths	8-hour teacher cultural competency training 8-hour parenting training Attend four local cultural events as part of intervention Develop Indian academic club at school with support from Native professionals
Self-efficacy	Youths doubt their ability to resist peer pressure Low self-esteem and self-efficacy due to racism and internalized oppression	Develop nonusing peer groups Reinstitute initiation rituals for youths	Native American youth societies in each town Weekly age- and gender-specific support groups in each town Skill-building workshops
Observational learning	There is a cadre of anti-drinking leaders in the community National Indian sobriety movement activities (e.g., National Association of Native American Adult Children of Alcoholics, Wellness Conference) High level of substance abuse among adults	Exposure to role models Exposure to consequences of excessive drinking	Attend one Indian men's and one Indian women's wellness conference Invite sobriety movement leaders to three community education events Invite Indian Alcoholics Anonymous speakers to two events
Reinforcement	There are more reasons to drink than not to drink	Increase community supports for ATOD-free behavior Develop tribal acknowledgments of success	Youth appointments to tribal council Youth "whip" persons at powwows Develop youth sobriety drum/dancing group Change school and tribal policy

NOTE: ATOD = alcohol, tobacco, and other drugs.

their own monies spent on activities, use of program funds, rules for overtime and travel out of the area, qualifications for community volunteers, supervision at events, parental permission for events, and so on. Clear-cut policies allow for equity of treatment for all staff and clients and for uniform training in the case of staff turnover. The need for specific policies and procedures will emerge as the program is implemented. Such policies are a useful and ever-evolving tool in program management.

Detailed implementation descriptions facilitate both implementation and evaluation. A matrix of key components and characteristics of the intervention is mapped out and might include responsible persons, the target group, activity, materials, a forum for activity, frequency/duration, and outcome expected (King, Lyons-Morris, & Fitz-Gibbon, 1987). Consider the balance, however, between the amount of creativity and spontaneity needed within community-based interventions and the amount of detail needed to ensure adequate program implementation. Implementation descriptions should be a "thick" description of what is actually happening on-site and not a bureaucratic straitjacket of micro-management.

EVALUATION IN NATIVE COMMUNITIES

Program evaluations of HPDP efforts in Indian Country are undertaken for a variety of purposes and, by nature of the heterogeneity of Indian life, in a variety of contexts. Evaluations conducted by tribal health programs and local IHS offices frequently have incremental program improvement as a key outcome, whereas demonstration and research projects funded by the federal government or national foundations usually focus on causal modeling, health service outcomes, and discovery. The theory of social program evaluation has progressed significantly during the past 10 years and warrants consideration here as the range of appropriate approaches for Indian Country are considered. Articulating the assumptions of various approaches allows us to conscientiously determine the best fit for the goals of Native communities.

Evaluation Theory Overview

Shadish, Cook, and Leviton (1991) have developed a useful three-stage topology of evaluation theory based on each stage's approach to five fundamental issues: (1) social programming, (2) knowledge construction, (3) valuing, (4) knowledge use, and (5) evaluation practice.

Stage 1 theory asserts that the purpose of evaluation is to determine causal relationships in an investigation of social problems. Positivistic methods are the only acceptable methodology. Experimental design, valid instrumentation, and bias control are key evaluative principles. Viewing evaluations as objective science, this approach urges practitioners to keep their distance from program stakeholders, advocates, and detractors.

The lack of direct fit between social interventions and social problem amelioration, combined with the difficulty of applying strict experimental methods to community-based projects, spawned a second stage of evaluation theory during the 1970s. The pragmatist approach of Stage 2 theory focuses on the manner in which evaluative information is used to design and modify social interventions and on the uses and perspectives of various stakeholders. This approach contends that rational choice is not an adequate model to explain how evaluation results are used or applied in policy making or in field practice. The evaluator should, conversely, think about the implications for his or her research beforehand and should plan research questions, design, and methods with an eye to the eventual use and potential influence of the research.

Stage 2 evaluation theory exchanges claims regarding the certainty of knowledge for emphasis on the utility of knowledge. Case studies, ethnographies, and other qualitative approaches are all acceptable. In contrast to the distance approach of the Stage 1 theorist, evaluation practice involves close contact with program plans and implementation.

Stage 3 theory retains the belief in rigorous methodology and the search for ultimate truth about program effectiveness while stressing the importance of descriptive knowledge and contextual fit. This approach advises a contingent strategy, specifying the conditions under which certain questions, designs, and methods make sense. Theories of social programming take a conceptual leap at this stage. In addition to incrementally improving existing programs, evaluation results are thought to inform future initiatives and, therefore, can yield bold program change. Toward this end, the Stage 3 theorist prescribes the use of rigorously evaluated demonstration projects that explore theoretical explanation and causal mediating processes.

Use of evaluation results in Indian Country often is dependent on the placement of the evaluator. The practitioner working at the local program level has responsibility to managers and government contract specialists, and he or she focuses on incremental change and program improvement. "Enlightenment" evaluations, those looking for root causes of social problems and amelioration approaches, are more appropriately responsible to national policy task forces, usually are very well funded, and rarely are expected to provide information needed for immediate decision-making.

With these theoretical considerations in mind, the selection of a relevant evaluation approach in Native communities is dependent on (a) an identification of stakeholders, (b) the potential uses of the produced knowledge, (c) the epistemological framework of the Native community, and (d) the values that will guide the assessment of program merit. Social science now recognizes that these concepts are culturally specific and not universal paradigms (Bernstein, 1988; Derrida, 1980; Foucault, 1972, 1973, 1980; Habermas, 1988; Lyotard, 1984; Marcus & Fischer, 1986; Said, 1993). Programs aspiring to postcolonial or empowerment practice must, therefore, include Native perspectives on the aforementioned elements to make real their emancipatory claims.

Managing the Evaluation

Evaluations often are contracted out to public health or other social science specialists. Management of the evaluation begins by developing a contract that defines resources, staffing, qualifications, timing, and other issues that are specific to the project and locale.

A primary concern is the adequacy of program resources for evaluation. A rigorous and thorough evaluation may consume up to 30% of total project costs and, likewise, a high percentage of staff time. The division of labor between the evaluation and the program staff is outlined before any activities begin. Program staff are routinely charged with collecting data from their participants and activities. The program director or manager is charged with governing the evaluation tasks of the program staff and ensuring that all staff-related data are collected and stored for use or review by the evaluator. Program administrators and the evaluator choose or develop the instruments, and the evaluator analyzes and reports process and outcome findings. Evaluation staff or other neutral parties administer instruments and satisfaction surveys. An adequate schedule for on-site visits and monitoring should be part of the contract. In the first 12 or 18 months of new projects, evaluation reports may be required more frequently, and evaluation visits may be required as well. A clear plan for regular meetings and a format to obtain and use process evaluation feedback are important contract items (DeJung, 1991).

Developing an Evaluation Protocol

Once these issues are considered and decisions have been made about how to proceed, the steps or components of the evaluation are delineated. A standard approach is to develop an evaluation protocol. This document is a detailed blueprint (20 to 25 pages) for evaluation practice and may include the following sections:

1. Significance of the problem addressed by the program
2. Description of the program
3. Program impact theory or model; the rationale that justifies the claim that the program will remedy the problem (the logic model is useful here)
4. Program objectives and measures
5. Evaluative research design; dimension to be evaluated (process and outcome) and methodological strategy to be used
6. Participant selection criteria
7. Data collection procedures
8. Methods and example of analysis
9. Anticipated use of results and implications for policy and practice
10. References (Rundall & Spigner, 1988)

The evaluator has the primary responsibility for developing the protocol, with approval from funders and program staff.

Process Evaluation

The process evaluation answers questions about the program's fit and implementation within the community's current context, program staffing, and the feedback mechanisms to improve or redesign the intervention. Some possible implementation questions include the staff's ability to articulate goals and objectives; a description and judgment about the quality of each intervention; the adequacy of dosage to individual clients; adequacy of documentation to record dosage and participant involvement; frequency of staff and management meetings; the cultural, age, and gender appropriateness of any curriculum or manuals used; ratio of staff to participants; staff prior experience, training, and current competency; and adequacy of staff and/or participant supervision (Green & Lewis, 1986). Evaluators should schedule ongoing observations of interventions to evaluate content, participant receptiveness, and staff competency.

Differing characteristics of primary prevention versus intervention programs are a concern in some Native communities. In youth programs particularly, stigmatization might be attached to either inclusion or exclusion, depending on the popularity of the HPDP effort and the intervention focus. In one example, youths who used any amount of alcohol or drugs were excluded from a primary ATOD prevention project. This created a perception that the project was labeling families as good or bad, and a division in the community ensued. This rule, and the project's rigid confidentiality regulation, created animosity and suspicion from those families excluded from participation in the program. In the process of changing norms and creating cohesive peer groups, some level of community upheaval can be expected.

Client record-keeping systems are important not only to ensure intervention quality but also for funding-reporting requirements. Process evaluation questions related to record keeping might include a review of standardized forms related to client confidentiality (particularly with computerized systems), release of information to other agencies or parents, documentation of group and individual contacts with participants, and community events records. Client confidentiality is crucial in bounded Indian communities, particularly when interventions collect data on sensitive issues such as ATOD use and sexual activity. Parental and community desires to know about interventions and participants must be weighed against individual and family rights to privacy and fear of rumor and gossip.

Monitoring the stability of administrative systems is an important consideration in the interpretation of HPDP outcomes. Because of generally low pay and the amount and severity of "life events" experienced by Native families, high staff turnover, even for administrative positions, may be common. Formal staff orientations and training plans help to keep the program running at optimal levels in the event of staff turnover. Appropriate evaluation questions for administrative systems might include the plans for staff development and training; board, other staff, and higher administrative support; a review of personnel and grievance procedures; staff credentialing and certification; and the adequacy of secretarial support.

Process evaluation activities should include an examination of facilities. Program environs affect participation both culturally and physically. Adequate space for meetings, training, and events attracts community members and maintains staff morale.

A review of community linkages is an important focus for process evaluation. A formalized memorandum of agreement and procedures should be established between agencies that exchange referrals. Other community issues for process evaluation include the staff's understanding of community linkages, delegation of responsibility to maintain and initiate contacts, and the availability of other agency resources for the HPDP client population.

Outcome Evaluation

In addition to the philosophical choices outlined here, the rigor and design of the outcome evaluation is, in many cases, dependent on funders' requirements. Evaluations conducted internally are by definition less rigorous and usually do not entail comparison or control groups. Nonexperimental designs such as the one-shot case study, the one-group pretest/posttest design, and the static-group design are common methods for internal outcome evaluation (Campbell & Stanley, 1963, p. 8). Qualitative methods such as case study, participant observation (Greene, 1994; Yack, 1992), and rapid ethnographic assessment (Murray, Tapson, Turnbull, McCullum, & Little, 1994) have been successfully used to provide thick description of program activities and outcomes. Qualitative methods are particularly useful when more information is needed about the population at risk, the determinants of the health problems under question, and/or their risk and protective factors.

Positivist approaches require experimental or quasi-experimental designs (Campbell & Stanley, 1963). Randomization into intervention and control groups often is a problem for reservation or other community-based interventions. School-based interventions are a popular way in which to overcome this problem; they allow for randomization of classrooms and for more thorough or systematic pre- and posttesting. In the authors' experience, comparison groups, rather than control groups, are the norm.

The use of standardized valid instruments is a concern for Native American populations, as with other populations of color. Some instruments, fortunately, are normed for Native populations. The Tri-Ethnic Center at the University of Colorado at Fort Collins and the Native American and Alaska Native Center for Mental Health Research at the University of Colorado at Denver both have produced valid and reliable mental health and cultural identification measures, as have other Native-specific research endeavors. A viable alternative to developing new outcome measures is to contract with one of the many commercial research institutes. These organizations not only supply prevention-related instruments but also will statistically analyze the data and provide detailed reports for a reasonable price.

Report Writing and Dissemination of Results

The evaluation staff have responsibility for process and outcome evaluation reports to funders. Refereed journal articles are the customary way in which program and evaluation knowledge is circulated to the professional community. The authorship of any journal articles or other papers on the intervention would be discussed in advance. Project staff significantly contributing to the evaluation should be included in the authorship.

Journal articles do not routinely reach a significant Native audience. Video documentaries or other video reports of intervention projects and outcomes are beginning to become popular in Indian Country (Rhine & Pierce, 1995). Video documentaries are an excellent medium in which to circulate knowledge about interventions and their results directly to Indian Country and also are a significant source of community pride.

CHAPTER SUMMARY

This chapter has attempted to review important issues and identify key resources in needs assessment, program planning, and evaluation in Indian Country. So long as Native communities suffer disproportionately from disease, trauma, and other social problems, HPDP efforts are indispensible. Conducting these efforts affords multiple pleasures and issues for all health professionals as well as multiple outcomes. HPDP programs accomplish cultural revitalization, empowerment, and self-reflection; increase local capacity; and raise health consciousness and status. The authors support a postcolonial approach to work in Native communities. This approach is inherently hybrid. It uses the latest that public health and other social science disciplines have to offer in assessment, planning, and evaluation while anchoring HPDP efforts with Native control and in Native cultural and spiritual knowledge.

The authors advocate more collaborative investigation into community-based assessment, planning, and evaluation for Indian Country. Although the prevention field has made great strides during the past 20 years, not enough is known about root causes of health problems or strategies for effective amelioration. Much of the work of the National Institutes of Health and the Centers for Disease Control and Prevention, unfortunately, still is far removed from the realities of life on the reservation or in urban Native communities. Native wisdom and methods of knowledge production need legitimation by mainstream social science not only to enhance intervention efforts and participation but also to grow and adapt to the changing postmodern society.

NOTES

1. In this chapter, *Indian Country* refers not only to the standard definition of land within a reservation and land outside the reservation that is owned by tribal members or the tribe and held in trust by the federal government (O'Brien, 1989, p. 198), but also to urban community-based organizations and corporate enterprises that are Native run and operated primarily for the benefit of Native peoples.

2. In this chapter, the term *Native peoples* refers to Native American Indians and Alaska Natives.

3. An example is the Navajo Area Office.

4. Some laudable examples include the National Cancer Institute's Native American Initiative projects, the IHS's Women's Alcohol and Other Drug Treatment Study, and the Native American perinatal needs assessment performed by the Western Consortium for Public Health in Berkeley, California.

REFERENCES

Beauvais, F., & LaBoueff, S. (1985). Drug and alcohol abuse interventions in American Indian communities. *International Journal of the Addictions, 20,* 139-171.

Beauvais, F., & Trimble, J. E. (1992). The role of the researcher in evaluating American Indian and other drug abuse programs. In M. A. Orlandi (Ed.), *Cultural competence for evaluators* (Publication No. [ADM] 92-1884). Washington, DC: U.S. Department of Health and Human Services, Office of Substance Abuse Prevention.

Berkhofer, R. (1979). *The white man's Indian.* New York: Vintage Books.

Bernstein, R. (1988). *Beyond objectivism and relativism: Science, hermeneutics, and praxis.* Philadelphia: University of Pennsylvania Press.

Campbell, D. T., & Stanley, J. C. (1963). *Experimental and quasi-experimental designs for research.* Boston: Houghton Mifflin.

Connell, J., Kubisch, A., Schoor, L., & Weiss, C. (Eds.). (1995). *New approaches to evaluating community initiatives: Concepts, methods, and contexts.* Queenstown, MD: Aspen Institute.

DeJung, J. (1991, October). *Evaluation guidelines.* Paper presented at the New Grantees Workshop, Rockville, MD.

Derrida, J. (1980). *Of grammatology.* Baltimore, MD: Johns Hopkins University Press.

Duran, B. (1996). Indigenous versus colonial discourse: Alcohol and American Indian identity. In E. Bird (Ed.), *Dressing in feathers: The construction of the Indian in American popular culture.* Boulder, CO: Westview.

Duran, E., & Duran, B. (1995). *Native American postcolonial psychology.* Albany: State University of New York Press.

Edwards, D., Seaman, J., Drews, J., & Edwards, M. (1995). A community approach for Native American drug and alcohol prevention programs: A logic model framework. *Alcoholism Treatment Quarterly, 13*(2), 43-62.

Fleming, C. M. (1992). American Indians and Alaska Natives: Changing societies past and present. In M. A. Orlandi (Ed.), *Cultural competence for evaluators* (Publication No. [ADM] 92-1884). Washington, DC: U.S. Department of Health and Human Services, Office of Substance Abuse Prevention.

Foucault, M. (1972). *The archeology of knowledge* (A. Sheridan, Trans.). New York: Pantheon Books.

Foucault, M. (1973). *The order of things: An archeology of the human sciences* (A. Sheridan, Trans.). New York: Vintage/Random House.

Foucault, M. (1980). *Power/knowledge: Selected interviews and other writings 1972-1977.* New York: Pantheon Books.

Glanz, K., Lewis, M. L., & Rimer, B. (1990). *Health behavior and health education, theory, research and practice.* San Francisco: Jossey-Bass.

Green, L. W., & Kreuter, M. W. (1991). *Health promotion planning: An educational and environmental approach.* Mountain View, CA: Mayfield.

Green, L., & Lewis, F. (1986). *Measurement and evaluation in health education and health promotion.* Mountain View, CA: Mayfield.

Greene, J. C. (1994). Qualitative program evaluation: Practice and promise. In N. Denzin & Y. Lincoln (Eds.), *Handbook of qualitative research*. Thousand Oaks, CA: Sage.

Habermas, J. (1988). *On the logic of the social sciences*. Cambridge: MIT Press.

Hodgkenson, H. (1990). *The demographics of American Indians: One percent of the people, fifty percent of the diversity*. Washington, DC: Center for Demographic Policy.

Institute of Medicine. (1988). *The future of public health*. Washington, DC: National Academy Press.

Keller, E. (1992). *Secrets of life, secrets of death: Essays on language, gender and science*. New York: Routledge.

King, J., Lyons-Morris, L., & Fitz-Gibbon, C. T. (1987). *How to assess program implementation*. Newbury Park, CA: Sage.

Kretzmann, J., & McKnight, J. (1993). *Building communities from the inside out: A path toward finding and mobilizing a community's assets*. Chicago: ACTA Publishers.

Krieger, N. (1994). Epidemiology and the web of causation. *Social Science and Medicine, 39,* 754-762.

Lincoln, Y., & Denzin, N. (1994). The fifth movement. In N. Denzin & Y. Lincoln (Eds.), *Handbook of qualitative research*. Thousand Oaks, CA: Sage.

Lyotard, J. (1984). *The postmodern condition: A report on knowledge*. Minneapolis: University of Minnesota Press.

Marcus, G., & Fischer, M. (1986). *Anthropology as cultural critique: An experimental moment in the human sciences*. Chicago: University of Chicago Press.

May, P. (1986). Alcohol and drug misuse prevention programs for American Indians: Needs and opportunities. *Journal of Studies on Alcohol, 47,* 187-195.

McKnight, J., & Kretzmann, J. (1990). *Mapping community capacity*. Chicago: Northwestern University, Center for Urban Affairs and Policy Research.

McLeroy, K., Bibeau, D., Steckler, A., & Glanz, K. (1988). An ecological perspective on health promotion programs. *Health Education Quarterly, 15,* 351-377.

Minkler, M., & Wallerstein, N. (1997). Improving health through community organization and community building. In K. Glanz, F. Lewis, & B. Rimer (Eds.), *Health behavior and health education* (2nd ed.). San Francisco: Jossey-Bass.

Murray, S., Tapson, L., Turnbull, L., McCullum, J., & Little, A. (1994). Listening to local voices: Adapting rapid appraisal to assess health and social needs in general practice. *British Journal of Medicine, 308,* 698-700.

O'Brien, S. (1989). *American Indian tribal governments*. Norman: University of Oklahoma Press.

Ong, A. (1987). *Spirits of resistance and capitalist discipline*. Albany: State University of New York Press.

Parker, L. (1990). The missing component in substance abuse prevention efforts: A Native American example. *Contemporary Drug Problems, 17,* 251-270.

Prakash, G. (1995). Postcolonial criticism and Indian historiography. In L. Nicholson & S. Seidman (Eds.), *Social postmodernism: Beyond identity politics*. Cambridge, UK: Cambridge University Press.

Rhine, G., & Pierce, C. (producers). (1995). *The red road to sobriety* [video]. San Francisco: Kifaru Productions.

Rundall, T., & Spigner, C. (1988). *Instructions for writing an evaluation research protocol*. University of California, Berkeley, School of Public Health.

Said, E. (1993). *Culture and imperialism*. New York: Knopf.

Schinke, S., Gilchrist, L., Schilling, R., & Walker, D. (1986). Preventing substance abuse among American Indian and Alaska Native youth: Research issues and strategies. *Journal of Social Science Research, 9*(4), 53-67.

Scott, J. (1990). *Domination and the art of resistance*. New Haven, CT: Yale University Press.

Shadish, W. R., Jr., Cook, T. D., & Leviton, L. C. (1991). *Foundations of program evaluation: Theories of practice*. Newbury Park, CA: Sage.

Siegel, L. M., Attkisson, C., & Carson, L. (1987). Need identification and program planning in the community context. In F. Cox, J. Erlich, J. Rothman, & J. Tropman (Eds.), *Strategies of community organization*. Itasca, IL: F. E. Peacock.

Slagle, L., & Weibel-Orlando, J. (1986). The Indian Shaker Church and Alcoholics Anonymous: Revivalistic curing cult. *Human Organization, 45,* 310-319.

Stanton, B., Black, R., Engle, P., & Pelto, G. (1992). Theory-driven behavioral intervention research for the control of diarrheal diseases. *Social Science and Medicine, 35,* 1405-1420.

Tesh, S. (1988). *Hidden arguments: Political ideology and disease prevention policy*. New Brunswick, NJ: Rutgers University Press.

Trimble, J., Padilla, A., & Bell, C. (1987). *Drug abuse among ethnic minorities* (Publication No. [ADM] 87-1474). Washington, DC: National Institute on Drug Abuse.

U.S. Department of Health and Human Services. (1990). *Breaking new ground for American Indian and Alaska Native youth at risk: Program summaries* (Technical Report No. 3, Publication No. [ADM] 90-1705). Rockville, MD: Author.

U.S. Department of Health and Human Services. (1991). *Healthy People 2000: National health promotion and disease prevention objectives* (Publication No. [PHS] 91-50212). Rockville, MD: Public Health Service.

U.S. Department of Health and Human Services. (1993). *Measurement in prevention: A manual on selecting and using instruments to evaluate prevention programs* (Publication No. [SMA] 93-2041). Rockville, MD: Public Health Service.

U.S. Department of Health and Human Services. (1995a). *Regional differences in Indian health* (annual report). Rockville, MD: Indian Health Service.

U.S. Department of Health and Human Services. (1995b). *Trends in Indian health.* Rockville, MD: Indian Health Service.

Weibel-Orlando, J. (1989). Hooked on healing: Anthropologists, alcohol and intervention. *Human Organization, 48,* 149-155.

Yack, D. (1992). The use and value of qualitative methods in health research in developing countries. *Social Science and Medicine, 35,* 603-612.

16

Traditional Approaches to Health Care Among American Indians and Alaska Natives

A Case Study

LARRI FREDERICKS
FELICIA SCHANCHE HODGE

Developing and implementing an educational program for American Indian and Alaska Native populations presents a formidable challenge for two reasons. First, the multiplicity of tribes creates a dilemma regarding which cultural approach to select in the development and implementation phase. There are more than 500 separate and distinct American Indian and Alaska Native tribes identified in the United States, and many of these tribes continue to practice their traditional ceremonies, languages, and beliefs. Second, there is a dearth of educational materials and knowledge that educators can use when trying to develop programs specifically for American Indians and Alaska Natives. The majority of educational approaches implemented in Indian and Native communities have been patterned after mainstream Western curricula, and the success rate of these models has been minimal.

The development of a culturally appropriate educational intervention requires consideration of the available resources and the important cultural themes of the target population. In spite of the multiplicity of American Indian and Alaska Native groups, there still are striking cultural similarities and concepts from which to draw. These include tribal values such as the importance of family and community, cooperation, sharing, harmony with nature, and an oral tradition that incorporates the lessons learned and values of the tribe in the form of story-telling. The following case study provides information on the development and implementation of a culturally designed cancer intervention program, the American Indian Women's Talking Circle (AIWTC). This intervention method, which was implemented in four American Indian communities in California, is fast becoming an acceptable and preferred method of communication and education within American Indian and Alaska Native communities (Moody & Laurent, 1984).

BACKGROUND

The word *cancer* strikes fear in all members of society. This is no less true for American Indian and Alaska Native cultures. Cancer is a disease with such negative connotations that it must be addressed in a culturally sensitive manner. There is no word for cancer in Indian languages; many tribal people think of cancer as a "white disease"; therefore, they do not perceive themselves to be at risk. Other Indians and Natives view cancer in a fatalistic manner, not realizing that many cancers can be prevented, treated, and cured (Black Feather, 1992; Harlan, Bernstein, & Kessler, 1991; Samet, Hunt, Lercehn, & Goodwin, 1988). Cultural taboos (e.g., those related to modesty and not bringing attention to oneself), coupled with confusion about what cancer is and how it can be treated, have added to this problem. These factors contribute to the inability of many American Indians and Alaska Natives to be active and vocal in their health and medical care. Such misunderstandings, related to culture and care, add to the failure of cancer education programs in many American Indian and Alaska Native communities.

FOCUS GROUPS

A series of focus groups held at the beginning of the AIWTC project revealed American Indian women's fears regarding cancer, barriers to cancer screening and treatment, and health care beliefs specific to American Indian and Alaska Native women and their cultures (Hodge, 1995a). A 50-year-old Miwok Indian woman shared her experience and fears regarding cancer: "My grandmother died of cancer. She never talked about it, never said a word. Cancer was not talked about in our family. It was a silent killer. We didn't know anything about it. After she died, we found out it was cancer. And even then, no one talked about it."

Others discussed how difficult it is for them to receive medical care. A Pomo woman stated, "I have five kids. What am I supposed to do with them? I can't leave them home alone. The clinic is okay, but I can't always make it to town." Lengthy delays between screening and follow-up referrals also were noted, as was the inability to obtain timely clinic appointments.

There also were misunderstandings about the Pap test and recommended treatment. For example, one American Indian woman said, "I got treated for an infection, and no one said I had cancer. I thought I was cured." Patients were reluctant to talk to the physician about the Pap smear, and they often did not know whether they ever had a Pap smear procedure; they knew they had a "pelvic," but they were unaware whether a Pap smear also had been performed.

Also, some Indian patients expressed fears concerning the use of radiation in treatment and screening, and they believed that surgery spread the cancer.

Traditional practices such as the use of native healers, ceremonies, and language were found to be important factors in the healing and treatment of disease or illness. Women reported that they often went to the clinic doctor and the native healer. Both providers helped them, each unaware of the other's role. The women also reported that they relied heavily on relatives' and elders' advice on treatment procedures. Some of these procedures included the use of herbs, teas, and cere-monial "sweats."

Cancer is a relatively "new" disease among Native people in the United States. At the turn of the century, it was a rare occurrence in the indigenous population. The main reason for this was that American Indian and Alaska Native people during this period were less influenced by the Western world. Many tribes were following more traditional and subsistence ways of living. A natural diet (low in fat) and an active lifestyle were major contributors to the absence of disease. Recent reports show that cancer is now the second leading cause of death in American Indian women over 45 years of age (Hampton, 1995). Among Alaska Natives, cancer ranks as the second leading cause of death. Although cancer incidence, mortality, and survival rates vary according to location and tribe (Jordan & Key, 1981; Michalek, Mahoney, Cummings, Hanley, & Snyder, 1989; Skubi, 1988), the 5-year survival rate for easily treatable cancers such as cervical cancer is poorer for American Indian and Alaska Native women than for any other ethnic group (Mahoney, Michalek, Cummings, Nasca, & Emrich, 1989). This is due, in part, to inadequate screening and follow-up care (AMC Cancer Research Center, 1991). Indian women often delay seeking medical treatment to attend to the needs of their families. Although this behavior is not unique to Indians, its consequences for this population are especially harmful.

Efforts to increase screening rates for breast and cervical cancer are producing less than desirable results. Barriers to increased cancer screening among Native women include nonfinancial obstacles such as lack of health and prevention in-formation, transportation difficulties, and cultural differences between Native patients and non-Native providers that may create misunderstandings, language, and gender-specific issues (privacy and modesty) related to the American Indian and Alaska Native cultures (Fredericks, 1990; Gordon, Campos-Outcalt, Steele, & Gonzales, 1994). The challenge for health care providers and health delivery systems is to provide culturally appropriate and culturally sensitive health care services that take into account both system barriers and cultural barriers facing Native peoples.

CULTURALLY APPROPRIATE APPROACHES TO MEANINGFUL INTERVENTION

Cancer prevention and screening programs generally build on the premise that if women are given adequate information, then they will follow recommended screening and treatment protocols (Marcus, Crane, Kaplan, & Reading, 1992).

These programs rely heavily on a strong patient education and referral strategy. What is lacking is an appropriate match between the culture and educational material so that these materials are set within the cultural context of the targeted population.

To address this need for developing a meaningful intervention model for American Indians and Alaska Natives, the first step was to develop educational materials that were culturally appropriate. This meant creating educational materials that would take into account the Native communities that were to use them. These educational materials needed to be set within the context of American Indian and Alaska Native cultures so that they were acceptable. This meant not only adding ethnic artwork to mainstream materials but also creating educational materials that would take into account the learning style and cultural values of the population being targeted for positive change.

In developing the educational materials for the AIWTC, it was recognized that in American Indian and Alaska Native cultures, education traditionally was provided through the telling of tribal stories by storytellers who were respected members of the tribal community. This was the preferred way of educating the young and refreshing the memories of older tribal members on how to do things, as they say, "in the people's way." These stories not only were entertaining and educational but also contained messages on what was valued and acceptable to the tribe. For these reasons, traditional tribal tales, storytelling, and the use of respected members of the Indian communities became important features of the AIWTC educational curriculum design.

It also was important that the educational material be presented in a familiar, comfortable, and culturally acceptable style. The talking circle format met all of these needs. Historically, talking circles have been used by most tribes as a vehicle in which to discuss and present important issues relevant to all members of the tribe. Through the use of American Indian stories and the talking circle format, the educational material was set within the cultural context of the American Indian and Alaska Native communities.

With these considerations in mind, the Center for American Indian Research and Education (CAIRE) in Berkeley, California, developed the AIWTC. Funded by the National Cancer Institute, the project was designed to increase the rate of cervical cancer screening and Pap smear-related follow-up care for American Indian women. The program consists of a series of talking circles organized to bring American Indian women together to talk about their fears and the barriers to cervical cancer screening. The talking circles also included a health curriculum aimed at increasing knowledge about cervical cancer and health in general. These talking circle sessions provide information about Pap smears, cancer risks, and other issues related to women's health.

The talking circles are designed to incorporate the spirit of Indian life into discussions about health by merging the tradition of oral storytelling with a contemporary education program about cervical cancer prevention, treatment, and control. Storytelling is a culturally appropriate educational technique because it uses an inside approach, working from within the cultural milieu rather than from outside it. This approach takes into consideration cultural factors and, therefore, is more comfortable and familiar to American Indian and Alaska Native participants. The approach also uses the well-tested strategy of employing tribal members and training them to act as talking circle group facilitators. These talking circle facilitators are the core and strength of the project. They are respected members of their communities who coordinate the sessions, deliver the curriculum lessons, and play the important role of storytellers.

We recognize the value of contemporary educational materials, especially in relation to serious medical conditions such as cervical cancer. These materials are more meaningful and readily acceptable, however, if conveyed in a nonthreatening, traditional manner. The talking circle model is a culturally sensitive and appropriate intervention that is able to reach an often invisible and forgotten population. Shaping the health message to the American Indian worldview makes it stronger, more understandable, and readily acceptable. This empowers Indian women to take control of their own health and become active in their own cervical cancer screening and follow-up care.

THE TALKING CIRCLE

The talking circle is composed of 5 to 15 American Indian or Alaska Native women who are recruited from the community participating in the project. The group meets once a week for 1 hour for 16 weeks (i.e., 4 months). These talking circle sessions have two purposes. First, they are educational in that they present a health topic and message, stressing the value of prevention and the positive role of cancer screening procedures. Second, they provide a caring and supportive environment in which American Indian women can talk openly about their concerns and issues related to their health and well-being. Organized in a comfortable setting, usually at the Indian clinic or another familiar Indian facility, the women gather to share information, give support, and solve problems.

Coordinating and conducting the talking circles takes time, commitment, and organizational skills. The talking circle facilitators are responsible for this task, and it is their dedication and hard work that is essential to making the talking circles a success. Their duties include the recruitment of all talking circle participants, securing the room for all 16 sessions of the talking circle in advance, inviting guest speakers on health issues, preparing refreshments for participants, and presenting the talking circle health curriculum. The facilitator position is key to the success of the talking circle and requires skills in leadership and teaching. The facilitator is active and respected in the community and is comfortable with the leadership role. She is responsible for presenting the talking circle educational curriculum and material, and she has gone through extensive training with the CAIRE training staff before going into the field. This facilitator training covers coordinating and recruiting for the talking circles and an in-depth overview of the health curriculum including role-playing and teaching presentation style.

The talking circle format is designed to make the group meetings run smoothly and to foster respect for the Indian women who participate. Typically, the chairs are arranged in a circle so that all are equal, and each session opens with an Indian prayer or a "smudging" of the room to cleanse it. At the first talking circle session, the facilitator introduces the AIWTC program and explains how the talking circle will be conducted. The participants are again told that the AIWTC is composed of 16 sessions, that each session is approximately 1 hour long, and that all participants are encouraged to attend all 16 sessions. Each session follows the same structural outline. After the opening Indian prayer or smudging of the room, the facilitator or a participant reads the American Indian or Alaska Native story and its health message to the group. The group may then discuss the story and health message.

Next, the facilitator presents the health education material from the AIWTC curriculum guide. Discussion is welcomed at any point. When a participant wishes to speak, she picks up the talisman (i.e., a feather or another object) from the center of the table or, if it is being passed around the circle, waits until it reaches her. Holding the talisman signals to the group that a participant wishes to speak without interruption. This type of educational talking circle is very informal, and bonding takes place very quickly. It is a place to learn, to share, and to help. It also is a place where each person is treated with respect, a key element in the talking circle tradition. When the discussion of the health topic is complete, the talisman is again passed around the talking circle. If no one wishes to speak, then the facilitator closes the talking circle and announces the date and time of the next meeting. She hands out the following week's American Indian or Alaska Native story and announces the health topic that will be presented.

A video developed by CAIRE for the AIWTC also is shown to the participants at the first talking circle session (Hodge, 1995b). This video discusses cervical cancer, emphasizes the importance of cancer screening, and demonstrates how talking circles are conducted in Indian communities. At the first meeting, the facilitator introduces herself and shares some of her personal background with the group. The participants then introduce themselves, and the talking circle begins. It is important that no new members are added after the second session, although there is a sign-up sheet for women who want to join future talking circles. This is done to ensure that the women form a support group and can feel comfortable sharing their experiences within the talking circle. The facilitator stresses confidentiality, and each member signs a confidentiality form pledging to keep confidential all names and information shared at group sessions.

An American Indian or Alaska Native story is recited at the opening of all 16 talking circle sessions. These stories set the theme and remind the participants of traditional Indian values such as caring, working together, sharing, and staying healthy in spirit and body. After the tribal story is read, the talking circle participants discuss the story and its value message. After the Indian story discussion, the facilitator presents the health educational topic from the AIWTC curriculum guide to the participants. Discussion on the educational material is welcomed at any time during the presentation. When the discussion is completed, the talking circle is closed. The facilitator then announces the health topic and Indian story for the following week's talking circle meeting.

The AIWTC specifically targets American Indian and Alaska Native women with the goal of increasing cervical cancer screening. However, the talking circle intervention can be used as a health education format for both men and women and with other health concerns such as nutrition, diabetes, and heart disease. The talking circle approach is very adaptable. The most important factor is the design of the educational curriculum so that it includes both health education material and cultural material relevant to the population being targeted. It is a design that can fit most American Indian and Alaska Native communities, whether they are urban or rural. The Native Nutritional Circles project, another CAIRE talking circle program, targets American Indian and Alaska Native heads of households and is designed to strengthen positive food habits and increase nutritional knowledge related to health and disease. Although this program has not been completed, it has been met with enthusiasm in California Indian communities. Preliminary data indicate that it is successfully meeting its goals.

CURRICULUM DEVELOPMENT

The curriculum developed for the AIWTC was formalized as an educational guide for the talking circle facilitators. It is comprehensive in that it includes all the information, both traditional Indian stories and health educational material, that the facilitators will need to conduct all 16 sessions of the talking circle. The first three chapters are introductory and cover three important areas: cervical cancer and the importance of prevention, the importance of the oral tradition of storytelling in American Indian and Alaska Native cultures, and coordinating and conducting the talking circles. These chapters provide essential background information for successfully implementing the talking circles.

The complete curriculum guide consists of 16 health educational sessions and presents an overview of topics that, in addition to cervical cancer screening, are important to women's health. Each session focuses on a specific issue such as the importance of early detection of cancer, the pelvic examination and barriers, the Pap test and results, breast cancer and the breast self-examination, menopause, using the health care system, building self-esteem, high-risk behaviors, sexually transmitted diseases, substance abuse, and community resources. These sessions provide educational health information in a supportive atmosphere for learning and discussion.

In the talking circle, hands-on learning by the Indian women also takes place. For each session, women receive educational materials such as booklets on the pelvic examination, Pap smear, breast self-examinations, and menopause. At the beginning of each session, each participant also is given a large folder that is divided into sections that follow the curriculum so that she can keep all her health materials together. Many of the health curriculum sessions have large flip charts and view models for the facilitators to use in their health presentations and for the participants to view. Guest speakers, such as clinic physicians, are invited to speak on issues such as the pelvic examination, Pap test results, and menopause.

In developing the AIWTC curriculum, one of the most important concerns was to create a useful and informative educational guide. It is designed to emphasize the importance of cervical cancer screening and to present health information to American Indian and Alaska Native women in an understandable form that empowers them to become active in the care of their bodies. Included in the curriculum guide was crucial information about how a Pap test is conducted, what a pelvic examination entails, what a positive Pap test indicates, and why follow-up treatment is so important. The 16 sessions also present an opportunity to discuss other important topics relevant to women's health such as information on AIDS, sexually transmitted diseases, breast cancer, menopause, and self-esteem. The AIWTC curriculum is designed so that all 16 sessions of the talking circle are interesting, educational, and important to the overall theme of the talking circle intervention.

Another consideration in the development of the curriculum guide was the requirement that the presentation or discussion of session topics (e.g., Pap test, breast cancer) take only 40 to 45 minutes. The other 15 to 20 minutes would be needed for the Indian story and a discussion of its message. CAIRE chose to limit the sessions to 1 hour because most participants have difficulty obligating more than that amount of time each week. Hence, the curriculum had to be concise. The talking circles also are enhanced by educational handouts and other educational tools such as charts, models, and videos. The take-home handouts are important because women have more time to look at the materials and are able to share them with their family and friends.

Because the facilitators are responsible for talking circle recruitment, coordination, and teaching, it is important that they be knowledgeable and part of the local American Indian or Alaska Native community. It also is important to keep the time schedule for the talking circles flexible. If five talking circles each with 16 sessions are held in one community, the times should vary. For example, one complete 16 session talking circle might be scheduled at noon on Sunday, the next for 6 p.m. on Monday, and so on. For each complete talking circle, it is important that the time remain the same for all 16 of the sessions. It also is important to change the times for new talking circles because American Indian and Alaska Native women have different scheduling needs. The facilitators should talk to the women in the community about these needs before scheduling future talking circles.

It is important to recruit facilitators from the area in which the talking circle takes place so that they have a working knowledge of the local Indian community. Facilitators also should have some health background because the curriculum is detailed and organized around health materials. Some of the facilitators have been nurses, community health representatives, health educators, and various other workers from Indian health clinics. Facilitators must be committed to the talking circle project and to the health of their community, and they must be willing to put time into learning the curriculum and the health topic. They also should be personable and responsible. Talking circle facilitators need to be not only good storytellers but also persons to whom the participants can turn for information and knowledge. Facilitators' workloads range from half- to full-time, depending on how many talking circles are being conducted in a given period.

The AIWTC facilitators are trained in two workshops. The first workshop takes place before the first talking circle begins and is related to confidentiality issues, human subjects protocol, emergency contacts, and the facilitators' protocol handbook, which covers in detail the responsibilities and duties of the facilitator. The second workshop deals specifically with the AIWTC curriculum guide. Each facilitator is given a complete curriculum guide that covers all 16 of the talking circle sessions. This guide provides an introduction to the health theme of the intervention (in this case, the importance of cervical cancer screening), a guide for telling the American Indian stories and discussing their importance to American Indian or Alaska Native culture, and a complete instructional guide for all of the health educational sessions of the talking circle. The curriculum guide also provides a list of educational handouts that are provided for each session and the educational aids that are available for topics. At this second training workshop, the trainers go over all 16 sessions of the curriculum as if they are conducting them at the talking circle. After the trainers finish, they assign each facilitator two talking circle sessions to present to the training group. After these practice sessions, the training group discusses how to be an effective facilitator, how to get people to talk and share, how to handle situations in which someone is talking too much, and general problem-solving techniques for possible situations that might occur in the talking circle.

When the two training workshops are concluded, the facilitators then conduct their first regular 16-session talking circles. On completing this, they attend one more workshop that is called the "debriefing," where they meet to compare and evaluate their experiences. The facilitators discuss the problems they confronted, what worked and did not work in the curriculum guide, and what changes they would make. After this workshop, the suggestions and ideas from the facilitators were immediately incorporated into the curriculum guide. These changes usually were on the health topic and involved including more or less information or providing new handouts for the health topic.

The three training workshops worked well. The facilitators reported that they felt prepared to go out into the field, felt at ease with the staff at the intervention site and at the main office, and felt a part of the larger program. In particular, they appreciated the opportunity to suggest changes in the program structure. AIWTC facilitators found their jobs challenging and rewarding and received high ratings by talking circle participants in the project evaluations.

USE OF STORYTELLING

The talking circles incorporate the sharing of a traditional American Indian or Alaska Native story at the beginning of each session, primarily as a means of reinforcing the positive traditional roles and values of American Indian and Alaska

Native cultures. These stories are drawn from creation stories, origin stories, and animal stories told and retold from generation to generation. Their themes incorporate the strength of Indian people, the importance of women, and the need for prevention, curing, and healing.

One favorite talking circle story is "Grandmother Spider Steals the Sun" (Erdoes & Ortiz, 1984, p. 154). This is the story of how daylight came into the world and the tale of the exploits of Possum, Buzzard, and Grandmother Spider, who all try to outsmart the people from the other side of the world, who are greedy and refuse to share their sun with them. In their attempts to steal the sun, Possum fails and burns the hair off his tail. Buzzard also fails and burns the hair off his head. Only Grandmother Spider succeeds. Now her side of the world has light, and everyone rejoices.

Grandmother Spider is strong and crafty, for she not only brought the sun to the Cherokee, but fire with it.

This story illustrates the value and strength of women in the Cherokee tribe. Grandmother Spider was able to outsmart the people from the other side of the world as she brought back the sun and fire. It also was Grandmother Spider who taught her people the art of making pottery. This story shows that women are strong, capable, and smart. They also are the carriers of their tribal traditions. The themes of this story reinforce the value of women and of taking control when necessary. These messages are easily woven into the cervical cancer screening curriculum to illustrate the need for Indian women to take control of their health by following recommended screening protocols.

Other origin stories explain how Native peoples were made and how human hands were selected. For example, "How Ah-ha'-le Created People" illustrates the importance of everyone working together (LaPena, Bates, & Medley, 1993). Coyote, who is often a trickster in other American Indian tales, is credited with organizing the animals as well as creating humans in this Miwok story. The importance of the story lies in its emphasis on the traditional values of community, cooperation, and working together for the welfare of all.

Other health-specific stories are used such as "The Origin of Curing Ceremonies" (Erdoes & Ortiz, 1984). This White Mountain Apache tale emphasizes the belief that for every sickness, there is a curing ceremony. It describes how curing ceremonies were needed and, therefore, how they began through belief and ritual given to American Indian people by the Creator. This is important because it shows the value placed on believing in oneself, the rituals of the tribe, and finding the strength to cure illness. Knowledge is available in the world; it only needs to be sought. Practicing prevention and staying healthy are important values for American Indians.

American Indian stories like these form the basis for the educational messages used in each of the sessions. The messages are reinforced by encouraging the talking circle members to discuss the stories and the associated health messages. They also are invited to tell their own tribal stories. All of the American Indian and Alaska Native stories shared in the AIWTC were made into an anthology and given as a gift to the Indian women at the final session of the talking circle.

These American Indian and Alaska Native stories are important to the program because they provide the thread that unites the Indian women with a sense of belonging and ownership of the talking circles. American Indian culture has endured through the telling of tribal tales. Ours is an oral tradition, and the spoken word is what gives life and meaning to Indian history and customs. Songs, chants, curing rites, prayers, jokes, personal narratives, and (most important) stories are the carriers by which traditions and values are passed from one generation to the next. Although Indian stories are meant to entertain, their primary purpose is to educate and instill tribal values (Caduto & Bruchac, 1994; Erdoes & Ortiz, 1984).

American Indian and Alaska Native stories address virtually every imaginable issue. They are emblems of living religions and often refer to a Great Creator or Spirit, who is assisted by animal helpers. They explain the origin of everything—the land, oceans, animals, people, plants, the sun, the moon, stars, fire, medicine, curing, and so on. Stories give concrete form to the values and practices that link current generations to their ancestors. They portray ancient social order and daily life, how families were organized, how political structure operated, how men hunted and fished, and how power was divided between men and women. Stories are indexes for appropriate and inappropriate behaviors. They provide examples to emulate or shun; they teach the children—and refresh the adults—on where they fit, what their society expects of them, how to live harmoniously with others, and how to be responsible, worthy members of their tribes.

Indian stories are effective when used in the talking circles because they present essential ideas and values in a simple, entertaining form. Many, but not all, of the characters in the stories are animals found within the tribe's natural environment. These creatures often have magical or supernatural powers. They usually speak and act as humans do, and sometimes they transform from animal to human and back to animal form again by taking off and putting on their skins, as in the Pomo Rattlesnake story (Margolin, 1993). Some animals provide positive role models, whereas others are negative. The good characters live well and fit happily into their surroundings; the bad characters break the rules and make life difficult for themselves and everyone else. Through their behavior, the animal characters may teach how to hunt, sing, dance, perform ceremonies, make houses and clothing, be good people, and seek supernatural guidance in their own lives.

Stories and characters vary a great deal from tribe to tribe. For example, the same type of animal can play a very different role in the myths of different tribes. Spider usually is very wise and helpful to people in Navajo stories, whereas it often is cunning and crafty in the stories of the Gros Ventre tribe. In spite of the regional variations, American Indian and Alaska Native traditional stories also have many common characteristics and themes. They generally emphasize communal welfare, the sacredness of language and traditions, and a concern with harmony with nature. These common themes reflect a universal concern with fundamental issues about humans and the world in which they live.

The American Indian and Alaska Native stories selected for the AIWTC project serve several ends. They bring the Indian women participants together, they teach and reaffirm Indian and Alaska Native cultural traditions and values, and they remind Indian women that women are valuable and that when they protect their health and well-being, they protect the health of their families and the Indian communities that depend on them.

All sessions of the talking circle curriculum begin with a traditional Indian story. These stories focus on many of the issues just mentioned—creation, community, cooperation, and sharing, among others. Each story is selected specifically to emphasize the value of health in traditional American Indian life and to motivate healthy behavior such as regular cervical cancer screening and follow-up care. These traditional stories are chosen to enhance the program's health education material by setting it within a strong and sturdy Native tradition to which participants feel they belong. The facilitator is the storyteller, and the Indian stories provide, as they have provided for countless years, the cultural lessons that continue to instruct and direct Indian people from all tribes.

EMPOWERMENT AS A MEANS OF CHANGE

Defining and measuring empowerment is a difficult and inconsistent task. In general, empowerment can be defined as a process by which individuals with lesser power gain control over their lives and influence the organizational and societal structures in which they live (Segal, Silverman, & Temkin, 1995). The AIWTC was designed as a cultural intervention to increase cervical cancer screening by empowering Native women through knowledge, support, and acknowledgment of their cultural worth and value to American Indian communities. This goal was to be met largely by providing health education information to Indian women in a culturally acceptable and usable manner, empowering them to change their behavior. The culture-nurturing American Indian stories, the talking circle design, and the all-Indian support group assisted in this achievement. The behavior change sought was that of increased cervical cancer screening to improve health and prevent cancer deaths. The preliminary results from the AIWTC data indicate that the talking circles are successful as a health intervention model and have a positive impact on American Indian women's health.

EVALUATION

The evaluation of the AIWTC is an important part of the project because it allows for understanding the impact of the intervention on cervical cancer screening and on the health of American Indian and Alaska Native women. It also identifies the parts of the intervention that are valuable and that could be used in the clinic setting. An emphasis in this project was placed on collecting uniform measures across the talking circle groups. Both qualitative and quantitative process data were used to track intervention activities on a day-to-day basis such as measuring the participants' satisfaction with the variables. A pre- and posttest questionnaire measured participants' changes in knowledge about cancer, changes in attitudes and behaviors, and quality of life measures. Medical chart reviews verified the behaviors (Pap tests) and provided information on other health problems for which the participants were seeking medical care. A diary kept by the facilitators recorded problems encountered in the talking circles that added to the process evaluation. The diary also was helpful because it highlighted the questions, concerns, and weekly group interactions. A record was kept of participants' attendance so that a ratio could be calculated related to outcome measures, adherence to screening guidelines, and follow-up of suspicious cancer screening findings.

At the final session of the AIWTC, the participants were asked to respond anonymously to a written questionnaire evaluating the project. The areas on which they commented the most were the American Indian and Alaska Native traditional stories, the health curriculum, and the talking circle support group. All of these responses were positive. Many individuals indicated that they enjoyed the stories so much that they did not want to miss a session. Others said that they shared the stories with their families and that the stories made them feel a sense of pride and belonging to the group. Many felt that the health curriculum helped them to better understand the importance of cervical cancer screening and following medical treatment. The talking circles also motivated them to make appointments for Pap smears and other health examinations. A few noted that they had, for the first time, asked their health providers questions about health and for clarification of terms or procedures that they did not understand. Some indicated a renewed interest in staying healthy. Several women stated that they wanted to continue the talking circles and were going to try to keep the group going. In general, the women's responses indicated that they felt more comfortable talking about their bodies and more knowledgeable about how to participate in their medical care.

Many women also indicated that it was difficult for them to attend all 16 sessions. However, they did not suggest that there should be fewer sessions. In fact, many suggested that the talking circles include more topics and that the session time be expanded to 2 hours.

The few unfavorable comments were not about the project design but rather about topics such as expanding the guest speaker list and including more alternative medicine choices and educational material handouts.

The numerous favorable evaluations of the AIWTC were motivated by the women's feeling that the talking circles belonged to them and the American Indian community. As they described it, the talking circles were by Indians and for Indians. This feeling of ownership was enhanced by the Indian facilitators, the use of American Indian and Alaska Native stories, and the talking circle design, which created an environment that encouraged learning and the acceptance of health and prevention materials.

CHAPTER SUMMARY

The evaluation of the AIWTC program by the Indian participants confirmed the importance of using acceptable cultural methods for educational programs. The participants indicated that the talking circle facilitates communication and provides a setting for individuals to change health behavior favorably. Although using storytelling to teach the importance of health and prevention is not a new technique, it is an exciting, revitalized means to motivate American Indian and Alaska Native women to adopt healthy lifestyles. The talking circle's primary message is that Indian women are valued and that their health and well-being are important for the future of their families and communities. The talking circles, reinforced with American Indian and Alaska Native stories, are valuable tools for improving the health of Native peoples.

REFERENCES

AMC Cancer Research Center. (1991). *Cancer prevention and control: Native Americans of the Northern Plains.* Denver, CO: Author.

Black Feather, J. (1992). Cultural beliefs and understanding cancer. *American Indian Culture and Research Journal, 16*(3), 139-144.

Caduto, M. J., & Bruchac, J. (1994). *Keepers of the night.* Golden, CO: Fulcrum.

Erdoes, R., & Ortiz, A. (Eds.). (1984). *American Indian myths and legends.* New York: Pantheon Books.

Fredericks, L. (1990). *Health care and health behavior: Alaskan Athabascan and contemporary medicine.* Unpublished doctoral dissertation, University of California, Berkeley.

Gordon, P. R., Campos-Outcalt, D., Steele, L., & Gonzales, C. (1994). Mammography and Pap smear screening of Yaqui Indian women. *Public Health Reports, 109,* 99-103.

Hampton, J. (1995). Cancer in Indian Country: Keynote address. *Alaska Medicine, 35,* 243-245.

Harlan, L. C., Bernstein, A. B., & Kessler, L. G. (1991). Cervical cancer screening: Who is not screened and why? *American Journal of Public Health, 81,* 885-890.

Hodge, F. S. (1995a). *American Indian women's focus groups.* Berkeley, CA: Center for American Indian Research and Education.

Hodge, F. S. (producer). (1995b). *American Indian Women's Talking Circle: Cervical cancer project* [video]. Berkeley, CA: Center for American Indian Research and Education.

Jordan, S. W., & Key, C. R. (1981). Carcinoma of the cervix in southwestern American Indians: Results of a cytologic detection program. *American Cancer Society, 47,* 2523-2532.

LaPena, F., Bates, C. D., & Medley, S. (Eds.). (1993). *Legends of the Yosemite Miwok.* Yosemite National Park, CA: Yosemite Associates.

Mahoney, M. C., Michalek, A. M., Cummings, K. M., Nasca, P. C., & Emrich, L. J. (1989). Cancer mortality in the northeastern Native American population. *Cancer, 64,* 187-190.

Marcus, A. C., Crane, L. A., Kaplan, C. P., & Reading, A. E. (1992). Improving adherence to clinic-based trial of three intervention strategies. *Medical Care, 30,* 216-230.

Margolin, M. (Ed.). (1993). *The way we lived: California Indian stories, songs and reminiscences.* Berkeley, CA: HeyDay Books.

Michalek, A., Mahoney, M. C., Cummings, M., Hanley, J., & Snyder, R. (1989, October). Mortality patterns among a Native American population in New York state. *New York State Journal of Medicine, 89,* 557-561.

Moody, L. E., & Laurent, M. (1984, January-February). Promoting health through use of storytelling. *Health Education, 15*(1), 8-10.

Samet, J. M., Hunt, W. C., Lercehn, M. L., & Goodwin, J. S. (1988). Delay in seeking care for cancer symptoms: A population-based study of elderly New Mexicans. *Journal of the National Cancer Institute, 80,* 432-438.

Segal, S. P., Silverman, C., & Temkin, T. (1995, June). Measuring empowerment in client-run self-help agencies. *Community Mental Health Journal, 31,* 215-227.

Skubi, D. (1988). Pap smear screening and cervical pathology in an American Indian population. *Journal of Nurse-Midwifery, 33*(5), 203-207.

17

Tips for Working With American Indian and Alaska Native Populations

ROBERT M. HUFF
MICHAEL V. KLINE

There are a variety of terms that often are used interchangeably when speaking or writing about American Indian and Alaska Native population groups. Kramer (1996) observes that Native peoples use their tribal names when referring to themselves but seem to prefer the use of the term *American Indian* over *Native American* when referring to all tribal groups. Thus, when working with American Indian and Alaska Native populations, it would be advisable for the health promoter to determine what term is preferred by the group or individual with whom he or she is working. It also will be important to recognize the diversity of cultural beliefs and practices that characterize the many distinct tribal communities living in North America. This brief "tips" chapter seeks to bring forward a few suggestions for working with American Indian and Alaska Native populations in health promotion and disease prevention (HPDP) activities. These recommendations have been culled from the preceding three chapters as well as from a number of other sources (Duran & Duran, Chapter 15, this volume; Fredericks & Hodge, Chapter 16, this volume; Hodge & Fredericks, Chapter 14, this volume; Huff, Chapter 2, this volume; Huff & Kline, Chapter 1, this volume; Joe & Malach, 1992; Kramer, 1996) and are offered as a starting point for consideration when engaging in HPDP activities with American Indian and Alaska Native populations.

CULTURAL COMPETENCE

As noted in Chapter 1 of this book, the need for health promoters to become culturally competent and sensitive to multicultural diversity is a critical skill to develop when working with any multicultural group. The following tips to the health promoter might help to begin that process:

► Seek to learn the history of the American Indian or Alaska Native population group with which you are working.

► Become familiar with the cultural values, beliefs, and ways of life of the people with whom you are working.

► Seek to incorporate the cultural beliefs, values, and traditions of the American Indian or Alaska Native group you are working with in the design, implementation, and evaluation of the HPDP program that is being developed. This can begin by including representatives of the target group in all phases of the program planning process.

► Remember that every American Indian or Alaska Native group will have its own unique traditions and patterns of life. These may be very different from that of the agency or individual with the responsibility for the HPDP project. Thus, it will be critical, on the one hand, to examine your own values, beliefs, and biases as these relate to those of the target group and, on the other, to work toward suspending your own issues to enter the culture of the target group with the respect and sensitivity to which it members are entitled.

► Take the time to make multiple visits to the community in which the target group resides. Talk with tribal leaders and members, attend local events that are open to the public, and otherwise seek to become familiar with the community's ways of life.

► Seek to develop early and continuing support from the community for any HPDP programs and services that are to be offered.

► Remember that among American Indian and Alaska Native groups, there is likely to be a range of acculturation levels from the very traditional to the fully acculturated. Therefore, assess the situation before making planning decisions to ensure that all members of the target group will benefit from the interventions planned.

► Seek to incorporate traditional values, beliefs, and ways of life into the design of educational materials while respecting differences among tribal groups.

► Seek to incorporate appropriate cultural visuals, directions, instructions, and culturally appropriate translators when providing HPDP services to American Indian and Alaska Native populations.

► Become familiar with acceptable and appropriate verbal and nonverbal communication patterns for the tribal group to which HPDP services are being provided.

► Become familiar with traditional values and practices related to gender, touching, religion, food preferences, and other related cultural differences because a failure to do so can lead to a failure of the program or service to achieve its desired aims.

▶ Respect tribal sovereignty when working with American Indian and Alaska Native population groups because not doing so can result in resistance or the collapse of support for programs being planned. Building community capacity to problem solve means respecting and learning to work from within rather than from outside the tribal group.

HEALTH BELIEFS AND PRACTICES

There are a variety of health beliefs and practices among the many diverse American Indian and Alaska Native tribal groups in North America. Thus, it is critical to develop some understanding and sensitivity to this diversity and to develop the flexibility to work within the traditional health practices of the group to which you are seeking to provide services. Thus, the health promoter should keep in mind the following:

▶ Identify and seek to understand the explanatory model(s) that the individuals within the community use to make sense of and deal with threats to their personal health and well-being.

▶ Expect that there will be a range of explanatory models that are employed across this broad multicultural population group, ranging from very traditional health beliefs and practices to those that are more reflective of the Western biomedical model.

▶ Where differences exist between the explanatory models of the target group and those of the health promoter, make efforts to ameliorate or otherwise find ways in which to work within these different frames of reference and perception.

▶ Remember that traditional ceremonies still are practiced that seek to promote balance and well-being among American Indian and Alaska Native tribal groups. Thus, you are encouraged to become familiar with these ceremonies and other health practices because they may provide opportunities to merge beneficial practices into the biomedical model and thereby extend the range of potential healing and health-promoting practices into the community.

▶ Remember that traditional healers, medicine men, and herbal remedies and medicine still are very important in many urban and rural areas.

▶ Consider that modesty, taboos, and traditional healing practices must be respected when providing HPDP services and programs.

▶ Consider consulting with and involving spiritual, cultural, and traditional healers within the community when beginning the program planning process.

▶ Seek to involve traditional healers where appropriate in the delivery of HPDP programs and services.

► Remember that *respect* is a strong central value of all American Indian and Alaska Native cultures. Thus, treating everyone with kindness, equality, and goodness is very important.

► Remember that cultural sensitivity is an important value held by American Indian and Alaska Native peoples. Thus, you must be open and willing to accept and work within other worldviews and interaction styles.

PROGRAM PLANNING CONSIDERATIONS

It has been stressed in many places throughout this text that program planning is a comprehensive and critically important process if the health promoter is to design and carry out high-quality and successful HPDP programs and services. Kline, in Chapter 4 of this volume, observed that it does not necessarily matter what planning model one uses so long as the basic elements of the planning process are involved, including adequate needs assessment, objectives setting, appropriate and culturally sensitive intervention planning, and evaluation to measure the efficacy of the program or service to meet its specified objectives. With this is mind, the health promoter is encouraged to identify and use a planning model and to consider the following suggestions and recommendations when beginning the planning process:

► Be aware that successful working relationships between American Indian and Alaska Native communities and those seeking to work with them are dependent on clarifying assumptions and overcoming misconceptions about these peoples and public health practices.

► Remember that many American Indian and Alaska Native peoples feel exploited and mistrustful of Westerners. Thus, patience, sensitivity, and respect will be important components of any HPDP effort. You must build credibility by working from *within* the tribal group rather than from *outside* the group. This will help build community capacity and foster a more trusting relationship.

► The ideal working relationship for you is one in which you are working directly under the supervision of the tribe or Native community agency.

► The community should be involved in all aspects of the program planning process, from needs assessment to evaluation.

► Be aware that tribal leaders often see HPDP and other outside funding as economic and employment opportunities for their tribe. It will be important to keep this in mind when considering staffing and other manpower needs of the HPDP program.

► Review all previous HPDP program efforts in the community to identify potential community resources and assets, interventions that have been found to enhance or impede the successful adaptation of programs in the community, and any other factors that might play a role in the new program or service to be developed.

▶ Be sure that the goals, objectives, and interventions of the HPDP program or service reflect the felt needs of the target group. Where community needs and interests are not in agreement with yours, seek ways in which to balance the needs of all concerned parties prior to launching a full-blown program or service.

▶ Above all, be sure that HPDP programs or services reflect the values, beliefs, and interests of the community to which they are targeted.

NEEDS ASSESSMENT CONSIDERATIONS

Carefully crafted needs assessment instruments and methodologies are critical to establishing accurate baseline data about a community's health needs and interests. The process must be rigorous and include not only the more usual information that is gathered (e.g., morbidity and mortality rates, demographics) but also the cultural factors that can affect the successful implementation of an HPDP program or service. Thus, the health promoter is encouraged to review the cultural assessment framework presented in Chapter 26 of this volume and to consider the following additional suggestions:

▶ Be aware that no matter what planning model is used for program development, it is essential to include a cultural assessment as part of the baseline data gathered about the target group.

▶ Needs assessment instruments will need to reflect the linguistic, literacy, and cultural symbols and values of the community.

▶ Remember that standardized needs assessment instruments designed for the mainstream culture often have little meaning for those who are not fully acculturated and assimilated into the mainstream. Thus, instruments will need to be shaped to reflect the community in which they are to be administered.

▶ Providing opportunities for Native communities to conduct their own needs assessments can help build community capacity by empowering community members to become more involved in defining and solving their own health and social problems.

▶ Community surveys, where conducted, are best undertaken with the support and direction of the tribal health department.

▶ Remember to include key informants such as political, spiritual, and cultural leaders in the community needs assessment process.

▶ Be aware that key informant information should be triangulated with other data from the assessment process to ensure that all the needs of the community are identified and considered as program planning efforts go forward.

▶ Be sure to include assessment of media resources and channels including informal channels of communication and information sharing that are used within the community. These may play a significant role in the marketing of the HPDP program or service when they are ready to go on-line.

▶ The PRECEDE model (see Chapter 4) can be a useful framework for identifying and describing health behaviors with respect to their predisposing, enabling, and reinforcing factors and can help frame the new knowledge, attitudes, and behaviors that will be the targets of intervention in the community.

▶ Focus groups can provide a useful way in which to assess knowledge, attitudes, and health behaviors of American Indian and Alaska Native peoples.

▶ Be sure that assessment and evaluation efforts reflect the needs, interests, and values of the stakeholders within the community.

INTERVENTION CONSIDERATIONS

Well-planned and appropriate interventions are key to the success of any HPDP program or service. This will involve tailoring interventions to the particular cultural characteristics of the target group (Pasick, D'Onofrio, & Otero-Sabogal, 1996), that is, by employing themes, values, and other important features of the culture in the intervention process. Therefore, the health promoter is urged to consider the following recommendations when planning program interventions:

▶ Remember that "one size fits all" is not a useful approach to intervention design. Programs must be tailored to each individual target group.

▶ Be aware that effective HPDP interventions build on the strengths, resources, and assets of the community. Seek to identify and involve these in the intervention design and implementation process.

▶ Linguistic, literacy, gender relevance, and other cultural factors must be considered in the design of the intervention to be implemented in the community.

▶ Be aware that the development of a culturally appropriate educational intervention requires consideration of available resources and the inclusion of important cultural themes of the target group.

▶ Educational materials must be culturally appropriate and set within the context of the American Indian or Alaska Native culture for which they are being designed. Remember, these tribal groups are very diverse and reflect different ways of looking at and relating to the world in which they live.

▶ As much as possible, educational materials also should reflect the learning styles and cultural values of the population for which they are being designed. This will require that these elements be included in the needs assessment process.

▶ Be aware that the use of "talking circles" in conjunction with the use of tribal stories has been found to be a very useful and culturally appropriate educational intervention for American Indian and Alaska Native populations.

▶ Be aware that storytelling is a culturally appropriate educational technique because it uses an insider approach rather than working from outside the cultural milieu.

▶ Always assess the cultural appropriateness of any pictures, models, dolls, or other educational materials prior to their inclusion in the program, because some materials might make the target group members uncomfortable.

▶ Employing and training tribal members to facilitate educational programs is a valuable approach for facilitating implementation of HPDP programs in American Indian and Alaska Native communities.

▶ Intervention design should employ relevant theory to support design efforts.

▶ Seek to develop interventions that focus on positive health changes rather than on those with negative or fear-arousing consequences.

EVALUATION CONSIDERATIONS

Evaluation is at the heart of all HPDP programs or services because this process provides validation for the activities that have been carried out, points to where the program or service can be improved, and lays the groundwork for ongoing support from funding agencies and the community itself. The health promoter should consider the following suggestions when planning evaluation activities:

▶ Seek to develop evaluation strategies, methods, and instruments that reflect an understanding of current theory and practice in the evaluation and research literature.

▶ Be aware that support for evaluation of HPDP programs for Native communities will be dependent on the needs of the stakeholders, the potential use of the knowledge to be gained, how the target group views and uses knowledge, and the values that have been used to guide program assessment.

▶ Remember that evaluation and assessment are processes that often are difficult to gain support for, even from the most sophisticated of groups. Thus, efforts to explain the underlying assumptions governing these processes, as well as the methods and anticipated outcomes from these activities, can help make explicit what often is unclear to those inexperienced with evaluation and assessment activities.

▶ Evaluation and assessment measures should be culturally relevant and tailored to the linguistic and educational capabilities of the target group. Thus, efforts to involve community members in identifying evaluation criteria important and meaningful to them are strongly suggested.

▶ Recognize that HPDP program participants might have limited test-taking abilities or skills. Thus, efforts to design evaluation methods should consider how best to measure participant gains from the program using approaches that are familiar, acceptable, and of interest to the community.

▶ Providing evaluation and assessment training for tribal members who are to be involved in program assessment, implementation, and evaluation activities can help promote input and support for these efforts.

▶ Wherever possible, provide opportunities for staff members from the community to be actively involved in all aspects of the program evaluation process.

▶ Be sure to design evaluation and assessment reporting and feedback mechanisms into the program to ensure that the community is made regularly aware of how well the program or service is functioning to improve the health issue or problem for which it was designed.

REFERENCES

Joe, J. R., & Malach, R. S. (1992). Families with Native American roots. In E. W. Lynch & M. J. Hanson (Eds.), *Developing cross-cultural competence: A guide for working with young children and their families*. Baltimore, MD: Paul H. Brookes.

Kramer, J. (1996). American Indians. In J. G. Lipson, S. L. Dibble, & P. A. Minarik (Eds.), *Culture and nursing care: A pocket guide*. San Francisco: UCSF Nursing Press.

Pasick, R. J., D'Onofrio, C. N., & Otero-Sabogal, R. (1996). Similarities and differences across cultures: Questions to inform a third generation for health promotion research. *Health Education Quarterly, 23*(Suppl.), S142-S161.

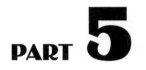

PART **5**

Asian American Populations

18

Asian American Health and Disease

An Overview of the Issues

JILLIAN INOUYE

Because the Asian American group is one of the fastest growing ethnic groups in the United States, and because of the diversity of history, language, and cultural practices, it is critical that health professionals be sensitive and responsive when working with the different subgroups. The purpose of this chapter is to provide an overview of the Asian American population and subpopulations in the United States, describe their health and disease patterns, and indicate important points and caveats to consider when working with them. This chapter is divided into three main sections. The first section addresses terminology, historical perspectives, sociodemographic characteristics, acculturation, integration, and growth. The second focuses on health and disease patterns, health beliefs and practices, and barriers to health promotion and disease prevention. The final section summarizes the chapter. This chapter is intended to provide helpful insights and dispel the myths of Asian Americans as a "model minority" group.

INTRODUCTION

Defining Terms and Describing Diversity

Ethnicity refers to groups whose members share a common social and cultural heritage passed on to each successive generation (Giger & Davidhizar, 1995), whereas *race* usually is related to biological features such as skin color and blood group. Ethnicity includes self-definition and identification with a culture such as

337

language, history and origins, education, religion, and occupation (Kitano, 1995). Sometimes, this distinction overlaps, and some (e.g., U.S. Census Bureau) refer to race while actually referring to ethnicity. The term *ethnicity* is used in this chapter.

The term *Asian American* refers to people of Asian descent who are citizens or permanent residents of the United States. The term encompasses at least 23 subgroups such as Asian Indian, Cambodian, Chinese, Filipino, Hmong, Japanese, Korean, Laotian, Thai, Vietnamese, and "other Asian," with 32 linguistic groups. Among this group, the Chinese and Filipinos are the two largest subgroups, followed by the Japanese, Asian Indians, and Koreans. The Chinese and Filipinos consist of 1.6 million and 1.4 million members, respectively, with the Japanese, Asian Indians, Koreans, and Vietnamese following with 848,000, 815,000, 799,000, and 615,000 members, respectively (Flack et al., 1995).

According to the 1990 census, Asian and Pacific Islander Americans (APIAs) are the fastest growing ethnic minority in the United States and stand at 8.4 million (U.S. Bureau of the Census, 1992b). Approximately 95% (6.9 million) Asians and 5% (365,000) Pacific Islanders make up the total APIA population, with Asian Americans comprising about 3.3% of the total U.S. population. It is projected that the APIA population will double in size by the year 2009, triple by 2024, and quadruple by 2038 and reach 41 million (or 10.7%) of the total U.S. population (U.S. Bureau of the Census, 1992a).

Despite the dramatic increase in the population, the APIA group often is neglected, poorly understood, and given little attention by the health care system and policymakers (Lin-Fu, 1993). Ignorance of the bipolar distribution and inconsistencies in coding for race/ethnicity in health statistics contribute to the myth of a healthy ethnic population. Because approximately 30 to 50 diverse ethnic groups of APIAs were combined in census counts, it is difficult to determine the exact numbers and ethnic-specific health problems. In addition, at birth, infants of mixed ethnicity were coded according to a hierarchy of categories. A child with Asian and African American parents would be classified as African American. According to Farley, Richards, and Bell (1995), correct coding of ethnicity might significantly increase infant mortality rates for Chinese, Japanese, and Filipinos. These inconsistencies and the tremendous diversity in immigration patterns, language, culture, religion, lifestyle, diet, health, and geographic distribution of this population make development of health policy and programs difficult for Asian Americans.

Sociodemographic Characteristics of Asian American Populations

According to Takeuchi and Young (1994), sociodemographic factors can provide a general assessment of a community's health status. These indicators usually are income status, per capita income, and employment. Stereotypical thinking about the "model minority" label for Asian Americans also has led to erroneous conclusions about their lack of health problems because of the economic success of one or two of the subgroups.

Changes in U.S. immigration policies contributed to differences in demographic characteristics of the Asian population. Before 1965, immigration policy often was exclusionary, racist, and xenophobic (Johnson et al., 1995). For example, the Chinese Exclusion Act of 1882 was the first to legally bar an ethnic group from immigrating to the United States. The Chinese population then declined until the repeal of the exclusionary act by the Magnuson Act of 1943, which set quotas of 105 individuals per year (Takeuchi & Young, 1994). This act was abolished in 1965, and with the fall of Saigon in 1975, the Asian population (especially from Vietnam, Cambodia, and Laos) has more than doubled in size each decade and now approaches 66% foreign born (U.S. Department of Commerce, 1993).

Fully 79% of the APIA population reside in the following 10 states: California, New York, Hawaii, Texas, Illinois, New Jersey, Washington, Virginia, Florida, and Massachusetts (Flack et al., 1995). After arrival in the United States, most Asian immigrants settled in areas with high concentrations of their own ethnic groups. These communities often have substandard housing, high unemployment, poverty, and crime (Johnson et al., 1995).

According to Yoon and Chien (1996), the education and income of APIAs formed a bipolar distribution, with a high percentage of older persons having at least 4 years of high school education and also a high percentage having only 0 to 4 years of elementary education, relative to the total population. Although the median family income was higher than the total population, a higher percentage lived in poverty (Lin-Fu, 1988).

Educational attainment and income levels often are used as measures for identifying high-paying jobs, status, and prestigious occupations. However, this has not always been the case for this group. In 1990, 12.2% lived below the poverty level, and one out of five (20.5%) full-time workers age 25 years or over made less than $15,000 per year (Lin-Fu, 1993). Results that highlight the possibility of erroneous conclusions and possible consequences on decision making for health care were reported by Takeuchi and Young (1994). They found that the average Asian American household income was lower than the U.S. average income and that 14 of 17 Asian American groups had poverty levels that exceeded the U.S. average (Laotians, Hmong, and Cambodians had levels above 45%). Unemployment rates for APIAs as a group were below the U.S. average, yet the Hmong, Laotians, and Cambodians had unemployment rates in double digits.

According to Lin-Fu (1994), a bipolar pattern of socioeconomic status has contributed to the myth that Asian Americans are a model minority. This is illustrated by the following educational percentages. In 1990, 39.1% of Asian Americans had a college education, significantly higher than the 21.5% for the total U.S. population. However, 5.3% were functionally illiterate, which was more than twice the rate for the total population (2.4%). For women, the rate was more than three times that of the total population (6.2% vs. 2.1%).

Historical Perspectives: A Brief Overview of Asian American History In the United States

Immigration has played the major role in the growth of the Asian American population. In 1990, 74% of APIAs were foreign born, and many were relatively recent arrivals (U.S. Bureau of the Census, 1992b). Approximately 4,451,200 people immigrated to the United States from Asian countries between 1971 and 1990. The immigration histories of Asians to the United States differ for the various subpopulations based on economic, political, and social factors in their originating countries. The migration patterns of a few of the larger Asian groups are highlighted in this section.

Chinese Americans. A significant number of Chinese Americans migrated between 1840 and 1882 with the California Gold Rush. Mainly males, they entered the country as laborers in the mines and railroads and then later in agriculture and service trades. Most had little education and were alone because families were not allowed to immigrate with them. After 1965 and the easement of immigration laws, better educated professionals and families from Taiwan, mainland China, and Hong Kong came to the United States. The Chinese comprise the largest group among Asian Americans, and 63% are foreign born (Takeuchi & Young, 1994). Fully 66% live in five states: California, New York, Hawaii, Illinois, and Texas (U.S. Department of Commerce, 1993).

Japanese Americans. Early immigration from Japan to the United States and Hawaii commenced around 1895 with a primary focus on farm work. The peak of immigration occurred between 1900 and 1910 (Shiba & Oka, 1996) but soon decreased after the National Origins Act of 1924 barred Asians from entering the United States. According to Takeuchi and Young (1994), this immigration pattern created a generational difference within the Japanese American community that has a unique effect on self-identification and social boundaries. Each generation had a unique sense of identification with its mother country and acculturation rates, unlike other Asian immigrant groups. In 1942, with Executive Order 9066, all persons of Japanese ancestry living in California, Washington, Oregon, and (to a small extent) Hawaii were forcibly moved to relocation camps. The internment experience disrupted families and had enormous financial implications because of loss of land and jobs. A large number of young men volunteered to serve in all-Japanese military units. The young, primarily second-generation Japanese American men used the GI Bill for higher education and upward mobility. These events assisted in the assimilation process, and this group often has been identified as a model minority because of its economic successes.

Filipino Americans. Immigrants of Filipino (or Pilipino, as there is no *F* in the Filipino alphabet) ancestry, like many of the other Asian immigrants, are distinguished by their arrival in waves. The first wave began in the early 1700s when Manila men deserted Spanish galleons in Mexico and emigrated to New Orleans (Cantos & Rivera, 1996). Between 1906 and 1934, male agricultural workers immigrated to Hawaii and the western United States. The Tydings-McDuffie Act of 1934 made the Phillippines a commonwealth with an annual quota of about 50. The second wave occurred between 1946 and 1965 because of citizenship awarded to Filipinos who joined the armed services in World War II and also because of war brides, students, and professional immigration. The third wave occurred after the Amended Immigrant Naturalization Act of 1965 relaxed quotas. On the average, this third wave appears to be better educated than the previous waves. Between 1980 and 1990, 31.6% of the Filipino Americans were foreign born (U.S. Department of Commerce, 1993). They were noted for high educational standards, and a high percentage held bachelor's degrees, 36.2% for males and 41.6% for females (U.S. Department of Commerce, 1993).

Korean Americans. Between 1898 and 1905, approximately 8,000 Koreans settled in Hawaii because of unstable conditions in Korea, including the Sino-Japanese War, the Tonghak Rebellion, a cholera epidemic, locust plagues, drought, and famine. They worked as laborers on Hawaii sugar plantations. Anti-Asian sentiments and the National Oriental Exclusion Act of 1934 banned all Asian immigration until after World War II. The second wave, during the period 1950 to 1953, consisted of wives of Americans who had fought during the war in Korea, picture brides, and students (Takeuchi & Young, 1994). The third wave after 1965 followed the opening of the Immigration and Naturalization Act and also occurred as a result of economic strife. Because of this situation, many nurses, pharmacists, dentists, and physicians came to the United States between 1965 and 1977 (Reardon, 1996). Many of the men followed their spouses (who were professionals) without adequate preparation for themselves. A major issue involving Korean American men is a loss of control and a sense of not belonging (Hurh & Kim, 1990). Individuals also faced problems of financial struggles, poor health care, difficulty with social interactions, and mental problems such as *Hwa Byung,* which is a Korean culture-bound syndrome of suppressed anger and depression (Pang, 1990). As in most Asian cultures, education is valued and children excel in school, particularly in science. They also are more likely to participate in the labor force.

Southeast Asian Americans. Prior to the early 1970s, immigration of Southeast Asians ranged from 1,500 to 4,700 per year. This figure increased considerably by the mid-1970s. Two waves occurred between 1975 and 1977 and between 1980 and 1986 because of war, internal political conflicts, and famine (Takeuchi & Young, 1994). Following the fall of Saigon, Vietnamese made up the first group of refugees with people who had higher education, professional skills, and families from wealthy backgrounds. The second wave of Vietnamese were known as "boat people." These individuals escaped to seek freedom and consisted of enlisted men in the armed forces, fishermen, and traders (Farrales, 1996). There also were many women and children, as well as unaccompanied children, in this wave.

The Hmong are a people found in areas of southern China, Laos, Vietnam, Burma, and Thailand. Many originally were from Laos but lived for many years in Thailand refugee camps. They fought for the U.S. Central Intelligence Agency against the Communists and were targeted for genocide when the war ended. The second migration of the Hmong consisted of families and clans attempting reunification with other members in the United States.

Cambodians who immigrated between 1975 and 1979 were well-educated professionals affiliated with the U.S. government or who escaped on their own. Between 1980 and 1985, larger numbers of rural agrarian individuals and families

TABLE 18.1 Oriental and Occidental Values

Oriental or Eastern Values	Occidental or Western Values
Harmony with nature	Mastery of nature
Tradition	Change
Hierarchy	Mobility (upward/downward)
Formality	Informality
Indirectness and subtlety	Directness and openness
Stoicism, suppression of emotional expression	Open display of emotional expression
Age/wisdom and virtue	Youth/physical vigor and appearance
Mutual consideration and self-depreciation	Assertiveness and self-determination
Modesty	Self-confidence
Family/group orientation and interdependence	Individualism and independence
Extended family	Nuclear family
Convergent thinking	Divergent thinking
Cyclical concept of time	Specific point, schedules, clocks
Past and present orientation	Future orientation
Rote learning	Discovery learning
Conformity	Competition

SOURCE: Adapted from Lin-Fu (1994) and Stauffer (1995).

arrived with many widows and orphans because of the brutal civil war. A large percentage lacked the skills necessary for life in the United States (Kulig, 1996). The poverty rates among Southeast Asian Americans are high.

Acculturation, Integration, and Growth of Asian American Populations in the United States

Beliefs and values play an important role in acculturation and integration of Asian Americans into Western culture. Although many immigrants came to the United States with the idea of economic advancement and intended to return to their home countries when those governments stabilized, some arrived as political refugees with the hope of integration into their new country. Thus, the process of integration differs for each of the Asian groups. In addition, differences in beliefs and values illustrate some of the possible areas of conflicts and frustrations experienced by new immigrants and sometimes later generations; these are highlighted in Table 18.1.

Immigration causes a number of adjustment and acculturation stresses that are related to overall health (Kuo & Tsai, 1986; Lin, Masuda, & Tazuma, 1984). People who were forced to leave their homes faced political exile and separation from family members. For a culture that values the nuclear and extended family, this can be devastating. Language adjustment was another stress that had to be overcome to function in a new country. Foods that were thought to be strengthening and health maintaining were difficult to acquire. Most Asians come from homogeneous ethnic countries and were thrust into heterogeneous surroundings where their self-identities were threatened. They often have to deal with this "differentness" as well as the prejudices and racial bigotry of others.

In addition, immigration policies, political climate, and economic factors at the time of immigration play a role in the acculturation process. Two subgroups are discussed to illustrate differences in geographic settlement and time of immigration and political climate.

Japanese Americans are the only Asian group to refer to generational differences according to their arrival and/or birth in the United States. The first generation was called *Issei* and immigrated during the first wave between 1890 and 1924. Because of language difficulties and prejudice these immigrants experienced, they formed relatively self-sufficient communities and maintained cultural values (Ishida & Inouye, 1995). Members of the second generation, or *Nisei,* were born in the United States and were largely influenced by the values of their parents. Many were bilingual but maintained the customs and beliefs of their parents. Education and acculturation were the roads to economic security and acculturation, and many families sacrificed for one or two of their children to achieve high occupational attainment. Nisei born during the pre-World War II era and their parents were subject to hostility and racial discrimination during the war with Japan. This climaxed with the evacuation and internment of Japanese Americans living on the West Coast and in Hawaii with Executive Orders 9066 and 9102. More than 120,000 citizens and noncitizens were imprisoned, with enormous financial implications such as loss of homes and businesses. Despite this dehumanizing experience, an overwhelming number of Nisei volunteered to fight in the war in an all-Nisei battalion and its larger unit of Japanese Americans in the 442nd Regimental Combat Team (Kakesako, 1993). This unit emerged as the most decorated unit in the history of the U.S. armed forces for its size and duration of service (Chang, 1993). Following the war, members of the Nisei generation identified more with their American background, used the GI Bill for educational attainment, and became active in the political arena in some states. Members of the third generation of *Sansei* and the fourth generation of *Yonsei* are less familiar with the language and customs of their ancestors. Approximately 50% have married outside the ethnic group, promoting further assimilation into American culture (Kikumura & Kitano, 1973).

Korean Americans represent 11% of the Asian American population and are scattered throughout the United States, but nearly half reside in three states: California, New York, and Hawaii. They are the fifth largest Asian ethnic population in the United States behind the Chinese, Filipinos, Japanese, and Asian Indians (Koh & Koh, 1993). A major reason prompting Koreans to immigrate to the United States was consideration for their children's futures. Because of this, many had difficulty leaving behind their cultural and social norms and adjusting to their new country (Earp, 1995). Men followed their spouses, many of whom were nurses or physicians, because it was easier for females to immigrate due to their professions. These men were inadequately prepared, and they suffered from loss of control and a sense of not belonging (Hurh & Kim,

1990). Many Korean immigrants still use traditional Korean health care practices with a belief in two contrasting forces: *Yang* and *Um* (similar to the Chinese Yin and Yang). Korean elders in Chicago still seek medical care from traditional providers (Yu, Huber, Wong, Tseng, & Liu, 1990). A survey of more than 6,000 Korean Americans in Los Angeles County found that about half of Korean Americans do not have health insurance and that nearly a quarter of all households have a family member who, at one time or another, failed to receive appropriate medical care because of an inability to pay, lack of time to visit a doctor, or not knowing where to go (California Korean Health Education and Information and Referral Center, 1989).

Caveats When Generalizing About Asian American Population Subgroups in the United States

The stereotypes that Asian Americans are hardworking, intelligent, successful, and mentally healthy have masked social, economic, and mental health problems of the Asian American populations. This type of thinking also has diverted attention away from how discrimination and prejudice have affected the lives of Asians, submerged within-group differences by applying the same labels to all Asians, fostered or created hard feelings and competitiveness between Asian Americans and other minority groups, and lowered research interest and priorities for this group (Sue, 1994). Stereotyping Asian Americans as having similar beliefs and health practices also leads health professionals to assume that programs for one Asian group will work for another Asian group. It would follow, then, that health care workers need to be careful not to apply care and programs indiscriminantly to all groups in the same manner.

Health data specific to Asians are either nonexistent or uninterpretable because of the convention of aggregating data. Therefore, there also is a lack of awareness of various disorders or problems specific to this population. According to Flack et al. (1995), methodological approaches in existing data sources have (a) led to less developed knowledge about morbidity risk and health care use unique to subgroups, (b) hampered the mainstream exploration of more rigorous study designs in health care research for APIAs, (c) trivialized the scientific significance of finding alternative data collection approaches and sampling procedures that would take into account the ethnic diversity within and the peculiar geographic distribution of Asian Americans, and (d) delayed the development of culturally appropriate measures that would enable health researchers to have a precise understanding of the health status, morbidity patterns, and health services use of these subgroups.

Yu, Liu, and Williams (1993) also present detailed limitations of the existing U.S. national data sources for APIAs and state that these weaknesses include (a) evidence of inaccuracy in the numerators and a serious undercount of the APIA population, (b) failure of conventional sampling techniques to capture small minority populations, (c) lack of studies on the cost efficiency of sampling rare populations of which APIAs are an example, (d) lumping of the diverse groups under the rubric of APIAs, and (e) failure to recognize the importance of language and culture in shaping the health and lifestyle of APIAs.

HEALTH AND DISEASE PATTERNS
AMONG ASIAN AMERICANS

An Overview of the Issues

Health and disease patterns among Asian Americans differ by generations and immigration dates. To a large degree, these patterns depend on the degree of acculturation. If individuals were born in the United States and have lived here for many generations, they are largely indistinguishable from the general population in their health care beliefs (Spector, 1996). However, new immigrants differ on many social and health-related issues. Chen (1996) determines that those at high risk would include individuals with the following characteristics: low socioeconomic status, uninsured, limited English proficiency and/or linguistically isolated, foreign born or recently immigrated, and rigid adherence to certain cultural health beliefs and traditions that might conflict with some proven effective Western practices.

Prior to 1985, it was felt that APIAs were at lower risk for death and illnesses. Findings since then suggest that the health status is worse than was initially believed (Chen & Hawks, 1995). It is now felt that APIA health status will deteriorate and perhaps exceed the mortality rates of other racial groups in certain diseases during the next 20 years (Chen & Hawks, 1995). Studies conducted mainly in California, with the largest APIA population, found specific differences in disease patterns for different Asian subpopulations. Poor health was found among many residents of Chinatown because of poor working conditions and lack of minimal and preventive health care (Li, Schlief, & Chang, 1972). These findings and others are categorized according to disease patterns in this section.

Cancer. The incidence rate for cancer of the liver among Asians living in the San Francisco Bay Area is 39%. In a study of Korean American men, it was thought to be eight times higher than that among U.S. white men (Koh & Koh, 1993). Korean American men also have a fivefold higher incidence of stomach cancer (Koh & Koh, 1993). The lung cancer rate is 18% higher among Southeast Asian men than among white males, and the liver cancer rate is more than 12 times higher among Southeast Asians than among the white population. Cancer of the stomach is ranked second in Japanese Americans, whereas in whites and blacks prostate cancer and lung cancer are ranked first and second (U.S. Department of Health and Human Services, 1994).

Tuberculosis. Reducing the tuberculosis incidence in Asian Americans per 100,000 population is an objective for *Healthy People 2000* (U.S. Department of Health and Human Services, 1990). Tuberculosis incidence increased by 15% from 1988 to 1992 in the general population. This increase was 28% among APIAs. The incidence of tuberculosis is 40 times higher among Southeast Asians than among the total population. In one county, approximately 75% of the tuberculosis cases are in the foreign born, many of whom developed multidrug-resistant tuberculosis. Tracing transmission and increasing compliance with treatment regimes will require improved community-based epidemiology and the provision of culturally and linguistically competent health care services.

Hepatitis B. Because of recent immigration status, many infectious diseases such as Hepatitis B virus infection and tuberculosis are common. Chronic carrier rates range from 5% to 15% for the Chinese, Koreans, Filipinos, and Southeast Asians, compared to 0.2% for the total U.S. population (Franks et al., 1989). What is disturbing is that among 661 U.S.-born infants, 4.3% had chronic Hepatitis B virus infection despite the fact that such infection is preventable through vaccination (Lin-Fu, 1994).

Reducing Hepatitis B cases in the year 2000 is another objective for *Healthy People 2000.* Baseline cases showed a 38% reduction from 1987 to 1992. Although immunization rates for Hepatitis B virus are good, follow-up coverage is poor. Providers need to be encouraged to offer Hepatitis B virus immunizations with added prevention and control efforts.

Diabetes. Myers, Kagawa-Singer, Kumanyika, Lex, and Markides (1995) report that Japanese Americans have twice the rate of diabetes (Type II) as white Americans and four times the rate of Japanese in Japan. The reason for this increased rate is unclear because obesity does not appear to be a prevalent problem in this population.

Smoking. The U.S. smoking average for adults is 30% and for Asian male smokers is 35% to 50%. In specific APIA groups, the rates are as follows: Japanese, 37%; Chinese, 28%; Filipinos, 20%; Laotians, 92%; Kampucheans, 70.7%; Chinese Vietnamese, 54.5% (Han, Kim, Song, & Lee, 1989; Levin, 1985; Rumbaut, 1989; Sasao, 1992). A report in *Healthy People 2000* states that the cigarette smoking prevalence rate for Vietnamese males declined from 55% to 35% in 1990. This still is higher than the 32% rate for U.S. males and the overall objective of 20%. This suggests that scientifically based, culturally appropriate prevention strategies and interventions for smokers need further study and more intervention programs.

Alcohol consumption. Although alcohol consumption among Asians overall is lower than that among white Americans, recent immigrants from Japan have a much higher proportion of heavy drinking than do white Americans (Higuchi, Parrish, Dufur, & Hartford, 1994). Later-generation Chinese consume more alcohol than do immigrant Chinese (Sue, Zane, & Ito, 1979). Zane and Kim (1995) summarize some of the substance use literature and state that although general drinking rates of Asians are lower than the national average, it appears that alcohol use has been underestimated, particularly for certain groups such as Japanese American and Filipino American males.

Suicide. Chinese and Japanese American women age 55 years or over commit suicide at a much higher rate compared to the non-Asian population, including whites, blacks, and American Indians (Griffith et al., 1989; Liu & Yu, 1985)

Genetic disorders. Lin-Fu (1994) reports that there are genetic disorders common to Asians such as alpha and beta thalassemia, Hemoglobin E, lactase deficiency, and G-6PD deficiency.

Cardiovascular problems. A study revealed that Southeast Asian refugee children in Minnesota had elevated risks for hypertension, with odds ratios of 1.64 for Vietnamese, 1.84 for Cambodians, 2.69 for Hmong, and 2.89 for Laotians (Munger, Gomez-Marin, Prineas, & Sinaiko, 1991). Noncompliance with Western prescription antihypertensive medications was very high in non-English-speaking Chinese with hypertension (Stavig, Igra, & Leonard, 1988). This combination of medication noncompliance and high disease rates forecasts dire results for selected Asian populations.

Other unusual and serious conditions include a high rate of coronary artery disease among Asian Indians (Enas & Mehta, 1995) despite their largely vegetarian diet. Sudden unexpected nocturnal death syndrome is especially prevalent among young Hmong men who seem to be at no apparent risk for cardiovascular incident (Frye, 1995). These conditions point to as yet unexplained, and thus difficult to treat, conditions for Asians.

Low birthweight. Yoon and Chien (1996) report that the incidence for low birthweight varies from 4.5% for Chinese to 7% for Filipinos. Inadequate prenatal care of Hmong women is present in Minneapolis, Minnesota, because providers are not properly addressing concerns about sexual modesty (Spring, Ross, Etkin, & Deinard, 1995).

Philip R. Lee, assistant secretary of health, and Moon Chen analyzed *Healthy People 2000* objectives for APIAs and found that for growth retardation in low-income children, there has been some progress (Chen, 1993; Lee, 1995). But the gap between Asian children and all other children has not been narrowed, and more progress is needed.

Mental health. Regarding the area of mental health and help-seeking behavior, there is widespread belief that Asians in the United States are the model minority with few mental health problems. Sue (1994) dispels the false images and stereotypes about mental health needs of Asian Americans in his review of three studies. Posttraumatic stress disorder, dissociation, depression, and anxiety are high in Cambodians because of their traumatic immigrant history (Calson & Rosser-Hogan, 1993). Kinzie, Fredrickson, Ben, Fleck, and Karls (1990) also found the rate for posttraumatic stress disorder to be high among all Indochinese refugee patients seen at their clinic.

In the Southeast Asian refugee families, Frye (1995) reported anecdotal evidence of the high incidence of domestic violence. This might be related to their settlement in urban communities quite different from their agrarian backgrounds, to response to violence in their new communities, to changes in kinship ties, and/or to the stresses in the family structure after immigration and settlement. Using a global ethnic category masks the heterogeneity of the different subpopulations and leads to erroneous conclusions about their health status.

A study by Uehara, Takeuchi, and Smuckler (1994) that examined the level of functioning of adults with serious mental illness in the state of Washington found that when using Asian Americans as an ethnic category compared to whites, Asian Americans had higher community functioning scores. When analyses were done on specific subpopulations (e.g., Chinese, Japanese, Filipinos, Laotians, Vietnamese), however, only the Chinese had higher scores than did whites.

Responses to psychotropic drugs for Asian Americans are different from those for their white counterparts on which blood levels have been normed. The thresholds for psychotropic drugs and alcoholism are different for APIAs where they have higher plasma or serum drug concentrations, even when controlling for differences in weight and body surface (Bond, 1990).

HIV/AIDS. Although the dominant "face of AIDS" is that of a gay white male or an intravenous drug user, it has been changing during the past few years. The state of Hawaii noted a steady rise in the numbers of HIV/AIDS cases among APIAs (Governor's Committee on HIV/AIDS, 1996). The APIA group has the highest rate of increase in reported AIDS cases in the San Francisco and Los Angles areas when compared to other racial/ethnic groups (Asian Pacific AIDS Education Project, 1990). This group is at great risk because its members tend to delay diagnosis and treatment based on lack of knowledge about availability of treatment, the fear of being identified with the disease, and the shame of their health status due to social and cultural taboos (Gock, 1994).

Health prevention and promotion. In the past, there has been a lack of specific health data for Asian American subgroups, and this has been equated with a lack of health problems or needs. Although the National Center for Health Statistics now reports health status for Chinese, Japanese, and Filipinos (Hahn, Mulinare, & Teutsch, 1992), this growing population still has received little attention. *Healthy People 2000* included few baseline data for this group, with only 8 targeted objectives for all APIAs combined, compared to 48, 31, and 27 for blacks, American Indians and Alaska Natives, and Hispanics, respectively.

One objective focuses on increasing the proportion of counties with culturally and linguistically appropriate community health promotion programs for racial/ethnic minority populations. Although there are insufficient data to evaluate progress, one report found that only 30% of the states have deemed bilingual or bicultural materials as important. Subsequently, definitions of culturally appropriate community health promotion programs need to be established with means to evaluate cultural and linguistic competencies of these programs.

Lee (1995) reports that APIAs received clinical preventive services in 1991 at a lower rate than that of the total U.S. population. Increasing the proportion of people with screening and immunization services, as well as at least one counseling service, is an important health objective. Lee states that 63% of the total U.S. population have their cholesterol checked, compared to 58% of APIAs. Rates of Pap tests for women age 19 years or over were 64% for APIA women, compared to 76% for all U.S. women in that age group. Regarding breast examinations for women age 50 years or over, 38% of APIAs were examined, compared to 51% of all U.S. women in that age group. Regarding influenza vaccine for women age 65 years or older, 29% of APIAs had it, compared to 42% of all U.S. women in that age group.

The development and implementation of a national process to identify significant gaps in disease prevention and health promotion data, and the establishment of mechanisms to meet these needs, is another important health objective. M. Chen (1993) summarizes the progress of the health objectives and comments that in addition to the health problems not being "on target," many other health parameters are not included in these objectives. These areas of neglect have seriously affected federal priority setting and resource allocations because of lack of data.

According to Yoon and Chien (1996), *Healthy People 2000* states that U.S.-born APIAs have no distinguishing health needs relative to the population as a whole, yet several investigators have demonstrated inconsistencies in the National Center for Health Statistics' coding for race/ethnicity. Newer findings of high prevalence rates for specific diseases also speak to the different health needs for different groups.

Health Beliefs and Practices: A General Overview

Health beliefs and practices often are shaped by cultural values in determining what is important in one's life. Although variations are the norm rather then the exception, Asian groups share some similarities based on their religious background and the influence of Chinese culture throughout Asia (Lasky & Martz, 1993). Two beliefs that are prominent in Asians, especially Southeast Asians, are those of kinship solidarity and equilibrium or balance (Frye, 1995). A general overview of these two beliefs in the context of ideology is provided in this section.

Beliefs. Kinship solidarity refers to the view that the individual is subservient to the kinship-based group or family. This kinship is reinforced by identifiable clan names for the Hmong (Rairdan & Higgs, 1992) or *kenjinkais* (prefectural associations primarily for social and cultural purposes) for the Japanese (Lee & Takamura, 1980). Most Asian family patterns are characterized by filial piety, male authority, and respect for elders. This pattern sometimes determines decision-making practices relating to health care for recent immigrants.

The prominence of Confucian ideology, Buddhism, and Taoism in Asian cultures focuses on upholding a public facade and sanctions against public admission of problems. Attitudes toward mental illness focus on it as evidence of personal weakness. Somatization of emotional problems is better accepted. Therefore, many Asians will seek help for "headaches" and other illnesses without revealing true emotional problems. Although they do not believe in a clear dichotomy between mental and physical illness, mental illness is seen as shameful and as a punishment for misdeeds (Lasky & Martz, 1993).

Health is defined in the United States as a state of complete physical, mental, and social well-being and not merely the absence of disease (World Health Organization, 1947). Asians view it as a state of harmony with nature or freedom from symptoms or illness (Lin-Fu, 1994). The concept of balance is related to health promotion, and the concept of imbalance is related to disease (Spector, 1996). This balance or equilibrium relates to temperature in foods, climate, and body elements and diet, and it influences people's daily activities of living and health promotion. To achieve health and avoid illness, the people must adjust to the environment in a holistic manner. Traditional practitioners assist people in achieving this balance through energy balance.

Practices. It often is assumed by health care workers that everyone embraces the Western biomedical model. Traditional or cultural beliefs of spiritual or super-natural forces and balance with nature often are overlooked. One's cultural beliefs and use of language influence how one conceptualizes etiology, symptoms, and treatment of illnesses and also how one is to interact with health care providers and organizations.

Because of language difficulties and cultural differences, many Asians, especially the newer immigrants, still might prefer the traditional forms of Chinese and native medicine and seek help from Chinatown "physicians" or "masters" who treat them with traditional herbs and other methods (Spector, 1996). Asians often do not seek help from the Western system at all because of lack of understanding of the use of many painful diagnostic tests and lack of information and understanding about what is being done to them and why.

Alternative, complementary techniques (also referred to as unconventional or unorthodox therapies) are health practices that do not conform to those of the Western biomedical community, are not taught widely in U.S. medical and nursing curricula, and are not generally available in an allopathic health care system (Spector, 1996). These include acupuncture, massage, chiropractic, and herbs and usually are referred to as therapies that are not a part of one's cultural heritage, as opposed to traditional therapies or those that are part of one's cultural heritage.

In a national survey, Eisenberg et al. (1993) reported results of a survey of 1,539 subjects and found that about one third of all American adults use some form of unconventional medical treatment. The most frequent users are educated, upper income white Americans ages 25 to 49 years living on the West Coast. These practices include relaxation techniques, chiropractic, massage, imagery, spiritual healing, commercial weight loss programs, lifestyle diets, herbal medicines, megavitamins, self-help groups, energy healing, biofeedback, hypnosis, homeopathy, acupuncture, folk remedies, exercise, and prayer. Although there was no breakdown for Asian respondents, one can assume that the use is much higher in this group.

Barriers to Health Promotion and Disease Prevention in Asian American Populations

Access and barriers to health care for Asian Americans are similar to those for other ethnic groups and focus on socioeconomic factors such as availability of health insurance, access and location of health care facilities, transportation, poverty, and unemployment (Mayeno & Hirota, 1994). Whereas Spector (1996) points to poverty as the major obstacle to the health care system, others (e.g., Williams, 1990) indicate that lifestyle and cultural factors outweigh socio-economic status in accounting for differences in health care status. Hawks (1996) identifies five barriers typical for Asian Americans: the label of a model minority, diversity and linguistic barriers, financial barriers, insufficient data, and lack of culturally competent health care providers.

The myth of the model minority. The greatest barrier perpetuating the inaccurate focus on this group is the myth that all APIAs are affluent and healthy. A study by Somani (1994) in Ohio found that 17% of Asians had incomes falling below the national poverty guidelines, with groups such as Laotians, Vietnamese, and others from Southeast Asia having poverty levels as high as 60%. Their risk factor for tuberculosis is the highest among all racial/ethnic groups, and Hepatitis B also is common. Fully 75% of Asian Indian females, 44% of Korean females, and 25% of Chinese females had never had a mammogram in their lifetimes. In addition, 17% of APIAs lack insurance. The small businesses in the ethnic ghettos do not provide health insurance, nor do most immigrants believe in insuring one's health given that preventive medical care is not a priority for Asian immigrants (Johnson et al., 1995).

Diversity and linguistic barriers. Ethnocultural barriers include differences in language and communication styles, cultural values different from mainstream health care, economic differences, and stereotypical thinking about Asian health care needs, knowledge, and practices. Louie (1995) states that APIAs underuse available health care services because of lack of health care access and insurance coverage and/or lack of linguistically appropriate and culturally competent services. Language was cited by 60% of the Southeast Asians in San Diego as a major problem in obtaining health care (Rumbault, Chavez, Moser, Pickwell, & Wishnik, 1988). Yi (1995) found that underuse of preventive health care by Vietnamese women was based on language acculturation and length of residence in the United States. Still other reasons for underuse might relate to Asian Americans' beliefs about health and disease and the use of traditional treatments for self-care. Some Asian cultures believe that stoicism and restraint of public display of emotion are valued and that suffering is a part of life. With this belief, many might postpone seeking treatment for symptoms until they become unbearable (Uba, 1992).

Insufficient data. Hawks (1996) discusses the lack of data as related to difficulties in accessing this population because of lack of bilingual researchers, undercounting by the census, problems in methodology, data systems, collection instruments, and analyses at all levels of data gathering systems. It is very difficult to treat and do program planning if comprehensive data on health needs are not available.

Lack of culturally competent health care providers. A final barrier is variations of health values and priorities between consumers and health professionals. Although Frye (1995) speaks about the profound ignorance of health care professionals about the customs, culture, and experiences of Southeast Asian refugees, this also is true for Asians in general. An example by Anderson (1990) illustrates this discrepancy in health care delivery. She gives an example of Chinese and white families who were taught prescribed treatments for their chronically ill children in their homes. The Chinese families did not always carry out these treatments, and although they attempted to do some of them, they stopped these exercises when any discomfort was displayed by their children. White families emphasized the treatment and tried to complete them even if their children showed discomfort. They were felt to be sharing the beliefs of the practitioners that treatment would help achieve normal functioning. Although the Chinese families also had a high priority on having normal children, the contentment and happiness of their children was paramount to their notion of "normal family functioning" (Anderson, 1990). Thus, the problem and solution from two different perspectives can lead to two different outcomes. What is necessary is sensitivity to culturally different priorities in health care and disease prevention by providers who are trained and culturally competent.

CHAPTER SUMMARY

The topics covered in this chapter revealed several common themes that emerge about Asian Americans. These themes have been reported before and also may be relevant to other ethnic groups discussed in other chapters of this book. These themes include (a) the issue of heterogeneity within groups and the difficulties it engenders regarding summary statements of health needs, priorities, and social policies; (b) the myth of Asian Americans being a model minority with disregard for heterogeneity and bipolar distribution of socioeconomic status and illness; (c) the differences related to length of immigration status on the different health and social needs as well as prevalent cultural beliefs; (d) the lack of provider sensitivity and information about the different groups; and (e) the lack of data on health status of individual Asian groups.

McAllister and Farquhar (1992) suggest that the health needs of the community might not be the same as those of health professionals. Based on the recurring themes supported in the literature, what is needed in the future for health professionals are details and statistics about subpopulations of Asian Americans, outreach programs, language assistance, and culturally sensitive health care delivery. The greatest need, however, is the sensitivity of health providers to identify this group as members of the human race with health needs the same as everyone else but for different conditions specific to the subgroups.

REFERENCES

Anderson, J. (1990). Health care across cultures. *Nursing Outlook, 38*(3), 136-139.

Asian Pacific AIDS Education Project. (1990). *Asian Pacific AIDS statistics, August, 1990.* Los Angeles: Author.

Bond, W. S. (1990). Ethnicity and psychotropic drugs. *Clinical Pharmacy, 10,* 467-470.

California Korean Health Education and Information and Referral Center. (1989). *1989 Korean Health Survey in Los Angeles County.* Los Angeles: Author.

Calson, E. B., & Rosser-Hogan, R. (1993). Mental health status of Cambodian refugees ten years after leaving their home. *American Journal of Orthopsychiatry, 63,* 223-231.

Cantos, A., & Rivera, E. (1996). Filipinos. In J. Lipson, S. Dibble, & P. Minarik (Eds.), *Culture and nursing care: A pocket guide.* San Francisco: UCSF Nursing Press.

Chang, T. (1993, March 21). A legacy of bravery: The 442nd comes home. *The Honolulu Advertiser* (special section), p. 4.

Chen, A. M. (1996). Demographic characteristics of Asian and Pacific Islander Americans: Health implications. *Asian and Pacific Islander Journal of Health, 4*(1-3), 40-49.

Chen, M. S. (1993). A 1993 status report on the health status of Asian/Pacific Islander Americans: Comparisons with *Healthy People 2000* objectives. *Asian American and Pacific Islander Journal of Health, 1*(1), 37-55.

Chen, M. S., & Hawks, B. L. (1995). A debunking of the myth of healthy Asian Americans and Pacific Islanders. *American Journal of Health Promotion, 9,* 261-268.

Earp, J. B. (1995). Koreans. In J. N. Giger & R. E. Davidhizar (Eds.), *Transcultural nursing: Assessment and intervention.* St. Louis, MO: C. V. Mosby.

Eisenberg, D. M., Kessler, R. C., Foster, C., Norlock, P. E., Calkins, D. R., & Delbano, T. L. (1993). Unconventional medicine in the United States: Prevalence, costs, and patterns of use. *New England Journal of Medicine, 328,* 246-252.

Enas, E. A., & Mehta, J. (1995). Malignant coronary artery disease in young Asian Indians: Thoughts on pathogenesis, prevention, and therapy. *Clinical Cardiology, 18,* 131-135.

Farley, D. O., Richards, T., & Bell, R. M. (1995). Effects of reporting methods on infant mortality rate estimates for racial and ethnic subgroups. *Journal of Health Care for the Poor and Underserved, 6,* 60-75.

Farrales, S. (1996). Vietnamese. In J. Lipson, S. Dibble, & P. Minarik (Eds.), *Culture and nursing care: A pocket guide.* San Francisco: UCSF Nursing Press.

Flack, J., Amaro, H., Jenkins, W., Kunitz, S., Levy, J., Mixon, M., & Yu, E. (1995). Panel I: Epidemiology of minority health. *Health Psychology, 14,* 592-600.

Franks, A. L., Berg, C. J., Kane, M. A., Browne, B. B., Sikes, R. K., Elsea, W. R., & Burton, A. (1989). Hepatitis B virus infection among children born in the United States to Southeast Asian refugees. *New England Journal of Medicine, 321,* 1301-1305.

Frye, B. A. (1995). Use of cultural themes in promoting health among Southeast Asian refugees. *American Journal of Health Promotion, 9,* 269-280.

Giger, J. N., & Davidhizar, R. E. (Eds.). (1995). *Transcultural nursing: Assessment and intervention.* St. Louis, MO: C. V. Mosby.

Gock, T. (1994). Acquired immunodeficiency syndrome. In N. Zane, D. Takeuchi, & K. Young (Eds.), *Confronting critical health issues of Asian and Pacific Islander Americans.* Thousand Oaks, CA: Sage.

Governor's Committee on HIV/AIDS. (1996). *HIV and AIDS in Hawaii: Status report and policy statement.* Honolulu: Hawaii Department of Health.

Griffith, E., Delgado, A., Foulks, E., Ruitz, P., Spiegel, J., Wintrob, R., & Yamamoto, J. (Eds.). (1989). *Suicide and ethnicity in the United States.* New York: Brunner/Mazel.

Hahn, R. A., Mulinare, J., & Teutsch, S. M. (1992). Inconsistencies in coding on racial and ethnic groups. *Journal of the American Medical Association, 267,* 259-263.

Han, E. E. S., Kim, S. H., Song, H., & Lee, M. S. (1998). *Korean Health Survey: A preliminary report.* Los Angeles: Korean Health Education Information and Referral Center.

Hawks, B. L. (1996). Barriers to health improvement for Asian Americans. *Asian American and Pacific Islander Journal of Health, 4*(1-3), 50-54.

Higuchi, S., Parrish, K. M., Dufur, M. C., & Hartford, T. C. (1994). Relationship between drinking patterns and drinking problems among Japanese, Japanese-Americans and Caucasians. *Alcoholism: Clinical and Experimental Research, 18,* 305-310.

Hurh, W., & Kim, K. (1990). Adaptation and mental health of Korean male immigrants. *International Migration Review, 24,* 456-470.

Ishida, D., & Inouye, J. (1995). Japanese Americans. In J. N. Giger & R. E. Davidhizar (Eds.), *Transcultural nursing: Assessment and intervention.* St. Louis, MO: C. V. Mosby.

Johnson, K. W., Anderson, N. B., Bastida, E., Kramer, B. J., Williams, D., & Wong, M. (1995). Panel II: Macrosocial and environmental influences on minority health. *Health Psychology, 14,* 601-612.

Kakesako, G. K. (1993, March 19). Nisei proved their loyalty on the warfront. *The Honolulu Star-Bulletin,* p. A1.

Kikumura, A., & Kitano, H. H. L. (1973). *Changing lives.* San Francisco: Jossey-Bass.

Kinzie, J. D., Bochnlein, J. K., Leung, P. K., Moore, L. J., Riley, C., & Smith, D. (1990). The prevalence of posttraumatic stress disorder and its clinical significance among Southeast Asian refugees. *American Journal of Psychiatry, 147,* 913-917.

Kitano, H. H. L. (1995). Ethnic identity. *Asian American and Pacific Islander Journal of Health, 3*(1), 5-7.

Koh, H. K., & Koh, H. C. (1993). Health issues in Korean Americans. *Asian American and Pacific Islander Journal of Health, 1*(2), 176-193.

Kulig, J. C. (1996). Cambodians. In J. Lipson, S. Dibble, & P. Minarik (Eds.), *Culture and nursing care: A pocket guide.* San Francisco: UCSF Nursing Press.

Kuo, W. H., & Tsai, Y. M. (1986). Social networking, hardiness, and immigrants' mental health. *Journal of Health and Social Behavior, 27,* 133-149.

Lasky, E. M., & Martz, C. H. (1993). The Asian/Pacific Islander population in the United States: Cultural perspectives and their relationship to cancer prevention and early detection. In M. Frank-Stromberg & S. Olson (Eds.), *Cancer prevention in minority populations.* St. Louis, MO: C. V. Mosby.

Lee, P., & Takamura, J. (1980). The Japanese-Americans in Hawaii. In N. Palafox & A. Warren (Eds.), *Cross-cultural caring.* Honolulu, HI: Transcultural Health Care Forum.

Lee, P. R. (1995). Progress report for Asian and Pacific Islander Americans. *Asian American and Pacific Islander Journal of Health, 3*(2), 63-64.

Levin, B. L. (1985, May). *Cigarette smoking habits and characteristics in the Laotian refugee: A perspective pre- and post-resettlement.* Paper presented at the Refugee Health Conference, San Diego.

Li, F. P., Schlief, N. G., & Chang, C. J. (1972). Health care for the Chinese community in Boston. *American Journal of Public Health, 62,* 536-539.

Lin, K. M., Masuda, M., & Tazuma, L. (1984). Adaptational problems of Vietnamese refugees. IV: Three year comparison. *Psychiatric Journal of the University of Ottawa, 9,* 79-84.

Lin-Fu, J. (1988). Population characteristics and health care needs of Asian/Pacific Americans. *Public Health Reports, 103,* 18-27.

Lin-Fu, J. (1993). Asian and Pacific Islander Americans: An overview of demographic characteristics and health care issues. *Asian American and Pacific Islander Journal of Health, 1*(1), 20-36.

Lin-Fu. J. (1994). Ethnocultural barriers to health care: A major problem for Asian and Pacific Islander Americans. *Asian American and Pacific Islander Journal of Health, 2*(4), 290-289.

Liu, W., & Yu, E. (1985). Ethnicity, mental health, and the urban delivery system. In L. Maldonaldo & J. Moore (Eds.), *Urban ethnicity in the United States.* Beverly Hills, CA: Sage.

Louie, K. (1995). Cultural considerations: Asian-Americans and Pacific Islanders. *Imprint, 42*(5), 41-46.

Mayeno, L., & Hirota, S. (1994). Access to health care. In N. Zane, D. Takeuchi, & K. Young (Eds.), *Confronting critical health issues of Asian and Pacific Islander Americans.* Thousand Oaks, CA: Sage.

McAllister, G., & Farquhar, M. (1992). Health beliefs: A cultural division? *Journal of Advanced Nursing, 17,* 1447-1454.

Munger, R. G., Gomez-Marin, O., Prineas, R., & Sinaiko, A. (1991). Elevated blood pressure among Southeast Asian refugee children in Minnesota. *American Journal of Epidemiology, 133,* 1257-1265.

Myers, H. F., Kagawa-Singer, M., Kumanyika, S. K., Lex, B. W., & Markides, K. S. (1995). Panel III: Behavioral risk factors related to chronic disease in ethnic minorities. *Health Psychology, 14,* 613-621.

Pang, K. Y. (1990). Hwa-byung: The construction of a Korean popular illness among Korean elderly immigrant women in the United States. *Culture, Medicine, and Psychiatry, 14,* 495-512.

Rairdan, B., & Higgs, Z. (1992). When your patient is a Hmong refugee. *American Journal of Nursing, 92*(3), 52-55.

Reardon, T. (1996). Koreans. In J. Lipson, S. Dibble, & P. Minarik (Eds.), *Culture and nursing care: A pocket guide.* San Francisco: UCSF Nursing Press.

Rumbaut, R. G. (1989). Portraits, patterns and predictors of the refugee adaptation process: Results and reflections from the IHARP panel study. In D. W. Haines (Ed.), *Refugees as immigrants: Cambodians, Laotians, and Vietnamese in America.* Totowa, NJ: Rowman & Littlefield.

Rumbault, R. G., Chavez, L. R., Moser, R. J., Pickwell, S. M., & Wishnik, S. M. (1988). The politics of migrant health care: A comprehensive study of Mexican immigrants and Indochinese refugees. *Research in the Sociology of Health Care, 7,* 143-202.

Sasao, T. (1992). *Statewide Asian drug service needs assessment.* Sacramento: California Department of Health.

Shiba, G., & Oka, R. (1996). Japanese Americans. In J. G. Lipson, S. L. Dibble, & P. A. Minarik (Eds.), *Culture and nursing care: A pocket guide.* San Francisco: UCSF Nursing Press.

Somani, P. (1994). Myth of a model minority. *Asian American and Pacific Islander Journal of Health, 2*(4), 284-289.

Spector, R. (1996). *Cultural diversity in health and illness* (4th ed.). Stamford, CT: Appleton & Lange.

Spring, M. S., Ross, P. J., Etkin, N. I., & Deinard, A. S. (1995). Sociocultural factors in the use of prenatal care by Hmong women, Minneapolis. *American Journal of Public Health, 85,* 1015-1017.

Stauffer, R. Y. (1995). Vietnamese Americans. In J. Giger & R. Davidhizar (Eds.), *Transcultural nursing* (2nd ed.). St. Louis, MO: C. V. Mosby.

Stavig, G., Igra, A., & Leonard, A. (1988). Hypertension and related health issues among Asians and Pacific Islanders in California. *Public Health Reports, 103,* 28-37.

Sue, D. (1994). Asian-American mental health and help seeking behavior: Comment on Solberg et al. (1994), Tata and Leong (1994), and Lin (1994). *Journal of Counseling Psychology, 41,* 292-295.

Sue, S., Zane, N., & Ito. J. (1979). Alcohol drinking patterns among Asian and Caucasian Americans. *Journal of Cross-Cultural Psychology, 10,* 41-56.

Takeuchi, D., & Young, K. (1994). Overview of Asian and Pacific Islander Americans. In N. Zane, D. Takeuchi, & K. Young (Eds.), *Confronting critical health issues of Asian and Pacific Islander Americans.* Thousand Oaks, CA: Sage.

Uba, L. (1992). Cultural barriers to health care for Southeast Asian refugees. *Public Health Reports, 197,* 544-548.

Uchara, E., Takeuchi, D., & Smuckler, M. (1994). The effects of combining disparate groups in the analysis of ethnic differences: Variations among Asian American mental health consumers in level of community functioning. *American Journal of Community Psychology, 22*(1), 83-100.

U.S. Bureau of the Census. (1992a). *Population projections of the United States by age, sex, race, and Hispanic origin: 1992-2050.* Washington, DC: Government Printing Office.

U.S. Bureau of the Census. (1992b). *Statistical abstract of the United States, 1992* (112th ed.). Washington, DC: Government Printing Office.

U.S. Department of Commerce. (1993). *1990 census of populations: Asian and Pacific Islanders in the United States* (Publication No. CP-3-5). Washington, DC: Government Printing Office.

U.S. Department of Health and Human Services. (1990). *Healthy People 2000: National health promotion and disease prevention objectives.* Washington, DC: Government Printing Office.

U.S. Department of Health and Human Services. (1994). *Chronic disease in minority populations.* Rockville, MD: Centers for Disease Control and Prevention.

Williams, D. R. (1990). Socioeconomic differential in health: A review and redirection. *Social Psychology Quarterly, 53*(2), 81-99.

World Health Organization. (1947). Constitution of the World Health Organization. *Chronicle of WHO, 1,* 1.

Yi, J. K. (1995). Acculturation, access to care and use of preventive health services by Vietnamese women. *Asian American and Pacific Islander Journal of Health, 3*(1), 30-41.

Yoon, E., & Chien, F. (1996). Asian American and Pacific Islander health: A paradigm for minority health. *Journal of the American Medical Association, 275,* 736-737.

Yu, E., Huber, W., Wong, S., Tseng, G., & Liu, W. (1990). *Survey of health coverage needs in Chicago's Chinatown: A final report.* San Diego: Pacific/Asian Mental Health Research Center.

Yu, E., Liu, H., & Williams, T. (1993). Methodological problems in collecting epidemiologic data on Asian Americans and Pacific Islanders. In D. Takeuchi & N. Zane (Eds.), *Asian American health.* Newbury Park, CA: Sage.

Zane, N., & Kim, J. H. (1995). Substance use and abuse. In N. Zane, D. Takeuchi, & K. Young (Eds.), *Confronting critical health issues of Asian and Pacific Islander Americans.* Thousand Oaks, CA: Sage.

19

Assessing Needs and Planning, Implementing, and Evaluating Health Promotion and Disease Prevention Programs Among Asian American Population Groups

JUNE GUTIERREZ ENGLISH
ANH LÊ

Asian Americans encompass many different groups with tremendous diversity in history, cultural practices, language, socioeconomic status, degree of acculturation, and generational differences. Inouye, in the preceding chapter, admonished health professionals to be sensitive and responsive when working with each ethnic subgroup. There will be considerable differences in the approach directed at highly acculturated groups with a long history of American residence compared to that directed at recent immigrants. In terms of generational differences and needs, Sabogal, Otero-Sabogal, Pasick, Jenkins, and Perez-Stable (1996) note that whereas Chinese American preadolescents might prefer a comic book in English, their parents might prefer a health magazine in the Chinese language. Planning health promotion and disease prevention programs requires systematic identification and selection of a particular course of action related to achieving

AUTHORS' NOTE: The authors extend their appreciation to, and acknowledge the assistance of, the *Suc Khoe La Vang!* (Health Is Gold!) Tobacco Education Project and the Pathways to Early Cancer Detection for Vietnamese Women Project, Vietnamese Community Health Promotion Project, Division of General Internal Medicine, University of California, San Francisco, for the use of their materials in preparing this chapter. The authors thank Stephen J. McPhee and Christopher N. H. Jenkins of *Suc Khoe La Vang!* The authors also acknowledge the editorial assistance provided by Michael V. Kline.

or improving desirable health-related behaviors. Because of the diversity among groups, issues, and topics, it would be an impossible task for this chapter to comprehensively cover the range of concerns related to planning and implementing health promotion and disease prevention programs for Asian Americans. Rather, its purpose is to provide the health practitioner with a basic program planning foundation and to selectively examine topics related to current and useful approaches. Specific elements of the planning process, including selected health issues and cultural concerns unique to the Asian American experience, also are considered. This chapter operates more heavily from a health education vantage point because health education is a primary mechanism for achieving health promotion goals. It is at the health education level, given the realities of financial support in most communities, where most current planning activities that target Asian Americans occur.

In the latter part of the chapter, the authors describe two different health education programs in the San Francisco Bay Area. Both are examined in terms of their differing educational strategies, methods, and interventions. Both programs share a common focus on that region's Vietnamese community. Because Southeast Asian countries contribute a sizable proportion of recent immigrants who require public health services, it was felt that these programs could serve as suitable examples from which to further discuss selected planning issues relevant to practitioners working with Asian Americans.

ASIAN AMERICAN HEALTH ISSUES

At a recent meeting of the Congressional Asian Pacific Caucus (1997), Susan Shinagawa, a breast cancer survivor, noted,

> It provided me no comfort when the doctors kept saying that I had nothing to worry about. . . . They said that Asian women don't get breast cancer. But I was soon to learn that statement to be an absolute fallacy perpetuated by inadequate and aggregate national statistics, which also perpetuated the myth of Asian/Pacific Islanders as the "model health minority." (p. 31)

Her declaration serves as a poignant example supporting Inouye's contention, in the preceding chapter, that health data specific to Asians are either nonexistent or uninterpretable because of the convention of aggregating data. There has been a blatant lack of awareness among health professionals concerning specific health and health-related problems of different subgroups of Asian Americans. Aggregating Asian American health data has masked differences in disease patterns for specific subpopulations and has resulted in portraying the overall Asian American population as healthy and at lower risk for death and illness. In reality, however, after data are separated by subgroup, studies have identified that there are specific differences in disease patterns for different Asian subpopulations (Chen &

Hawks, 1995; Inouye, Chapter 18, this volume; U.S. Department of Health and Human Services, 1990).

The U.S. Department of Health and Human Services (1990), in its report titled *Healthy People 2000,* notes the difficulties in defining health status, behaviors, and risks specific to each Asian American group, including concerns with diabetes, hypertension, tobacco use, heart disease, stroke, and cancer. More recent and disturbing data show that the "absolute number of cancer deaths among all Asian American and Pacific Islanders [has increased] at the fastest rate among all racial/ethnic populations," especially among women (Chen & Koh, 1997). "Low utilization of health care services" by Asian Americans also creates problems for those involved in program planning and design (Myers, Kagawa-Singer, Kumanyika, Lex, & Markides, 1995, p. 615). For example, Lin's (1978) study of the use of mental health services in an immigrant Chinese community shows that care seeking is not simply an autonomous choice on the part of an individual but rather is controlled by others (i.e., caregiver service agencies or the family unit).

These difficulties and oversights regarding the identification of health problems in the target group must be taken into account during the initial assessment phase of the program planning process. Health promotion planners working in Asian American populations must not assume that health education programs designed for one specific Asian group will similarly work for another.

DESIGNING HEALTH PROMOTION PROGRAMS FOR ASIAN AMERICAN POPULATIONS

Kline, in Chapter 4, noted that the task of developing and implementing a health promotion program requires planners and participants to work together to accomplish a complex range of activities. These include assessment of needs of the target population, development of appropriate objectives, tailoring target group-specific strategies and interventions, implementing and monitoring the interventions, evaluating the results, and refining approaches toward greater program effectiveness and efficiency. The planner needs to operate from a rational planning framework and not on the basis of pragmatic, empirical, or expediency considerations. Although there are no perfect health education and health promotion planning models, several have been widely used over time and have served as established frameworks for planning. Regardless of which model is used in planning Asian American health promotion programs, the planner must build a cultural assessment component into the planning process (e.g., see Huff & Kline's cultural assessment framework in Chapter 26).

The reader is encouraged to review Kline's earlier chapter in this book (Chapter 4) for an intensive discussion of the health promotion planning process and various planning frameworks including the PRECEDE-PROCEED framework (Green & Kreuter, 1991; Green, Kreuter, Deeds, & Partridge, 1980). The authors of the present chapter feel that the approach advocated in the PRECEDE planning framework can have major value to the practitioner working with Asian

Americans. Recently, the Pathways to Early Cancer Detection project (Hiatt et al., 1996) in the San Francisco Bay Area incorporated portions of the PRECEDE framework (Green & Kreuter, 1991) and its modification for cancer screening (Walsh & McPhee, 1992) in its integrated program to increase the use of breast and cervical cancer detection practices in four different ethnic populations. Two of these populations were Chinese and Vietnamese women.

SPECIFIC CONCERNS IN COMMUNITY ASSESSMENT AND THE IMPORTANCE OF SOCIOCULTURAL ISSUES IN PLANNING HEALTH EDUCATION PROGRAMS FOR ASIAN AMERICANS

Conducting a thorough needs assessment is critical to identify community issues and problems, to formulate relevant objectives, and to determine what educational interventions are appropriate. PRECEDE can be helpful because it guides planners to consider relationships between and among particular health behaviors and their predisposing, enabling, and reinforcing factors (Green & Kreuter, 1991). The Pathways project found that certain predisposing factors among recent Asian immigrants, lacking a preventive orientation and having difficulty understanding medical treatment procedures, can hinder early cancer detection (Hiatt et al., 1996). This level of target group assessment can provide convincing evidence regarding the need for early educational interventions designed to positively affect these factors.

Another major consideration of the needs assessment process is development of valid and reliable instruments for obtaining information about the target group. The Pathways project provides some valuable guidelines for the practitioner based on its experiences in developing a 101-item core instrument covering demographics, health beliefs and practices, and cultural values in four different languages for four different racial/ethnic groups (Pasick, D'Onofrio, & Otero-Sabogal, 1996). Among the guidelines emphasized are the need to recognize that translation and adaptation is a complex process requiring at a minimum (a) an understanding of each language and culture, (b) a commitment to research objectives by everyone involved, and (c) iterative pretesting in all groups and subgroups (by age, language, ancestry, etc.).

Needs assessment information should seek to identify local mores and customs. This is particularly true if the target group is located within an ethnic enclave, as in the case of many new Asian immigrants. At the very least, outreach workers who are involved (e.g., lay health advisers) in obtaining assessment information, and who may ultimately introduce the health education program to the community, should be perceived as nonthreatening and nonintrusive. They should be drawn from the same ethnic group and preferably be from that community.

Contacts during the assessment process should be linguistically appropriate when working in established communities or with recent immigrants. For some groups, such as Chinese or Filipinos, the assessment process might lead to staff having to deal with more than one language or several dialects. For example, the official language of the Philippines, Pilipino, is not necessarily the language of choice for all Filipinos (especially those from the southern islands) because it is based on a northern dialect.

Within a single Asian American ethnic group (e.g., Japanese, Korean, Chinese, Vietnamese), health-related attitudes and behaviors may differ between generations. The assessment must identify such differences and the possible impact of acculturation and biculturalism on persons in a specific community, and it must design interventions accordingly. Survey or interview data with community members of the appropriate demographic breakdown may reveal a significant "generation gap" in values or expressed health beliefs and behaviors. (According to C. Jenkins of the Pathways project discussed in this chapter, the project attempted to assess acculturation in its preintervention survey of immigrant women by asking each respondent the approximate percentage of her lifetime spent in the United States.)

Acculturation has occurred when a person participates in the dominant culture, with the corresponding loss of other elements of ethnic culture. Biculturalism occurs when a person participates in both the dominant or majority culture and a subculture. The impact of acculturation on Asian American health behavior is shown in intergenerational differences in rates of smoking (Asian and Pacific Islander Tobacco Education Network and Asian and Pacific Islander American Health Forum, n.d.). Heavy advertising of tobacco use in Third World countries has resulted in cultural acceptance and high prevalence rates of smoking among Asian male immigrants—especially Vietnamese, Chinese Vietnamese, and Cambodians—that significantly exceed the 21% rate of "the adult male Californian" (Chen & Koh, 1997). The American-born second and third generations' lower rates of tobacco use more closely reflect the decline in tobacco use and the influence of prevailing values about tobacco found in the dominant American culture.

Intergenerational differences in health beliefs and behaviors due to biculturalism need to be further explored for Asian American groups, particularly in the area of breast health. Chavez, Hubbell, McMullin, Martinez, and Mishra's (1995) study of how women of different ethnic groups perceive risk factors for breast cancer shows that U.S.-born women of Mexican descent exhibited a collection of beliefs about breast and cervical cancers that were intermediate between the views held by Anglo women and those held by immigrant Mexican women. Unfortunately, similar study data for Asian American women are not yet available despite high mortality rates due to breast cancer in women belonging to some of the largest Asian American groups.

Continued affirmation of an Asian American ethnic identity or group affiliation is not predictive of the second (U.S.-born or -raised) generation's degree of belief or participation in traditional folk medicine. Capps (1994) notes that the effect of abrupt cultural changes among an exclusively Protestant Hmong community in Kansas City has been to introduce medical pluralism, an eclectic medical culture that blends "influences from biomedicine, Christianity, and Chinese medicine" (p. 172), with selective loss of such Hmong medical/religious concepts (including soul loss, shamanism, and animal sacrifice) and practices that no longer "fit" their new situation and collective identity. The local community must be viewed for any unique changes or characteristics during the needs assessment portion of program planning.

There also might be a discrepancy between what the health professional and what the community perceives as a "problem behavior" in need of change. This also is due to cultural beliefs. Culture may be loosely defined as shared understandings among members of a corporate group about a wide range of critical life areas including health and illness issues. These beliefs, values, and practices may be embedded in the traditional social structure and social support system or religion. Thus, illness and pain, in part social constructions, may be viewed or treated as a "moral process" by group members in ways not congruent with that of biomedicine (Good, Delvecchio, Brodwin, Good, & Kleinman, 1992). One example is the Vietnamese folk cold remedy, *cao gio*. Because this process may result in some skin discoloration, this folk tradition often has been misinterpreted by the dominant society (Dean, 1996).

It also may be difficult to introduce an intervention involving conditions that might be stigmatized in a traditional Asian culture. Various studies of community mental health services for Asian Americans suggest that low rates of use might be due in part to such stigmatization. Survey or interview data with community members from similar generations might reveal generation gaps in values or expressed health beliefs and behaviors.

The planner must be able to identify such unique changes or characteristics during the needs assessment process as well as their impact on health education program design. An effective program must address the health needs of the specific segment of the population targeted (e.g., senior smokers, young smokers, women smokers) in the Asian American community. In these instances, program planners also must deal with these specific issues.

TWO HEALTH EDUCATION PROGRAMS IN THE VIETNAMESE COMMUNITY

The *Suc Khoe La Vang!* (Health Is Gold!) program within the Vietnamese Community Health Promotion Project, Division of General Internal Medicine, University of California, San Francisco, has been involved in several community-based health education and disease prevention activities. These activities include a tobacco education program targeted at Vietnamese male smokers (Jenkins et al., 1997) and the National Cancer Institute-funded 4-year Pathways to Early Cancer Detection program in four ethnic groups (Pasick et al., 1996). Although the overall Pathways program includes four ethnic groups of women, the breast and cervical cancer detection program targeting Vietnamese women is of main interest in this chapter. The overall program involves a multidisciplinary, multicultural team of investigators concerned with increasing breast and cervical cancer screening among underserved low-income women in the San Francisco Bay Area. The two health prevention and education projects to be discussed structure their design and interventions to the different needs of the target groups they intend to reach. Both deal with similarly located geographic communities in San Francisco, but in some ways, the programs are as different as the health issues on which they focus.

Initially, it is helpful to review the background of this San Francisco community of recent Vietnamese immigrants. Between the end of the war in Vietnam in 1975 and 1990, more than 615,000 refugees and immigrants arrived in the United States from the countries of Indochina (McPhee et al., 1996). Among these arrivals, more than 280,000 have settled in California. Many came directly to California from Vietnam; others moved to California after settling in other states. The Vietnamese comprise the fastest growing Asian and Pacific Islander group in California. According to the 1990 census, 1 of every 100 Californians was Vietnamese (U.S. Bureau of the Census, 1991). It is predicted that by the year 2030, Vietnamese will number nearly 1.8 million and constitute the largest Asian and Pacific Islander population within the state, surpassing the respective numbers of Chinese, Japanese, and Filipinos (Bouvier & Agresta, 1987).

The Vietnamese community in the San Francisco Bay Area constitutes an ethnic enclave. However, it reflects diversity in age, education, exposure to urban life and degree of prior acculturation or Westernization, English proficiency, and health status. More recent poorer immigrants tend to be less well educated, in poorer health, and less familiar with Western concepts. They also are more likely to experience poverty, cultural conflict, and barriers to the health care system (McPhee et al., 1996).

The traditional family structure is patriarchal (dominated by adult males), with clear role delineation by gender. This attribute affects health-related behaviors including male smoking. For the most part, only the men smoke. Immigrant Vietnamese men, like many other recent Asian immigrants, have a strikingly high rate of tobacco use, with corresponding health risks. Vietnamese women in the San Francisco Bay Area have a low rate of screening for breast and cervical cancers. Unfortunately, these are their two most common cancers. The Pathways project for Vietnamese women sought to increase breast and cervical cancer screening and detection in this group by improving its members' preventive health behavior.

Program 1: The *Suc Khoe La Vang!* (Health Is Good!) Tobacco Education Program

Community Needs Assessment

The mainstream American population has benefited from health education messages against cigarette smoking since the first U.S. surgeon general's warnings were issued more than 30 years ago. Many communities in the United States have lagged far behind in gaining this important knowledge. One such community has been the Vietnamese population.

The Vietnamese Community Health Promotion Project has conducted anti-tobacco health education intervention programs in the San Francisco Bay Area since 1989. These were initiated with a 15-month pilot program that developed an anti-tobacco, media-led education campaign targeting Santa Clara County, site of the largest Vietnamese community in California, as well as San Francisco and Alameda counties. The *Suc Khoe La Vang!* program conducted eight research surveys documenting the seriousness of the problem (McPhee et al., 1996). The most current survey interviews were conducted in San Francisco and Alameda counties. One of the authors (Lê) was closely associated with this program. The surveys were developed in English, translated into Vietnamese, back translated, and pilot tested using Vietnamese interviewers (Jenkins et al., 1997). Smoking prevalence rates of about 36% among Vietnamese men were identified in 1992, a rate about 1.5 times that of the general population in California. For Vietnamese women, smoking prevalence rates ranged from less than 1% to 9%. Surveys conducted earlier disclosed that about one quarter of the Vietnamese population did not know that cigarette smoking can cause cancer (Jenkins, McPhee, Bird, & Bonilla, 1990).

Needs assessment survey results indicated that among Vietnamese men, those most likely to smoke were between 25 and 44 years of age, had less than a college education, had limited English capability, and were more recent immigrants (Jenkins et al., 1997; McPhee, Jenkins, & Lê, 1993). Further data regarding the incidence of the most common cancers among San Francisco Bay Area Vietnamese men showed that lung cancer was the leading type (B. Topol, California Cancer Registry, personal communication, May 15, 1995). This information also suggested the need to consider the health consequences of exposure to environmental tobacco smoke for children and spouses in Vietnamese households where smoking occurs. Such consequences may, for example, include higher incidence in the development of otitis media, asthma, and lung disease in children as well as cervical and lung cancers in women.

Program Design, Methodology, and Interventions

The *Suc Khoe La Vang!* program was designed to lower smoking prevalence among Vietnamese men in the San Francisco Bay Area. The intervention was conducted in the atmosphere of the passage of a recent statewide tobacco control initiative (California Proposition 99) that included an increased cigarette excise tax, a general State Department of Health education campaign, and new ordinances restricting smoking.

From 1990 to 1992 in San Francisco and Alameda counties, the Suc Khoe La Vang! project mounted a 2-year media-led campaign that it evaluated in a controlled trial. Prior to this period, an uncontrolled 15-month pilot anti-tobacco media program was conducted. The current intervention targeted recent male Vietnamese immigrants because earlier needs assessments disclosed that they were more likely to smoke. Houston, Texas, served as the comparison community.

The project published anti-tobacco news articles in Vietnamese-language newspapers and magazines, resulting in 465,000 print media exposures. It produced a Vietnamese-language videotape, which was broadcast on Vietnamese-language television, and several Vietnamese-language health education materials including a New Year's calendar, bumper stickers, lapel buttons, three posters, two brochures (*Thuoc La Va Benh Tat* [Tobacco and Disease] and *Thuoc La Va Gia Dinh* [Tobacco and the Family]), and a 32-page, four-color, self-help, smoking cessation booklet (*Lam The Nao De Bo Hut Thuoc* [How to Quit Smoking]) (Lê, 1998). The first brochure focused on the dangers of smoking and targeted the Vietnamese smoker. The second brochure, which addressed the issue of exposure to secondhand smoke and its effects on family members, targeted both the Vietnamese male smoker and the Vietnamese woman in the household. The booklet included discussions of topics such as methods of quitting, testimonials from former smokers and Vietnamese physicians, stress management, exercise, and diet. More than 15,000 copies of the brochures and 4,600 copies of the "quit kit" were distributed.

An anti-tobacco, Vietnamese-language counteradvertising campaign was conducted that included three different types of billboards, print media advertisements, and paid television advertisements. Project staff gave anti-tobacco health education presentations at community events. A continuing medical education course on smoking cessation counseling methods for 68 Vietnamese physicians was conducted because many Vietnamese visit Vietnamese physicians for their health care. Anti-tobacco education programs also were organized at two Vietnamese-language Saturday schools in San Francisco and Oakland (Balderson, 1992: Lê et al., 1994). Vietnamese-language "no smoking" signs and brochures on smoking ordinances were distributed to Vietnamese restaurants and businesses in the community.

Evaluation

To determine whether there was a reduction in smoking prevalence following the intervention and whether the proportion of smokers who quit during the intervention would be higher in the target community (San Francisco Bay Area) than in the comparison community (Houston), telephone surveys were conducted. A total of 1,200 randomly selected Vietnamese men in each community were contacted at preintervention and postintervention. The sampling frame consisted of telephone numbers chosen randomly from the 23 most common Vietnamese surnames listed in area telephone directories (Jenkins et al., 1997).

The survey instrument (mentioned earlier) was developed in English, translated into Vietnamese, back translated, and pilot tested. Respondents were asked whether they had ever smoked cigarettes and whether they had smoked a cigarette during the prior week. Respondents were considered *never* smokers if they answered no to the first question. They were considered *current* smokers if they responded yes to both questions. Current smokers were queried as to the amount and duration of their smoking, how much they wanted to quit smoking and how difficult they thought it would be to quit, whether they had ever tried to quit, and if so, on how many occasions. Both former and current smokers were asked whether they had ever been advised by a physician to quit (Jenkins et al., 1997).

The project also wanted to measure exposure to intervention activities and asked respondents whether they had ever read, seen, or attended any of the five elements of the media intervention. Survey questions included demographic items such as age, year of immigration to the United States, educational level, English-language proficiency, employment status, and poverty status.

The project reported modest success of the anti-smoking intervention directed at Vietnamese men. The intervention produced both a significant decrease in smoking prevalence and a significant increase in quitting among men in the intervention community relative to men in the comparison community. The reader is strongly encouraged to review Jenkins et al. (1997) for an in-depth discussion of the evaluation results and processes.

Program 2: Pathways to Early Cancer Detection for Vietnamese Women

This program involved cancer screening among Vietnamese women and took place during approximately the same time frame as Program 1 in an inner-city neighborhood of San Francisco. Unless otherwise noted, information used in this section is drawn from "Pathways to Early Cancer Detection for Vietnamese Women" (McPhee et al., 1996). Emphasis focuses on the neighborhood-based intervention aspects of the project dealing with Vietnamese women rather than the methodological and evaluative aspects of the overall project design. The reader can find this information in the report of the comprehensive 4-year study, "Pathways to Early Cancer Detection in Four Ethnic Groups" (Pasick et al., 1996). At the time of this writing, the Pathways projects still are in progress, but information concerning baseline design and data collection activities is available.

Community Needs Assessment

At the outset of a health education or promotion intervention effort, program baseline data for establishing the scope and seriousness of the problem are not readily available. In this instance, such information about breast and cervical cancers among Vietnamese women in the study community was limited. The community needs assessment was based in part on demographic data and preliminary California Cancer Registry data for the years 1988 to 1992 concerning age-adjusted incidence rates of breast and cervical cancers among Vietnamese women as well as key informant information. Several previous statewide and area-specific studies conducted between 1987 and 1992 helped to establish that Vietnamese women were less likely to have had recommended screening procedures for breast and cervical cancers (McPhee et al., 1996).

An extensive baseline survey was later developed (after the intervention had been conducted). The survey, consisting of 101 core questions covering demographics, health beliefs and practices, and cultural values, was administered to each specific project group after an exhaustive effort was made to ensure the appropriateness of each question to that group. Although information from the survey would have been helpful in the formulation of the project intervention, it was administered later to be used for evaluation of the intervention and comparison of differences between the project groups.

Program Design

Hiatt et al. (1996) describe the development of the Pathway's conceptual framework, using foundations from the PRECEDE-PROCEED framework (Green & Kreuter, 1991) and modifications of that framework for cancer screening including factors impinging on the patient and physician that could affect cancer screening (Walsh & McPhee, 1992). The framework was used in the needs assessment analysis, as were other theories including the transtheoretical model of health behavior change in the data analysis (Freudenberg et al., 1995; Prochaska & Velicer, 1997). Bowen, Kinne, and Urban (1997) expand this model to assess community readiness to adopt or support higher levels of the target behavior. Each project associated with Pathways activities made an intensive effort to apply elements of theories appropriate to each particular population differences and its goals (Hiatt et al., 1996).

According to the PRECEDE-PROCEED framework (Green & Kreuter, 1991), possible influences on the cancer screening behavior of Vietnamese women were reviewed and analyzed prior to choice of methodology. These included strong social solidarity (reinforcing factors) and cultural and demographic characteristics of the immigrants that contributed to maintaining a social enclave and retention of some traditional values such as modesty (predisposing factors) and knowledge and access issues (enabling factors) (McPhee et al., 1996). Because of these challenges, the program was designed to use the social bonds among women of the community through recruitment and training of 10 indigenous lay health workers who would serve as neighborhood leaders for facilitating outreach and educational strategies.

The goal of this Pathways study for Vietnamese women was to determine whether a neighborhood-based intervention fosters adoption of a preventive health care orientation and increases acceptance and use of screening tests for early cancer detection among Vietnamese women in San Francisco (McPhee et al., 1996). Prior to implementation of the intervention, the Pathways survey developed earlier was administered as described earlier in the evaluation section.

Intervention and Methods

A three-phased multifaceted intervention was used to raise the women's awareness concerning the importance of preventive care and breast and cervical cancer screening and then to motivate them to seek screening. The investigators sought to use neighborhood connections because they could provide behavioral modeling and social reinforcement through familiar communication channels (McPhee et al., 1996).

The specific methods selected were informal small group educational events in private homes and a community health fair centered around the traditional Vietnamese New Year (*Tết*) festival. A multitude of linguistically and culturally appropriate educational materials conveying the desired messages about the need of preventive care and screening included a special training manual for the lay health workers for use in presentations and the subsequent discussions, videotapes, and materials for the participants and Vietnamese physicians (McPhee et al., 1996). The small group events were organized around the informal educational sessions led by the previously trained neighborhood leaders and similarly recruited individuals.

Evaluation

The primary evaluation tool was the household survey described earlier in the needs assessment section. Project investigators intended to administer the survey, by oral interview, before and after the interventions to assess whether there was an increase in screening behaviors following participation in program activities and whether there was a similar positive change in women's knowledge, attitudes, and intentions toward preventive care behaviors (McPhee et al., 1996). At the time of this writing, only the preintervention results had been reported. A control group in a similar Vietnamese community in Sacramento, California, also received the survey. The reader is encouraged to review the project's data analysis methods and baseline survey results (McPhee et al., 1996).

COMPARISON OF APPROACHES OF THE TWO PROGRAMS

It is useful for the practitioner to examine some of the differences in planning approaches taken by the tobacco education and cancer education and screening programs just described. Owing to differing health needs and different program goals of the respective target groups, there was a need to develop and employ different techniques. Common elements in both programs included the use of pre- and postintervention surveys and a control group for evaluation, the use of trained Vietnamese community members and Vietnamese health care professionals in outreach, and the development and use of culturally appropriate educational tools and materials in Vietnamese. Educational materials included brochures, posters, and videotapes. Surveys provided baseline changes in variables associated with the desired health behaviors. For men, these were smoking and quitting; for women, the Pathways project standardized survey questions assessed plans for health screening, acculturation, and insurance. The survey of a sample of male smokers was conducted by telephone. The survey of the much smaller sample of women was conducted face to face by persons visiting households, which presumably enhanced the willingness of the women to participate. The Pathways staff also suggested the use of volunteers to save time and funds.

The Tobacco Education program used a higher profile approach with more channels of communication than did the neighborhood-based cancer education program, which was intended to reach the more socially insulated women of the enclave. Vietnamese-language media were designed to complement a concurrent statewide media program for the general public. This 2-year program provided messages tailored for the community and included billboards, newspapers, and paid television advertisements (Jenkins et al., 1997), complete with videotape. Although this project had the funding to procure paid television advertising, it often is quite costly. Community cable television stations often will run materials at no charge owing to public access requirements, but they might not reach the desired target group. Radio spots can be had at less expense or for free if public service announcements are prepared and sent out with an appealing cover letter. Media (print, radio, and television) geared toward serving an Asian American market will, of course, be more receptive and should be the first contacted. Staff arranged presentations to community groups, provided education on smoking cessation techniques to local Vietnamese physicians, conducted anti-tobacco activities for youths at Vietnamese-language schools, and distributed Vietnamese-language "no smoking" signs and smoking control ordinances to restaurants and businesses (Jenkins et al., 1997).

The techniques used by the cancer education program were more personal and centered on traditional characteristics of social solidarity and mutual assistance. Neighborhood-based small group events conducted by trained neighborhood leaders provided short and informal home presentations on preventive health care topics. Health fairs coordinated with community festivities also were used to introduce new concepts in a nonthreatening way. Like the face-to-face survey used in the project, the small group intervention does require more time and effort than do mass media or large presentations but serves as a better way in which to contact and draw out a cloistered group of individuals. An interpersonal approach, which reinforces information through training or modeling, is much more effective than simply handing out brochures full of information that may be perceived as irrelevant or simply discarded.

Both projects employed a pre- and posttest survey, with a control group, as the principal means of evaluation. Evaluation was based solely on the survey, outcome data, and attendance at events or process information (e.g., number attending meetings). Although ideally one obtains an objective evaluation of an educational presentation by using a written pre- and posttest to obtain a determination of efficacy in changing knowledge, in reality this can be difficult outside of the classroom setting. For informal situations such as the small group events described here, where participants might have limited test-taking skills, literacy skills, or time or might have physical difficulties such as poor eyesight or uncomfortable testing conditions, it probably is more appropriate to forgo an evaluation of process beyond a simple head count until such problems can be overcome.

However, evaluation is necessary, and not just to refine the program process (delivery of services). Evaluation must be done to determine the impact and long-term outcome of the program on an individual's health behaviors and to determine whether objectives are being met. For these two projects, collecting this information by means of an oral survey (via telephone or face-to-face conversation) before and after the intervention proved to be a technique acceptable to the participants and the community, if somewhat labor intensive. This survey constituted the primary evaluation tool and provided the data necessary to assess the behavioral results of the intervention strategy and, therefore, its efficacy in meeting program objectives and mitigating the targeted health concern.

CONCLUDING THOUGHTS

Pasick et al. (1996) cite the need to differentiate between the terms *tailoring* and *targeting*. Targeting implies the need to clearly identify the specific population subgroup that will be exposed to the intended intervention. The authors of the present chapter want to stress to the practitioner the need during all segments of the planning process to recognize that Asian Americans encompass many different groups including Chinese, Japanese, Koreans, and those from several countries in Southeast Asia. They reside in many communities, mainstream to small and isolated enclaves. The planner must be acutely aware of the groups' and sub-groups' diversity in history, cultural practices including health beliefs and practices, language, socioeconomic status, and generational differences. All of the groups represent varying degrees of acculturation and assimilation in their current country of residence. Once the planner has targeted, he or she also needs to be able to tailor. Tailoring, as espoused by Pasick et al. (1996), implies the need for the planner to be able to adapt the intervention and/or total design to fit the needs and characteristics of a target audience. *Cultural tailoring,* then, urges the planner to develop the interventions, strategies, methods, messages, and materials to be adaptable to the specific cultural characteristics of the target group (Pasick et al., 1996). In short, then, the health promotion planner working within an Asian American population cannot *tailor* until he or she has correctly *targeted*.

The basic strategies and interventions employed in the two Vietnamese health education programs described in this chapter can provide some practical ideas for the health professional concerning how to conduct two different types of health education campaigns. The specific activities employed are geared toward an urban Asian American community of recent immigrants with limited language skills. However, a general understanding of these methods can enable the adaptation of these types of interventions to other types of programs for Asian American community groups in various settings, assuming that careful and culturally sensitive planning and implementation processes are conducted. Use of the PRECEDE-PROCEED framework in the process of community assessment should assist the planner in designing appropriate services to meet the needs in each community. Health education and promotion programs can play a vital role in helping individuals address health needs, be they from aging, relocation, or concerns arising from a myriad of other changes that everyone faces in life. Given the diverse circumstances under which Asian Americans now live and work, the challenge for the health care provider is to appreciate the impact that ethnic and social ties might have on health behavior choices and to use these factors effectively in developing programs for communities.

Health promotion professionals working in minority communities need to encourage cultural competence among staff working in community health promotion programs. Although staff might possess the language skills and knowledge of the basic customs and cultural beliefs of those they serve, program results may be enhanced if there is a concerted effort to integrate the services into the social framework of the community (Congressional Asian Pacific Caucus, 1997). Steckler et al. (1995) view the use of social networks as an intervention that can increase access to services among disenfranchised groups through the recruitment of socially significant community members to help convey the program message.

Members of the community for which the program is intended should participate, either as staff or as volunteers, in the assessment, planning, and implementation process whenever possible. They can help provide an insider's perspective on issues and insights into local social norms and structure. This participation increases the likelihood that the project will not conflict with any fundamental cultural values and that it will be credible and well received. At the very least, educational materials and tools such as survey and interview questions should be linguistically and culturally appropriate. Be aware that key informants might not have knowledge or represent all elements in the community or group. If these persons represent the intended program users (or targeted group) or already provide services to the desired users, then so much the better. In designing a new outreach program to increase use of mammography services by uninsured and underinsured Asian American (primarily Filipino) women in a suburban southern California county, one of the authors (Gutierrez English) had to decide whether to concentrate on soliciting information and support from the community's physicians or from its nurses. The decision was made to work closely with the larger nurses' group rather than with the physicians, primarily because of considerations of gender, status, and general similarity to the targeted subgroup. Based on their recommendations, new informants also will be drawn from senior groups and fraternal clubs based on provincial origin in addition to the group's "town council," a somewhat misleading term considering the geographic dispersion of this community.

A formal community advisory board, which was used in both of the Vietnamese health education programs discussed in this chapter, also can provide valuable information, feedback, support, and resources for program activities. For example, the media-led Tobacco Education program included Vietnamese community members from the fields of media, social work, academia, and medicine on its board.

An important function of these community representatives is to help identify persons in the community already recognized by other community members as sources of assistance and support regarding issues and problems. According to Jackson and Parks's (1997) review of a number of community health promotion programs, the recruitment of indigenous workers based on the collective wisdom of the community and who will serve as the program's lay health advisers taps into the existing social networks and enhances the distribution of the health promotion message to the community. Bowen et al. (1997) used a similar networking technique to obtain informants for the community needs assessment of the mammography project. The Pathways to Early Cancer Detection for Vietnamese Women project used the indigenous model in setting up its small group interventions among Vietnamese women by using neighborhood leaders as lay health advisers, who in turn drew other women into the project.

REFERENCES

Asian and Pacific Islander Tobacco Education Network and Asian and Pacific Islander American Health Forum. (n.d.). *Facts on Asians and Pacific Islanders and tobacco*. San Francisco: Author.

Balderson, A. (1992, July-August). Xin Dung Hut Thuoc, Suc Khoe La Vang! (Please Don't Smoke, Health Is Gold!). *UCSF Newsbreak*, p. 2.

Bouvier, L. F., & Agresta, A. J. (1987). The future Asian population of the United States. In J. T. Fawcett & B. V. Carino (Eds.), *Pacific bridges: The new immigration from Asia and the Pacific Islands*. Staten Island, NY: Center for Migration Studies.

Bowen, D., Kinne, S., & Urban, N. (1997). Analyzing communities for readiness to change. *American Journal of Health Behavior, 21,* 289-298.

Capps, L. L. (1994). Change and continuity in the medical culture of the Hmong of Kansas City. *Medical Anthropology Quarterly, 8,* 161-177.

Chavez, L. F., Hubbell, F. A., McMullin, J. M., Martinez, R. J., & Mishra, S. J. (1995). Structure and meaning in models of breast and cervical cancer risk factors: A comparison of perceptions among Latinas, Anglo women, and physicians. *Medical Anthropological Quarterly, 9,* 40-74.

Chen, M. S., & Hawks, B. L. (1995). A debunking of the myth of healthy Asian Americans and Pacific Islanders. *American Journal of Health Promotion, 9,* 261-268.

Chen, M., & Koh, H. (1997). The need for cancer prevention and control among Asian Americans and Pacific Islanders. *Asian American and Pacific Islander Journal of Health, 5*(1), 3-6.

Congressional Asian Pacific Caucus. (1997). Proceedings of the forum: Cancer crises among Asian/Pacific Islanders as articulated by Asian/Pacific Islanders. *Asian American and Pacific Islander Journal of Health, 5*(1), 7-36.

Dean, P. (1996, December 13). Culture at the crossroads. *Los Angeles Times,* pp. E1, E4.

Freudenberg, N., Eng, E., Flay, B., Parcel, G., Rogers, T., & Wallerstein, N. (1995). Strengthening individual and community capacity to prevent diseases and promote health: In search of relevant theories and principles. *Health Education Quarterly, 22,* 290-306.

Good, M. J., Delvecchio, G., Brodwin, P., Good, B., & Kleinman, A. (1992). *Pain as human experience*. Berkeley: University of California Press.

Green, L. W., & Kreuter, M. W. (1991). *Health promotion planning: An educational and environmental approach*. Mountain View, CA: Mayfield.

Green, L. W., Kreuter, M. W., Deeds, S., & Partridge, K. B.(1980). *Health education planning: A diagnostic approach*. Mountain View, CA: Mayfield.

Hiatt, R. A., Pasick, R. J., Perez-Stable, E. J., McPhee, S. J., Engelstad, L., Lee, M., Sabogal, F., Bird, J. A., D'Onofrio, C. N., & Stewart, S. (1996). Pathways to early cancer detection in the multiethnic population of the San Francisco Bay Area. *Health Education Quarterly, 23*(Suppl.), S10-S27.

Jackson, E. J., & Parks, C. P. (1997). Recruitment and training issues from selected lay health advisor programs among African Americans: A 20-year perspective. *Health Education and Behavior, 24,* 418-431.

Jenkins, C. N. H., McPhee, S. J., Bird, J. A., & Bonilla, N.-T. (1990). Cancer risks and prevention practices among Vietnamese refugees. *Western Journal of Medicine, 153,* 34-39.

Jenkins, C. N. H., McPhee, S., Lê, A., Pham, G. Q., Ngoc-The, H., & Stewart, S. (1997). The effectiveness of a media-led intervention to reduce smoking among Vietnamese-American men. *American Journal of Public Health, 87,* 1031-1034.

Lê, A. (1998). Tobacco control and education efforts among members of four racial/ethnic minority groups. In *Tobacco use among U.S. racial/ethnic minority groups: African Americans, American Indians and Alaska Natives, Asian Americans and Pacific Islanders, and Hispanics—A report of the Surgeon General*. Atlanta, GA: Centers for Disease Control and Prevention.

Lê, A., McPhee, S. J., Jenkins, C. N. H., Fordham, D., Ha, N. T., & Pham, G. Q. (1994, October). *Tobacco prevention and cessation among Vietnamese: Youth as couriers of new information*. Paper presented at the annual meeting of the American Public Health Association, Washington, DC.

McPhee, S. J., Bird, J. A., Ha, N.-T., Jenkins, C. N. H., Fordham, D., & Lê, B. (1996). Pathways to Early Cancer Detection for Vietnamese Women. *Health Education Quarterly, 23*(Suppl.), S60-S75.

McPhee, S. J., Jenkins, C. N. H., & Lê, A. (1993). *Smoking prevention and cessation among Vietnamese in Northern California: Final report*. Sacramento: Report submitted to the Tobacco Control Section, Department of Health Services, State of California.

Myers, H., Kagawa-Singer, M., Kumanyika, S., Lex, B., & Markides, K. (1995). Panel III: Behavioral risk factors related to chronic diseases in ethnic minorities. *Health Psychology, 14,* 613-621.

Pasick, R. J., D'Onofrio, C. N., & Otero-Sabogal, R. (1996). Similarities and differences across cultures: Questions to inform a third generation for health promotion research. *Health Education Quarterly, 23*(Suppl.), S142-S161.

Prochaska, J., & Velicer, W. (1997). The transtheoretical model of health behavior change. *American Journal of Health Promotion, 12*(1), 38-48.

Sabogal, F., Otero-Sabogal, R., Pasick, R. J., Jenkins, C. N. H., & Perez-Stable, E. J. (1996). Printed health education materials for diverse communities: Suggestions learned from the field. *Health Education Quarterly, 23*(Suppl.), S123-S141.

Steckler, A., Allegrante, J. P., Altman, D., Brown, R., Burdine, J. N., Goodman, R. M., & Jorgensen, C. (1995). Health education intervention strategies: Recommendations for future research. *Health Education Quarterly, 22,* 307-328.

U.S. Bureau of the Census. (1991). *Statistical abstract of the United States, 1990.* Washington, DC: Government Printing Office.

U.S. Department of Health and Human Services. (1990). *Healthy People 2000: National health promotion and disease prevention objectives.* Washington, DC: Government Printing Office.

Walsh, J. M. E., & McPhee, S. J. (1992). A systems model of clinical preventative care: An analysis of factors influencing patient and physician. *Health Education Quarterly, 19,* 157-175.

20

Promoting Health Among Asian American Population Groups

A Case Study From the Field

DIANNE N. ISHIDA

The Charles Fujimoto family is a three-generation Japanese American family whose members live together in an urban community on the West Coast. The family consists of Charles and his wife, Ruth, and their three children ranging from ages 16 to 21 years. Charles is the oldest son. When his second-generation Japanese American father died, his 76-year-old widowed mother, Helen, moved in with them. Charles' father had started his own store, which Charles expanded and now runs as a family business. Until recently, all extended family members helped with the business. The elder Mrs. Fujimoto, who is of petite build and has osteoporosis and Parkinson's disease, had been responsible for keeping the store adequately stocked. She was an active member of a Buddhist temple and a member of its senior group. Helen provided child care to her three grandchildren when they were younger. Following a recent fractured hip, she has limited mobility, requiring assistance with some of her activities of daily living. Family members have arranged their work and school schedules to cover both business and assisting Helen. Although a home care service provides weekly physical therapy and periodic nursing assessment, family members assume the bulk of the care and are being stretched to their limits. The elder Mrs. Fujimoto has expressed guilt in being a burden to her family.

This case study depicts a multigenerational Japanese American family in an urban community on the West Coast. Since the early immigration during the late 1800s and early 1900s, many generations of Japanese Americans live in the United States. They refer to their generational differences according to the arrival or birth in the United States (Hashizume & Takano, 1993). Currently, there are sixth- and seventh-generation Japanese Americans. The different generational groups are distinguishable by the individuals' ages, experiences, languages, and values and are briefly described here. The reader is encouraged to review Inouye's earlier chapter in this book (Chapter 18). The *Issei,* the first generation, immigrated from Japan during the late 1800s to 1924. They experienced racial prejudice, a language barrier, and a lack of knowledge about their new country. They kept to themselves and formed relatively self-sufficient communities. They were able to retain most of their cultural values. The second generation, the *Nisei,* were the first generation of Japanese born in the United States. They were U.S. citizens but held many of the cultural beliefs and practices of their parents. They were more fluent in the English language and had higher educational levels than their parents. They were strongly influenced by the effects of World War II and the evacuation and internment experience. Most were forced to submerge their Japanese culture. Young men of this generation felt compelled to demonstrate their loyalty in the strongest way possible—by fighting for the country of their birth, the United States. The well-decorated 100th Infantry Battalion and its larger unit, the 442nd Regimental Combat Team, were all-Nisei units (Daniels, Taylor, & Kitano, 1991; Kakesako, 1993, Yoshishige, 1993). The GI Bill offered many Nisei veterans the opportunity for an education. As a whole, Japanese Americans have been extremely successful in assimilating in certain states. The *Sansei,* the third generation, tended to be more acculturated, frequently adopting child-rearing practices and attitudes of contemporary middle-class Americans. Third and succeeding generations of Japanese Americans are more typical of their American-born counterparts while maintaining a viable ethnic community and identity. Approximately 50% of the Japanese in the United States marry outside their ethnic group, further promoting assimilation into the American culture (Kikumura & Kitano, 1973).

Although outwardly a Japanese American family might seem quite acculturated, intergenerational relationships are close among most Japanese Americans. There is a continuous flow of goods, money, and services between generations. Family contacts with the elderly are frequent. Generally, one child, often the oldest son or an unmarried child, assumes responsibility for the care of elderly parents (Kobato, 1979). There appears to be more reliance on the family structure and less dependence on outside individual agencies and organizations.

ISSUES ADDRESSED IN THE CASE STUDY

Care of the Elderly at Home

A major issue being addressed in the case study is caring for an elderly parent who no longer can live independently. The aging population of elderly Asian Americans is a problem that needs to be addressed because their numbers are increasing. Between 1980 and 1992, the population of Asians and Pacific Islanders increased by 124%, making this group the fastest growing minority group in the United States, compared to an approximate 9% growth rate for the overall

U.S. population (O'Hare, 1992). Although within this population 9.3% were age 60 years or over compared to approximately 12.6% of all Americans who were age 65 years or over (Strumpf & Kauffman, 1994), the life expectancies of the former might be greater. For instance, life expectancy data from the state of Hawaii show that Chinese, Japanese, and Filipinos have longer life expectancies than do Caucasians (Yang, Braun, Onaka, & Horiuchi, 1996). This has both social and economic implications. Frequently, working age adults in Asian American families need employment to be able to maintain manageable lifestyles. As a whole, Asian Americans tend to have larger families than do other ethnic groups (U.S. Department of Commerce, 1993), which can lead to more crowded living arrangements that interfere with accommodating elders, especially those who have become incapacitated. (Interestingly, Japanese Americans, on whom the case study focuses, have smaller families than do most other Asian American population groups.). This can lead to family conflict. The value placed on respecting and caring for one's elders might not correspond to the ability to meet this responsibility within the family.

Decision making. Decision making on crucial matters might necessitate extended family involvement when a parent is involved. Although one adult, frequently the oldest son in Japanese American families, might be the spokesperson for the family, all members may voice their opinions. It is important for health professionals to provide assistance that supports the family members' efforts to care for their elderly at home if this is their desire—or at least to make them feel comfortable with the decision they have made. Exploring the family's resources should be done prior to providing the family with information on other available resources and possible options that are available. These discussions should be timed sufficiently early to allow ample time for family members to get together, weigh their choices, and anticipate the outcomes before making their decision.

Communication styles. Posing questions that allow for an elaboration of the family's views and beliefs is more important than posing questions that require only a "yes or no" response. Asking family members what they see as viable options also will help the health care provider focus on workable solutions. If this is not done, then family members might be hesitant to share opinions they believe could be contrary to what the health professional is proposing. They might feel that it would be impolite to disagree with the health care worker or with any professional whom they should hold in esteem.

Filial piety. Like many other Asian Americans (Bagley, Angel, Dilworth-Anderson, Liu, & Schinke, 1995; Bethel, 1992; Chang, 1995; Stauffer, 1995; Vance, 1995), the Fujimoto family holds to a strong belief and sense of duty to care for elderly family members within the household. Traditionally, family members respect and obey their elders (Bethel, 1992; Ishida & Inouye, 1995; Lasky & Martz, 1993; Shiba & Oka, 1996). Charles and Ruth realized that they needed outside help to care for the elder Mrs. Fujimoto at home, so they agreed to the home care service. This was the least disruptive choice for the elderly Helen. It is both Helen's and the family's desire to be able to continue keeping the elder Mrs. Fujimoto at home. The Fujimoto family prides itself in being able to sufficiently care for and provide for each of its members. There is a strong family orientation and interdependence among family members and between generations. Family members would feel as though they had not met their responsibility if they placed the elder Mrs. Fujimoto in an institution. That option would be the very last resort. Charles' other siblings, who live out of town, would be involved if institutionalization were to be considered. It is important for health care workers to realize that any decision to institutionalize a family member is very difficult and not taken lightly by any Asian American family.

Support to Primary Caregivers

To maintain the incapacitated elderly at home, support to primary care providers frequently is needed. Because women are the primary caregivers in the Japanese American family (Ishida & Inouye, 1995; Shiba & Oka, 1996), both Ruth and her two daughters have been taking turns in providing any personal care that is needed to the elder Mrs. Fujimoto while Ruth's son and husband have assisted with being on hand and helping with bed-to-chair and chair-to-bed transfers. Family members go out of their way to serve foods that Helen enjoys and are traditionally given to maintain good health such as soft-boiled rice, *miso* soup (a soup made from fermented soybean paste), and sushi. Helen's church friends visit regularly and provide an additional social outlet for her as well as culinary treats.

Social support. The Fujimoto family, like other Asian American families that care for elders at home, needs health services that support its ability to maintain its members at home.

Ethnic-specific community resources. The family needs to be made aware of the range of services available in its community (e.g., elder care, respite, senior companion, day care, hospice) and how to access these services should the need arise. Although third- and later generation Japanese Americans might be open to community services, elders might be reluctant to accept any public or private social services (Lee & Takamura, 1980). This might place the children caring for them in a dilemma. Respite care for family members might be needed to allow members time to meet their own needs and maintain family harmony. Health care workers need to monitor the primary caregivers' level of stress and fatigue and should convince them to take the needed time for themselves if they are to continue in that role. Resources in the form of available extended kin and close friends and neighbors might need to be tapped at this time. Traditionally, Japanese Americans relied on trusted family, close neighbors, or community organizations such as churches to provide mutual assistance during crises (Lee & Takamura, 1980). The Fujimoto family could depend on church members and neighbors to provide some respite for family members.

Health Promotion of All Family Members

The elder Mrs. Fujimoto needs to be kept active physically, mentally, and socially. She also needs to feel that she is contributing to the family to lessen her feeling of being a burden. Encouraging family members to include her in the normal family activities such as meals, family get-togethers, outings, and informal discussions serves to validate her as an integral part of the family while keeping her active. The health care worker can explore with the Fujimoto family how to accommodate Helen so that she may still participate and feel a part of the family business. The Fujimoto family decided to implement an idea its members had discussed a few years ago—to fully computerize their family operations and to maintain a mini office at home. In this way, both Mrs. Fujimotos, Ruth and Helen, could assist the family business while at home. Once the store inventory was computerized, the elder Mrs. Fujimoto still could assist with purchasing using the computerized inventory lists and a fax machine.

Social support networks. The needs of various family members also should be considered. Frequently, individual needs are secondary to family obligations. Family members become overextended and often ignore their own health and social needs. Attention to their own diet, exercise, and sleep and rest needs might lag. Family members might need to be reminded to care for themselves to continue caring for the elder Mrs. Fujimoto. Because family members might not seek health care until there is a medical problem, regular health checkups for all family members need to be encouraged. Both Charles' wife and the couple's daughter may be prone to osteoporosis in the future and should be encouraged to maintain the recommended calcium intake for their age and to do weight-bearing exercises. When the elder Mrs. Fujimoto did her daily exercises, Ruth or her children used this time to exercise themselves.

Traditional foods. Traditional foods made with tofu (soybean) can provide the needed calcium. Families need to be made aware of new information such as how phytoestrogens in soybean products also can be helpful for cardiovascular and bone strength. Many foods traditionally served on New Year's Day, an important celebration for the Japanese, are believed to promote health. New Year's staples include rice, millet, beans, fresh vegetables, fruits, and fish. Frequently, *mochi* (pounded glutinous rice cakes) are eaten, and specially made ones are offered to the gods (Brandon & Stephan, 1994).

Communication Dynamics

The health care provider needs to be aware of the dynamics within the Asian American family. Because problems are generally handled within the confines of the family, concerns might not be shared with the health care provider unless there is a trusting relationship established. The health care worker needs to establish an ongoing relationship with the family for trust to be established. Because the oldest son traditionally is responsible for looking after his parents (Bethel, 1992;

Ishida & Inouye, 1995; Shiba & Oka, 1996), the health provider needs to maintain communication with him. He probably would be the family spokesperson and primary decision maker, although any decision affecting the family would generally be discussed with his wife and other adult family members (Ishida & Inouye, 1995; Shiba & Oka, 1996). Interestingly, in the United States, providing care in these instances seems to fall on the natural daughters rather than on the oldest son's wife. Again, it is important for health workers to be aware of this dynamic.

The health care provider needs to show respect for Asian American beliefs and values. The reader is encouraged to review the earlier chapter of Inouye (Chapter 18), which deals in some depth with the subject of beliefs and values. Engaging in active listening (rather than talking) and being alert to nonverbal cues are important (Ishida & Inouye, 1995). Japanese Americans tend to avoid conflict and embarrassment to maintain harmony; therefore, they tend not to openly disagree with health service providers. The nodding of heads might mean that they are hearing but not necessarily agreeing with what is being said. Being alert to the congruency of verbal and nonverbal behaviors, asking how comfortable they are with the available choices, and asking open-ended questions that elicit what they think about the situation, resources, or suggestions provide a better idea of what they want and can live with. Paying attention to nonverbal signs of stress also is important. These could include nodding, inattention, avoidance of the topic, and short or noncommittal answers.

Actions must be directed to support the family's need to care for its members at home if that is what the family wants. The health care worker needs to allow the family to explore its own resources as it considers options for the future. Providing accurate and clear information on other community resources and options in a timely manner is important to allow the family time for its own deliberation and discussion. The health care worker needs to prepare the family to anticipate future needs for the elder Mrs. Fujimoto such as day care, elder care, and possibly nursing home placement when her care is beyond the family's capability.

OUTCOMES OF CARE

Home care services eventually were stopped as the elder Mrs. Fujimoto increased her mobility and the family was able to supervise her exercises and activity. To maintain their own health, various family members joined in the exercise regime for Helen and were trying to maintain a more balanced diet that included calcium-rich foods. They appreciated the information concerning possible resources should Mrs. Fujimoto need them in the future, and they had discussed these options with Helen. They agreed that they would care for the elder Mrs. Fujimoto at home for as long as they could, using whatever support services were available if need be, but would not completely rule out institutionalization if home management became impossible for them. The home environment was assessed for safety hazards to avoid further falls. Safety bars and ramps were added to the home. A daily exercise regime for the family members became part of their regular family activity. By reassessing the elder Mrs. Fujimoto's diet, all members also began eating in a healthier manner.

REFERENCES

Bagley, S. P., Angel, R., Dilworth-Anderson, P., Liu, W., & Schinke, S. (1995). Adaptive health behaviors among ethnic minorities. *Health Psychology, 14,* 632-640.

Bethel, D. L. (1992). Life on Obasuteyama, or inside a Japanese institution for the elderly. In T. S. Lebra (Ed.), *Japanese social organization.* Honolulu: University of Hawaii Press.

Brandon, R. M., & Stephan, B. B. (1994). *Spirit and symbol: The Japanese New Year.* Honolulu: Honolulu Academy of Arts.

Chang, K. (1995). Chinese Americans. In J. N. Giger & R. E. Davidhizar (Eds.), *Transcultural nursing: Assessment and intervention* (2nd ed.). St. Louis, MO: C. V. Mosby.

Daniels, R., Taylor, S. C., & Kitano, H. H. L. (Eds.). (1991). *Japanese Americans: From relocation to redress.* Seattle: University of Washington Press.

Hashizume, S., & Takano, J. (1993). Nursing care of Japanese American patients. In M. S. Orque, B. Bloch, & L. S. A. Monrroy (Eds.), *Ethnic nursing care: A multicultural approach.* St. Louis, MO: C. V. Mosby.

Ishida, D., & Inouye, J. (1995). Japanese Americans. In J. N. Giger & R. E. Davidhizar (Eds.), *Transcultural nursing: Assessment and intervention* (2nd ed.). St. Louis, MO: C. V. Mosby.

Kakesako, G. K. (1993, March 19). Nisei proved their loyalty on the war front. *The Honolulu Star-Bulletin,* p. A1.

Kikumura, A., & Kitano, H. H. L. (1973). *Changing lives.* San Francisco: Jossey-Bass.

Kobato, F. (1979). The influence of culture on family relations: The Asian American experience. In P. K. Ragan (Ed.), *Aging parents.* Los Angeles: University of Southern California, Ethel Percy Andrus Gerontology Foundation.

Lasky, E. M., & Martz, C. H. (1993). The Asian/Pacific Islander population in the United States: Cultural perspectives and their relationship to cancer and prevention and early detection. In M. Frank-Stromborg & S. J. Olsen (Eds.), *Cancer prevention in minority populations: Cultural implications for health care professionals.* St. Louis, MO: C. V. Mosby.

Lee, P., & Takamura, J. (1980). The Japanese Americans in Hawaii. In N. Palafox & A. Warren (Eds.), *Cross-cultural caring: A handbook for health care professionals in Hawaii.* Honolulu, HI: Transcultural Health Care Forum.

O'Hare, W. P. (1992). *America's minorities: The demographics of diversity* (Population Bulletin 47). Washington, DC: Population Reference Bureau.

Shiba, G., & Oka, R. (1996). Japanese Americans. In J. G. Lipson, S. L. Dibble, & P. A. Minarik (Eds.), *Culture and nursing care: A pocket guide.* San Francisco: UCSF Nursing Press.

Stauffer, R. Y. (1995). Vietnamese Americans. In J. N. Giger & R. E. Davidhizar (Eds.), *Transcultural nursing: Assessment and intervention* (2nd ed.). St Louis, MO: C. V. Mosby.

Strumpf, N. E., & Kauffman, K. S. (1994). Long-term care: Meeting obligations to the elderly. In J. C. McClosky & H. K. Grace (Eds.), *Current issues in nursing* (4th ed.). St. Louis, MO: C. V. Mosby.

U.S. Department of Commerce. (1993). *We the American . . . Asians* (Economic and Statistics Administration, Publication No. WE-3). Washington, DC: Government Printing Office.

Vance, A. R. (1995). Filipino Americans. In J. N. Giger & R. E. Davidhizar (Eds.), *Transcultural nursing: Assessment and intervention* (2nd ed.). St. Louis, MO: C. V. Mosby.

Yang, H., Braun, K. L., Onaka, A. T., & Horiuchi, B. (1996). *Life expectancy in the state of Hawai'i, 1980-1990* (Issue No. 63). Honolulu: Hawaii Office of Health Status Monitoring.

Yoshishige, J. (1993, March 21). Wartime heroics: A Nisei history. *The Honolulu Advertiser* (special section), p. 5.

21

Tips for Working With Asian American Populations

MICHAEL V. KLINE
ROBERT M. HUFF

The term *Asian Americans* refers to people of Asian descent who are citizens or permanent residents of the United States. They reside in many communities, mainstream to small and isolated enclaves, and consist of approximately 23 subgroups, such as Asian Indians, Cambodians, Chinese, Filipinos, Hmong, Japanese, Koreans, Laotians, Thais, Vietnamese, and "other Asian," with 32 linguistic groups. Among this group, the Chinese and Filipinos are the two largest subgroups. There has been a lack of awareness of various health-related problems specific to this population, owing to the convention of aggregating health data. The stereotypes that Asian Americans are hardworking, intelligent, successful, and mentally healthy have masked social, economic, and mental health problems of the Asian American populations. It is critical for the health promoter to recognize the great diversity in cultural beliefs and practices, history, language, and generational differences characterizing each subgroup.

This brief "tips" chapter provides some fundamental information, suggestions, and recommendations for working with these different groups in health promotion and disease prevention (HPDP) activities. These tips have been distilled from the preceding three chapters and other sources (English & Lê, 1999, Chapter 19, this volume; Frankish, Lovato, & Shannon, Chapter 3, this volume; Green & Kreuter, 1991; Hiatt et al., 1996; Huff, Chapter 2, this volume; Huff & Kline, Chapter 1, this volume; Inouye, Chapter 18, this volume; Ishida, Chapter 20, this volume; Kline, Chapter 4, this volume; McPhee et al., 1996; Pasick, D'Onofrio, & Otero-Sobogal, 1996; Pasick, Sabogal, et al., 1996; Sobogal, Otero-Sobogal, Pasick, Jenkins, & Perez-Stable, 1996). They are offered as general starting points that need to be considered for those involved in assessing, designing, implementing, and evaluating HPDP programs for Asian American population groups.

CULTURAL COMPETENCE

The health promoter needs to develop cultural competency skills for working across multicultural population groups. This is an especially important issue to be considered when working with Asian American populations characterized by such great diversity and differences connected to health practices and health-related problems. The following tips for the health promoter can help facilitate processes that will contribute to more effective HPDP programs:

▶ Seek to learn the history and immigration patterns of the specific ethnic group you will be targeting for HPDP interventions.

▶ Be aware that most new immigrants come from homogeneous ethnic countries and have been thrust into heterogeneous surroundings where their self-identity may be threatened and where they often must deal with this "differentness" as well as prejudices and racial bigotry.

▶ Become familiar with the particular target group's specific cultural values, beliefs, and ways of life. These include forms of address and other verbal and nonverbal communication patterns, food preferences, attitudes toward health and disease, and related cultural characteristics that differentiate this group from other Asian American populations.

▶ Become familiar with the language differences within each group and how language adjustment was another stress that had to be overcome to function in a new country.

▶ Engage in active listening (rather than talking) and be alert to nonverbal cues because some Asian American populations tend not to disagree openly with health service providers, thereby avoiding conflict and embarrassment so as to maintain harmony. The nodding of heads might mean they are hearing but not necessarily agreeing with what is being said.

▶ Be alert to the correspondence between verbal and nonverbal behaviors, being careful to ask open-ended questions that elicit what the individuals or groups think about the situation, resources, or suggestions as well as how comfortable they are with the available choices in terms of what they want and can live with.

▶ Be aware that although in many Asian American families one adult might be the spokesperson for the family, all members should be encouraged to voice their opinions.

▶ Be aware of the dynamics within the Asian American family. Because problems are generally handled within the confines of the family, concerns might not be shared with the health care provider unless there is a trusting relationship established.

▶ Seek to incorporate or assist planners in incorporating these cultural values, beliefs, and ways of life into the HPDP program or service where appropriate.

▶ Be aware that many different Asian American groups refer to their generational differences according to the arrival or birth in the United States and are, with your exploration, distinguishable by their various ages, experiences, languages, beliefs, and values.

▶ Recognize that acculturation is a critical factor in explaining risk behavior and health status. The more traditional the individual or group, the less likely the individual or group is to know about, understand, or practice Western approaches to HPDP.

▶ Be aware that for many Asian American subgroups, immigration caused a number of adjustment and acculturation stresses that might be related to their overall health and health practices such as being forced to leave their homes, facing political exile, or being separated from family members.

▶ Seek to learn how differences in beliefs and values among different subgroups may help identify some of the possible areas of conflict and frustration experienced by new immigrants and sometimes later generations.

▶ Be aware that all of the groups represent varying degrees of acculturation and assimilation in their current country of residence.

▶ Be aware that beliefs and values play an important role in acculturation and integration of Asian Americans into Western culture and that the process of integration differs for each of the Asian groups.

▶ Acknowledge that the measurement of acculturation is an important activity for understanding how traditional, acculturated, and assimilated a specific ethnic group might be. There are a variety of scales that can be used, and the reader is urged to read Chapters 1, 6, 7, 8, and 26 for a more detailed discussion of this process.

▶ Be aware that two beliefs that are prominent in Asians, especially those from Southeast Asia, are *kinship solidarity* and *equilibrium or balance*. Kinship solidarity refers to the view that the individual is subservient to the kinship-based group or family.

▶ Be aware that most Asian family patterns are characterized by filial piety, male authority, and respect for elders and that this pattern sometimes determines decision-making practices relating to health care for recent immigrants.

▶ Appreciate that family and family support is one of the most important core values among Asian American population groups. Be aware how devastating separation from family members can be to a culture that values the nuclear and extended family.

▶ Remember that decisions associated with seeking medical care and/or participating actively in a prescribed treatment or health program might involve the head of the household or other family members, whose decisions will be based on what they feel is best for the family.

▶ Be aware that avoiding conflict and achieving harmony in interpersonal relationships is a strong cultural value among Asian Americans.

▶ Show respect for Asian American beliefs and values because they are an extremely important factor in all relationships and especially in HPDP encounters.

▶ Recognize that the diverse circumstances under which Asian Americans live and work require you to appreciate the impact that ethnic and social ties might have on health behavior choices and the need to use these factors effectively in developing HPDP programs or services.

HEALTH BELIEFS AND PRACTICES

There are a variety of health beliefs and practices that characterize the many different Asian population groups residing in the United States. The health promoter needs to understand and be sensitive to the differences he or she is likely to encounter. The health promoter needs to be aware of how to use this knowledge and how to incorporate these differences into HPDP programs or services. The health promoter should keep the following tips in mind:

▶ Recognize that belief in folk illnesses still is a strong cultural characteristic among many traditional Asian population groups. Developing an understanding of some of these illnesses and their traditional treatments can help you to be more effective in the design of specific HPDP intervention and treatment services.

▶ Remember that it often is assumed by health care workers that everyone embraces the Western biomedical model. However, within Asian cultures, traditional or cultural beliefs of spiritual or supernatural forces and balance with nature often are overlooked, and traditional practitioners may assist the individual in achieving this energy balance.

▶ Understand that there are a number of explanatory models used to make sense of health and disease and that these are generally associated with the social, psychological, and physical domains. Recognize that although health is defined in the United States as a state of complete physical, mental, and social well-being and not merely the absence of disease, Asians view it as a state of harmony with nature or freedom from symptoms or illness.

▶ Remember that the need to achieve a harmonious relationship with nature might be a central concept of the traditional health care system still used today. This system often is the first one used when an illness or other disorder is detected in a family member, and those who use this system are generally not inclined to discuss this with a Western health care practitioner.

▶ Be aware that beliefs and expectations about health care treatment may enhance or impede Asian groups' participation in the health program or service. There is a need to explore these beliefs and expectations in the assessment or initial health care encounter phase.

▶ Be aware that although there are wide variations in health beliefs and practices shaped by cultural values in determining what is important in one's life, many Asian groups may share some similarities based on their religious background and the influence of Chinese culture throughout Asia.

▶ Recognize that the prominence of Confucian ideology, Buddhism, and Taoism in Asian culture focuses on the upholding of a public facade and against public admission of mental or physical illness or any admission of personal weakness.

▶ Be aware that to a large extent, culture and language influence how one conceptualizes etiology, symptoms, and treatment of illnesses and may influence how one is to interact with health care providers and organizations.

▶ Recognize that because of language difficulties and cultural differences, many Asians, especially the newer immigrants, still might prefer the traditional forms of Chinese and native medicine and seek help from Chinatown "physicians" or "masters" who treat them with tradition herbs and other methods.

▶ Be aware that Asians often do not seek help from the Western system of medicine because of painful diagnostic tests and lack of information and understanding about what is being done to them.

▶ Be sensitive to the effect of abrupt cultural changes among an immigrant community introduced to medical pluralism. An eclectic medical culture that blends influences from biomedicine, Christianity, and Chinese medicine could result in a selective loss of medical or religious concepts and practices that no longer "fit" their new situation and collective identity.

PROGRAM PLANNING CONSIDERATIONS

The health promoter must be aware that planning HPDP programs or services for Asian American population groups, given their tremendous diversity, requires systematic identification and selection of tailored courses of action related to achieving or improving health-related behaviors. Such programming also will require the planner to be culturally competent and sensitive to the differences in how the planner views and operates in the world and how his or her target group sees this same process. Thus, the health promoter should consider the following comments and suggestions relevant to the program planning process:

▶ Be sensitive to indiscriminately applying health care and programs to all groups in the same manner. Also, recognize that because all Asian Americans do not have similar beliefs and health practices, health professionals cannot assume that programs for one Asian group will work for another similar group.

▶ Be sure that the program or service being developed will be culturally acceptable to the target group and will not come into conflict with the target group's values, beliefs, attitudes, or knowledge about the problem.

▶ Clearly identify potential barriers that might be encountered that would impede participation in the HPDP program or service and identify how you might overcome these.

▶ Wherever possible, seek to eliminate obstacles to participation in the HPDP program or service. This may involve simplifying how the target group enrolls in or accesses the service or program, bringing the program or service to the target group, making sure that the program or service is offered in the language of the target group, and making sure that any follow-up activities participants might need to do are simplified, relevant, and easily understood.

▶ Consider employing the principles of *relevance* and *participation* when designing the program or service, that is, starting your program or service where the target group is and involving its members' active participation throughout the entire process, from design through evaluation.

▶ Make sure that the organization or agency involved in designing the program or service has a mission, policies, procedures, an organizational structure, and staff that reflect a sense of cultural competence and sensitivity to the target group on which the program or service is being focused.

NEEDS ASSESSMENT

The extensive data that serve as the foundations of Asian American HPDP programs and services serve to help the HPDP planner to better understand and address the specific health needs and interests of the planner's target population. It is critical that the health promoter take the time to adequately determine the characteristics of the target group he or she will be serving including factors such as morbidity and mortality, historic and immigration patterns, specific cultural characteristics, demographics, health care access and use patterns, and related variables. Huff and Kline, in Chapter 26, present a cultural assessment framework that can help provide guidelines for the assessment areas that should be considered when preparing to develop the needs assessment component of the program planning process. In addition, the following suggestions may be useful in the needs assessment process:

▶ Remember that conducting a thorough needs assessment is critical to identify community issues and problems in Asian American communities, to formulate relevant objectives, and to determine what educational interventions are appropriate.

▶ Be aware that regardless of the planning model used (e.g., PRECEDE-PRO-CEED) for Asian American health promotion programs, you must be extremely conscious of and sensitive to the need for building a cultural assessment component into the planning process.

▶ Be aware that aggregating Asian American health data might mask differences in disease patterns for specific subpopulations and could result in an erroneous portrayal of the overall Asian American population as healthy and at lower risk for death and illness.

▶ Remember that needs assessment information should seek to identify local mores and customs. This is particularly true if the target group is located within an ethnic enclave, as in the case of many new Asian immigrants.

▶ Where possible, involve community representatives who can function to help identify persons in the community already recognized by other community members as sources of assistance and support regarding issues and problems.

▶ Where possible, train and use community members to assist in the data collection process because this can help facilitate community ownership of the program or service being developed and can provide perspectives that might have otherwise been missed by a noncommunity member.

▶ Recognize that, at the very least, outreach workers (e.g., lay health advisers) who are involved in obtaining assessment information and who may ultimately introduce the health education program to the community should be perceived as nonthreatening and nonintrusive. They should be drawn from the same ethnic group and preferably be from that community.

▶ Be aware that contacts during the assessment process should be linguistically appropriate when working in established communities or with recent immigrants. For some groups such as Chinese and Filipinos, the language of the assessment process might have to deal with more than one language or several dialects.

▶ Be sure to include key community members (both formal and informal) in the community needs assessment process.

▶ Recognize that survey or interview data with community members from similar generations may reveal "generation gaps" in values or expressed health beliefs and behaviors.

▶ Consider including acculturation measures in the needs assessment instrument.

▶ Be sure to assess the types of media used within the community because this might be a critical factor when the program or service is ready to go on-line and marketing activities are being planned. It also relates to acculturation levels in the community.

▶ Be sure that assessment and evaluation efforts reflect the needs, interests, and values of the stakeholders within the community.

▶ Be aware that at the outset of an HPDP program, baseline data for establishing the scope and seriousness of the problem might not be readily available. Initial assessment information might need to be based in part on demographic data, on morbidity and mortality data, and (in large part) on key informant information.

▶ Be aware that key informants might not have knowledge of or represent all elements in the community or group. If these persons represent the intended program users (or targeted group) or already provide services to the desired users, then so much the better.

▶ Understand that an extensive baseline survey consisting of core questions covering demographics, health beliefs and practices, and cultural values might need to be administered to target groups after an exhaustive effort is made to ensure the appropriateness of each question to that group.

▶ When designing questions for survey instruments or interviews to be administered to Asian American subgroups in a language other than English, recognize that translation and adaptation is a complex process that requires an understanding of each language and culture and might require iterative pre-testing in all groups and subgroups (by age, language, ancestry, etc.).

▶ Focus groups can be a useful and effective approach to determining the knowledge, attitudes, behaviors, and felt needs of the community.

▶ The PRECEDE model can be helpful because it guides you to consider relationships between and among particular health behaviors and their predisposing, enabling, and reinforcing factors and can provide convincing evidence regarding the need for early educational interventions designed to affect these factors positively.

INTERVENTION CONSIDERATIONS

Well-planned and culturally appropriate interventions are critical to the successful implementation of HPDP programs and services for Asian American population groups. *Cultural tailoring* urges the planner to develop the interventions, strategies, methods, messages, and materials to be adaptable to the specific cultural characteristics of the target group (Pasick, D'Onofrio, & Otero-Sabogal, 1996). The health promoter might wish to consider the following comments and suggestions as he or she begins the design phase of the program planning process:

▶ Be aware that new immigrants may differ on many social and health-related issues. You also should be aware that those at high risk will more likely include individuals with the following characteristics: low socioeconomic status, uninsured, limited English proficiency and/or linguistically isolated, foreign born or recently immigrated, and rigid adherence to certain cultural health beliefs and traditions that might conflict with some proven effective Western practices.

▶ Understand that an effective program must specifically address the health needs of the segment of the population targeted (e.g., women at risk for cervical or breast cancer, male smokers) within the Asian American community. You also need to deal with these needs as they result from the target group's diversity and collective history and culture.

▶ Recognize that the development of culturally appropriate interventions requires consideration of available community resources and inclusion of important cultural themes of the target group. For example, *family* is one of the strongest core values of traditional Asian culture, so interventions that have a family focus might prove more effective than those that focus on the individual.

▶ Remember that members of the community for whom the program is intended should participate and can help to provide an "insider's" perspective on issues and insights into local social norms and structure. This participation increases the likelihood that the project will not conflict with any fundamental cultural values and that it will be credible and well received.

▶ Recognize that a formal community advisory board used earlier in the planning stages also can provide valuable information, feedback, support, and resources during the educational intervention activities.

▶ Be aware that program results may be enhanced if there is a concerted effort to integrate the services into the social framework of the community.

▶ Be aware that interventions such as role modeling and use of community social networks may be useful approaches for demonstrating and reinforcing individual behavior change.

▶ Consider that developing partnerships with local media (e.g., radio, television, newspapers) for the dissemination of health education and health promotion information can be a valuable and effective approach for both marketing programs or services and reinforcing the successes of program participants who may be recruited as role models for the community in which the program or service has been targeted.

▶ Be aware that the use of behavioral theory to guide development of intervention approaches is central to well-conceived and appropriately designed intervention strategies (Frankish et al., Chapter 3, this volume).

▶ Be aware that a multiphased and multifaceted intervention might need to be used, for example, (a) to initially raise the awareness concerning the importance of preventive care and screening, (b) to motivate the target group to seek screening, and (c) to use neighborhood connections because they can provide behavioral modeling and social reinforcement through familiar communication channels.

▶ Recognize that the recruitment and training of a group of community peer networkers who can distribute program materials and reinforce messages can be an extremely effective method for maintaining community involvement and support for the HPDP program or service.

▶ Recognize that employing and training community members to facilitate educational programs in the community is a valuable and effective approach for implementing an HPDP program or service.

▶ Seek to develop interventions that focus on positive health changes rather than on negative or fear-arousing consequences.

▶ Remember that development of educational materials must reflect relevant cultural values, themes, and learning styles of the target group for which they are designed.

▶ Recognize that all materials used in the HPDP program that are written in a language other than English must be *back translated* and pilot tested to ensure that they say what was meant and that the messages are clear and understandable to the target group.

▶ Always assess the cultural appropriateness of any pictures, models, dolls, manuals, videotapes, messages tailored for the community (e.g., billboards, newspapers, radio and paid television advertisements), or other educational materials prior to their inclusion in the program because some materials might make the target group uncomfortable.

▶ Be aware that special training manuals can be developed for participating physicians and lay health workers for use in presentations and the subsequent discussions, videotapes, and other materials for the participants and physicians. These should be linguistically and culturally appropriate.

▶ Consider selecting methods and events led by trained neighborhood leaders or similarly recruited individuals. Such events could involve informal and small group educational events in private homes and community health fairs centered around the traditional New Year's festivals.

▶ Consider techniques that are more personal and centered on traditional characteristics of social solidarity and mutual assistance.

EVALUATION CONSIDERATIONS

Evaluation is central to understanding how well a program or service is doing in meeting the needs of the clientele it is serving. For this reason, the health promoter is urged to consider the following recommendations:

▶ Evaluation of HPDP programs and services should include culturally relevant measures for evaluating the impact of the program or service on the target group.

▶ Assessment and evaluation items must be tailored to the educational and linguistic capabilities of the target group for which they are intended. Here again, back translation of items will be an important consideration in the development of the assessment and evaluation instruments.

▶ Be aware that evaluation and assessment are processes that frequently are difficult to gain support for, even from the most sophisticated of groups. Efforts to explain underlying assumptions governing these processes, as well as the methods and anticipated outcomes from these activities, can help make explicit what often is unclear to those inexperienced in evaluation and can help motivate increased interest and support for evaluation and assessment methods and procedures.

▶ Providing evaluation and assessment training for community members who will be involved in the provision of the HPDP program or service can help promote increased input and support for evaluation efforts. This also can extend the number of staff and community supporters who can be involved in data collection activities related to assessment and evaluation activities.

▶ Consider administering surveys or conducting oral interviews before and after the interventions to assess whether there was an increase in screening or other target behaviors following participation in program activities or there were positive changes in target group knowledge, attitudes, and intentions toward the target behaviors. In reality, this can be difficult outside of a classroom setting.

▶ Be aware that participants might have limited test-taking skills, literacy skills, or time or might have physical difficulties such as poor eyesight or uncomfortable testing conditions. Thus, it might be more appropriate in some instances to forgo a time- and item-intensive evaluation of outcomes and process until such problems can be overcome.

REFERENCES

Green, L. W., & Kreuter, M. W. (1991). *Health promotion planning: An educational and environmental approach*. Mountain View, CA: Mayfield.

Hiatt, R. A., Pasick, R. J., Perez-Stable, E. J., McPhee, S. J., Engelstad, L., Lee, M., Sabogal, F., Bird, J. A., D'Onofrio, C. N., & Stewart, S. (1996). Pathways to early cancer detection in the multiethnic population of the San Francisco Bay Area. *Health Education Quarterly, 23*(Suppl.), S10-S27.

McPhee, S. J., Bird, J. A., Ha, N. T., Jenkins, C. N. J., Fordham, D., & Lê, B. (1996). Pathways to early cancer detection for Vietnamese women: Suc Khoe La Vang (Health Is Gold). *Health Education Quarterly, 23*(Suppl.), S60-S75.

Pasick, R. J., D'Onofrio, C. N., & Otero-Sabogal, R. (1996). Similarities and differences across cultures: Questions to inform a third generation for health promotion research. *Health Education Quarterly, 23*(Suppl.), S142-S161.

Pasick, R. J., Sabogal, F., Bird, J. A., D'Onofrio, C. N., Jenkins, C. N. J., Lee, M., Engelstad, L., & Hiatt, R. A. (1996). Problems and progress in translation of health survey questions: The Pathways experience. *Health Education Quarterly, 23*(Suppl.), S28-S40.

Sabogal, F., Otero-Sabogal, R., Pasick, R. J., Jenkins, C. N. J., & Perez-Stable, E. J. (1996). Printed health education materials for diverse communities: Suggestions learned from the field. *Health Education Quarterly, 23*(Suppl.), S123-S141.

PART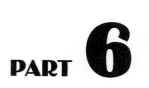

Pacific Islander Populations

22

Pacific Islander
Health and Disease

An Overview

JOHN CASKEN

This chapter is designed to introduce the health practitioner to the current health status of Pacific Islander Americans (PIAs) in the United States. For the health professional, these populations can be unknown territory, primarily because their numbers are so small. There is the tendency to lump the various subpopulations together, making the assumption that all PIAs have the same problems and can be expected to respond to the health concerns in similar ways. This chapter examines the overall problems that can be encountered when dealing with these populations, lays out some specific health and medical problems, and discusses pitfalls to be avoided when dealing with these populations.

PACIFIC ISLANDER AMERICANS IN THE UNITED STATES

Defining Terms and Describing the Diversity of Subgroups

Turning the globe to the Pacific Ocean reveals the small specks of land that create the island territories that make up the Pacific Islands, the home base of the PIAs from which most Pacific Islanders moved to become PIAs. Just as finding the individual specks of land on the face of the Pacific Ocean can be a difficult task, so too can be finding the small groups of PIAs who have moved to take up residence in the continental United States. The term *continental United States* is used among many Native Hawaiians who see the expression *the mainland* as reinforcing the "colonialist" approach of the non-Native Hawaiians (Trask, 1985).

If it is difficult to find each island in the Pacific Ocean, so too can it be even more difficult to find PIAs in the United States. The problem of small, widely scattered numbers is one of the key issues encountered when examining the health status of PIAs. In effect, there are practically no data about these populations. Prior to the 1980 census, all PIAs except Native Hawaiians were included in the Asian and Pacific Islander (API) classification. Since the 1980 census, PIAs have been separated out from the API group. Native Hawaiians have been separated out since the 1960 census. However, apart from the census, most other data sets continue to include PIAs among APIs. Even in the state of Hawai'i, which has the largest population of PIAs in the United States, only Samoans and Native Hawaiians are separated out by ethnicity. All other PIAs are included under the category "other" in Hawai'i State Department of Health statistics.

A related issue is that even within groups of PIAs, there can be confusion as to what the name implies. How representative of a specific PIA community is any individual PIA? This confusion arises from the current fashion of determining ethnicity. Just as in the 18th and 19th centuries, any drop of African American blood was sufficient to label a person as a member of that racial/ethnic group, now the current fashion often is to describe as a PIA anyone who has even the slightest blood claim to that designation. The fashion has been legalized, as one can see in the definition of Native Hawaiian that is used in this chapter. Public Law 100-579, the Native Hawaiian Health Care Act of 1988, states,

> The term *Native Hawaiian* means any individual who has any ancestors who were Natives, prior to 1778, of the area that is now the state of Hawai'i as evidenced by (a) genealogical records, (b) *Kupuna* (elders) or *Kama'aina* (long-term community residents) verification, or (c) birth records of the state of Hawai'i. (Section 8.3, emphases added)

With this, as with other ethnic definitions, there is a caution. In many cases, demographic information in the data sets that are used for health purposes includes self-definition of ethnicity. This permits those who have no blood line claim or title to appropriate an ethnic designation to which other members of that ethnic group might not feel they are entitled. Such an approach has been legitimized by the 1980 and 1990 censuses, which allowed self-identification. Naturally, there also have been changes in how ethnicity was defined in the 1980 and 1990 censuses, which further complicates the problem of who is part of an ethnic group.

As discussed in Chapter 1, there often is confusion between the terms *race* and *ethnicity*. There are more differences within a given population than between populations that claim distinction (Young, 1994). Other authors have suggested that ethnicity is, in fact, a useless variable because it never can be clear exactly what is meant by the term. The argument goes that it is better to use socio-economic descriptors that can be quantified (Navarro, 1989).

A subtheme of this chapter is to raise this issue of ethnicity as a variable, even though it appears that ethnicity will continue to be used as a descriptor for some time to come despite the fact that errors in ethnic classification can affect health data (Dearing, 1996). The reason for raising this issue is that if, for example, a person is classified as a Samoan, then what does that mean? To the individual, it means one thing; to the observer, it means something else. However, it is rare for the observer to clearly lay out the parameters of the description. Does the term *Samoan* include Western Samoans as well as American Samoans? Does it include recent immigrants to the United States as well as those who were born in the United States? Obviously, it includes those who were born in Samoa. Implicit in the use of ethnic variables, it seems, is that ethnicity can be the basis of the health status of the person. Yet, the four groups just mentioned, although classified as Samoans, probably would exhibit different health status, based not so much on their ethnicity as on their socioeconomic status. Having raised the issue, however, for the present this chapter will continue to accept the descriptor. Still, it is important for the health professional to be aware of the discrepancies involved in data and not accept data at face value but rather recognize that what includes also excludes (Stone, 1988).

As noted earlier, it is difficult to determine in general the PIA population. The difficulties are compounded when examining the health problems specific to the PIA population. Pacific Islanders who have moved from their home islands to the continental United States, as opposed to moving to the state of Hawai'i, begin a subtle process of transformation as they adopt the habits of their neighbors (Barringer, Gardner, & Levin, 1993). Although ties are kept with the islands—for some, the remittances at home form an important part of the home island's economy—diets change, approaches to education change, jobs change, recreational activities change, and housing situations change, all of which can lead to major changes in health outcomes (Hall, 1990: Pouesi, 1994).

Origins of Pacific Islander Americans

PIAs come from the Polynesian, Micronesian, and Melanesian groupings of islands in the North and South Pacific. This tripartite division is based primarily on genetic, linguistic, and sociocultural analysis (Bellwood, 1979). The 1990 census reported a total of 365,042 PIAs (Figure 22.1). Among the Polynesians in the 1990 census, the largest group numerically was Native Hawaiians (211,014), followed by Samoans (62,964), Tongans (17,606), and Tahitians (1,098). Among the Micronesians, the largest group was Guamanians (49,345) (the indigenous inhabitants of Guam are more correctly called *Chammoros*), Northern Mariana Islanders (1,142), and Palauans (1,461), with Micronesians (politically divided in Yapese, Trukese, Pohnpeians, and Kosraeans) and Marshallese being too few to include, according to 1990 census figures. Melanesians are represented primarily by the Fijians, with a 1990 population of 7,036. The Fijian population also includes Indians from the Asian subcontinent, many of whom had immigrated to Fiji during the late 19th and early 20th centuries and then emigrated from Fiji following the Fijian constitutional changes designed to

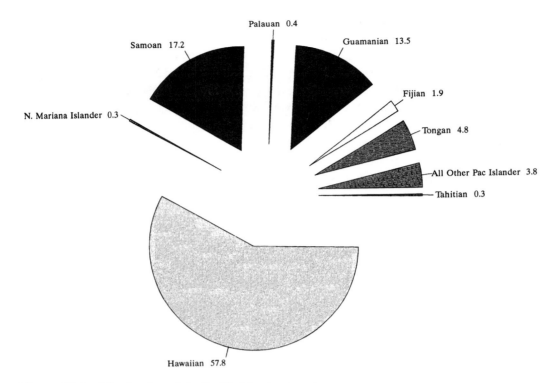

Figure 22.1   Distribution of the Pacific Islander American Population: 1990 (percentages)
SOURCE: U.S. Bureau of the Census (1993).

give more political power to the ethnic Fijians. All other PIA populations totaled 13,974 in 1990 (U.S. Bureau of the Census, 1993).

Because the Native Hawaiian population forms 57.8% of the PIA population, this chapter concentrates on this subpopulation. Reasons other than size also suggest such an emphasis. For starters, the Native Hawaiian population's health status has been more thoroughly researched than has that of the remaining subpopulations (Wegner, 1989). Then, too, there is the consideration that PIAs genetically not only could be considered as three different subgroups but also could have major ethnic differences even within the subgroups. This would include the ethnic differences between the Tahitians, who have been dominated by the French for nearly 200 years, and the Tongans, who remained under British rule for more than 100 years. Most important, there are political issues that affect approaches to health between Native Hawaiians and other PIAs. Many Native Hawaiians are seeking to redefine the political structure in Hawai'i with calls for sovereignty, and Native Hawaiian health status is being linked with these calls (Blaisdell, 1993; Trask, 1993).

As might be expected, the majority of PIAs live in the state of Hawai'i, primarily because the state is home to approximately 180,000 Native Hawaiians, a number that included nearly 9,000 pure Hawaiians in 1990. The state also is home to many of the other PIA groups, partly because the climate and lifestyle are similar to those of the other Pacific Islands. However, no PIA group

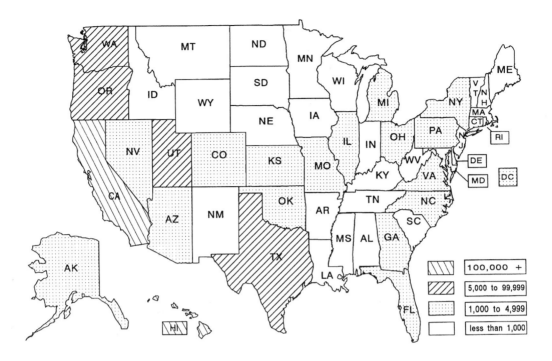

Figure 22.2 Distribution of the Pacific Islander American Population: 1990
SOURCE: U.S. Bureau of the Census (1993).

has more than 50% of its numbers living in Hawai'i (Figure 22.2). As of 1990, approximately 50% of Samoans and Guamanians lived in California, 80% of Fijians also lived in California, and Utah was home to approximately 20% of Tongans living in the United States, reflecting the missionary influence in the South Pacific of the Church of the Latter Day Saints. In the continental United States, PIAs are found predominantly in Seattle, the San Francisco Bay Area, Los Angeles, and San Diego on the West Coast. Using statistics on live births in 1992 as an indicator of where the majority of PIAs live in the continental United States, 983 Samoan live births were recorded for the state of California, compared to 588 Samoan live births in Hawai'i. In the same year, there were 390 Guamanian live births in California, compared to only 47 in Hawai'i. For the same year, Guamanian live births totaled 70 in Washington, 29 in New York, and 25 in Texas, whereas Samoan live births totaled 133 in Washington and 20 in Texas (Centers for Disease Control and Prevention, 1995; U.S. Bureau of the Census, 1993).

A final reason for placing emphasis on Native Hawaiians is that Hawai'i is the first outside destination for many of the other Pacific Islanders as they begin their journey to the continental United States. The state also provides the closest medical assistance for the Pacific Islands in a cultural context that feels more familiar to the Pacific Islanders. Janes (1990) suggests that in Hawai'i, it is easier for PIAs to retain their familiar lifestyles and traditions. For example, Samoans keep Samoan habits and traditions while they are in Hawai'i, but when they move to California, the typical traditional patterns disappear.

It would be appropriate here to note that the U.S. citizenship status of PIAs varies, depending on the political relations between the United States and the individual territory. For example, Native Hawaiians are full citizens. American Samoans carry U.S. passports and can freely take up jobs in the United States, but they are classified as U.S. nationals, not U.S. citizens. American Samoa also sends a representative to the House of Representatives in the U.S. Congress. Western Samoa is an independent state with close political links to New Zealand and close familial links to American Samoa.

Since the Organic Act of Guam in 1950, Guamanians have been full U.S. citizens. Guam is now seeking commonwealth status similar to that of Puerto Rico. After spending a number of years under U.S. political control, many of the other Polynesian and Micronesian territories have become independent states, although they still have very close connections to the United States politically and also to the state of Hawai'i through family and medical support. With this independence came the loss of U.S. citizenship and, in many cases, fiscal support. No Melanesian state has been under the direct control of the United States.

Historical Perspectives: A Brief Overview of Pacific Islander Americans in the United States

PIAs' history of interaction with the United States is very different from that of most of the population groups discussed in this book. There was no large-scale immigration of Pacific Islanders for specific purposes such as the importation of West Africans to work as slaves on plantations or the importation of Chinese to work on the California railroads. This was partly because of the small population base in all of the islands, which ruled out such a move. Also, these populations were believed to be incapable of hard work; Japanese, Chinese, and Filipinos were imported to work on the sugar plantations in Hawai'i because the Hawaiians were not considered sufficiently industrious to work on the plantations (Daws, 1968).

As the small number of PIAs indicates, there has been very little permanent immigration from the Pacific Islands into the continental United States. Key routes for many have been through the military and education (Barringer et al., 1993).

From a Hawaiian viewpoint, it would be more historically correct to talk about the history of the United States in Hawai'i (Kame'eleihiwa, 1992). At the time the Declaration of Independence was being signed in the United States, King Kamehameha I, from the Big Island of Hawai'i, was embarking on a set of conquests designed to bring all the inhabited islands of the Hawaiian chain under his rule, a task he had effectively accomplished by the time of his death in 1819 (Howe, 1984). From then until the overthrow of Queen Lili'uokalani in 1893 (Budnick, 1992; Dougherty, 1992), Hawai'i remained a separate kingdom that signed formal treaties with the United States and various European powers. In 1898, the islands were annexed by the United States. In 1959, Hawai'i became the 50th state (Daws, 1968).

During the past 10 years, the calls for sovereignty for Native Hawaiians have become increasingly strong. It is now generally accepted that Native Hawaiian sovereignty will become a reality, although there is a wide variety of opinions among the Native Hawaiians as to the form that sovereignty should take. The state of Hawai'i funded and set up a Hawaiian Sovereignty Elections Council to ask the following question of Native Hawaiians: "Shall the Hawaiian people elect delegates to propose a Native Hawaiian government?" This seemingly simple procedure was challenged by many of the groups seeking sovereignty on the grounds that it should be the Native Hawaiians themselves who should decide what questions should be asked in this matter as well as when and how they should be asked, rather than the state (even with some Native Hawaiian input) trying to determine those issues.

Sociodemographic Characteristics of Pacific Islander Americans in the United States

Age

Based on the 1990 census, it is clear that PIAs are a young population group, with 10.6% of the population being under 5 years of age, compared to 7.4% for the U.S. population overall. Only 63.8% of PIAs are age 18 years or over, compared to 74.4% for the U.S. population overall. The largest difference is found in the population age 65 years or over—4.0% for PIAs versus 12.6% for the U.S. population overall. The median age of the U.S. population overall is 32.9 years, compared to 25.0 years for PIAs. The youthfulness of the PIA population group has important considerations, especially for maternal and child health areas. For example, 18.3% of Native Hawaiians, 16.4% of Guamanians, and 10.7% of Samoans have children between the ages of 15 and 19 years, compared to 5.3% for the U.S. population overall (Centers for Disease Control and Prevention, 1995; U.S. Bureau of the Census, 1993).

Education

Western education is highly respected among most PIA population groups (Barringer et al., 1993). In 1990, PIAs had a higher percentage of the population with high school diplomas than did the U.S. population overall (76.1% vs. 75.2%). That advantage is quickly dissipated, however, as the figures were reversed at the undergraduate level. That is, only 10.8% of PIAs had undergraduate degrees, compared to 20.3% for the U.S. population overall. By contrast, despite the downward drag of the PIA figures, the total API figure was 36.6%.

As suggested earlier, even though PIAs comprise a small population group, these overall figures hide specific problems such as the extremely low numbers among Native Hawaiians living in rural areas. One such area is the Wai'anae Coast of Oahu, which has a high concentration of Native Hawaiians living in the four census tracts that make up the district. According to 1990 census data for Native

Hawaiians living on the Wai'anae Coast, only 42% of Native Hawaiians age 35 years or over had high school diplomas, compared to 80.8% for the state population overall. At the undergraduate level, the picture is equally bleak. Only 2.9% of Native Hawaiians age 18 years or over had bachelor's degrees, compared to 20.4% for the state population overall. The overall figure for Pacific Islanders on the Wai'anae Coast was 3.8% (U.S. Bureau of the Census, 1993).

Even the figure of 10.8% of PIAs holding undergraduate degrees suggests an imbalance tied to other low socioeconomic indexes including jobs and housing. Health problems for low socioeconomic status groups, regardless of their ethnic backgrounds, can be considerably different from those for other members of the same ethnic group who have a higher socioeconomic status (Montgomery, Kiely, & Pappas, 1996).

Ability to Use the English Language

The ability to use the English language is a crucial predictor of employment status and is useful for activities of daily living that can affect overall health. The ability to use English also is critical in terms of health promotion activities, especially when much of the material is based in English. Even when educational material is prepared in another language, the amount of such material normally is very restricted. It also can be difficult to find a native speaker who can correctly deal with health promotion and disease prevention (HPDP) activities in another language. Thus, it is critical that PIAs have an ability to use English. The 1990 census data suggested that approximately one third of Pacific Islanders could not speak English very well. Given that people's judgment on this matter might well err on the high side, a secondary finding is perhaps more relevant—that of linguistic isolation. This refers to households in which no one age 14 years or over speaks only English and no one who speaks a language other than English speaks English very well. Among Pacific Islanders, only Tongans had a problem in this category, with 21.6% claiming to be linguistically isolated. Samoans were the next highest at 9.3%. These percentages should be expected given the high proportion of PIAs who completed their high school educations (normally conducted in English) (U.S. Bureau of the Census, 1993).

Occupational Status

Figure 22.3 shows that PIAs are more likely to be in service, manufacturing, and laboring positions than are members of the U.S. population overall. Because job status is a critical component of a person's socioeconomic status, the health problems of PIAs would be expected to differ more on occupation and overall socioeconomic status than on membership in a specific ethnic population group (Navarro, 1989).

The managerial and professional specialty figure of 18.1% for PIAs is not too far from the 26.4% for the U.S. population overall. Again, however, the overall figure hides problem areas. For example, on the Wai'anae Coast, only 16.9% of

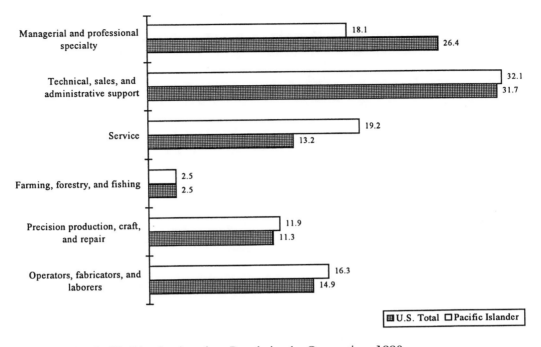

Figure 22.3 Pacific Islander American Population by Occupation: 1990
SOURCE: U.S. Bureau of the Census (1993).

the people who live there are employed as managers or professionals, compared to 38.3% for the state population overall.

Income and Poverty Status

Income, although used as a general indicator of economic status, is a limited tool because it fails to take into account wealth, which provides the basis on which so many other demographic variables depend (Greenberg, 1989). Income also can give a false reading if one looks at total family income rather than at per capita income because for PIAs the family income can include the amounts from the extended family as well as a variety of entitlements, as Figure 22.4 shows.

Per capita income figures do give a broad indication of the economic status of a group, especially when considered against figures showing percentages of families below the poverty level, although many (e.g., Schram, 1995) argue that the poverty level index is totally arbitrary and does not fully indicate the real extent of poverty, as Figure 22.5 shows.

A key issue to bear in mind when dealing with these demographic data is that the socioeconomic status of a person can have a major effect on his or her health status. Looking at the data examined in this section can be more revealing about a person's health status and possible health problems than can looking at specific health data. If a person's income level is known, and if his or her job, living situation, housing, and educational level also are known, then it will be relatively easy to predict what the person's health status will be like (Marmot & Thewell, 1997).

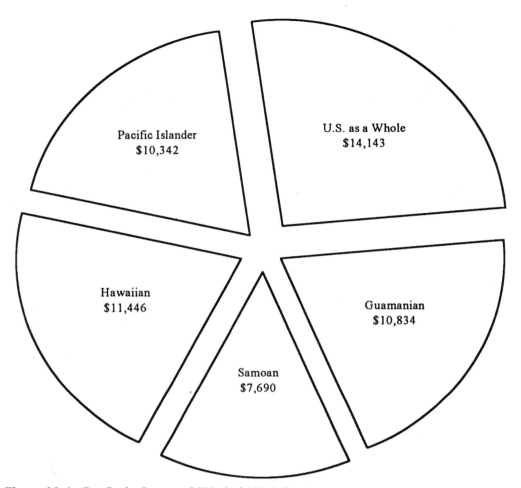

Figure 22.4 Per Capita Income: 1990 (in 1989 dollars)
SOURCE: U.S. Bureau of the Census (1993).

Acculturation, Integration, and Growth of Pacific Islander Americans in the United States

This section begins with one major caveat. As suggested earlier, the history of Native Hawaiians demonstrates that the health professional must exercise caution in presuming that all ethnic groups came to the United States and are now becoming acculturated to the mainstream culture and growing as a population group within the United States. Native Hawaiians, American Indians, and Alaska Natives claim that they are the indigenous inhabitants, and we should not be examining how they have acculturated. The health professional must be cautious not to inhibit access to health care because of an attitude suggesting that they should meet *our* standards.

Having recognized what for some is a critical issue, we can now look at the growth and acculturation of other PIAs in the United States. As always for this group, it is difficult to document any growth until recently. With a total popula-

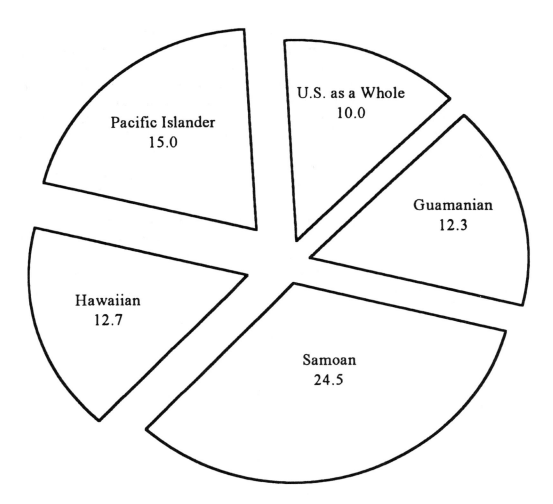

Figure 22.5   Poverty Rates for Families: 1989 (percentages in poverty)
SOURCE: U.S. Bureau of the Census (1993).

tion in the 1990 census of only 365,042, of whom 211,014 were Native Hawaiians (most of whom resided in the state of Hawai'i), the growth obviously is not going to be spectacular. In addition, with the recent attempts at the federal and state levels to reduce legal and illegal immigration, the prospects of more rapid growth are not good. The 1990 census count of 365,042 was approximately a 41% increase over the PIA population count of 259,566 in the 1980 census (U.S. Bureau of the Census, 1993).

Part of the reason for this growth is natural fertility of these young populations and the overall decrease in deaths during that period. Part of the growth also came from the way in which the 1990 census rephrased the race question on the census form as well as from improvements in the collection and processing procedures in the 1990 census. Individual immigrant groups also were very active in 1990, ensuring that all of their members completed the application, with the knowledge that the key to more resources was in increased numbers.

Because only about 13% of Pacific Islanders were "foreign born" using the 1990 census language, acculturation is a relatively easy process for this group. For Native Hawaiians, at nearly 58% of the population, acculturation is not the big deal it might be for, say, the Asian American population (after all, only 1% of the Native Hawaiian population are foreign born), and Hawai'i had been a territorial possession of the United States for about three generations before statehood in 1959. Samoans (at 23%) and Guamanians (at 11%) also had low percentages of members who were foreign born, suggesting that for them, as well, acculturation should be a relatively easy process. Because the Tongan population in 1990 was approximately 61% foreign born, acculturation has been a more difficult process. Embedded in the concept of acculturation, however, is the suggestion that the new arrivals take on the culture of the established population. When a Samoan travels to the continental United States but settles in with family members who already have established themselves, questions arise as to what culture is adopted. The new arrival might pick up only the minimal skills necessary to survive in the United States but continue to follow most aspects of the Samoan culture of the new Samoan group he or she has joined (Barringer et al., 1993). Acculturation also is more difficult if the move to the United States is not seen as a permanent move and there is a constant returning to the islands as the real home. Thus, acculturation is a very difficult concept to measure for PIAs.

For most Pacific Islander populations, such as Samoans, the move to live in the continental United States has led to a change in attitude toward work and the workplace (Filoialli, 1980). The reality of living in a cash-based economy forces changes that can be avoided in the homeland, even when the cash economy there is powerful (Bousseau, 1993). The ties of the family ensure that no one goes hungry or homeless. However, even though relationship ties still are very strong, it is becoming increasingly difficult for Samoans living in large cities in a cash economy to support relatives in the way they would be supported in Samoa (Franco, 1991).

Caveats When Generalizing About Pacific Islander Americans in the United States

The main caveat has been repeated many times in this and other chapters of this book; that is, *any generalizations about an ethnic group should be avoided.* Ethnicity as a variable is too ill defined to be used with precision.

Another major caveat that has been emphasized early and will be dealt with again is the suggestion that PIAs are, on the whole, healthier than the general population and so do not need any special care. As will be seen, it is a myth that APIs are healthier than the U.S. population overall (Chen, 1996; Chen & Hawks 1995), and it is even more of a myth that PIAs are healthier than the U.S. population overall.

A third caveat, which might almost fall into the realm of myths, is that PIAs are too tied to their traditional health beliefs to be concerned with Western medicine, so any approach to these population groups must be done only in a traditional form. As will be seen, PIA populations do have very specific traditional beliefs about health practices, but these are primarily for illnesses that are vague and ill defined. For illnesses that are clearly Western in nature, such as accidents, surgical procedures, and AIDS, help usually is sought from Western practitioners, although help also can be sought from traditional healers in the same way as folk remedies also will be used by many people in urban America (MacPherson & MacPherson, 1990).

HEALTH AND DISEASE

Health and Disease Patterns Among
Pacific Islander Americans: An Overview of the Issues

Myths and Historical Background

The 1985 report of the Secretary's Task Force on Black and Minority Health suggested that the "Asian/Pacific Islander minority in aggregate is healthier than all other racial/ethnic groups in the United States, including whites" (p. 6). It naturally led to the general idea that API populations had no health problems that needed special attention—the myth of healthy APIs (Chen & Hawks, 1995). Even worse, the Asian population treated as one whole was seen as superior to the white population on a wide variety of sociodemographic indicators, as can be seen, for example, in the varying attempts to limit the number of Asian Americans obtaining entrance into the University of California. Even though the PIA population has been separated from the Asian American population since 1980, the myth of a healthy population still persists, partly because the numbers of Pacific Islanders are so small that, when they are disaggregated, it is difficult to paint a clear picture of their strengths and weaknesses. When we disaggregate the PIA population from the Asian American population, the former comprise only about 5% of the API category (Aiu, 1996). The base conclusion has to be that because of the weighting of Native Hawaiians and their poor health indexes, PIAs have some of the poorest health statistics in the United States (Blaisdell, 1996).

If it is a myth today that the Pacific Islander population is unhealthy, this certainly was not the case when Captain Cook first landed on the Big Island of Hawai'i in 1778. He described the Hawaiians in words that he could not have used about his own crew or his own countrymen at that time:

> The Native men are above middle size, strong, muscular, well made of dark copper colour . . . who walk gracefully, run nimbly, and are capable of great fatigue. . . . The women . . . have handsome faces . . . are very well made . . . very clean, have good teeth, and are perfectly void of any disagreeable smell. (quoted in Beaglehole, 1967, pp. 1178, 1180)

Similar statements from the eyewitness accounts of the earliest travelers to Hawai'i, including physicians on board the ships of Cook, Vancouver, and Perouse, all comment on the excellent health status of Hawaiians.

Although for many years the Hawaiian population in 1778 had been estimated at approximately 300,000, new approaches have estimated that the population in 1778 could have been around 1,000,000 (Stannard, 1989). Despite Hawaiians' excellent health in 1778, by the 1840s their demise was being predicted. This claim is becoming increasingly more real, as demonstrated by the small number of pure Hawaiians. The Office of Technology Assessment report attached to the Native Hawaiian Health Care Act of 1988 predicted that pure Hawaiians would die out during the early 21st century and that Native Hawaiians, with an increasing percentage of Hawaiian blood, also would decline (U.S. Congress, Office of Technology Assessment, 1987).

Although none of the other Pacific Islander populations that were investigated by Europeans during the 18th century could claim to be as healthy as Cook and other early visitors found the Native Hawaiians to be, most of the Pacific Islander populations certainly were at least as healthy as the European populations at that time, and the status of the lowest members of the Pacific Island societies undoubtedly was better than that of similarly placed Europeans (Howe, 1984).

E Ola Mau: The Native Hawaiian Health Needs Study (Native Hawaiian Health Research Consortium, 1985) was commissioned by Senator Inouye to respond to the 1984 report on the poor health of Native Hawaiians. Although the five-volume study recognized the part played by poor access to health and medical resources, the study stressed throughout that the emphasis should be placed on the role played by the loss of land, literature, religion, culture, and sovereignty and concluded that

> the historical and cultural basis for our health plight must be the major consideration, and not merely concern for proximal causal factors such as specified in the currently fashionable government model of lifestyle, environmental, health care, and biological factors, with problems only in terms of physical health promotion, disease prevention, and intervention. (p. HC-4)

The Native Hawaiian Health Care Act of 1988 was designed to respond to the issues raised by the E Ola Mau study. Instead, using the framework of *Healthy People: The Surgeon General's Report on Health Promotion and Disease Prevention* (U.S. Department of Health, Education, and Welfare, 1979), the act placed nearly all of its emphasis on the HPDP aspects of *Healthy People* rather than on dealing with issues of loss of land, sovereignty, religion, and culture (Casken, 1994). Similarly, McCubbin's (1983) culture loss/stress hypothesis suggests that the current maladaptive behaviors of Native Hawaiians are due to the rapid and severe loss of culture by Native Hawaiians with Westernization and Western values.

The latest aggregation of health status data on Native Hawaiians was presented to Papa Ola Lokahi in March 1996 and was the third in a series conducted by many of the same group of researchers. These health data on Native Hawaiians are being presented here not to suggest that these figures are representative of all PIAs but rather to emphasize the health status of the largest group of PIAs in the United States. Also included are some data on Samoans in Hawai'i. To echo a theme that has been voiced throughout this chapter, there are essentially no data available on PIAs as a group except in very limited circumstances, and there are even less data on individual subgroups of PIAs. Discussion of these Native Hawaiian data also could promote, among other groups of PIAs, the approaches to improving health status that are being used among Native Hawaiians.

Chronic Health Conditions

Using data through 1992 collected through the Hawai'i State Department of Health and the Hawai'i Health Surveillance Program, the overall conclusion is that chronic disease patterns for Native Hawaiians are similar to those for the rest of the population. Diseases that are of increasing concern to Native Hawaiians are malignant neoplasms, circulatory disease, heart disease, cerebrovascular disease, and chronic obstructive pulmonary disease. Of decreasing concern are atherosclerosis, congenital abnormalities, perinatal conditions, and hypertension. Diabetes has increased among Native Hawaiian males by 28%, compared to a 15% increase for the U.S. population overall. For women, however, there has been a decline of 10% among Native Hawaiians, compared to an increase of 21% among the U.S. female population overall.

Acute and Infectious Conditions

Two conditions are of importance here for the PIA population. The first would be AIDS, and the second would be injuries and accidents. Discussions with Hawai'i State Department of Health officials suggest that the potential problem with tuberculosis is primarily among the Asian populations and not Pacific Islanders. Officials did caution, however, that some of the housing conditions for PIAs could indeed be seen as a danger for this population.

When the data for AIDS are examined, one can see a repeat of the pattern noted previously in terms of keeping ethnic groups separate. The state of Hawai'i STD/AIDS Prevention Branch keeps data on 23 subgroups in the API category, which in theory should at least allow researchers to make predictions about the populations under study. Part of the difficulty is that although the data are broken down by these 23 subgroups, regulations forbid dissemination of the data on any ethnic group where there are four or fewer entries in a particular ethnic cell. Thus, apart from noting that the new cases coming into the system in 1994 and 1995 total 50 for Native Hawaiians, the Polynesian count cannot be broken down among the other Pacific Islander groups, and one can say only that there have been four new cases reported during the years 1994 and 1995 among Micronesians and none among Melanesians in the state. The count cannot be broke down further because the numbers in the individual ethnic cells are four or less; to report them could lead to a breach of confidentiality lawsuit. The California data are simply broken down into the usual Office of Management and Budget 15 five-part categories.

Accidental falls for Native Hawaiians increased by 119% during the periods 1980 to 1986 and 1989 to 1991, whereas the pattern for the general population showed a decrease of 73%. Similarly, during the same period, firearm accidents among Native Hawaiians increased by 300%, compared to an increase of only 100% among the U.S. population overall (Johnson, Oyama, & LeMarchand, 1996).

All of these issues are amenable to a variety of interventions. One issue, however, is whether the attempts to improve the health status of Native Hawaiians and other PIAs by simply using standard Western approaches, even those that are culturally acceptable, can fully answer the question of land and sovereignty raised by Blaisdell (1993). Blaisdell agrees with the standard of a *Maori* (Polynesian) physician, Mason Durie, who notes, "More effective utilization of land and retention of tribal lands as health measures in the broad sense may prove more effective in the long run [to improve Maori health] than advice about diet or early cancer detection" (Dure, 1987, p. 212).

Health Beliefs and Practices: The Effects of Pacific Islander American Diversity on Access and Use of Health Resources in the United States

Just as data on individual ethnicities are difficult to obtain, so too is information on health beliefs not as widespread as statisticians and authors would like. One difficulty with health beliefs is in pinpointing what is original and what is the result of an interweaving of customs and beliefs (Linnekin, 1983).

Blaisdell (1989), Bushnell (1993), and Chun (1994) all have documented Native Hawaiian health beliefs that were operational prior to 1778. The key belief was the spiritual aspect of a sickness and the relationship between sickness and the breaking of rules (*kapu*). Second was the link between the sickness of the individual and the community; sickness was not the Western individual focus but rather involved the whole community. These beliefs have been carried down through today. It is difficult, however, to clearly demonstrate how these beliefs affect the practice of medicine and people's access to health care. With the resurgence of all things Native Hawaiian, there has been a resurgence too in Native Hawaiian approaches to health and medical care, especially in the Native Hawaiian health care system. E Ola Mau, an organization of Native Hawaiian health professionals, has been organizing workshops and forums to investigate the extent of traditional healing practices. One of the key issues, however, has been the question of reimbursement. Native Hawaiian health beliefs suggest that the healer cannot be reimbursed directly for his or her healing work. Such skill is not a question of learning but rather a question of righteousness (Blaisdell, 1989). However, some healers have been seeking compensation, and insurance companies are interested in reimbursement. Discussions with Native Hawaiians suggest that, as in most cultures, traditional health beliefs are used along with standard allopathic medical practices.

The issue of determining what is truly a traditional health belief also can be clearly seen in the Samoan medical beliefs and practices. In contemporary Samoa, there are two coexisting systems, traditional and Western, based on a determination as to whether the sickness is indigenous (*ma'i Samoa*) or foreign (*ma'i Palagi*) (MacPherson & MacPherson, 1990). Depending on the sickness, treatment is sought from a traditional healer (*fofo*) or an allopathic practitioner. MacPherson and MacPherson (1990) suggest that these sytems will continue because there are many illnesses that continue to be regarded as indigenous. They suggest, however, that as Samoan communities assimilate in the United States, these differences will disappear. This approach of dealing with indigenous sickness with indigenous care and dealing with introduced sickness with Western care is found in nearly all of the other PIA groups.

There is no simple generic description that covers health beliefs. It is essential to know the geographic area one is dealing with as well as the ethnic group. Even the assertion that beliefs are subordinate to economics is debatable. If a PIA is living in what might be called a typical middle-class situation, with a regular job that carries health insurance, this does not ensure that he or she is going to find it easier to access standard Western professionals for all health care. Health beliefs and practices held by that individual will continue to play a role in determining whether Western medical care is accessed.

Tied in with the individual's health beliefs and practices will be his or her opinion of the appropriateness of access to available medical care services. If the person believes that he or she will be given inferior service because of the negative way in which the medical care providers might perceive the person (in spite of having the economic means to successfully complete the medical care encounter), then the person might not complete the encounter. The principle or strategy for improving this situation is based on providing medical care through professionals who are of the same ethnicity as the patient so as to make the patient feel more comfortable in the Western medical model. Two issues fall out from this solution. The first is that finding the appropriate professionals often is very difficult. Even if one finds the appropriate professionals, there often is very little with which to persuade the professionals to serve in that medical setting. The second is the more precise question of what constitutes an appropriate professional. Is it simply being ethnically linked to that clinic in the broadest sense? For example, will any Pacific Islander be appropriate for a Samoan population-based clinic, must it be someone who was born in American Samoa of the correct family but whose knowledge of Samoan may be very limited, or should it be someone who speaks Samoan well and has some understanding of Samoan beliefs and practices regarding health and disease but might not have been born there (or, indeed, might not even be a Pacific Islander by ethnicity)? As the Indian Health Service discovered, simply being an American Indian did not necessarily mean that an American Indian health professional would be welcomed in a specific medical clinic. Of course, the key difficulty with this approach to access for Pacific Islanders is again the small, scattered numbers that make it very difficult to provide appropriate medical care in easily accessible areas.

Finally, there is the economic issue hinted at earlier but made more direct in the words of the director of the Native Hawaiian Health Clinic, Hui Malama Ola Na 'Oiwi. In an interview in 1994, he remarked that the only Native Hawaiians who had used his clinic were those who had no jobs or no health insurance (Casken, 1994). Ethnically based clinics that appear to be primarily designed to provide medical care to those who cannot afford to receive it through their family physicians will become segregated institutions that have appeal only to members of that ethnic group who do not have other resources.

Barriers to Health Promotion and Disease Prevention Among Pacific Islander Americans in the United States

Faced with Western medicine and a health care system that is unfamiliar, Americans of Asian and Pacific Island heritage experience unique access barriers to primary care. In addition to linguistic and cultural differences, financial problems beset many subgroups, especially recent immigrants and refugees. (U.S. Department of Health and Human Services, 1990, p. 37)

The barriers to HPDP have been touched on throughout this chapter and in many ways repeat the problems faced by all ethnic groups discussed in this book. An immigrant family, unless well provided with economic resources, will be in a second-class situation with regard to medical care and health activities (Mokuau, 1996). Although the family's or individual's economic situation in the natal territory might have been no better than that in the immigrant territory, the lack of viable economic resources were more than compensated for in the former by the invisible social commitments that support communities in their home territories.

Coming to the United States, especially to the continental United States, is a radical change for many PIAs (Wong, 1996). In addition to the obvious barriers, the more subtle barrier is the political and socioeconomic climate of the United States. In contrast to all the Pacific Islander jurisdictions, the United States is basically a classical liberal society (Greenberg, 1989). It is a society that prizes the rights of private property above the property rights of the community, that stresses that the individual is responsible for himself or herself rather than being part of a responsible community, that views the free market as the best way in which to distribute goods and values as opposed to the needs of the community, and that believes the government should play a very limited role and should not try to control the free market, should not try to level the playing field, and should not take over an individual's own responsibilities. PIAs thus have to contend with a social system that, although it initially might seem familiar, is in reality a social system that is a contradiction to the one in which they were raised. When one thinks of the role of individual responsibility that has been built into HPDP activities since the first publication of *Healthy People* (U.S. Department of Health, Education, and Welfare, 1979), the barriers to successful implementation of these activities among most PIAs are immense.

CHAPTER SUMMARY

The health professional who is working with or plans to work with PIAs must consider a number of key issues as he or she designs an approach. The overall understanding must be that it is a myth that this is a healthy population. The myth has arisen in part because of the extremely limited amount of data available on this population. We know very little about the size of the population, the exact locations, the health needs, and the overall socioeconomic status. We do know that the population is extremely small in comparison to the rest of the U.S. population or, indeed, in comparison to any other ethnic group within the U.S. population. As noted earlier, PIAs form only about 5% of the Office of Management and Budget API classification and thus are totally swamped in any data that are used to describe that population.

It was suggested that even within this comparatively small population, there are major differences among the three main groups: Polynesians, Micronesians, and Melanesians. Perhaps even more noticeably, within those subgroupings, there are further differences based on socioeconomic status. Thus, the task of the health professional working with these populations becomes increasingly difficult. An additional factor is that the definitions that are used to determine who is a member of each subgroup are so vague that almost anyone could claim to be a member of any subgroup.

Because Hawai'i is the state in which the majority of PIAs live, this chapter has suggested that one approach should be to examine the situation in Hawai'i as a first step in approaching other PIA populations. At least two of the subpopulations are broken down within the Hawai'i State Department of Health's data reports. Yet even in Hawai'i, the same problems present in the continental United States are present in the state as well.

Temporary solutions would be to ensure that more of the data collected are broken down into sets that are applicable to this population. As we saw in the Hawaiian data, results that suggest that PIAs are reasonably healthy can hide major problems for those PIAs at the lower end of the socioeconomic scale. Perhaps the first charge of the concerned health professional would be to deal with issues of education, language use, and employment because these can be key to improving a person's health status.

Paraphrasing Pukui (1983), perhaps today one could say that now is the right time to work for the good health of PIAs.

REFERENCES

Aiu, P. D. (1996). Data dilemmas for API community-based organizations. *Asian American and Pacific Islander Journal of Health, 4*(1-3), 112-118.

Barringer, H., Gardner, R., & Levin, M.(1993). *Asians and Pacific Islanders in the United States.* New York: Russell Sage.

Beaglehole, J. C. (Ed.). (1967). *The journeys of Captain Cook on his voyages of discovery, 1776-1780.* Cambridge, UK: Cambridge University Press.

Bellwood, P. (1979). *Man's conquest of the Pacific: The pre-history of Southeast Asia and Oceania.* New York: Oxford University Press.

Blaisdell, R. K. (1989). Historical and cultural aspects of Native Hawaiian health. In E. Wegner (Ed.), *Social process in Hawai'i, Vol. 32: The health of Native Hawaiians: A selective report on health status and health in the 1980s.* Honolulu: University of Hawai'i Press.

Blaisdell, R. K. (1993). The health status of Kanaka Maoli (indigenous Hawaiians). *Asian American and Pacific Islander Journal of Health, 1*(2), 116-160.

Blaisdell, R. K. (1996). 1995 update on Kanaka Maoli (indigenous Hawaiians') health. *Asian American and Pacific Islander Journal of Health, 4*(1-3), 160-165.

Bousseau, S. J. (1993). *Fa'a Samoa: Yesterday and today—A resource guide.* Sacramento: California Office of Criminal Justice Planning.

Budnick, R. (1992). *Stolen kingdom: An American conspiracy.* Honolulu, HI: Aloha Press.

Bushnell, O. A. (1993). *The gifts of civilization: Germs and genocide in Hawai'i.* Honolulu: University of Hawai'i Press.

Casken, J. (1994). *Bringing culture into health? The Native Hawaiian Health Care Act of 1988.* Unpublished doctoral thesis, University of Hawai'i.

Centers for Disease Control and Prevention. (1995). *Monthly Vital Statistics Report, 43*(10). (Supplement DHHS Publication No. [PHS] 95-1120 5-0025)

Chen, M. A. (1996). Demographic characteristics of Asian and Pacific Islander Americans: Health implications. *Asian American and Pacific Islander Journal of Health, 4*(1-3), 40-49.

Chen, M. S., & Hawks, B. L. (1995). A debunking of the myth of healthy Asian Americans and Pacific Islanders. *American Journal of Health Promotion, 9,* 261-268.

Chun, M. N. (Trans.). (1994). *Native Hawaiian medicine.* Honolulu, HI: First People's Productions.

Daws, G. (1968). *Shoal of time.* Honolulu: University of Hawai'i Press.

Dearing, E. G. (1996). Asian American and Pacific Islander identity and classification. *Asian American and Pacific Islander Journal of Health, 4*(1-3), 82-87.

Dougherty, M. (1992). *To steal a kingdom.* Waimanalo, HI: Island Style Press.

Durie, M. H. (1987). Implication of policy and management decisions on Maori health. In M. W. Raffel & N. K. Raffel (Eds.), *Perspectives on health policy; Australia, New Zealand, and the United States.* New York: John Wiley.

Filoialii, L. A. (1980). *Attitudes towards the traditional Fa'a Samoa as a problem of adjusting to urban life in America.* Unpublished master's thesis, Pepperdine University.

Franco, R. W. (1991). *Samoan perceptions of work: Moving up and moving around.* New York: AMS Press.

Greenberg, E. (1989). *The American political system: A radical approach* (5th ed.). Boston: Little, Brown.

Hall, S. (1990). Cultural identity and diaspora. In J. Rutherford (Ed.), *Identity: Community, culture, difference.* London: Lawrence & Wishart.

Howe, R. K. (1984). *Where the waves fall: A new South Sea Islands history from first settlement to colonial rule.* Honolulu: University of Hawai'i Press.

Janes, C. R. (1990). *Migration, social change, and health: A Samoan community in urban California.* Stanford, CA: Stanford University Press.

Johnson, D., Oyama, N., & LeMarchand, L. (1996, March). *Papa Ola Lokahi Hawaiian health update: Mortality, morbidity, morbidity outcomes, and behavioral risks.* Report presented to Papa Ola Lokahi, MEDTEP Research Center, Honolulu, HI.

Kame'eleihiwa, L. (1992). *Native lands and foreign desires.* Honolulu, HI: Bishop Museum Press.

Linnekin, J. S. (1983). Defining tradition: Variations on the Hawaiian identity. In *American ethnologist.* Lake Forest, IL: American Ethnological Association.

MacPherson, C., & MacPherson L. (1990). *Samoan medical belief and practice.* Auckland, New Zealand: Auckland University Press.

Marmot, M., & Thewell, T. (1997). Social class and cardiovascular disease: The contribution of work. In P. Conrad (Ed.), *The sociology of health and illness: Critical perspectives* (5th ed.). New York: St. Martin's.

McCubbin, H. (1983). Cultural loss and stress among Native Hawaiians. In *Native Hawaiian Educational Assessment Project.* Honolulu, HI: Kamehameha Schools/Bernice Pauahi Bishop Estate.

Mokuau, N. (1996). Health and well-being for Pacific Islanders: Status, barriers and resolutions. *Asian American and Pacific Islander Journal of Health, 4*(1-3), 55-67.

Montgomery, L. E., Kiely, J. L., & Pappas, G. (1996). The effects of poverty, race, and family structure on U.S. children's health: Data from the NHIS, 1978-1980 and 1989-1991. *American Journal of Public Health, 86,* 1401-1406.

Native Hawaiian Health Research Consortium. (1985). *E Ola Mau: The Native Hawaiian health needs study* (5 vols.). Honolulu, HI: Alu Like.

Navarro, V. (1989). Race or class or race and class. *International Journal of Health Services, 19,* 311-314.

Pouesi, D. (1994). *An illustrated history of Samoans in California.* Carson, CA: KIN Publications.

Pukui, M. K. (1983). *Olelo No'eau.* Honolulu, HI: Bishop Museum Press.

Schram, S. F. (1995). *Worlds of welfare: The poverty of social science and social science's poverty.* Minneapolis: University of Minnesota Press.

Secretary's Task Force on Black and Minority Health. (1985). *Executive task force on black and minority health* (Vol. 1). Washington, DC: U.S. Department of Health and Human Services.

Stannard, D. (1989). *Before the horror: The population of Hawai'i on the eve of Western contact.* Honolulu: University of Hawai'i Press.

Stone, D. A. (1988). *Policy paradox and political reason.* Glenview, IL: Scott, Foresman.

Trask, H. K. (1985). Hawaiians, American colonization and the quest for independence. In G. Sullivan & G. Hawes (Eds.), *Social process in Hawai'i, Vol. 31: The political economy of Hawai'i.* Honolulu: University of Hawai'i Press.

Trask, H. K. (1993). *Notes from a native daughter: Colonialism and sovereignty in Hawai'i.* Monroe, ME: Common Courage Press.

U.S. Bureau of the Census. (1993). *Census of the population and housing: Summary of social, economic, and housing characteristics: Hawai'i, 1990* (CPH-5-13). Washington, DC: Government Printing Office.

U.S. Congress, Office of Technology Assessment. (1987). *Current health status and population projections of Native Hawaiians living in Hawai'i.* Washington, DC: Government Printing Office.

U.S. Department of Health, Education, and Welfare. (1979). *Healthy people: The surgeon general's report on health promotion and disease prevention.* Washington, DC: Public Health Service.

U.S. Department of Health and Human Services. (1990). *Healthy People 2000: National health promotion and disease prevention objectives* (DHHS Publication No. [PHS] 91-50213). Washington, DC: Government Printing Office.

Wegner, E. (Ed.). (1989). *Social process in Hawai'i, Vol. 32: The health of Native Hawaiians: A selective report on health status and health care in the 1980's.* Honolulu: University of Hawai'i Press.

Wong, D. (1996). Access, barriers, and problems of present working models of API community health centers. *Asian American and Pacific Islander Journal of Health, 4*(1-3), 88-96.

Young, T. K. (1994). *The health of Native Americans: Toward a biocultural epidemiology.* New York: Oxford University Press.

23

Health Promotion Planning in Pacific Islander Population Groups

GREGORY P. LOOS

There are numerous groups of Pacific Islanders, and although they might share certain commonalities (e.g., value orientations, colonization experiences, migration and development patterns), use of the collective term *Pacific Islander* is in no way meant to imply that these populations or communities are homogeneous in nature. Realizing this, complex concepts such as health and its promotion and disease and its prevention will vary across and within Pacific Island societies. Within this and other logical restrictions to Pacific Islander uniformity and comparability, this chapter discusses general approaches to the topics of health promotion and disease prevention (HPDP) that the author believes to be accurate based on his own circumscribed familiarity with the many different Pacific Islander populations.

This chapter is directed at Pacific Islanders in the aggregate. That is, the focus of HPDP is on social action for health rather than on individual behavior change. Furthermore, although the author's experience with Pacific Islander populations is limited to specific culture groups in the Pacific Basin and Pacific Rim jurisdictions, the approaches to health behavior change advocated herein are applicable to most Pacific Islander groups including migrant populations from the islands of the Pacific that have relocated to the U.S. mainland and elsewhere outside their home jurisdictions.[1]

To be effective among Pacific Islander populations, social actions that contribute to HPDP must use a variety of strategies including (a) advocacy that generates public interest in, and political and economic support for, health; (b) social systems that encourage healthy lifestyles as a social norm and that foster community action for health; and (c) the instillation in Pacific Islander communities of attitudes, knowledge, and skills that enable them to act effectively within culturally accepted parameters to prevent health problems (Stevenson & Burke, 1992). To make these strategies operational, it is clear that socially appropriate health communication and social mobilization strategies are required to foster community action for health.

The approaches to community-based health behavioral change discussed in this chapter rely heavily on aspects of well-known models of behavior change such as the importance of predisposing, enabling, and reinforcing factors espoused by Green (Green, Kreuter, Deeds, & Partridge, 1980), health belief models (Becker & Rosenstock, 1975; Fishbein & Ajzen, 1975), and frameworks for stages of behavioral change proposed by Andreasen (1995) and others (DiClemente & Prochaska, 1985; Rogers, 1983). The HPDP methods discussed in this chapter help operationalize these theories for the practitioner in an effort to facilitate more effective health interventions among Pacific Islander populations. Three approaches are distinguished and presented in some depth: community involvement/empowerment, foldback analysis, and social marketing.

Used individually or in sequence, each of these approaches is culturally appropriate for HPDP work with Pacific Islander communities. For example, because clan groupings are central to Pacific Islander cultures, community empowerment can be used effectively throughout the HPDP campaign process (i.e., from needs assessment, to HPDP campaign planning and intervention, to evaluation). On the other hand, foldback analysis, although useful throughout, is particularly valuable in reducing outsider bias and, therefore, is most functional at the front and tail ends of campaigns (i.e., to assess needs and to plan and evaluate interventions). Finally, given the geographic and increasing socioeconomic and intergenerational variations across Pacific Islander groupings, social marketing is recommended as the best approach for tailored interventions with targeted groups of Pacific Islanders.

In the professional literature, the breadth of HPDP planning may be comprehensive, incremental (Lindblom, 1977), or a mix in scope (Etzioni, 1977); planning also may be systems based or take an epidemiological perspective (Rothman, 1974). In this chapter, no one focus is championed more than another. What is advocated, no matter which planning perspective is used, is that the views of the Pacific Islander community must be engaged throughout if the HPDP campaign is to be successful. That is, no intervention planned and imposed in Pacific Islander communities will achieve the desired ends unless it is self-imposed. As such, it is more important to invest time to involve the Pacific Islander community from the onset than to rush into planning interventions that will not be supported or sustained.

This may be referred to as an indigenous planning model. Such an approach is emphasized for all phases of HPDP programs—assessment, planning, intervention, and evaluation. Each phase is discussed separately in what follows. To appreciate the recommendations made, however, it is necessary to establish some parameters for Pacific Islander populations as a whole and as they are discussed in this chapter.

EMPOWERMENT AS A PREMISE FOR HEALTH PROMOTION AND DISEASE PREVENTION AMONG PACIFIC ISLANDERS

Emerson states that "the secret of education is respecting the pupil" (quoted in Peter, 1980, p. 162). A fundamental principle of HPDP planning and activity is the need to keep in mind the perspectives of the target community and to evaluate people's health behavior in terms of a holistic concept of health. In this context, this chapter considers possible strategic parameters designed to improve HPDP efforts with Pacific Islander populations through methods that are politically, economically, and socioculturally acceptable to Pacific Islander populations.

Included in most models analyzing health behavior is a consideration of health beliefs and attitudes (e.g., the seriousness and causes of disease and one's degree of perceived susceptibility). In addition, health behavior models often include structural parameters such as the availability of resources and social factors known to influence service use such as demographic differences (e.g., income, age, ethnicity, sex). In a like manner, these same factors also are hypothesized to influence Pacific Islander health behavior and readiness to use formal health services. That is, for Pacific Islanders, multiple internal and external influences combine to determine health behavior, health status, and the potential for positive outcomes resulting from HPDP interventions. As presented in this chapter, health is not only a biomedical status but also one influenced by demographic, economic, and political parameters related to Pacific Islanders as well as to more conventional medical factors.

In addition to being easier to perceive population, political-economic, and material differences within and across Pacific Islander groups, perceptions of health and achieving qualitative standards of life for Pacific Islanders also are inclined to differ and to be influenced significantly by several distinct but interrelated psychosocial and cultural dimensions. Some of the more important of these, when considering Pacific Islander populations, include (a) a historical dimension (e.g., cultural heritage, colonial legacy, predominant religion), (b) a political-ideological dimension (e.g., organization of social rank, social value differences, different views about the importance of material or spiritual goods, different metaphysical interpretations of human life), (c) a psychological dimension (e.g., self-concept and roles of individuals in society, attitudes toward authority and cooperation, different readiness for change and experiment, the importance of "secondary" virtues such as punctuality and hygiene), and (d) a cognitive dimension (e.g., the perception, interpretation, and labeling of reality; the ability to express complex concepts in purely symbolic form as abstract, linguistic, logical, or mathematical principles that can be used without concrete objects or imagery).

An added overlay is the growing difference between traditional values and social structures and the expectation to share the benefits and enticements of modern consumption-oriented lifestyles. Differences in these views are creating increasingly dualistic societies in Oceania. This is particularly evident in those island communities with close and migrational relationships with former colonizing nations and/or advanced communication media (e.g., television, the Internet). Young adults and youths, seduced by consumption orientations and vestiges of wanting to emulate lifestyles of former colonizers, are torn most by these dichotomous circumstances.

This situation can create health-related concerns in the islands that differ between generations. Among Cook Islanders, for example, many teens wanting to migrate to New Zealand make the economic decision to give birth to children whom they can leave behind with their parents. The teens then feel capable of leaving the islands to pursue employment and experiential opportunities elsewhere. In exchange, the grandparent-caretakers receive social services from the New Zealand government to care for the children who remain behind and are left with emotional surrogates for the departed children. The result is a high teen pregnancy rate, the youngest population in the Pacific (50.1% under 15 years of age), and the potential for intergenerational psychosocial problems (World Health Organization [WHO], 1990, p. 2).

From another perspective, population growth, economic growth, and the increasing use of more technology-intensive production methods are threatening to result in a serious degradation of the fragile physical environment of the islands. As a result, direct and indirect environmentally related health problems will likely escalate. For example, the continued sale of old growth timber by the Solomon Islanders to purchasing agents from Asian countries such as Malaysia and Japan threatens sustainable development and the health of the people through loss of native flora and fauna as well as indirectly through the loss of topsoil for crop production.

Although the economic need in the islands is easy to intuit for most Pacific Islanders, the actual and potential negative environmental impacts, along with the possible concomitant impacts on health and nutrition, might be less easy to comprehend because they frequently are without precedent in the islands. Such negative impacts also might threaten Pacific Islanders' harmonic accord with the land that is central to their health belief system and psychic balance.

To address such complex issues effectively requires forethought and the development of intersectoral preventive health strategies. Such strategies, however, might compete for political priority with economic necessity in many of the island nations.

At a minimum, fostering successful HPDP strategies will require the ability of Pacific Islanders to visualize abstract concepts such as the long-term impacts of development and its potential negative influence on their social, health, and psychological welfare, that is, the ability not only to solve problems but also comprehend problems before they occur.

Development of such well-functioning and advanced cognitive capacities (i.e., the ability to understand abstract issues without prior experience) might not be fully possible among individuals in societies that are grounded in concrete life circumstances (e.g., the gathering, farming, and fishing societies found on many of the islands) and that lack precedent experiences of a similar type.

Furthermore, it is proposed (Arlin, 1975) that the ability to find health problems before they occur is an advanced cognitive ability that can only build on a history of sophisticated "problem solving." Such "sophistication" might not be established in many of the island jurisdictions that only now encountering complex environmental and health problems for the first time or that have little understanding of Western causative theories of health, relying more on animistic or fatalistic explanations for disease and environmental catastrophes.

Therefore, effective social action for HPDP in the islands will require both basic and advanced health literacy, which in turn will depend on culturally effective health communication strategies. To accomplish these ends, social culture must be considered and local vocabulary must be employed rather than professional health jargon and Western values (Loos, Hatcher, & Shein, 1994).

Many Pacific Islanders, however, might not have the means to establish communication and trust with health care providers and, because of this lack of trust, might be hesitant to share their traditional beliefs (Kumabe, Nishida, & Hepworth, 1985). Kim (1990) conducted focus group interviews in Hawai'i with several ethnic groups (e.g., Hawaiians, Filipinos, Samoans) regarding prenatal care. Men and women in this study complained that doctors did not speak their languages, did not verify their statuses, and did not share the same explanatory models for pregnancy.

Similar results (i.e., identifying cultural insensitivity among health care workers and language barriers for Pacific Islanders) have been found repeatedly in other studies (Loos et al., 1994). Thus, a major access barrier to health service use for Pacific Islanders is the general lack of health professionals who come from these ethnic groups, who comprehend their cultural values, and who can speak their languages.

Outside health workers' ignorance of Pacific Islander cultures can interfere with effective communication. Furthermore, "communication," for Pacific Islander populations, must be considered in a broad context including language and choice of illustrations used as well as tone, topic and context, body language, eye contact, and order of speaking (or when not to speak).

In addition, Pacific Islander deterministic attitudes toward health and disease (i.e., that poor health is a naturally occurring integral part of life resulting from a variety of forces) can cause Pacific Islanders not to seek health care or take part in HPDP strategies based on the Western view of health. Many Pacific Islanders lack familiarity with Western diagnostic techniques and treatments and, therefore, are apprehensive or outright disbelieving.

Information-seeking behavior also is different for Pacific Islanders. It frequently is less direct than that of Westerners; this is especially true when the information is coming from an "outsider." Relevance of the HPDP message to the beliefs, needs, and desires of the target audience is vitally important to engage Pacific Islander interest in an HPDP campaign.

Furthermore, investigation of certain subjects is inappropriate for Pacific Islanders, whereas investigation of other subjects is not only appropriate but expected. Therefore, fundamental cultural characteristics must be kept in mind during the introduction, design, and administration of HPDP assessments; the implementation of interventions; and the conduct of evaluation, not only out of consideration for the people but also for accuracy in the interpretation of their responses.

For these many reasons, for HPDP interventions across Pacific Islander culture groups to be successful, they must be based on a bio-psychosocial model of health that includes consideration of the origins and causes of health behavior in relation to economic, demographic, social, and cultural changes affecting health. As such, the primary goal of HPDP planning and intervention with Pacific Islander populations must be to engage the target community through the promotion of participatory processes.

Success in HPDP for Pacific Islanders will require both "bottom-up" and "top-down" planning and action. That is, learning from people, valuing their views, and listening rather than lecturing will be essential for successful community-based health promotion among Pacific Islanders. For these people, the methods selected must empower the target community to be centrally involved in the entire HPDP campaign process (Wallerstein, 1992).

Empowerment is a concept, a philosophy, a set of organized behavioral practices, and an organized program (Raeburn, 1992). As a concept, empowerment is the vesting of decision making or approval authority in members of the target Pacific Islander community. Empowerment as a philosophy and set of behavioral practices means allowing the members of the community to be in charge of their own lives while working on a cooperative basis for the betterment of the community. Empowerment as an organizational program involves providing the framework and giving permission to all members of the community to unleash, develop, and use their skills and knowledge to their fullest potential for the good of the community. Given this perspective of empowerment, the following should be kept in mind regarding Pacific Islanders:

- It is necessary to have community participation, not merely representation, throughout the HPDP process.
- The community must share responsibility in defining the HPDP problem and for its solution.
- For the HPDP campaign process to be successful, all influential stakeholder publics in the Pacific Islander community must be consulted and, to the degree possible, engaged to work together (Cronbach, 1982).
- This social connectedness is very important to the integrative dimension of a comprehensive approach to HPDP and to continued community support for the planned intervention.
- Although the HPDP project focus should consider long-term effects, it is more important to stress interim short-term objectives. The immediacy of short-term success will better ensure the Pacific Islander community participation in the HPDP process and sustain its members' interest in the longer-term horizon.
- HPDP interventions under consideration must be relative to a historical understanding of the specific Pacific Islander community. In this way, the selected HPDP

campaign will work through existing community structures and in congruence with the people's ways of operating. That is, it is important to focus on the context of the target population and to be aware of the conditions that will inhibit or facilitate HPDP interventions as these may exist in individual communities.

For Pacific Islanders, *empowerment* of people and community also implies an interconnected worldview with nature and the larger cosmos.

PACIFIC ISLANDER WORLDVIEW AND NOTIONS OF HEALTH AND DISEASE

A well-known *Maori* proverb says,

> If you tear the heart from the flax bush, where will the bellbird sing from?
> If you ask me, "What is the most important thing in the world?"
> I will say to you, "It is people, it is people, it is people."

Perhaps the most valuable result of all HPDP is the ability to make people do what they should do to preserve health when it ought to be done, whether they like it or not. As such, then, the aim of HPDP activity is not the knowledge of fact but rather the knowledge of values. When working cross-culturally to promote health and prevent disease, especially (perhaps) with Pacific Islander groups, it is important to determine where in their life views "health" is considered as well as what their beliefs are about, and their attitudes are toward, preserving health (Kamehameha Educational Research Institute, 1983).

Before suggesting new knowledge, attitudes, and behaviors, HPDP personnel need to empower Pacific Islander groups to express what health and disease mean to them. That is, how do Pacific Islanders define illness, what disorders do they recognize and which do they feel are susceptible to cure using modern methods, what are their notions of prevention and cause, what knowledge do they have of curing techniques, and how is illness tied to other aspects of culture? Such knowledge is gained during project assessment and planning and is foundational to the acceptance and success of HPDP interventions among Pacific Islanders.

To understand the minds of Pacific Islanders, Western notions of selfhood and individualism must be replaced with "a contextual perspective in which person, family, nature, and spiritual world are interconnected and interdependent" (Marsella, Oliveira, Plummer, & Crabbe, 1994, p. 12). That is, there is a "psychic unity" that binds the physical, mental, emotional, social, and spiritual being of the person with the ecological and cosmological, and the well-being of the individual (e.g., health) cannot be ensured unless the individual parts and the greater firmament are in harmony.

The distinguishing feature of indigenous island cultures is that they think of themselves as an integral part of the natural order that is a balanced relationship of people, Earth and its resources, and the greater infinite whole. In this context, the occurrence of disease signals disharmony that could be taking place at any point in the overall balance, and the promotion of health can best be achieved by redressing identified imbalances. For Pacific Islanders, becoming ill often is viewed as a naturally occurring process for redressing a social wrong as part of a larger cosmic order (Kinloch, 1985).

For example, among Hawaiians, the word *ola* alternately means *life, health, well-being, livelihood, salvation, curable, healed, saved, to save,* and *to heal* and is expected to be a way of living (i.e., in total life harmony). *Ma'i* (the wrong way of living) is the opposite of *ola. Ma'i* can be caused by bacteria or a virus, by an accident or injury, by by spirits or ghosts, or through retribution or revenge by someone else or the supernatural.

The Hawaiian word *lokahi* means healthful harmony and refers to overall equilibrium among all life forces and entities. *Ho'ola* (to do *ola*) refers to all of the healing arts including salvation, consultation, cure, and convalescence. As such, the concepts of HPDP align with *lokahi,* whereas health care services align more with *ho'ola.* Within most Pacific Islander groups, there are concepts and words similar to *ola, ma'i, lokahi,* and *ho'ola* (Hawai'i State Department of Health, 1991).

HPDP for the Pacific Islander never is an individual situation but always is a collective concern. Among Pacific Islander groups, the family is the basic unit of social structure, consisting of several nuclear families related by blood or marriage as well as adopted members (Kamehameha Educational Research Institute, 1984; Kamehameha Schools, 1985). The extended family system usually is headed by a designated "chief." This chief is sought for counsel, advice, and approval on any familial or personal matter, and the family as a whole typically is involved in both disease prevention and disease cure (Palafox & Warren, 1980; Pan Asian Parent Education Project, 1982).

Obedience to the family as a whole, family heads, and elders is a primary responsibility of all family members. The family is the key to the "island way" and has structure, meaning, duties, and pervasiveness that go beyond the meaning of family held in much of the West. The values of the family unit have retained their importance with Pacific Islander populations even as they migrate (Ablon, 1971; Janes, 1990). Because of this kinship allegiance, there is a sense of cooperation and responsibility among members to support and assist new migrants among expatriate populations (Labarthe, Reed, Brody, & Stallones, 1973; Prior, 1974, 1977; WHO, 1975).

For Pacific Islanders, ecological and cosmic harmony and reliance within the kinship group are central to the maintenance of health and are core to their belief systems. As such, these concepts must be incorporated throughout HPDP activity with Pacific Islander groups, from assessment to intervention and including evaluation. Fortunately, the communal focus of all activities among Pacific Islanders affords a basis for social action for health. Unlike many Western populations, in which the notion of "community" has to be created, the basis for healthy community initiatives is well established among Pacific Islanders.

COMMUNITY ANALYSIS FOR HEALTH PROMOTION AND DISEASE PREVENTION PLANNING

The process of analysis used to plan and prepare HPDP campaigns should consider multiple perspectives of need from key data sources to determine where the different perspectives converge and where the greatest consensus can be established (Bradshaw, 1977). The professional health community typically relies on normative perspectives of need such as those prescribed by professional health service and epidemiological standards (e.g., the *Healthy People 2000* objectives for the nation [U.S. Department of Health and Human Services, 1990]). Health professionals usually collect data related to these standards (e.g., vital statistics, mortality, morbidity, service use rates) to compare relative need across communities and to select targets for HPDP activity.

Although professional perspectives of need are important to identify health issues and target communities requiring HPDP activity, they are not necessarily adequate to explain how best to intervene, especially when the health professional and target community differ culturally. To empower and involve the Pacific Islander population in the HPDP process, means must be employed to also assess the felt needs of the community. Whereas some criteria of need for the layperson might be consistent with professional values, others might not be and still others might be outside the range of professional interests (Kamehameha Educational Research Institute, 1985).

For lay members of any target community, there are multiple life issues of importance, and where—or even if—"health" falls among competing priorities should be a starting point for HPDP investigations. Given the particular worldview and deterministic perspectives related to health and disease held by Pacific Islanders, HPDP might not be a high-ranked life issue (Hawai'i State Department of Health, 1988).

In an effort to determine whether the value structures of Hawaiians and other ethnic groups living in Hawai'i differ significantly, the author developed and compared three-dimensional value maps for Hawaiians and Caucasians/Japanese (non-Hawaiians) living in Hawai'i in response to the question, "What are the important things in life?" (the study methodology, foldback analysis, is discussed later) (Loos, 1998). Figure 23.1 presents these two maps.

For illustration of the value differences between Hawaiians and non-Hawaiians, it is interesting to note the dissimilarities in the two value maps. The important life issues for Hawaiians, generated by the community itself, tend to cluster together more than for non-Hawaiians. Indeed, the largest Hawaiian cluster joins five life issues ("me [1], knowing self [2], setting goals [4], close family [10], and belief in God [15]"). For non-Hawaiians, the largest cluster couples only two items ("safe neighborhoods [11] and community involvement [14]"). These visual cluster differences may epitomize the interconnectedness of life issues for Hawaiians (Pacific Islanders) more than for non-Hawaiians.

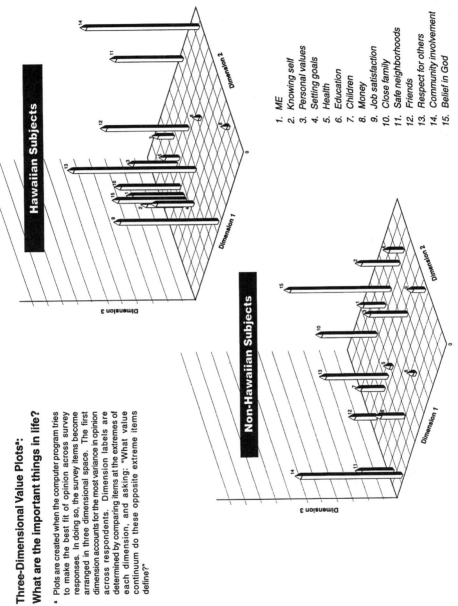

Three-Dimensional Value Plots[a]:
What are the important things in life?

[a] Plots are created when the computer program tries to make the best fit of opinion across survey responses. In doing so, the survey items become arranged in three dimensional space. The first dimension accounts for the most variance in opinion across respondents. Dimension labels are determined by comparing items at the extremes of each dimension, and asking: "What value continuum do these opposite extreme items define?"

Hawaiian Subjects

Non-Hawaiian Subjects

1. ME
2. Knowing self
3. Personal values
4. Setting goals
5. Health
6. Education
7. Children
8. Money
9. Job satisfaction
10. Close family
11. Safe neighborhoods
12. Friends
13. Respect for others
14. Community involvement
15. Belief in God

Figure 23.1   Three-Dimensional Value Plots: What are the important things in life?

These value maps also locate the relationship of "health (5)" among other identified "important things in life" for both groups. Determining this relationship, as we will see, provides vital information for the HPDP planner to design interventions that will be effective to influence community attitudes toward health.

For now, what is important to note is that the worldviews and connectedness of health *are* likely very different for Pacific Islander and non-Pacific Islander populations. To empower Pacific Islanders, HPDP methods must be used that will accurately record and precisely measure the study population's health values and beliefs without them being distorted by the biases of an outsider. This is the precise value of foldback analysis.

Foldback analysis is multimethod research that interweaves qualitative data collection and data analysis strategies to develop and explain survey research and community value maps (Loos, 1995). The method includes open-ended interviewing, nominal group dialogue, survey and attitude scaling techniques, and multidimensional and cluster analyses (see Figure 23.2).

These study methods are used in sequence where each procedure is "folded back" into the interpretation of results from the other methods. This sequenced approach combines the assets and helps to overcome the weaknesses of each method. As such, it is useful for cross-cultural studies in which inadvertent misinterpretation of data must be minimized.

The combination of techniques into a single, combined approach affords both a richer and a more usable database than does any of the procedures used alone. Therefore, it is recommended that the individual techniques be used in full sequence rather than in part. When this is not possible, segments of the overall sequence may be used; however, the full benefit of foldback analysis will be compromised.

Although the entire foldback process might require time upfront in the analysis phase of HPDP planning, it is time well spent because it (a) serves to engage and empower the Pacific Islander community in assessment, planning, and (later) evaluation; (b) provides guidance for HPDP campaigns and social marketing messages; and (c) reduces the chance of developing misguided HPDP interventions that will not be used or sustained by the Pacific Islander community. It is possible to adapt the foldback process for rapid analysis by replacing the large random sample (Step 4 in Figure 23.2) with a representative sample of key informants.

The statistical processes for foldback analyses are not complex and are available with several commercial software programs that are affordably priced.[2] These programs are available for use with personal computers, thus permitting greater use for the field health practitioner. The result is a bountiful database of community perception that can be used throughout all phases of the HPDP process.

Foldback Data Collection Process

The analysis of issues key to the local community is started during initial interviews (Step 1 in Figure 23.2) and then targeted, developed, and refined

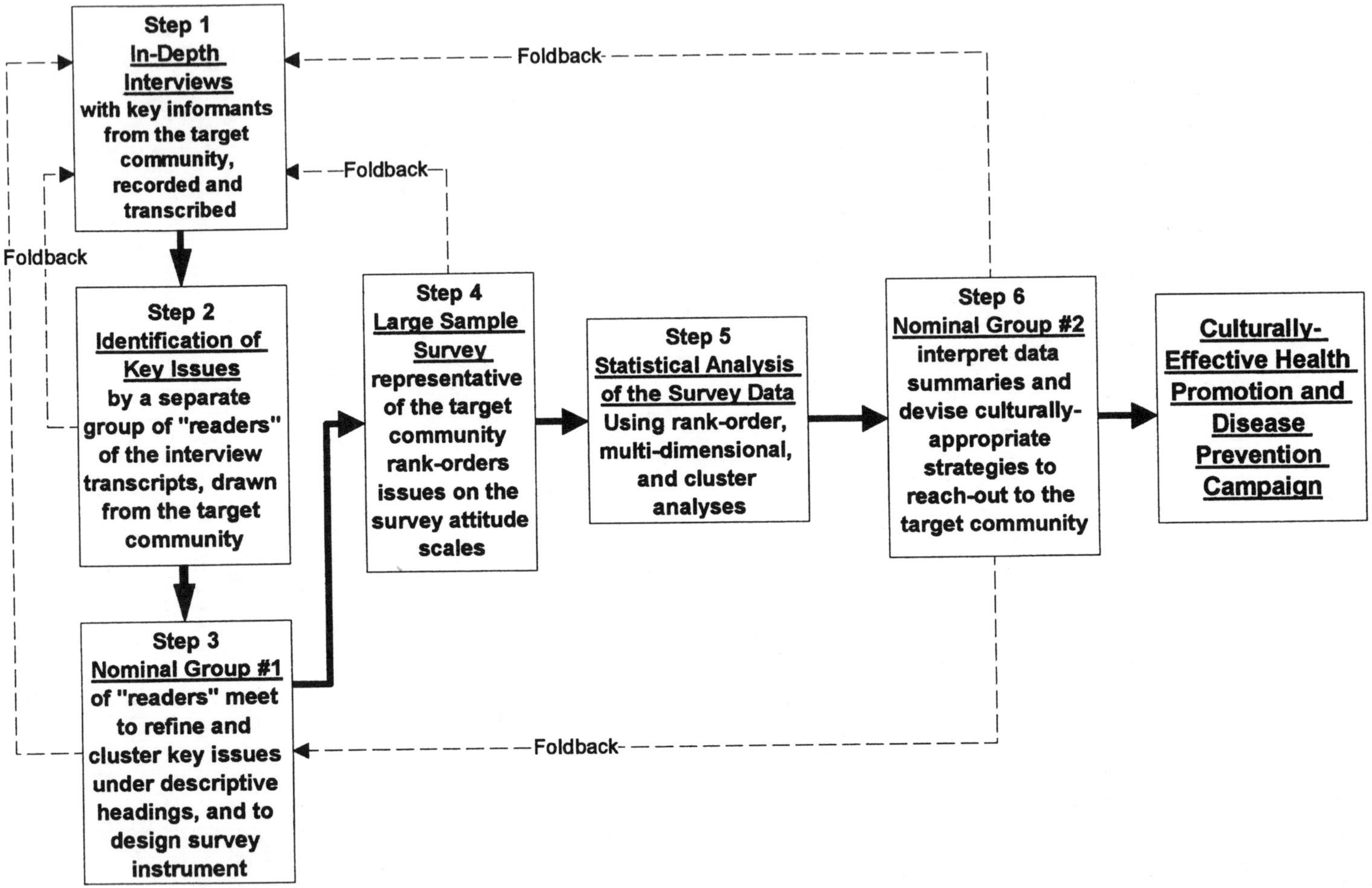

Figure 23.2 Sequence of Direct and "Foldback" Processes Involved in Foldback Analysis

during the first nominal group process (Steps 2 and 3). This information provides the foundation for the development of the survey instrument used with a larger sample of community respondents (Step 4) and later for the interpretation of survey results and value maps developed from survey data (Steps 5 and 6).

The survey instrument is formed by the community in large part using vernacular drawn directly from the original interview transcripts and nominal group dialogue. The target community also defines the sampling frame for the survey and helps to collect the data.

The survey instrument is constructed using attitude scales in whole or in part. Rank-order and modal score data are then made available to a second nominal group to analyze. These data also are submitted for further analysis using multidimensional scaling and cluster analysis.

Multidimensional scaling (MDS) is a procedure for transforming community ratings of similarity among, or preference for, identified "key issues" into a multidimensional graph or map (see Figure 23.1). In this manner, large and complex data sets can be reduced to two- and three-dimensional images for easier comprehension and interpretation.

Cluster analysis, on the other hand, groups key issues according to how similar or near in preference survey respondents scored them across the sample (see Table 23.1). In so doing, it permits the HPDP planner to identify which issues frequently cluster with which other issues and to determine concepts that are connected in thought among the target population.

Using Foldback Analysis for Planning Health Promotion and Disease Prevention Campaigns

Because the foldback process begins with a series of open-ended interview questions, it is important to direct these questions toward the HPDP issues of concern from the onset. Generally, however, it is productive to initiate interview responses with very general questions that most people can easily answer (e.g., "In your opinion, what are the important things in life?" "Tell me about a typical day").

Answers to such questions generally afford opportunities to explore more specific questions that might be crucial to HPDP intervention planning (e.g., community health beliefs about the target issue, barriers to HPDP use, HPDP interests and concerns, preferred channels of and locations for communication, how to craft messages to be most effective). Subsequent use of the nominal group and survey data can confirm community preferences among alternative HPDP strategies raised during the interviews.

All of the issues identified on the survey instrument and analyzed in Step 5 of the process (Figure 23.2) are important because they arose from interviews with members of the target community (Step 1) and were singled out for in-depth attention by them (Steps 2 and 3). Rank-order survey data, however, permit researchers to distinguish issues of higher and lower lesser importance among all the community-identified key issues.

TABLE 23.1 Cluster Analysis: What Are the Important Things in Life?

(a) Hawaiian Subgroup

Cluster 1	Cluster 2	Cluster 3	Cluster 4	Cluster 5
Me [1]	Me [1]	Knowing self [2]	Close family [10]	Safe neighborhood [11]
Knowing self [2]	Knowing self [2]	Personal values [3]	Job satisfaction [9]	Friends [12]
Setting goals [4]	Personal values [3]	Setting goals [4]	Respect for others [13]	Community involvement [14]
Job satisfaction [9]	Setting goals [4]	Health [5]	Belief in God [15]	
Close family [10]	Health [5]	Education [6]		
Respect for others [13]	Close family [10]	Children [7]		
Belief in God [15]	Friends [12]	Money [8]		
	Belief in God [15]			

(b) Non-Hawaiian Subgroup

Cluster 1	Cluster 2	Cluster 3	Cluster 4	Cluster 5
Me [1]	Me [1]	Setting goals [4]	Personal values [3]	Belief in God [15]
Knowing self [2]	Health [5]	Education [6]	Children [7]	
Personal values [3]	Education [6]	Money [8]	Close family [10]	
Close family [10]	Children [7]	Job satisfaction [9]	Safe neighborhood [11]	
Respect for others [13]	Safe neighborhood [11]		Friends [12]	
	Friends [12]		Respect for others [13]	
			Community involvement [14]	

NOTE: Table shows inclusive items and item numbers, as in Figure 23.1.

On the other hand, MDS permits HPDP planners to visualize the structure of community values that underlie the identification of key issues and the rank ordering in importance of these issues by the community. MDS value maps afford multiple insights into community values that underlie and shape decision making in the target population and that will be vital to planning successful HPDP campaigns (see Figure 23.1).

First, MDS provides an estimate of how much variance in community opinion underlies each dimension in the value map. Therefore, by labeling, understanding, and stressing these value dimensions in HPDP campaigns, the planner can better reach more of the target community.

For example, the first dimension in Figure 23.1 (left to right, contrasting "knowing self [2] and money [8]") accounts for 57.9% of the variance in opinion among Hawaiians.[3] Therefore, HPDP messages focused on this dimension alone could, in theory, attract the interest of three out of five residents in the Hawaiian community.

Second, interpretation and labeling of dimensions, and how best to use this information for HPDP communication within the target community, should be undertaken by the community itself. The planner should merely facilitate the process. Labeling dimensions is accomplished, first, by considering the items at the extremes of each dimension (e.g., "knowing self [2]" vs. "money [8]") and deciding what opposing constructs these items might represent (in this study, they were viewed as contrasting the "subjective" and the "material") and, second, by using these and other items along the same dimension but progressively less at the extremes (e.g., "belief in God [15], close family [10], and setting goals [4]" on the left and "community involvement [14], safe neighborhoods [11], and education [6]" on the right), the process of labeling tries to determine what common factor links all of these items in their displayed progression from one end of the continuum (dimension) to the other.

In this study, the Hawaiian community labeled the first dimension "the good and successful life." By emphasizing this motto in outreach messages, the planner could better secure the interest of the Hawaiian community in the HPDP message being delivered.

Third, MDS permits the planner to understand more how individual value subsets (e.g., "health" and "belief in God") are juxtaposed in the community's overall structure of values.

To increase the importance of a targeted issue (e.g., "health"), HPDP campaign messages should link the target issue with other issues of high importance to the community (e.g., "belief in God" was the highest ranked issue by Hawaiians in this study). By developing HPDP messages that discuss the target issue ("health") and the high-ranked issue ("belief in God") in the same communication, the target issue will increase in importance.

In addition, by using interconnecting items that lie between the target and the high-ranked issues on the value maps (e.g., "personal values [3]" and "close family [10]") (i.e., a line connecting "belief in God" to "health" would pass nearest these two intermediate items on the value map displayed in Figure 23.1), the importance of a lesser valued issue ("health") can be edged progressively toward the higher valued issue ("belief in God") and elevated in importance.

For example, by using HPDP messages that couple first *personal values*-"health," then *close family-personal values*-"health," and finally "belief in God"-*close family-personal values*-"health," the concept of "health" is aided gradually toward higher importance ("belief in God") among Hawaiians.

Fourth, together with MDS, cluster analysis permits researchers to understand best how to connect most effectively issues key to the community in HPDP campaign messages. Together with the MDS results, this information can be used to tailor further HPDP outreach messages to generate maximum interest in the target community.

Cluster data also can be used to locate HPDP services (e.g., at sites in the community delivering services appearing in the same cluster as "health." For example, in Table 23.1, "health" for Hawaiians is alternately clustered with "education" and "belief in God." Therefore, to reach the Hawaiian community, it might be preferable to locate HPDP services in church and educational facilities.

Fifth, the process of creating health campaign messages that are important to the community can be enhanced further by rereading the original interview transcript data for more in-depth understanding of the rank-order survey, MDS, and cluster analyses data. That is, by using the precise words and phrases of the target community drawn from the interview transcripts, culturally tailored HPDP messages can be created.

Sixth, by conducting a second follow-up survey after intervention as part of the HPDP impact evaluation, it is possible to determine whether the targeted issue (e.g., "health") did increase in importance (i.e., was higher ranked) and move in the preferred direction on the MDS value map.

Rank-order survey data, MDS, and cluster analyses all provide means to better understand the values of the Pacific Islander community (Carroll & Green, 1997). For the second nominal group, these data are more interpretable by returning to the original focus group interview transcripts and the work of the first nominal group. Using all of the foldback data, effective HPDP campaigns can be planned efficiently to have the greatest impact.

Strengths and Weaknesses of Foldback Analysis for Health Promotion and Disease Prevention

HPDP planning grounded in the values of the target community promises to have great potential for improving health promotion research, theory, and practice. Unfortunately, commonly used quantitative community assessment methods (e.g., aggregate rates of disease occurrence; knowledge, attitude, and practice survey research) seldom include in-depth "felt need" data from the subjective experience of the target population (Eakin & Maclean, 1992).

What is needed is a study approach that marries the cold preciseness of quantitative data with the richness of qualitative data in a systematic manner, that is, a study method that will focus on culturally sensitive HPDP interventions.

This is particularly crucial in developing countries and with minority populations in which health service resource allocations are limited and health status needs often are greater.

Foldback analysis offers both information-rich qualitative data and objective and measurable quantitative categories that can be easily manipulated to establish priorities and to assess, plan, and evaluate HPDP outcomes from the perspective of the service community. The foldback process engages (empowers) the target population throughout HPDP interventions and in the design, implementation, and analysis of the results. To date, however, the process has had limited use among Pacific Islander populations (e.g., with Hawaiians and Samoans in several studies).

The foldback analytical research model explains health behaviors in rational terms with minimal external bias but with no lack of procedural rigor. The analytic results are rich with information useful for crafting culturally appropriate campaign messages to plan improved HPDP interventions; and follow-up use of foldback analysis can serve as part of the evaluation process.

Conduct of all steps in the foldback process, however, does require an investment of time and resources. This is especially true at the front end of the project. Although possible, the adaptation of foldback analysis for rapid assessment has not yet been tested.

Although not a quick solution to HPDP planning, foldback analysis does afford a wealth of information and permits numerous opportunities for the planner to integrate with the target community. To date, the process has been used very successfully with some Pacific Islander populations.

PLANNING TARGETED PACIFIC ISLANDER HEALTH PROMOTION AND DISEASE PREVENTION CAMPAIGNS

Identification of Health Promotion and Disease Prevention Intervention Goals and Objectives

Because of the variation in economic, social, educational, and intergenerational parameters across and within Pacific Islander groups (e.g., between the main and outer islands, between home and migrant groups), it is best to tailor HPDP interventions for the greatest impact. Generally speaking, given the cognitive simplicity and heavier use of emotive strategies, it is believed that social marketing techniques would be more effective than detailed health education campaigns. Furthermore, social marketing, in addition to tailoring the message of the HPDP campaign, can use alternate delivery media and information dissemination media tailored to the infrastructure of the community and interests of the target group.

Most importantly, social marketing messages can be modified to the different stages of behavior change found across groups for the greatest progressive impact (Belinoff, 1996). Social marketing provides a framework for looking at health decisions from the point of view of the client and enables the design of interventions that address particular issues from the client's perspective, particularly because it employs (a) population segmentation and (b) a staged approach to behavioral change (see Table 23.2).

Social marketing, in contrast to other HPDP intervention approaches, employs more emotional (e.g., making the individual "feel good" about the message) than cognitive parameters. Given the likely great variability in cognition (e.g., worldview that can vary by location, social influence, income access, and other factors) among Pacific Islander populations, emotive continuity might be greater across publics. The author believes this to be true based on the continuity of value maps he has created using foldback analysis across several Pacific Islander groups (Loos, 1994).

Furthermore, because social marketing is based on classical marketing strategies, the intention is to repeatedly capture the attention of the community segment with short, succinct fragments of information rather than long-term engagement in detailed educational strategies. Given the community segment selected, different informational outreach tactics can be employed across settings (e.g., multiple communication media used more by the target group, in places frequented regularly such as church, work, and school) in an effort to reach the target group repeatedly and "drive home" the HPDP message.

Such announcements can be crafted from the information provided by foldback analysis and developed by the community segment itself. Short, culturally appropriate, catchy informational bits would be easier for the lay Pacific Islander public to develop and digest than would detailed HPDP educational curricula or other more cognitive-based approaches.

The hallmark of social marketing responsiveness is the needs, issues, and unique situations of consumers in creating programs or interventions, because otherwise there is a risk of developing programs that are not effective. Putting the consumer first (i.e., empowerment) on a continuing basis is what separates social marketing from health education or information programs. In fact, if consumers are kept in the center of the program with continuing dialogue (e.g., by using ongoing focus group processes), then the results always are a program built from the bottom up.

At the onset of the project, HPDP personnel, in collaboration with the Pacific Islander community, can target health issues of importance to the community and determine which segments of the community are at greatest risk. Once these are identified, representatives from those community segments can be engaged in a foldback analysis to identify their HPDP parameters of importance and preferred social marketing strategies.

Foldback analysis also can be used to determine the target group's current stage of behavior change, so intervention objectives and goals can be identified (see Table 23.2). The objective of social marketing is to move the behavior of the community segment from its members' current stage of behavior to the next (more preferred) stage of behavior, with the long-term goal that HPDP behavior is sustained in an ongoing manner.

TABLE 23.2 Schematic Overview of Stages of Behavioral Change and Social Marketing Strategic Issues

Stage	Precontemplation	Early Contemplation	Later Contemplation	Preparation to Act	Action Initiated	Commitment to Act	Maintenance of Action
Message issue	Make TP aware of new behavioral possibility and that it is not antithetical to TP's values	Persuade and motivate selected TP market segments to undertake new behavior by stressing its benefits	Persuade and motivate selected TP market segment to undertake new behavior by stressing its lower costs compared to status quo	Encourage self-efficacy of target and heighten social desirability of and support for new behaviors	Orchestrate TP opportunity for successful first experience	Determine whether new behavior is a one-time or repeated but finite action, situational action, or permanent lifestyle change	Anticipate what might thwart continued use and expansion of new behavior
Marketing goal	Increase TP awareness and interest; change TP values; identify barriers; overcome TP ignorance and presumed irrelevance for TP	Create TP's perception of benefits and positive consequences of new behaviors and negative consequences of status quo	Create TP's perception of lower personal costs associated with new behaviors and higher costs for continuance of status quo	Instill TP's personal belief that its members have the capacity to change and that TP's social milieu will support new behaviors versus the status quo	Make TP's first experience as rewarding as possible	Make continued action possible (i.e., reduce task complexity and time required); increase TP's priority for new behavior among competing behaviors	Create a win-win experience (e.g., prescribed social behavior change is adopted, and target is happy with change)
Prime Strategy	Provide education and propaganda to increase TP's perceived personal risk for status quo	Create a superior exchange of new behavior for old behavior that TP finds socially desireable, is easily undertaken, and affords TP added benefits	Create belief that perceived costs related to new behaviors are less than status quo costs and/or are manageable costs	Overcome TP's perceived lack of personal capacity and presumption of social opposition	Organize external environment to permit behavior to occur; it is urgent to get TP commitment to desired action on the spot	Make opportunities for behavior continuance as convenient and painless as possible for TP	Afford constant reminders and TP-appropriate reinforcers
Study caution	Consumers see few benefits and many costs at this stage	Use a single core strategy; emphasize benefits, not costs; focus on likelihood that benefits will occur and their value and importance to TP	Focus on short-term costs and cost reduction and efficiency-enhancing strategies TP can use	Cultural norms and values will differ for different TP segments	For major changes in behavior or lifestyle, "sequential approximation" of the ideal, repeated steps that are socially reinforced, might be required for TP to adjust slowly	Make the complex simple; success breeds success; some outcomes are less wonderful than TP imagined or are hard for TP to detect	Old habits die hard, especially when new behaviors are not as easy, convenient, and rewarding as TP expected (i.e., negative consequences can become excessive)
Research questions	What are TP's preferred media for communication?; times, places, and circumstances TP is receptive to message?; Do different TP segments require different messages?	What benefits does TP believe will occur?; How important are these things to TP?; focus on precise benefits and values, not benefit attributes or long-term outcomes	What are perceived costs related to new behavior, and why is each cost important to TP?; What are TP's preferences among combinations of benefits and costs?	Who are TP's opinion leaders?; identify TP's social networks and who its members turn to for advice; Who are TP's role models?	What are TP's personal rewards?; Is TP's locus of control internal or external?	What are TP's barriers and triggers to action?; What are new behavior's intrinsic and extrinsic rewards?	How can one improve delivery system, enlist social support, make benefits more visible, control TP expectations, and provide TP with skill training as needed?

SOURCE: Adapted from Andreasen (1995).
NOTE: TP = target population.

Selecting Appropriate Implementation Strategies

In order to implement strategies successfully in any culture group, it is important to be sensitive to its members' life view and learning and teaching styles. The need for such sensitivity is no less true for Pacific Islanders. How these people project, accept, and react to new ideas being proposed by "health experts" is filtered through their values, which influence how they perceive issues and what to seek, avoid, or ignore. Pacific Islander values may be subject to modification, provided that new ideas are presented through accepted social channels and processes. Therefore, these mechanisms must be identified and employed appropriately if HPDP campaigns are to be effective.

The ideas that follow, in large part, are drawn from (and might be limited by) the author's 20 years of professional experience in the areas of education and public health in the Pacific Basin and Pacific Rim. They are not meant to be fully inclusive.

Conceptions of Knowledge

In many Pacific Islander cultures, illness is considered the result of some moral transgression or the "hot" or "cold" nature of things. Presented without sensitivity, modern disease theory does not make sense to people with such beliefs.

Thus, it is crucial that the HPDP change agent understand that his or her advice might be misunderstood or ignored by people who operate with another concept of reality and understanding for cause and effect. The change agent also must appreciate that his or her values (e.g., the high value placed on good health and the maintenance of personal and environmental cleanliness) might not be mutually or similarly held across publics.

For Pacific Islanders, the learning of knowledge must incorporate both intellect and emotion—both head and heart. The power of the word must go hand-in-hand with a wholeness and connectedness to life. This final point is very different from the compartmentalization of Western thought.

Furthermore, among Pacific Islanders, knowledge is viewed as precious, something that should be aspired to but not too easily attained. Barriers to learning knowledge should be high enough to test learners' commitment and perseverance as well as appreciation once knowledge is attained. Holders of knowledge deserve respect so long as they earn it and deserve to be abandoned if they do not.

Knowledge also belongs to the group, not to the individual. As repositories of knowledge, individuals are (as trustees) expected to use it for the good of all. On the other hand, experts should not teach all that they know, thus forcing learners to hypothesize and invent as they learn. As such, the "problem-based" approach to teaching often is productive with Pacific Islander groups because of its heuristic aspects, in contrast to instruction that is solely didactic.

Traditional communities have numerous opinion leaders whom the change agent should engage in his or her HPDP efforts. For many Pacific Islander communities, these opinion leaders include family chief, church, and village leaders; traditional healers and birth attendants; or even local schoolteachers and postal workers. Less formal leaders might include local area recognized storytellers, market hawkers, and any area vendors where select publics might congregate (e.g., barber).

Furthermore, it is important to remember that many island cultures are matriarchal and that women remain important, although perhaps less formal, leaders of community opinion. It also should be remembered that socialization in many Pacific Islander communities, more than in the West, still is centered on strong gender-related roles in domestic and select public domains and that some topics might be taboo by gender.

Learning Styles

Whereas individuation and individual performance is fostered early in life in most Western cultures, communal behavior and learning is fostered early in the lives of Pacific Islanders. During the formative years, families assign chores to sibling groups, the eldest child usually taking the lead. This group approach to learning remains pervasive throughout life and across Pacific Islander groups.

For example, in controlled studies (Kamehameha Schools, 1985) conducted at the Kamehameha Early Education Program during the early 1980s, it was discovered that Hawaiian children taught using Western and indigenous study methods differed in performance. Both groups of children performed equally and on par with other ethnic groups on entry to the study. The children who were permitted continued use of group learning strategies, similar to child-rearing strategies found in Hawaiian homes, performed much better throughout their early academic years. By contrast, students who were required to adopt the Western instructional style (e.g., individualized seating, performance, and grading) fell behind progressively.

These studies suggest that group assessment, intervention, and evaluation strategies (e.g., focus group interviews) are apt to be more successful than is work with individuals. Furthermore, individualized assessments (e.g., testing such as the use of questionnaire forms) typically are less palatable to Pacific Islanders.

Much learning for Pacific Islanders is informal and semiconscious (e.g., through observation or embedded in the ongoing life of the community). Many lessons are conveyed indirectly in the course of doing something else (e.g., during chance social encounters or meetings of groups for entirely other purposes such as women's weaving).

For example, quilt making is popular among many Pacific Islander women, and successful HPDP communication can occur during such times. The Kamehameha Educational Research Institute used designs created by the target community and related to child growth and development as panels for quilts; as each quilt was constructed, the quilters discussed the importance of the information depicted in each panel.

Typically, prospective learners are put into group activity situations with a range of expertise and are "seeded" with experts, where participation is required. Newcomers are given assistance to develop skills and understanding but are largely left to observe, "pick things up," and hone their capacities for themselves.

Sometimes, apprentice-like or tutorial strategies are employed such as when a more competent worker is paired with someone less skilled and they work on projects together.

As such, there is much emphasis on the learners looking, listening, and imitating with a minimum of verbal exchange. Groups of learners work side by side learning by demonstration, trial and error, and joint effort. Moreover, certain things should be done only in context and for real rather than just practiced (i.e., learning by doing tasks in their proper setting). Therefore, learning work site injury prevention is done on the job rather than discussed in a classroom removed from the work site.

Among Pacific Islanders, the "medium *is* the message" because it helps shape and control the search and form of their associations and actions. Considering the isolation and lack of utilities on many of the Pacific Islands, especially the outermost ones, use of advanced media (e.g., television, videos, the Internet) is less prudent. Instead, "talk story" in "under the tree" small groups, radio broadcasts, the use of folk media (e.g., music, song, drama, dance, storytelling, proverbs), role-playing, and the use of pictorial presentations (e.g., wood carvings, paintings, shaded drawings [National Development Service, 1976, pp. 12-18], cartoons, comic books [Simonson & Sasaki, 1989]) all are accessible and acceptable communication modes and media (Abbatt, 1992, pp. 150-170).

Appropriate learning materials are essential tools for community health promotion and health communication. The just listed ways of conveying health messages to island publics also are good ways in which to involve the local community. That is, local composers, musicians, dancers, artists, actors, storytellers, and comedians should be involved in developing culturally appropriate health messages.

The best promotional materials should combine expert knowledge presented by peer instructors and materials producers. The risk of stating a message using incorrect "phraseology" and/or in terms that appear condescending or preachy is lessened when peer language and peer art are used.

Selection of credible spokespersons and recognized artists also strengthens the message. In addition, it is prudent to deliver HPDP messages at locations typically frequented by Pacific Islander groups (e.g., churches, sports clubs, community festivals) rather than more formal settings (e.g., clinics).

It is best to reinforce general or abstract ideas with specific, concrete examples or illustrations. Indeed, it often is best to use learners' own statements and productions in the promotional materials (e.g., these can be drawn from foldback interview transcripts).

Be specific and concise; do not use idioms unless they are well known (e.g., soda and chips vs. junk foods). Use common terminology rather than professional jargon (e.g., baby shots vs. vaccinations). Use direct, positive statements rather than complex, negative sentences (e.g., "You get Vitamin A and fiber when you eat fruits and vegetables" vs. "Studies show that if you don't eat fruits and vegetables, then needed nutrients and roughage required for good health will be absent").

Teaching Styles

Several "lessons" often are imparted at once (e.g., through storytelling that may or may not be directed at participants but rather at eavesdroppers nearby). Those who have knowledge to depart frequently make it difficult for learners to comprehend easily. For example, snippets of information are "thrown out," often without context or detail.

Pacific Islander trainers often refuse to give reasons or explanations for why things must be done and generally discourage questions. Stress is laid on memorization of the "right" way in which to do something. The responsibility for learning is placed on learners rather than teachers.

Sometimes, teachers tease learners for mistakes, but praise and blame typically are addressed to the group, and singling out of individuals in public is avoided. Disciplining is shared; it is done by whoever is closer. Correction can be heated, even physical, but sustained punishment is not condoned.

"Experts" favor the modest and withhold instruction from the arrogant. More important than individual attainment is learning to work with others and the skills of interpersonal relations and cooperation.

The teaching of certain types of knowledge is restricted on the basis of gender, descent, ability, and maturity, and these parameters can vary across Pacific Islander groups. It is best to permit the community to select the appropriate type of trainer for each topic taught.

EVALUATION OF HEALTH PROMOTION AND DISEASE PREVENTION STRATEGIES

Strengths and Weaknesses of Current Evaluation Methods

One obstacle to successful evaluation has been the way in which many HPDP activities are planned using an orientation to problems (instead of strengths) and that emphasize the medical model (e.g., natural sciences in the study of illnesses, which isolates individuals from their environment). The medical model is appropriate for linking a certain behavior to a specific disease (justifying the demand for HPDP), but its focus is too narrow to understand the social, economic, and cultural factors that underlie the behavior.

Increasingly, health promotion planning frameworks (e.g., the PRECEDE model [Green & Lewis, 1986]) direct attention at solutions (not just problems) and at intervention processes (not just program inputs). These same models correctly focus on intervening parameters (e.g., predisposing, enabling, and reinforcing factors) that can influence beliefs and attitudes and behavioral outcomes. As advocated throughout this chapter, these models must extend this same focus to program implementation strategies and the evaluation of program outcomes among Pacific Islanders.

What is essential to evaluation processes for Pacific Islanders is the participation of the community. Such participation is strongly encouraged by WHO and the American Public Health Association "in order to enable individuals [and communities] to determine for themselves the means to achieve optimal health" (Stoto, Behrens, & Rosemont, 1990, p. 12).

Disaggregative and reductionist views created by Western models of medicine are not adequate to assess HPDP programs for Pacific Islanders given their all-inclusive ecological, cosmic view of health and disease. To evaluate the contribution of HPDP initiatives, the opinion of lay publics of Pacific Islanders should be included using criteria of import to the Pacific Islanders themselves.

Good HPDP results among Pacific Islanders will require careful preparation to account properly for socioeconomic or cultural factors and variations. To accomplish this, the community must be involved. Indeed, the direct involvement of the target group in all HPDP project phases—assessment, planning, implementation, and evaluation—might be the most crucial aspect for project success. This is true because only Pacific Islanders can accurately view their HPDP issues holistically. This advocacy is appropriate regardless of whether a target population resides in the islands or has migrated.

Provided that the targeted Pacific Islander community segment has been involved throughout the HPDP process (e.g., from analysis to intervention), its members should determine the evaluation process as well. That is, it is *their* determination of HPDP need, HPDP project goals and objectives, and intervention design that is being evaluated. Therefore, it is best that they should determine how well these needs, goals, and objectives were met and how well intervention processes were conducted.

Process and Summative Evaluation Strategies

Community involvement may be critically important to successful HPDP among Pacific Islanders and is advocated throughout this chapter. Suggestions previously presented have related to culturally sensitive HPDP analysis, and intervention strategies apply equally to the development of process and summative evaluation methods.

Because HPDP initiatives with Pacific Islanders *must* include community involvement throughout, it also is crucial to evaluate the community's acceptance of these processes of involvement (e.g., the nature and scope of community participation, how it was initiated and sustained, whether it was productive and satisfying to the participants). Process evaluations among Pacific Islanders are better conducted using action-participatory research (e.g., employing ongoing focus group and talk-story strategies more than using paper-and-pencil activities).

Summative aspects of the project (e.g., the improvements in health awareness, policy and advocacy, health status, and health services use) can employ community participation as well. For example, a follow-up foldback assessment can be used to demonstrate whether targeted attitudes and values changed in the preferred direction, and observation strategies can be used to evaluate targeted behavior change.

The use of objective secondary analysis of extant data and project records by the researcher also can be employed because it need not involve the target community to gather and tabulate the data. The interpretation of these data, however, should be discussed with the community to better understand the meaning behind the numbers.

Health Promotion and Disease Prevention Materials Evaluation

Specific to printed materials used for HPDP campaigns (e.g., text, pictorial), it is recommended that they be tested using the Cloze Test (Folmer, Moynihan, & Schothorst, 1992, pp. 37-39). By deleting every *n*th word or picture segment, the Cloze Test ascertains how much of the message still is understood by the target population. That is, the more familiar the target population is with the subject, the easier it is to convey messages.

When materials are written in the native language, deleting every 5th through 7th word is suggested; when the materials are in a second language, it is recommended that every 10th through 12th word be left out.[4] A modified approach can be used for pictorial information (e.g., leaving out selected lines in a drawing).

Readability analysis also should consider the number of syllables per word and the number of words per sentence. Text that uses fewer syllables and words is generally easier to read.[5]

Finally, it is crucial to assess the materials directly, through solicited feedback from the target audience, by questionnaire or (preferably) by focus group interviews.

CHAPTER SUMMARY

To achieve significant improvements in the health status of Pacific Islanders, HPDP must become a priority. Although Pacific Island groups are sensitive to maintaining health and staving off disease, their perceptions of how best this is accomplished might be based on belief patterns and value structures that are uniquely their own.

For Pacific Islanders, the design, conduct, and evaluation of HPDP intervention strategies will be most successful when they employ "local" involvement in the production, implementation, and analysis. For Pacific Islanders, it is crucial for communities to make and follow up on their own conclusions.

Consumer-oriented perspectives, such as those provided by community empowerment, foldback analysis, and social marketing, are viewed as crucial to promoting health and preventing disease among Pacific Islanders. This is especially true because these methods are focused on and employ social groups as a whole and facilitate social action that is fundamental to the willing engagement of Pacific Islander populations.

To achieve healthy outcomes in the islands themselves and among expatriate populations of Pacific Islanders, it is essential that they be empowered to direct the HPDP process throughout (i.e., from assessment and planning, to intervention, to evaluation). Otherwise, Pacific Islanders will not engage HPDP concepts or sustain HPDP practices if they are not their own. Perhaps this is true for other ethnic groups as well, but it is central to Pacific Islander cultures.

Historical deductive methods, popular with the professional health community, cannot guarantee that they will identify needs and prescribe interventions that are supported by the Pacific Islander community. These methods emphasize professional hypothesis testing, with little attention devoted to inductive approaches aimed at generating culturally based health and disease hypotheses and concepts.

Foldback analysis, as a method of behavioral research, is particularly appropriate for engaging Pacific Islander communities in their own behavioral health analyses. Because foldback processes use the target community throughout—employing the researcher as a process facilitator—the results are highly meaningful locally.

The foldback process empowers the community in its own behavior analysis. To the extent possible, the researcher also becomes a participant and is viewed less as an outsider because he or she works *with* the community to assess HPDP needs and to plan and evaluate HPDP interventions.

Because of its tailored and paced approach to change based on the wants of the target audience and involving its members centrally throughout, social marketing HPDP intervention strategies are apt to work best with Pacific Islander populations. This is particularly true when considering the great variability of Pacific Islander group context, individual circumstance, and diversity of experiences found among the different groups and across subgroups. Because social marketing emphasizes stages of behavior change, HPDP strategies may be refined for different population segments and paced for progressive success.

On many of the islands, especially those of the South Pacific, the traditional collective responsibility system remains vital to the delivery of community services. This system also should be effective for promoting healthy community HPDP habits and lifestyles encouraged in this chapter (WHO, 1993).

The fundamental essence of HPDP for Pacific Islanders lies in community involvement for social action. The community empowerment, foldback assessment, and social marketing frameworks presented in this chapter should help create a receptive environment among Pacific Islanders for HPDP materials and programs.

NOTES

1. Relatively speaking, among cultural groups, there is strong continuity of social practices across Pacific Islander populations and consistency across settings within groups. Even when Pacific Islander populations relocate, social protocols and practices remain very much intact—even if other populations (e.g., co-workers, non-Pacific Islander groups) are engaged as surrogates for the familial and

social groups left behind. See Ablon (1971); Hanna, Fitzgerald, Pearson, Howard, and Hanna (1990); and Loos, Hatcher, and Shein (1997).

2. Most common statistical software packages (e.g., SPSS) include the appropriate analyses for foldback analysis procedures. One very affordable package, however, is by Borgatti (1992).

3. The first dimension for the non-Hawaiian group accounted for only 42.1% of the variance in opinion, implying that (a) this group is significantly less collective in its opinion (this makes sense given that its members are less uniform culturally) and (b) more dimensions would have to be considered to craft health promotion messages to reach as much of the non-Hawaiian community (i.e., the first dimension, at more than 40%, could address the primary value structures of only two of every five non-Hawaiians).

4. To calculate a readability score, the number of missing words correctly identified by the test population is divided by the total number of words deleted and then multiplied by 100. When 60% or more of the missing words are correctly identified, the language is correct. Scoring lower than 60% suggests that the text should be rewritten.

5. One approach, the Rudolph Flesch method, uses the following formula: Reading Ease = 206.835 − (.846 × Average Number of Syllables per 100 Words) − (1.015 × Average Sentence Length). Scores under 60 are increasingly difficult, scores 60 to 70 are standard, and scores over 70 are increasingly easy.

REFERENCES

Abbatt, F. R. (1992). *Teaching for learning*. Geneva: World Health Organization.

Ablon, J. (1971). Retention of cultural values and differential urban adaptation: Samoans and American Indians in a west coast city. *Social Forces, 49,* 385-393.

Andreasen, A. R. (1995). *Marketing social change: Changing behavior to promote health, social development, and the environment.* San Francisco: Jossey-Bass.

Arlin, P. (1975). Cognitive development in adulthood: A fifth stage. *Developmental Psychology, 11,* 602-606.

Becker, M. H., & Rosenstock, I. M. (1975). Comparing social learning theory and the health belief model. In W. B. Ward (Ed.), *Advances in health education and promotion* (Vol. 2). Greenwich, CT: JAI.

Belinoff, R. (1996, August). *Social marketing and its myths.* Paper presented at the Social Marketing in Public Health annual conference, Clearwater Beach, FL.

Borgatti, S. P. (1992). *ANTHROPAC 4.0.* Columbia, SC: Analytic Technologies.

Bradshaw, J. (1977). The concept of social need. In N. Gilbert & H. Specht (Eds.), *Issues, models, and tasks: Planning for social welfare.* Englewood Cliffs, NJ: Prentice Hall.

Carroll, J. D., & Green, P. E. (1997). Psychometric methods in market research. II: Multidimensional scaling. *Journal of Marketing Research, 34,* 193-204.

Cronbach, L. J. (1982). *Designing evaluations of educational and social programs.* San Francisco: Jossey-Bass.

DiClemente, C. C., & Prochaska, J. O. (1985). Process and stages of self-change: Coping and competence in smoking behavior change. In S. Shiffman & T. Wills (Eds.), *Coping and substance use.* Orlando, FL: Academic Press.

Eakin, J. M., & Maclean, H. M. (1992). A critical perspective on research and knowledge development in health promotion. *Canadian Journal of Public Health, 83*(Suppl.), S72-S76.

Etzioni, A. (1977). Mixed-scanning: A third approach to decision-making. In N. Gilbert & H. Specht (Eds.), *Issues, models, and tasks: Planning for social welfare.* Englewood Cliffs, NJ: Prentice Hall.

Fishbein, M., & Ajzen, I. (1975). *Belief, attitude, intention and behavior.* Reading, MA: Addison-Wesley.

Folmer, H. R., Moynihan, M. N., & Schothorst, P. M. (1992). *Testing and evaluation manuals: Making health learning materials more useful.* Amsterdam: Royal Tropical Institute.

Green, L. W., Kreuter, M. W., Deeds, S. G., & Partridge, K. B. (1980). *Health education planning: A diagnostic approach.* Mountain View, CA: Mayfield.

Green, L. W., & Lewis, F. M. (1986). *Measurement and evaluation in health education and health promotion.* Mountain View, CA: Mayfield.

Hanna, J. M., Fitzgerald, M. H., Pearson, J. D., & Howard, A. (1990). Selective migration from Samoa: A longitudinal study of pre-migration differences in social and psychological characteristics. *Social Biology, 37,* 204-214.

Hawai'i State Department of Health. (1988). *Timely prevention: The key to healthy children.* Honolulu, HI: Department of Health, Office of Research and Statistics.

Hawai'i State Department of Health. (1991). *Ka Papahana O Ka 'Ohana Ola Hawai'i.* Honolulu, HI: Department of Health, Office of Research and Statistics.

Janes, C. R. (1990). *Migration, social change, and health: A Samoan community in urban California.* Stanford, CA: Stanford University Press.

Kamehameha Educational Research Institute. (1983). *Life views of Hawaiians and non-Hawaiians: What are the important things in life?* Honolulu, HI: Author.

Kamehameha Educational Research Institute. (1984). *The "important things in life," for Hawaiians and non-Hawaiians.* Honolulu, HI: Author.

Kamehameha Educational Research Institute. (1985). *The perceived service needs of pregnant and parenting teens and adults on the Wai'anae Coast.* Honolulu, HI: Author.

Kamehameha Schools. (1985). *Developmental risk indicators and early childhood education services for Native American Hawaiians.* Honolulu, HI: Author.

Kim, U. (1990). *Culture, health care system and prenatal care: An analysis of three ethnic communities in Hawai'i.* Unpublished manuscript, University of Hawai'i.

Kinloch, P. (1985). *Talking health but doing sickness: Studies in Samoan health.* Wellington, New Zealand: Victoria University Press.

Kumabe, K. T., Nishida, C., & Hepworth, D. H. (1985). *Bridging ethnocultural diversities in social work and health.* Unpublished manuscript, University of Hawai'i.

Labarthe, D., Reed, D., Brody, J., & Stallones, R. (1973). Health effects of modernization in Palau. *American Journal of Epidemiology, 98,* 161-174.

Lindblom, C. E. (1977). The science of "muddling through." In N. Gilbert & H. Specht (Eds.), *Issues, models, and tasks: Planning for social welfare.* Englewood Cliffs, NJ: Prentice Hall.

Loos, G. P. (1994). A blended qualitative-quantitative assessment model for identifying and rank-ordering service needs of indigenous people. *Journal of Evaluation and Program Planning, 18,* 237-244.

Loos, G. P. (1995). Foldback analysis: A method to reduce researcher bias in health behavior research. *Qualitative Inquiry, 1,* 465-480.

Loos, G. P. (1998). *Value differences among Hawaiians and non-Hawaiians.* Unpublished manuscript, National Institute for Occupational Safety and Health.

Loos, G. P., Hatcher, P., & Shein, T. (1994). *Preventive health behaviors of Samoans in Hawai'i and American Samoa: A behavioral health research study.* Unpublished manuscript, University of Hawai'i.

Loos, G. P., Hatcher, P., & Shein, T. (1997). Health behavior strategies to improve rates of immunizations among Samoans. *Pacific Health Dialog, 3*(2), 166-177.

Marsella, A. J., Oliveira, J. M., Plummer, C. M., & Crabbe, K. M. (1994). Native Hawaiian (Kanaka Maoli), culture, mind, and well-being. In H. McCubbin & E. Thompson (Eds.), *Stress and resiliency in racial and ethnocultural minority families in America.* Madison: University of Wisconsin Press.

National Development Service. (1976). *Communicating with pictures in Nepal.* Kathmandu, Nepal: United Nations Children's Fund.

Palafox, N., & Warren A. (Eds.). (1980). *Cross-cultural caring: Transcultural health care forum.* Honolulu: University of Hawai'i, John A. Burns School of Medicine.

Pan Asian Parent Education Project. (1982). *Pan Asian child rearing practices: Filipino, Japanese, Korean, Samoan, Vietnamese.* San Diego: Author.

Peter, L. J. (1980). *Ideas for our time.* New York: Bantam Books.

Prior, I. A. (1974). Cardiovascular epidemiology in New Zealand and the Pacific. *New Zealand Medical Journal, 80,* 245-252.

Prior, I. A. (1977). Migration and physical illness. In S. Kasl (Ed.), *Epidemiologic studies in psychosomatic medicine.* Basel, Switzerland: S. Karger.

Raeburn, J. (1992). Health promotion research with heart: Keeping a people perspective. *Canadian Journal of Public Health, 83*(Suppl.), 20-24.

Rogers, E. S. (1983). *The diffusion of innovation.* New York: Free Press.

Rothman, J. (1974). Three models of community organization practice. In F. M. Cox (Ed.), *Strategies of communication organization.* Itasca, IL: F. E. Peacock.

Simonson, D., & Sasaki, P. (1989). *Bloodstream follies.* Honolulu, HI: Life Foundation.

Stevenson, H. M., & Burke, M. (1992). Bureaucratic logic in new social movement clothing: The limits of health promotion research. *Canadian Journal of Public Health, 83*(Suppl.), S47-S52.

Stoto, M. A., Behrens, R., & Rosemont, C. (Eds.). (1990). *Healthy People 2000: Citizens chart the course.* Washington, DC: Institute of Medicine.

U.S. Department of Health and Human Services. (1990). *Healthy People 2000: National health promotion and disease prevention objectives.* Washington, DC: Government Printing Office.

Wallerstein, N. (1992). Powerlessness, empowerment, and health: Implications for health promotion programs. *American Journal of Health Promotion, 6,* 197-205.

World Health Organization. (1975). *The prevention and control of cardiovascular disease.* Manila, the Philippines: World Health Organization, Western Pacific Regional Office.

World Health Organization. (1990). *Western Pacific region data bank on socioeconomic and health indicators.* Manila, the Philippines: World Health Organization, Western Pacific Regional Office.

World Health Organization. (1993). *Implementation of the global strategy for health for all by the year 2000* (Vol. 7). Manila, the Philippines: World Health Organization, Western Pacific Regional Office.

24

Promoting Health in Pacific Islander Populations

Case Studies

D. WILLIAM WOOD
CLAIRE K. HUGHES

The dramatic improvements in health care and social conditions in many developed countries have resulted in the near eradication of many infectious diseases. This epidemiological transition has meant that these nations are now faced with new diseases as the focus of attention for their health systems. These chronic diseases do not respond as did the infectious diseases; Dr. Ehrlich's "magic bullets" (Brandt, 1987, p. 40) seem ineffective in fighting these diseases, leaving both the medical system and the patients powerless to attain cures. With improved understanding of the etiology of these chronic conditions, prevention becomes the first line of defense against the pandemic.

As a chronic disease, Type II diabetes (non-insulin-dependent diabetes mellitus [NIDDM]) is a particularly insidious condition.

> The complications of Type II diabetes take root long before diagnosis is made. Type II diabetes is a "silent disease" that does not have the dramatic clinical onset characteristic of Type I diabetes. Several studies show that among Type II [diabetes] patients, 10%-20% already have complications such as retinopathy or neuropathy. (Zimmet & McCarty, 1995, p. 8)

Often taking as long as 10 or 20 years to manifest, the sequela of the untreated condition are devastating to the patient. The peripheral neuropathies often lead to amputations, retinopathies often lead to blindness, and renal failure often leads to end stage renal disease, with dialysis and death the all-too-common outcome of the disease. In part because of the insidious nature of the condition, its lack of initially clear signs and symptoms, and the fact that the preparation of medical practitioners often has less focus on chronic diseases than perhaps it should, it is estimated that the best of prevalence rates underestimate the condition by more than 50%.

Paul Zimmet, an internationally noted expert in diabetes, reports,

> By the year 2010, the global number of people with diabetes could have risen from 100 million to 240 million. . . . We expect the prevalence of diabetes in Latin America to double to 19 million. . . . The numbers could increase to 28 million in Europe and to 14 million in the former U.S.S.R., but the regions with the greatest potential increase by far are Asia and Africa. (Zimmet & McCarty, 1995, p. 16)

Data for the islands of the Pacific are less reliable but suggest similar patterns. In Hawai'i, no seroprevalence studies have been completed, but a recent monograph on diabetes suggests that not only are the rates increasing, they are doing so differentially across ethnic groups (Wood, 1994). Evidence from the islands of the Pacific also points to a rapid change in prevalence and a serious problem emerging with the disease (Federated States of Micronesia, 1997).

In fact, a suspected problem exists across the Pacific and among most indigenous peoples of the world. As is evidenced elsewhere—Native Americans, Aborigines in Australia, Chamorros in Guam, Samoans in both American Samoa and Western Samoa—all are affected. This chapter focuses on diabetes prevention among Pacific Islanders in their natural settings with the hope that interpretation of what seems to work "at home" will be possible for those Pacific Islanders resident in the continental United States.

The authors' expectation, within any of the literature searches performed for this chapter, was that many discussions about cultural competence and health programs for minority groups would emerge. This turned out, in general, not to be the case, meaning that discussions of minority populations did not necessitate discussions about cultural competence for health programs. Because the authors' initial review of the literature did not yield all of the information in which they were interested, the authors broadened the search to include cultural competence issues that were not necessarily associated with health activities.

What are the factors that the health promoter must consider if he or she were to develop a culturally sensitive health promotion program for minorities? The recent literature suggests the following:

Sinclair (1991) suggests that when considering minorities, age, education, economics, and community also should be considered or controlled in the development of a culturally sensitive program that is to be effective. Avila and Hovell (1994) found that exercise and diet modification training among Latinas was effective for decreasing obesity and increasing fitness within the targeted group, low socioeconomic status Mexican American women ($N = 44$). The Shintani et al. and Hawai'i-based Traditional Hawaiian Diet (THD) programs represent a Native Hawaiian, community-based activity developed as a response to the high rates of obesity and chronic illness associated with this ethnic affiliation (Shintani, Beckham, O'Connor, Hughes, & Sato, 1994). The THD is a 3-week program that relies on eight interventions: a noncaloric restricted weight loss program, dietary clinical intervention, cultural sensitivity, a transition diet, a whole person approach, group support, community intervention, and role modeling.

Obesity often is associated with NIDDM. Auslander, Haire-Joshu, Houston, and Fisher (1992) worked with African Americans with lower socioeconomic status and obesity, as one example. Their intervention was community based, focusing on four community organization strategies: integrating community values into health messages, facilitating neighborhood decision making, making use of formal and informal networks, and empowering.

In addition, outreach strategies are suggested to reach the African American population, as shown by Nakyonyi's (1993) work in Canada. A community-based outreach AIDS information program was presented that relies on educational material and media contacts. Educational material was suggested on various subjects including misconceptions, marriage, sexuality, confidentiality, basic HIV/AIDS information, condoms, homophobia, and the use of videos.

Other health promotion programs also are culturally sensitive. Whereas Auslander's et al. (1992) and Nakyonyi's (1993) previous efforts focused on the African American population, the work of Samolsky, Dunker, and Hynak-Hankinson (1990) focused on the major health problem associated with the Hispanic population. Their work included energy, fat and salt diet modification, and suggested that it is important to consider both cultural and demographic influences in helping this population. Heath, Wilson, Smith, and Leonard (1991) state that cardiovascular disease also is a problem for the Zuni Indians and suggest participation in a community-based exercise program and benefits associated with weight loss competitions.

Forety (1994) observed in a study that the Mexican American participants in their family-oriented approach were divided among three groups: a booklet-only comparison group, an individual group that received the booklet and a year's worth of classes, and a family group that received the booklet and a year's worth of family classes. Their unsurprising results were that those in the individual and family year-long group sessions had greater weight losses than did those in the pamphlet-based information-only group.

Alternatively, Rogler, Cortes, and Malgady (1994) suggest that a culturally sensitive program for Puerto Ricans (in New York City) would reflect and consider idiomatic phrases associated with anguish. Their work started with focus groups, then solicited important volunteers from the community, and finally compared the information obtained with the views of community-based mental health professionals. Their work suggested that sensitivity to idiomatic expressions more often was associated with an increase in use of services.

Similarly, de Leon Siantz's (1990) work, predominantly with Mexican American migrant farm workers (but also with Cubans and Puerto Ricans), emphasized lifestyle, problems, and strengths and needs often associated with depression. Important cultural characteristics included religion, familial perspective, male dominance, machismo, and the roles of women and children. de Leon Siantz suggests that for an assessment to be culturally sensitive, it has to include health status, education level, a measure of acculturation, degree of participation in traditional culture, and length of stay in the United States.

Schwab, Meyer, and Merrell (1994) report interesting work in their effort to design a culturally sensitive instrument that measured health beliefs and attitudes of Mexican Americans with diabetes. This is of special interest because of the well-acknowledged relationship between diabetes and diet. They relied on the health belief model because of its potential predictive value regarding health behaviors. Their work suggests that the model was effective for two of the five subscales: barriers and benefits. To ensure cultural sensitivity they added acculturation and fatalism subscales.

Alternatively, Castro de Alvarez's (1990) work in AIDS prevention among Puerto Rican women considered the cultural factors that contribute to the perception of risk and associated behavioral changes in examining culturally sensitive AIDS prevention programs. Castro de Alvarez suggests that such programs need to be culturally sensitive to gender role expectations and the role of motherhood. These Latinas may benefit from a health promotion program that assists them in executing self-protective behaviors. Such a program would consider that a Latina population expects a program to be sensitive to respect and modesty; therefore, suggestive clothing in a heterogeneous exercise class would be difficult for such a population.

What is the relationship between health promotion and empowerment? McFarlane and Fehir (1994) relied on the concepts often associated with empowerment—unity, validation of key health promoters, and the acceptance of a community's ability to identify and reestablish its own health needs. In this case, volunteer mothers were paired with mothers vis-à-vis community coalitions (with health clinics, social service agencies, local businesses, schools, churches, elected officials, and the media) to facilitate increasing access to health care.

From a more general perspective, Braithwaite, Bianchi, and Taylor (1994), relying on ethnographic procedures, suggest advocating for empowerment for disadvantaged populations by participating in the planning, assessment, and implementation of community-based health initiatives that have been identified as necessary for health promotion and disease prevention programs. Their research suggests that we rely on the intersection of three concepts: development of community-owned plans, community organizations, and ethnographic procedures. They suggest that consideration of these concepts is the most effective way in which to plan health intervention programs.

One of the problems among minority groups is a question of access and stage of diagnosis. When cancer is detected in its earlier stages (Stages 1 and 2), the survival rates are much greater than with the diagnosis of more advanced cases (Stages 3 and 4). Michielutte, Sharp, Dignan, and Blinson (1994) report that cancer is the third leading cause of mortality among Native Americans. They note that the presently existing intervention programs for Caucasians are not culturally relevant for the American Indian population. Their work explores fundamental differences in both behaviors and values between Caucasians and American Indians. Furthermore, van Breda (1989) notes that Native American children are products of their surrounding society, in this case often associated with poverty and alcoholism and its associated problems—diabetes, gastroenteritis, accidents, and fetal alcohol syndrome.

What are the issues and difficulties associated with culturally sensitive exercise programs? Lewis, Raczynski, Heath, Levinson, and Cutter (1993) and Lewis, Raczynski, Heath, Levinson, Hilyer, and Cutter (1993), among others, note that low-income and minority groups, in this case African American communities, tend to be less physically active than the general population. To facilitate participation, Lewis and colleagues collected data by focus groups and then conducted a random survey of Alabama residents' exercise practices, beliefs, and barriers to and facilitators of physical activity. They found that trained community leaders with intervention expertise were more likely to be associated with participation in physical activity.

More broadly, Campinha-Bacote (1994) suggests that we consider a culturally sensitive model, the culturally competent model of care, which includes awareness, knowledge, skill, and encounter as critical parts of a culturally sensitive model for those considering psychiatric nursing. The model views competence as a process, not as a static characteristic that ought to be incorporated into the provision of services.

In general, the culturally sensitive literature has focused on the groups mentioned heretofore, although the authors did find some interesting work by Watt, Howel, and Lo (1993) for the Chinese population. These researchers suggest that the Chinese have a lack of knowledge about health care possibilities in England. They asked this sample of 30 Chinese who frequented shops to fill out a questionnaire about their knowledge, use, and experiences that were associated with primary health care and health promotion. With a 71% return rate, it was determined that the Chinese are not making optimal use of health services. This population uses some services inappropriately (e.g., emergency clinics), whereas they underuse preventive health programs. The suggested reasons for either the inappropriate use or the underuse of services were language and communication difficulties.

What role does health promotion play among immigrant populations? The Levin-Zamir, Lipsky, Goldberg, and Melamed (1993) case study of Ethiopian immigrants to Israel found that the immigrants relied on an anthropological approach to bridge the gap between the skills brought from the existing country and the skills expected in Israel. Their work relied on educating the immigrant population about health services, nutrition, medication, the prevention of accidents, first aid, and the use of personal hygiene. Their program relied on visual tools, similar to the concern about the development of module tools, and was well accepted.

Jeffery's (1991) work best summarizes the section of literature focusing on culturally relevant health promotion programs for minority groups. He argues that the obesity among minority groups is better understood and intervened from a larger cultural theme perspective. The environment is assumed not to provide the necessary access of appetizing food at a low cost for underserved populations, and one needs to understand that for many underserved populations, exercise is not a sought after activity.

PROPOSALS FOR PREVENTION

In examining the potential of various interventions for Type II diabetes, several factors emerge that need to be examined. First, tradition in health education would suggest that for this type of condition (asymptomatic), some sort of health belief model (Rosenstock, 1974) based intervention would be appropriate. Unfortunately, many programs designed around these theoretical parameters (e.g., American Diabetes Association Prevention programs) have been unsuccessful among minority populations. Interestingly, the literature has been especially silent on the fact that for many minority populations, the salience of the threat for the disease is considerably lower than that for more immediate life threats from other external stimuli (e.g., violence, poverty, drugs). In fact, in reviewing the many theoretical proposals for the modification of human behavior with respect to disease, one finds the issue of overall or global risk and the salience of the particular risk to be avoided and sadly missing.

This chapter does not deal with the theoretical development of health promotion and disease prevention programs. However, as can be seen in several case studies that follow, the theme of multiple risk and intervention is continued.

LEVELS OF PREVENTION

Because of the long and complex etiology of most chronic diseases, the fact that the disease goes undiscovered for many years, and the fact that many of the sequelae of the disease often do not manifest for many years after diagnosis, prevention programs must differentially focus on several distinct population groups, each with specific prevention needs. For the asymptomatic, undiagnosed, high-risk population, awareness of the disease as a "real" life threat that can be avoided and controlled is essential; for these individuals, the adoption of healthy diets, lifelong exercise programs, and the periodic monitoring of blood glucose and general health is needed. For those diagnosed but as yet without the serious sequelae of the disease evident (e.g., neuropathy, retinopathy, renal dysfunction), the regimen for prevention shifts to one of more direct actions that will reduce the risk of the diabetes-related outcomes. More rigid control of diet, compliance with drug regimens, increased exercise, controlled weight loss programs, and (above all) regular monitoring of blood sugar and monitoring for the signs of advancement of the disease are essential. Finally, for those already symptomatic with the sequela of the disease, the regimen shifts to one of attempting to slow the inevitable processes. Close monitoring of the blood sugar levels, more

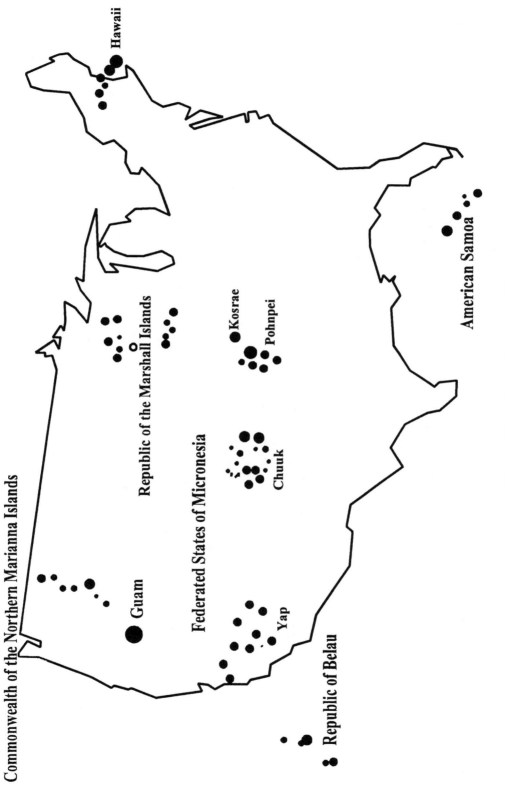

Figure 24.1   The Pacific Islands of Micronesia

aggressive drug therapy, and increased emphasis of dietary control, exercise, and weight loss usually are an essential part of the effort. All of these levels of prevention are amply infused with education about the disease, its etiology, and the ways in which the individual can alter the course of the disease.

DESCRIPTION OF CASE STUDIES

The case studies that follow are brief descriptions of efforts by local people to solve local problems. They are this way because this is what has been shown to work best in the islands of the Pacific. For the reader intent on adopting and adapting these programs to his or her own local setting on the mainland, a note of caution is in order. These programs were not externally derived. They arose from the bottom up, from seeds sown over the years, and finally began to bloom after local people acquired the necessary skills to make them happen. They are the essence of community development and community participation. They are "from the people."

As a general description, the Kosrae Gardening Project and the THD program are presented in two different ways. First, each is described on the basis of its central features as a sort of overview of the project. Then, each is presented systematically across the same variables to allow for comparison of the two projects.

In the Pacific, distances are enormous. The many island states and nations cover a portion of the Earth that is equivalent in size to the continental United States but with virtually no land and few people (Figure 24.1). With Hawai'i anchored as the easternmost point, the distance to Guam and Palau is approximately the same as that from Boston to Los Angeles. The population of this entire region (including Hawai'i), however, is well under 1.5 million. Island life creates special demands on the health systems of the region. Prevention, although logically beneficial to the health of the people, is not always well defined by the various health departments. This section of the chapter speaks to the role of the community in developing culturally appropriate disease prevention strategies and to promoting them in Micronesia.

The Kosrae Gardening Project

Summary

The island of Kosrae has seen the occurrence of many cases of Type II diabetes, with the negative sequelae resulting in the island population having a burden of disease costing more than the inhabitants can meet using conventional treatment paid by local resources. For those who have been medically referred to other islands or to Hawai'i for renal dialysis, the cost is so prohibitive that it cannot be borne in the long run. The Department of Health in Kosrae state always has had a strong public health program using public health nurses as both educators and outreach workers as well as for the provision of care in the community. From within this group, a simple plan to make affordable a better diet for those with diabetes and their families was begun.

The Kosrae Gardening Project has no official sanction from the government or health department, and it has essentially no budget—just people caring for people. The administrator for public health is a nurse in the Department of Health and was the instigator of the project, starting with patients who seemed amenable to taking some sort of concrete action to control their diabetes and eventually expanding that net to those families with an interest in learning about gardening and diabetes prevention at the same time.

The structure of the program is simplicity at its finest in that it calls on the basic cultural values of the population of Kosrae, namely independence and respect for the land. The skills development phase was quite short in that the initial participants were older and had previous experience with gardening. The health education phase began immediately with choice of produce to grow and followed through with preparation tips and actual demonstrations. The program had a natural duration, one cycle of growing (about 3 months), and allowed for ample discussion time with the public health nurse regarding diabetes control, dietary exchange, and the importance of exercise. In addition, the program duration was sufficient to establish the extent to which the diabetes was in control in the participants.

The second round of the project used those already participating in the project to work with others with minimal public health nurse intervention. Materials were provided for the educational component, and several special sessions also were held by the nurse; however, in general, the project was self-operating. Initially, 6 individuals participated. The second round saw 4 more join in. After 3 years, a total of 14 persons with diabetes had participated in this community project.

The Setting

Kosrae is the easternmost state in the Federated States of Micronesia (FSM), located about 2,500 miles west of Hawai'i at approximately 5′ 19″ North Latitude and 163° East Longitude. It is the smallest of the four states of the Federal States of Micronesia, with a land mass of 43.2 square miles, a population of 7,435, and no outer islands. Because of the size and the fact that Kosrae is the only state within the federation without outer islands, accessibility to health is ideally excellent. The economy is rural subsistence, with an annual average per capita domestic product of $1,989 (U.S.).

The population of Kosrae increased from about 4,305 in 1973 to 7,354 in 1994, an increase of 70% over the past two decades. The age and gender composition of the population also has changed over the past two decades. In general, the gender ratio has remained in excess of 100, indicating that there are more males than females in Kosrae. However, as is shown in the following population pyramids, the reverse (more females than males) is true for the 15- to 19-year, 20- to 24-year, and 55- to 59-year age groups (State of Kosrae, 1996).

The proportion of the younger generation has shown a gradual decline, whereas that of the adult population has gradually increased. For example, the proportion of the population under 10 years of age declined from a high of 34.4% to a low of 27.3%, whereas the proportion of those age 15 years or over increased from 63.3% to a high of 72.6%. The median age increased from 15.9 years in 1973 to 18.8 years in 1994, about a 3-year increase over the past two decades. These figures indicate that the population is gradually getting older. The reason for this gradual aging is mainly due to a decline in fertility, a continued low level of mortality, and age-selective migration.

This sets the stage in which the epidemiological transition (Gribble & Preston, 1993) found in many developing countries should be occurring, and in Kosrae we see a rapid increase in chronic disease while the burden of infectious disease remains. Over the past two decades, the causes of both morbidity and mortality have changed from essentially sanitation-based problems to more chronic and lifestyle-related problems (State of Kosrae, 1996, Appendix B). Over the same two decades, dependence on imported food has become very high, with canned goods being the main source of produce and protein. Type II diabetes is a major concern for the population of this small island. In 1994, there were no patients abroad for renal dialysis, but there were an estimated 277 individuals identified as diabetics on the island.

Kosreans are a proud people with a strong religious affiliation (Ridgell, 1988). The island is without bars and without dancing. On Sundays in Kosrae, there is no shopping, no television, no beachgoing, and no parties; there is only church attendance. Alcohol is consumed by permit only, with visitors required to obtain a permit after 3 days if they wish to purchase and consume alcohol. With the traditional culture almost destroyed through the diseases of modernization during the late 19th and early 20th centuries, the missionaries recreated the culture using their own interpretation. Thus, while more stringent and appearing more traditional than some, the real Kosraen culture is weak and poorly recalled.

Nonetheless, as one seeks culturally relevant interventions, those of Kosrae are appropriate to include in the listing because they have been derived from local traditions by local practitioners to be used with local people. Because of fiscal constraints, the government of Kosrae reduced the number of weekly hours for employment to 32 hours a few years ago. The day on which people (except emergency staff) were without work was to be used for agricultural activities and fishing for food for their families. About a year later, the people of Kosrae started a venture—that of agricultural self-sufficiency. Beginning with poultry, bananas and other fruits, and then vegetables, the efforts underway in Kosrae today target the year 2000 as the one in which major signs of progress will be visible to the people in terms of locally raised, locally appropriate foods being readily available. This project is set within that context as well as within the fact that Type II diabetes, primarily a nutrition- and lifestyle-related disorder, has become a problem of significance to this small island state.

The Objectives

Within the constraints of the culture of Kosrae, and in keeping with the goals and objectives of the government's self-sufficiency program while supporting positive diabetes education and control, this project attempts to assist persons with Type II diabetes in living better lives, more healthfully and with more stringent glycemic control.

The Design

The project has a startup phase in which some skill building occurs in terms of choice of crop and methods of cultivation and soil preparation. The next phase has to do the actual planting and to begin growing the gardens. Here, exercise such as weeding and turning the soil is promoted to ensure good crops. At the same time, the public health nurse begins some diabetes education efforts with the diabetics and their families. Beginning with the importance of maintaining glycemic control and the processes of testing for glucose levels, the importance of exercise and a proper diet, the importance of good foot and eye care, and dietary exchanges all are part of the education provided. As the gardens grow, the educational emphasis transfers to preparation of the produce and the use of fresh fruits and vegetables along with poultry and fish at the dinner table. The problems with canned goods, such as bully beef, and turkey tails, also are emphasized.

The final phase of the project involves instilling pride to the participants through photographs of produce grown, awards, and the like. At this time, the most successful gardeners are recruited to assist in the next group to be brought into the process.

The Issues Around Implementation

The initial recruiting of participants was thought to be a problem for the Department of Health. However, after the effort got under way, that concern quickly disappeared as individuals with Type II diabetes came forward to volunteer. The second concern was that of attrition. Here, the community itself served as a social pressure force, encouraging and recognizing the efforts that were being made. The gardens were used as examples of people taking initiative on their own, without government money, to solve their own food problems. Finally, concerns were expressed about sustainability of the process. Here, the jury is still out. The project has been operational for only about 3 years, and it is too early to see whether things will revert to former times or whether they can be maintained in the Kosrae of the future.

The Evaluation

A very real problem exists with the evaluation of this project. Ideally, the measures for evaluation should target the objectives of the project. However,

Kosrae is a very poor state, often having few (if any) medications at the hospital and having equipment that is outdated and not able to be maintained or repaired locally. Thus, assessing the glucose levels of participants, although an easy task in Hawai'i or on the mainland, is an impossibility because the Department of Health cannot afford the test strips or the meters with which to do the testing.

Assessment can be made of the success of the gardens; the photographs do that. And success can be measured on the basis of participants, both their numbers and their duration and subsequent participation as trainers/educators. The major evaluation of the effort, however, will come over time as one sees whether the Kosrae Gardening Project will be sustainable.

Results and Discussion

The fact that the project has remained operational for 3 years is a suggestion that it seems to be working. The years of abuse to which the endocrine systems of the people on Kosrae have been subjected cannot be expected to show immediate improvement. However, for what it is worth, the gardeners appear to have lost weight (this is a sensitive subject, and data are not readily available), appear to be more fit, and (according to the public health nurses) are healthier.

The likelihood that this intervention will be sustainable is quite high. It is a variation on a popular theme in the culture—living off the land. It also is in harmony with other community efforts and, while targeting a specific subgroup of the population, allows these individuals to take a leadership role within the community. The key to everything with the program will be the success it is able to generate in transferring the knowledge, attitudes, and practices of one group of participants to another.

Hawai'i: The Traditional Hawaiian Diet

Summary

The THD program is now well established as part of the health resources available to providers within the state of Hawai'i. It is used under medical supervision and otherwise and has been amply described in two separate publications (O'Connor, Teixeira, Tan, Beckham, & Shintani, 1995; Shintani & Hughes, 1992). This diet program, however, is more than just a diet designed to assist people in managing their hypertension and diabetes. It is essentially a plea to the people for a lifestyle change.

The initial work for the diet came from Moloka'i, where a 1985 cardiovascular risk study (Curb et al., 1991) of 247 Moloka'i homesteaders was completed. The results revealed a population with significant diseases present including high cholesterol (45% of sample), obesity (60%), hypertension (36%), and diabetes (23%). The subsequent dietary intervention led researchers to believe that the use of traditional Hawaiian foods (e.g., taro, fish, sweet potato, poi, banana) resulted in a reduction in nearly all indicators of the diseases mentioned.

As time has passed, the THD (the packaging of the Moloka'i Diet), with its additional features of exercise and health education, has been adopted by many in the state. In 1997, the state governor and 20 colleagues went on the diet for a 3-week period. The results were similar, and the publicity greatly assisted in spreading the word about a "local way" in which to manage some of the most devastating of diseases in Hawai'i.

Setting

Hawai'i is known as the "Aloha State" and more recently has become known as the "Health State" (Figure 24.2 and Table 24.1). Longevity is the greatest of any state in the union, and the health status indicators are, in general, better than U.S. average. With a warm healing climate and ready access to medical care (96% of the population have some form of health insurance), the people of the state boast short lengths of stay in hospitals for most conditions as well as the lowest admission rates.

However, in examining the situation further, one finds that within this generally healthy population there are subgroups for whom life is not so healthy. Most notable of these is the indigenous Hawaiian population. Initially resulting from studies of Native Hawaiians completed in 1985 (Native Hawaiian Health Research Consortium, 1985), the picture of the health of Native Hawaiians has become more clear over the past decade. With that clarity has come the Native Hawaiian Health System, funded by Congress in 1988 and now present on all major islands of the state.

It has been well established in the literature that Westernization of Native populations of the Pacific has caused deleterious effects on their health status (Blaisdell, 1988, 1993; Hankin & Dickinson, 1972; Prior, 1971; Reed, Labarthe, & Stallones, 1970; Ringrose & Zimmet, 1979; Shintani & Hughes, 1994; Taylor et al., 1992; Taylor & Zimmet, 1981; Zimmet, Arblaster, & Thoma, 1978). Similar declines in health conditions have occurred in Native Americans and immigrants to the continental United States (Boyce & Swinburn, 1993; Flegal et al., 1991; Howard, Abbot, & Swinburn, 1991; Kumanyika, Morssink, & Agurs, 1992; Swinburn, Boyce, Bergman, Howard, & Bogardus, 1991). Dietary change is the most prominent factor among the environmental and urbanization adaptations that negatively affect these populations, followed by decreased exercise and qualitative aspects of diet (Prior, 1971; Taylor et al., 1992; Taylor & Zimmet, 1981; Zimmet et al., 1978). The change from traditional diets to high-fat, high-calorie, low-fiber, refined and canned foods has resulted in an increasing prevalence of overweight, obesity, cardiovascular disease, and glucose intolerance and the eventual occurrence of Type II diabetes in these groups (Blaisdell, 1988, 1993; Flegal et al., 1991; Howard et al., 1991; Reed et al., 1970; Ringrose & Zimmet, 1979; Shintani & Hughes, 1994; Sloan, 1963; Taylor et al., 1992; Taylor & Zimmet, 1981). Ethnic Hawaiians exhibited alarming diabetes prevalence rates in 1963, when full-blooded Hawaiians were found to have a prevalence rate of 48.8% and part Hawaiians a rate of 26.6%, compared to the overall state rate of 18.4% (Sloan, 1963). Recent screening programs

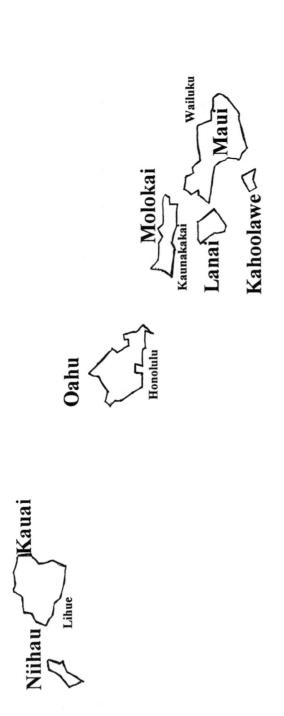

Niihau

Lihue

Kauai

Oahu

Honolulu

Molokai

Kaunakakai

Lanai

Wailuku

Maui

Kahoolawe

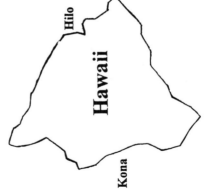

Hilo

Hawaii

Kona

State of Hawaii

Figure 24.2   State of Hawaii

TABLE 24.1 General Health Data for Hawaii: All Ethnicities

(a) Ten Leading Causes of Death by Sex, 1993

Condition	Total	Male	Female
1. Heart disease	2,204	1,287	917
2. Malignant neoplasm	1,717	1,006	711
3. Other diseases	741	389	352
4. Cerebrovascular disease	546	276	270
5. Influenza/pneumonia	303	163	140
6. Accidents	272	204	68
7. Chronic obstructive pulmonary disease	259	166	93
8. Other infective diseases	255	199	56
9. Diabetes mellitus	175	81	94
10. Suicide	123	104	19

(b) Chronic Conditions, 1992

Condition	Total	Rate per 1,000
1. Hypertension	92,182	80.9
2. Impairment of back/spine	72,017	63.2
3. Hayfever	63,853	56.1
4. Chronic sinusitis	57,805	50.8
5. Asthma	53,863	47.3
6. Hearing impairment	50,882	44.7
7. Arthritis	47,125	41.4
8. Skin condition	44,558	39.1
9. Heart disease	35,197	30.9
10. Diabetes	25,448	22.3

SOURCE: *State of Hawaii Data Book, 1995* (State of Hawaii, 1996).

among Native Hawaiians, using newer technology and standards, have established a diabetes prevalence rate of 18.5% and an impaired glucose tolerance rate of 34% (Beddow & Arakaki, 1997; RCMI: The Native Hawaiian Research Project, 1994). This impaired glucose tolerance rate is nearly twice the overall U.S. rate (Beddow & Arakaki, 1997). In the Native populations of Micronesia and Polynesia, rural Natives were leaner and healthier compared to urbanized Natives and were much healthier than the highly modernized Native Nauruans and Hawaiians (Taylor et al., 1992; Taylor & Zimmet, 1981; Zimmet & Whitehouse, 1981). Diabetes prevalence ranged from 4.6% in rural Samoans to 42.1% in urbanized Nauruans (Prior, 1971; Taylor et al., 1992; Taylor & Zimmet, 1981).

Whereas the negative health status of urbanized Native populations is well documented, information about health interventions and prevention efforts is noticeably lacking in the literature. Medically competent providers who are culturally uninformed and thus treat clients ineffectively (Aluli, 1991; Blaisdell, 1993; Hughes & Aluli, 1991; Mokuau, Hughes, & Tsark, 1995; Zimmet & Whitehouse, 1981), and the prevailing lack of knowledge about the relationship between chronic health conditions and lifestyle choices within Native populations, are frequent obstacles to care (Aluli, 1991; Aluli & Hughes, 1994; Blaisdell, 1993; Curb et al., 1991; Hughes & Aluli, 1991; Hughes, Tsark, & Mokuau,

1996; Mokuau et al., 1995). Other serious health care barriers are the accessibility to health services, including geographic distances and cost, and the acceptability or compatibility of health programs to the cultures they serve (Blaisdell, 1993; Mokuau et al., 1995).

The community-based THD program is an innovative, culturally competent approach to improving the health status among Native Hawaiians who suffer from diet-related chronic conditions such as obesity, hypertension, hyper-cholesterolemia, hyperlipidemia, diabetes, and other cardiovascular conditions (Blaisdell, 1993; Mokuau et al., 1995). The THD program integrates traditional foods, cultural values, and components of the traditional lifestyle of Hawai'i into a 3-week group intervention (Aluli & Hughes, 1994; Blaisdell, 1993; Hughes & Aluli, 1991; Hughes et al., 1996; Mokuau et al., 1995; Shintani et al., 1994). Traditional values such as spirituality, outreach to others, and unique cultural communication style are incorporated into the THD programs along with cultural preferences for group-focused affiliation, developing close bonds among peers, and reliance on personal networks in coping with problems (Blaisdell, 1993; Hughes & Aluli, 1991; Hughes et al., 1996; Mokuau et al., 1995; Pukui, Haertig, & Lee, 1972). THD program participants are self-selected and agree to participate fully in the 21-day program, which includes a diet of traditional foods, dining at a congregate site for breakfast and dinner, packing a take-out lunch and snacks, participation in health and cultural education, and monitoring by a physician and trained health personnel (Blaisdell, 1993; Hughes et al., 1996). The Moloka'i Diet study in 1987, sponsored by Na Pu'uwai (a Native Hawaiian advocacy organization), implemented the first THD program to study the remediation of hyperlipidemia as a cardiovascular risk factor in Native Hawaiians and employed the traditional communication style for health and cultural education (Aluli, 1991; Aluli & Hughes, 1994; Blaisdell, 1988, 1993). The THD meals incorporate traditional foods including mainly fish with occasional chicken, taro (a starchy tuber), sweet potato, yams, breadfruit, seaweed, bananas, taro leaves, and several Native greens (Mokuau et al., 1995; Shintani et al., 1994). Since 1987, numerous community-based THD programs have been sponsored by a variety of agencies, schools, and individuals, many in collaboration with the Hawai'i State Department of Health (1992, 1993a, 1993b; see also Hawai'i State Department of Education, 1994; Kamehameha Schools/Bernice Pau'ahi Bishop Estate, 1993).

Evaluation

The Wai'anae Diet Program (WDP), which started in 1989, is the best known of the THDs (Blaisdell, 1993; Shintani et al., 1994). It is customary for 20 individuals who are obese, based on body mass index (at least 27.2 for men and 26.9 for women), to participate for a 21-day period. Among the first WDP group of 10 men and 10 women, the average body mass index was 39.6 and ranged from 27.7 to 49.7 (Blaisdell, 1993; Shintani et al., 1994). The participants were encouraged to eat to satiety ad libitum amounts of pre-Western contact Hawaiian foods, except for protein foods, which were controlled at 5 ounces per day for each participant (Blaisdell, 1993; T. Shintani, personal communication, November 5, 1997; Shintani et al., 1994). This traditional diet is low in fat (7%), high in complex carbohydrates (78%), and moderate in protein (15%). The major protein foods were fish and occasionally chicken. The energy intake decreased from about 10.85 microjoules (2,594 kilocalories) pre-WDP to 6.57 microjoules (1,569 kilocalories) during the WDP (Blaisdell, 1993; Shintani et al., 1994).

The average weight loss experienced by the first group was 7.8 kilograms, and the average serum cholesterol decrease was 0.81 millimoles per liter from 5.76 to 4.95 millimoles per liter. The group blood pressure decreased an average of 11.5 millimeters hemoglobin systolic and 8.9 millimeters hemoglobin diastolic (Blaisdell, 1993; Shintani et al., 1994). Diabetic medications were cut dramatically for some within the first few days of the THD program, and eventually two of the six diabetics gave up all medication, maintaining dietary control of serum glucose levels (T. Shintani, personal communication, November 5, 1997). Another unexpected health benefit noted was a marked improvement among asthmatic participants (T. Shintani, personal communication, November 5, 1997). The health status improvements noted in the first program have been repeated in the 14 WDPs that have followed. The other community-based programs have mirrored these impressive results (Hawai'i State Department of Education, 1994; Hawai'i State Department of Health, 1992, 1993a, 1993b; Kamehameha Schools/Bernice Pau'ahi Bishop Estate, 1993).

There is great similarity in the nutrient composition of the diets of early American Indians, Pacific Islanders, and Asians (Blaisdell, 1988, 1993; Boyce & Swinburn, 1993; Shintani & Hughes, 1994; Swinburn et al., 1991). Although the THD is slightly lower in protein (Blaisdell, 1988), the nutrient composition is very similar to the traditional Pima Indian diet, which has been estimated to be 70% to 80% carbohydrates, 8% to 12% fat, and 12% to 18% protein (Boyce & Swinburn, 1993; Howard et al., 1991; Swinburn et al., 1991). The traditional diet of Hawaiians has been assessed at 78% carbohydrates, 12% to 15% protein, and 8% to 10% fat (Blaisdell, 1988). The Pima diet has changed to one that is about 47% carbohydrates, 35% fat, 15% protein, and 3% alcohol (Boyce & Swinburn, 1993; Howard et al., 1991). The adapted diets of Pacific Islanders reflect changes in percentages of nutrients similar to those of Westernization (Taylor et al., 1992; Zimmet et al., 1978). Researchers consistently have suggested that it is this shift in dietary nutrient and food composition, along with decreasing physical activity, that is responsible for increases in diabetes, hypertension, and other cardiovascular conditions that previously were rare in these populations (Blaisdell, 1993; Flegal et al., 1991; Howard et al., 1991; Reed et al., 1970; Ringrose & Zimmet, 1979; Taylor & Zimmet, 1981).

The THD approach of modeling and demonstrating healthy food choices, appropriate serving sizes, cooking methods, and cultural food customs and values is a culturally competent teaching method for the Native Hawaiian community (Pukui et al., 1972). For diabetics, the THD method reduces the stress and frustration of using measuring spoons and cups to serve each meal and memorizing correct serving sizes from the diabetic diet exchange lists to manage dietary intake. This culturally appropriate THD supplants the regimen of rigidly controlled daily living, adherence to a restrictive diet, and compliance with a controlled medication schedule demanded by Western treatment methods. Prescribed exchange diets can be confusing and tedious to plan and execute and are frustratingly limiting. THD participants take part in group meals at least twice a day and in evening educational sessions that foster bonding and group support and, by the end of the 3-week period, behavior change success and improved self-esteem among participants. Some community THD programs encourage family participation and offer three group meals daily. This fosters a family support system for dietary change. The THD programs, with their holistic approach, treat the whole individual (spiritual, emotional, and physical self), validate the importance of traditional practices and cultural values, and demonstrate an understanding and acceptance of cultural health practices such as *lomilomi* (massage) and *ho'oponopono* (a family-centered problem solving) (Blaisdell, 1993; Hughes & Aluli, 1991; Hughes et al., 1996; Mokuau, 1990; Pukui et al., 1972). The contrast between the THD programs (Aluli, 1991; Blaisdell, 1993; Hughes & Aluli, 1991; Mokuau, 1990) and Western treatment methods reflects the vast difference between these cultures (Prior, 1971; Zimmet et al,, 1978).

The THD program is one that is locally driven. The impetus to do something has come from within the culture and is promoted as part of the rediscovery of the culture in which Hawaiians have been participating for the past two decades. The fact that the program is locally planned and implemented removes many of the barriers of acceptability. The program is a natural fit with the Native Hawaiian Health System and is medically linked to obesity-related diseases.

EVALUATION

Analysis of the Case Studies

Although the Kosrae Gardening Project and the THD project both are about nutrition and at least partially focused on better dietary lifestyle and diabetes control, they differ in their levels of sophistication and application. The former is elegant in its simplicity. People used to grow gardens, and with the advent of the latter 20th century, modern foods and beverages such as Coca-Cola, Pringles potato chips, and frozen turkey tails (to name but three) now line the shelves of the local market. With a return to former ways, the people affected by Type II diabetes as well as by hypertension and other lifestyle-related diseases live healthier lives.

The THD project, on the other hand, focuses attention not on the growing of the foods but rather on the preparation and composition of the diet itself. Here, a relatively traditional Hawaiian diet is resurrected along with the culture in which it was used. The results of the diet are tracked and monitored intensively to see what effects occur within the diabetic and hypertensive populations participating. In both cases, the lessons are from the past, and the applications and implications clearly are for a healthier future.

Recommendations

Although it is important that programs at the community level be scientifically valid and do no harm to the participants, it is equally important that the programs have roots that are firmly entrenched within the community. The Kosrae Gardening Project and the THD project both are of this type. In examining these two projects, the following recommendations are made.

The roots of the program need to be in the community and its culture to ensure investment on the part of potential participants. The contents of the program need to be of relevance to those who will participate, and the health benefits of the program need to be recognized as valid by the health professionals in the community and those associated with the program. The predefined and desired health outcomes of the program should be explicit and known to participants. Participants should be involved in establishing those desired outcomes, again to enhance the quality and commitment of participation.

The levels of complexity of the programs are not as important as the levels of clarity in what is to be done and with what expected outcomes. The notion of comfort, of harmony with program methods and objectives, is the essential ingredient for success. Although important, cost is of somewhat lesser importance. In considering cost, the broadest of definitions must be used. That is, participant time, inconvenience, discomfort, and the like all must be considered.

From the two case studies examined, as well as from the literature reviewed, community participation in the planning, implementation, and evaluation of disease prevention interventions is a critical element in the process of development of these strategies. Focusing attention on discrete segments of the population seems a wise strategy as well. Finally, drawing from the familiar—that which is recalled from the past—affords each program an "instant history."

Implication

The fact that, in spite of Hawai'i's multicultural society, the THD project focuses efforts toward Hawaiians is not accidental. This population is at extreme risk for the many conditions outlined in this chapter, and because much of this risk is reduced with improved diet and weight loss, the intervention is appropriate. That others are not excluded and in fact are encouraged to participate, and have participated, in the program suggests that it has a multicultural potential for application.

Kosrae, on the other hand, is the antithesis of a multicultural society. Here, the focus of the program is on the activity and process and on its relevance to Kosreans.

As more of America becomes multicultural, and as immigration from the Pacific continues, models such as these might become even more important as models to adapt to local populations. That they have risen from within the cultures of the Pacific makes them competent in terms of their cultural content. That they seem to work makes them of value to those trying to prevent disease and promote the health of the population.

REFERENCES

Aluli, N. E. (1991). Prevalence of obesity in Native Hawaiian population. *American Journal of Clinical Nutrition, 53,* S1556-S1560.

Aluli, N. E., & Hughes, C. K. (1994, Spring). Cardiovascular risk and Native Hawaiians. *NIH-NHLBI Heart Memo,* pp. 19-21.

Auslander, W. F., Haire-Joshu, D., Houston, C. A., & Fisher, E. B., Jr. (1992). Community organization to reduce the risk of non-insulin-dependent diabetes among low-income African-American women. *Ethnicity and Disease, 2,* 176-184.

Avila, P., & Hovell, M. F. (1994). Physical activity training for weight loss in Latinas: A controlled trial. *International Journal of Obesity and Related Metabolic Disorders, 18,* 476-482.

Beddow, R., & Arakaki, R. (1997). Non-insulin-dependent diabetes mellitus: An epidemic among Hawaiians. *Hawaiian Medical Journal, 56,* 14-17.

Blaisdell, R. K. (1988, July). Ka ho'ok 'ai: Mokuna 'elua. *Ka Wai Ola OHA,* p. 28.

Blaisdell, R. K. (1993). The health status of Kanaka Maoli (indigenous Hawaiians). *Asian American and Pacific Islander Journal of Health, 1*(2), 117-162.

Boyce, V. L., & Swinburn, B. A. (1993). The traditional Pima Indian diet. *Diabetes Care, 16*(Suppl.), 369-371.

Braithwaite, R. L., Bianchi, C., & Taylor, S. E. (1994). Ethnographic approach to community organization and health empowerment. *Health Education Quarterly, 21,* 407-416.

Brandt, A. M. (1987). *No magic bullet: A social history of venereal disease in the United States since 1880.* New York: Oxford University Press.

Campinha-Bacote, J. (1994). Cultural competence in psychiatric mental health nursing: A conceptual model. *Nursing Clinics of North America, 29*(1), 1-8.

Castro de Alvarez, V. (1990). AIDS prevention program for Puerto Rican women. *Puerto Rican Health Science Journal, 9*(1), 37-41.

Curb, D. J., Aluli, N. E., Kauz, J. A., Petrovitch, H., Knutsen, S. F., Knutsen, R., O'Conner, H. K., & O'Connor, W. E. (1991). Cardiovascular risk factor levels in ethnic Hawaiians. *American Journal of Public Health, 81,* 164-167.

de Leon Siantz, M. L. (1990). Maternal acceptance/rejection of Mexican migrant mothers. *Psychology of Women Quarterly, 14,* 245-254.

Federated States of Micronesia. (1997). *Healthy Nation 2001: A five year plan.* Palikir, Pohnpei State: Government of the Federated States of Micronesia, Department of Health and Human Services.

Flegal, K., Ezzati, T. M., Harris, M. I., Haynes, S. G., Juarez, R. Z., Knowler, W. C., Perez-Stable, E. J., & Stern, M. P. (1991). Prevalence of diabetes in Mexican Americans, Cubans and Puerto Ricans from the Hispanic Health and Nutrition Examination Survey, 1982-84. *Diabetes Care, 14*(Suppl.), 628-638.

Forety, J. P. (1994). The impact of behavior therapy on weight loss. *American Journal of Health Promotion, 8,* 466-469.

Gribble, J. N., & Preston, S. H. (Eds.). (1993). *The epidemiological transition: Policy and planning implications for developing countries.* Washington, DC: National Academy Press.

Hankin, J. H., & Dickinson, L. E. (1972). Urbanization, diet, and potential health effects in Palau. *American Journal of Clinical Nutrition, 25,* 348-353.

Hawai'i State Department of Education. (1994). *Ho'oulu Kailua 'opio: Kailua traditional Hawaiian eating experience.* Honolulu, HI: Author.

Hawai'i State Department of Health. (1992). *The Kaua'i Native Hawaiian diet program: An evaluation.* Honolulu, HI: Author.

Hawai'i State Department of Health. (1993a). *Maui Traditional Hawaiian Diet program* (La'au no ka mea 'ai: Summary report). Honolulu, HI: Author.

Hawai'i State Department of Health, School Health Nursing Branch. (1993b). *Native Hawaiian Traditional Diet project at Kaimuki Intermediate School.* Honolulu, HI: Author.

Heath, G. W., Wilson, R. H., Smith, J., & Leonard, B. E. (1991). Community-based exercise and weight control: Diabetes risk reduction and glycemic control in Zuni Indians. *American Journal of Clinical Nutrition, 53*(Suppl.), S1642-S1646.

Howard, B. V., Abbot, W. G. H., & Swinburn, B. A. (1991). Evaluation of metabolic effects of substitution of complex carbohydrates for saturated fat in individuals with obesity and NIDDM. *Diabetes Care, 14,* 786-795.

Hughes, C. K., & Aluli, N. E. (1991). A culturally sensitive approach to health education for Native Hawaiians. *Journal of Health Education, 22,* 387-390.

Hughes, C. K., Tsark, J. A., & Mokuau, N. K. (1996). Diet-related cancer in Native Hawaiians. *Cancer, 78,* 558-563.

Jeffrey, R. W. (1991). Population perspectives on the prevention and treatment of obesity in minority populations: *Americal Journal of Clinical Nutrition, 53*(Suppl.), S1621-S1624.

Kamehameha Schools/Bernice Pau'ahi Bishop Estate. (1993). *Hawaiian cultural foods athletic project.*

Kumanyika, S. K., Morssink, C., & Agurs, T. (1992). Models for dietary and weight change in African-American women: Identifying cultural components. *Ethnicity and Disease, 2,* 166-175.

Levin-Zamir, D., Lipsky, D., Goldberg, E., & Melamed, Z. (1993). Health education for Ethiopian immigrants in Israel, 1991-92. *Israeli Journal of Medical Science, 29,* 422-428.

Lewis, C. E., Raczynski, J. M., Heath, G. W., Levinson, R., & Cutter, G. R. (1993). Physical activity of public housing residents in Birmingham, Alabama. *American Journal of Public Health, 83,* 1016-1020.

Lewis, C. E., Raczynski, J. M., Heath, G. W., Levinson, R., Hilyer, J. C., Jr., & Cutter, G. R. (1993). Promoting physical activity in low-income African-American communities: The PARR project. *Ethnicity and Disease, 3,* 106-118.

McFarlane, J., & Fehir, J. (1994). De Madres à Madres: A community, primary health care program based on empowerment. *Health Education Quarterly, 21,* 381-394.

Michielutte, R., Sharp, P. C., Dignan, M. B., & Blinson, K. (1994). Cultural issues in the development of cancer control programs for poor, underserved American Indian populations. *Journal of Health Care, 5,* 280-296.

Mokuau, N. (1990). A family-centered approach in Native Hawaiian culture. *Families in Society: Journal of Contemporary Human Services, 71,* 607-613.

Mokuau, N., Hughes, C. K., & Tsark, J. U. (1995). Heart disease and associated risk factors among Hawaiians: Culturally responsive strategies. *Health and Social Work, 20,* 46-51.

Nakyonyi, M. M. (1993). HIV/AIDS education participation by the African community. *Canadian Journal of Public Health, 84*(Suppl.), S19-S23.

Native Hawaiian Health Research Consortium. (1985). *'E Ola Mau: The Native Hawaiian Health Needs Study.* Honolulu: Author.

O'Connor, H. K., Teixeira, R. K., Tan, M., Beckham, S., & Shintani, T. (1995). *Wai'anae Diet cookbook: 'Elua.* Wai'anae, HI: Wai'anae Coast Comprehensive Health Center.

Prior, I. A. M. (1971, July-August). The price of civilization. *Nutrition Today,* pp. 2-11.

Pukui, M. K., Haertig, E. W., & Lee, C. A. (1972). *Nana I Ke Kumu* (Look to the Source) (Vol. 2). Honolulu, HI: Queen Lili'uokalani Children's Center.

RCMI: The Native Hawaiian Research Project. (1994). Diabetes mellitus and heart disease risk factors in Hawaiians. *Hawaiian Medical Journal, 53,* 340-364.

Reed, D., Labarthe, D., & Stallones, R. (1970). Health effects of Westernization and migration among Chamorros. *American Journal of Epidemiology, 92,* 94-112.

Ridgell, R. (1988). *Pacific nations and territories: The islands of Micronesia, Melanesia, and Polynesia.* Honolulu, HI: Bess.

Ringrose, H., & Zimmet, P. (1979). Nutrient intakes in an urbanized Micronesian population with a high diabetes prevalence. *American Journal of Clinical Nutrition, 32,* 1334-1341.

Rogler, L. H., Cortes, D. E., & Malgady, R. G. (1994). The mental health relevance of idioms of distress: Anger and perceptions of injustice among New York Puerto Ricans. *Journal of Nervous and Mental Disorders, 182,* 327-330.

Rosenstock, I. M. (1974). The health belief model and preventive health behavior. *Health Education Monographs, 2,* 354-386.

Samolsky, S., Dunker, K., & Hynak-Hankinson, M. T. (1990). Feeding the Hispanic hospital patient: Cultural considerations. *Journal of the American Dietary Association, 90,* 1707-1710.

Schwab, T., Meyer, J., & Merrell, R. (1994). Measuring attitudes and health beliefs among Mexican-Americans with diabetes. *Diabetes Education, 20,* 221-227.

Shintani, T., Beckham, S., O'Connor, H. K., Hughes, C., & Sato, A. (1994). The Wai'anae Diet Program: A culturally sensitive, community-based obesity and clinical intervention program for the Native Hawaiian population. *Hawaiian Medical Journal, 53*(5), 136-147.

Shintani, T., & Hughes, C. (Eds.). (1992). *The Wai'anae book of Hawaiian health: The Wai'anae Diet Program manual.* Wai'anae, HI: Wai'anae Coast Comprehensive Health Center.

Shintani, T. T., & Hughes, C. K. (1994). Traditional diets of the Pacific and coronary heart disease. *Journal of Cardiovascular Risk, 1,* 16-20.

Sinclair, M. A. (1991). A revised weight loss program in Manitoba Native communities. *Arctic Medical Research* (Suppl.), 97-98.

Sloan, N. R. (1963). Ethnic distribution of diabetes mellitus in Hawai'i. *Journal of the American Medical Association, 183,* 419-424.

State of Hawai'i. (1996). *The state of Hawai'i data book, 1995: A statistical abstract.* Honolulu, HI: State Department of Business, Economic Development, and Tourism.

State of Kosrae. (1996). *Healthy Kosrae 2001: State health plan.* Kosrae, Federal States of Micronesia: Department of Health.

Swinburn, B. A., Boyce, V. L., Bergman, R. N., Howard, B. V., & Bogardus, C. (1991). Deterioration in carbohydrate metabolism and lipoprotein changes induced by modern, high fat diet in Pima Indians and Caucasians. *Journal of Clinical Endocrine Metabolism, 73,* 156-165.

Taylor, R., Badcock, J., King, H., Pargeter, K., Zimmet, P., Fred, T., Lund, M., Ringrose, H., Bach, F., Wang, R., & Sladden, T. (1992). Dietary intake, exercise obesity and noncommunicable disease in rural and urban populations of three Pacific island countries. *Journal of the American College of Nutrition, 11,* 283-293.

Taylor, R. J., & Zimmet, P. Z. (1981). Obesity and diabetes in Western Samoa. *International Journal of Obesity, 5,* 367-376.

van Breda, A. (1989). Health issues facing Native American children. *Pediatric Nursing, 15,* 575-577.

Watt, I. S., Howel, D., & Lo, L. (1993). The health care experience and health behaviour of the Chinese: A survey based in Hull. *Journal of Public Health and Medicine, 15,* 129-136.

Wood, D. W. (1994). *Diabetes: A monograph on prevalence rates in Hawai'i.* Honolulu: University of Hawai'i, International Center for Health Promotion and Disease Prevention Research.

Zimmet, P., Arblaster, M., & Thoma, K. (1978). The effect of Westernization on Native populations: Studies on a Micronesian community with a high diabetes prevalence. *Australia and New Zealand Journal of Medicine, 8*(2), 141-146.

Zimmet, P., & McCarty, D. (1995). The NIDDM epidemic: Global estimates and projections—A look into the crystal ball. *IDF Bulletin, 40,* 8-16.

Zimmet, P., & Whitehouse, S. (1981). Pacific islands of Nauru, Tuvalu and Western Samoa. In H. C. Trowell & D. P. Burkitt (Eds.), *Western diseases: Their emergence and prevention.* Cambridge, MA: Harvard University Press.

25

Tips for Working With Pacific Islander Populations

ROBERT M. HUFF

MICHAEL V. KLINE

There are numerous groups of Pacific Islander peoples living in the continental United States and on islands scattered throughout the Pacific. As might be expected, these groups do share some common characteristics but also reflect significant diversity with respect to cultural beliefs, values, and ways of life. Thus, the term *Pacific Islander or Pacific Islander American* (PIA) in no way adequately begins to describe this diversity. In fact, the use of this term as a category for describing peoples in census tract and health databases often functions to obscure this diversity by lumping and combining the specific issues, health problems, and needs of these PIA population groups into one overall category. In addition, PIA groups often are combined under the much more broad category of *Asian or Pacific Islander,* which further serves to mask specific issues and problems of each of these PIA groups. Thus, as a general rule of thumb, the health promoter is encouraged to use the descriptor that is used by the particular PIAs in describing themselves and to learn as much as possible about the specific populations groups with whom the health promoter may be working. This "tips" chapter, although intentionally broad, seeks to provide some general considerations and tips for working with PIAs in health promotion and disease prevention (HPDP) programs. These tips have been drawn from the preceding three chapters (Casken, Chapter 22; Loos, Chapter 23; Wood & Hughes, Chapter 24) and other sources (Huff, Chapter 2, this volume; Huff & Kline, Chapter 1, this volume; Ishida, Toomata-Mayer, & Mayer, 1996; Kline, Chapter 4, this volume; Mokuau & Tauilu'ili, 1992) and are meant only as a starting point for the practitioner involved with providing HPDP programs or services to PIA population groups.

CULTURAL COMPETENCE

As has been noted in all the "Tips" chapters, the need to develop increasingly higher levels of cultural competence with respect to the many multicultural groups we are confronted with today is of paramount importance. Thus, the health promoter should heed the following tips:

▶ Devote time to learning the history and patterns of migration and immigration of the specific PIA population with which you will be working.

▶ Seek to discover the specific cultural values, beliefs, and traditions of your target group.

▶ Remember that every PIA group will have its own unique traditions and patterns of life and that these might be very different from yours and those of the agency that is providing the HPDP program or service to this group. It will be critical to develop the skill of suspending your own judgments, biases, and stereotypes because these can act to block sensitive and mutually respectful interpersonal relationships among all involved parties.

▶ Remember that there is likely to be a range of acculturation levels from the very traditional to the very acculturated. Therefore, there is a need to assess these levels before beginning the planning process for delivering the HPDP program or service to the target group. Do not assume that because your target group is residing in the continental United States, its members are acculturated and assimilated into the mainstream culture.

▶ Be very cognizant of both the verbal and nonverbal communication patterns and the cultural taboos of your target group.

▶ Take the time to make multiple visits to the community in which the target group resides. Talk with community leaders and members, visit important sites in the community where appropriate, sample local cuisine, participate in local events where the public is invited, and otherwise become familiar with the community's ways of life.

▶ Seek to establish early and continuing support from the community for any HPDP program or service that is to be offered.

▶ Be aware that there might be major discrepancies in the health data that are available about the target group. Here again, assessment of your target group using available data from the agency providing the program or service to your specific target group, as well as information derived from the community in question, will be essential.

HEALTH BELIEFS AND PRACTICES

An understanding of the health beliefs, practices, and health care use patterns of any cultural group is an essential component of the formative evaluation process one would use to increase his or her understanding of a specific target group. The following tips might prove useful to the health promoter in this early needs assessment process:

▶ Identify the explanatory model(s) used by the target group to define health and disease including preferences for traditional, Western, or a combination of both types of health care services when seeking help with illness or sickness states.

▶ Expect that there will be a range of explanatory models that are employed across this broad multicultural population group, ranging from very traditional folk beliefs and practices to those reflective of the current biomedical model.

▶ Seek to ameliorate and work with differences in explanatory models where these are in opposition between the target group and yourself.

▶ Seek to become more familiar with traditional healing practices of the community because these may provide opportunities to bring beneficial health practices into the biomedical framework.

▶ Identify perceptions related to personal control and responsibility for promoting individual health and well-being, that is, locus of control, interest, needs, and activities used for promoting or maintaining one's health.

▶ Identify the health care access issues, including usual patterns of use, types of care generally sought, barriers to care, social assistance services accessed by the target group, and other sources related directly or indirectly to the target group.

▶ Be aware that, in general, PIA population groups recognize that there are indigenous illnesses that must be treated with traditional remedies and Western illnesses that are more amenable to treatment using Western medical approaches.

▶ Recognize that there is no simple generic description for describing the health beliefs and practices of a PIA group. You must know the geographic locale and ethnic group to begin to understand these differences.

▶ Recognize that in matters of disease prevention and illness management, the whole family will likely be involved in the process.

▶ Consider that modesty, taboos, and traditional healing practices must be respected when providing the HPDP program or service.

▶ Consider involving traditional healers in the planning and delivery of the HPDP program or service.

▶ Where the HPDP program or service is focused on specific Western clinical conditions, be sure to identify and compare both your expectations and those of the PIA individual or group to ensure that both sides understand and agree with what is to be provided for that particular problem or condition.

▶ Recognize that cultural sensitivity to other points of view about health and disease will be a critical factor to consider when learning about your target group's health beliefs and practices.

PROGRAM PLANNING CONSIDERATIONS

Comprehensive and well-informed program planning is one of the most important tasks for designing a high-quality and successful HPDP program or service. Planning will require that the health promoter be culturally competent and sensitive to the differences in worldviews and ways of life of the target group. Keeping in mind the suggestions that have been made by others in this book, the health promoter also is encouraged to consider the following recommendations:

▶ Review all previous and current programs or services offered to the target group to identify intervention strategies and resources that have been found to enhance or impede the successful adaptation of programs or services by the target group.

▶ Develop positive alliances with the leadership of the community as you begin the program planning process.

▶ Be sure to include traditional healers as well as spiritual, cultural, and other important community members in the planning, implementation, and evaluation process.

▶ Be sure that the goals, objectives, and intervention processes target the felt needs of the target group and not just those of the sponsoring agency. Otherwise, this becomes a case of *doing to* rather than *doing with* the target group.

▶ Remember that successful HPDP programs for PIAs will employ a top-down and bottom-up approach to the planning and implementation process, that is, starting where the people are and involving them in every aspect of program development and delivery.

▶ Be aware that the program or service must fit within the cultural context of the community's values, beliefs, and health practices.

▶ Consider incorporating an indigenous model for planning, implementation, and evaluation of the HPDP program, that is, employing members of the target group to help plan, implement, and evaluate the program or service to be offered to the target group.

NEEDS ASSESSMENT CONSIDERATIONS

Needs assessment is the foundation of any successful HPDP program or service and never should be overlooked or minimally conducted. The data from this process are what will be used to identify the real and potential health issues and problems as well as the felt needs of the target group. Huff and Kline, in Chapter 26, present a cultural assessment framework that can be used for identifying information and health data about the target group under consideration. In addition to the assessment areas and questions presented in this framework, the following suggestions also might prove useful to the health promoter:

▶ Be aware that most census and health data lump the many diverse PIA groups together under the broad heading of *Asian Pacific Islander.* It will be critical to try and tease out the data directly applicable to the specific target group with which you will be working.

▶ Where possible, provide opportunities for PIA communities to conduct or be as involved as possible in conducting their own needs assessments because this can help build community capacity and a sense of community empowerment with respect to defining and solving their health and social problems.

▶ Recognize that needs assessment instruments need to reflect the linguistic, literacy, and cultural symbols and values of the community.

▶ Be aware that standardized needs assessment instruments designed for the mainstream culture might have little meaning for some PIA population groups. Thus, instruments will need to be shaped to reflect the community in which they are to be used.

▶ Consider including acculturation measures in the community assessment process.

▶ Consider that foldback analysis, as described by Loos in Chapter 23, may be a very effective approach to defining the real and felt needs of the community.

▶ Remember that any needs assessment process conducted with PIA population groups should employ a variety of approaches including interviews with key informants, focus groups, community surveys, and other approaches that actively involve the target group in defining its members' health issues and concerns.

▶ Be sure to include assessment of the media resources and channels that are used by members of the community because these might play an important role in the marketing of the HPDP program or service to be offered in the community.

▶ Be sure that questions to be asked of the target group reflect appropriate and relevant cultural values and expectations, and be aware that some question areas might not be appropriate based on cultural taboos and other social conventions.

INTERVENTION CONSIDERATIONS

As has been demonstrated throughout this book, well-planned interventions that employ behavioral theory in association with cultural themes, values, beliefs, and other cultural characteristics are key to the successful implementation of any HPDP program or service. The health promoter is encouraged to consider these factors as well as the following suggestions in the planning of intervention strategies:

▶ Remember that the most effective HPDP interventions are built on the community's strengths, resources, and assets and include significant involvement of the target group in the design process.

▶ When designing interventions, focus on the family system rather than on the individual. This recognizes the value and interpersonal dynamics of the family, which is very important to PIA groups.

▶ Be aware that because many island cultures are matriarchal, involving women in all aspects of the planning, implementation, and evaluation process can be a very effective strategy.

▶ Remember that intervention planning must start where the people are and fit within the context of the community's values, beliefs, and cultural practices.

▶ Remember that HPDP learning experiences for PIA populations should reflect concepts of wholeness and interconnectedness because these are central features of the cosmology of many PIA population groups.

▶ Be aware that the use of theory to support intervention design is an important feature of successful HPDP programming.

▶ Be aware that social marketing approaches can be highly effective in working with PIA population groups.

▶ Recognize that professional health jargon and Western values can impede HPDP processes among PIA population groups. Seek to include the cultural values and vocabulary of the target group because these have been found to enhance the potential for successful HPDP programs or services.

▶ When designing HPDP interventions, use short and culturally appropriate messages that present new ideas through accepted social channels and processes.

► Consider developing partnerships with local media to disseminate information about the HPDP program or service being planned by and for the community.

► Consider that "talk-stories," folk media (e.g., music, dance, song), role-playing, and pictorial presentations are very culturally acceptable and appropriate strategies to employ in HPDP programs or services for PIA population groups.

► Recognize that using multiple channels for the communication of HPDP messages such as through churches, schools, and work settings is an effective way in which to work with PIA populations. This also should include family chiefs, church and village leaders, and traditional healers as message sources for HPDP activities.

► Focus health messages on the positive health benefits of change rather than on the negative or fear-arousing consequences of the issue being addressed.

► Where possible, employ and train peer educators from the target community because this can help to enhance the credibility and acceptance of the HPDP program or service within the community in which it is being offered.

EVALUATION CONSIDERATIONS

As has been stressed in many of the chapters in this book, evaluation and assessment throughout the planning and implementation of HPDP programs or services are vital to understanding how well these activities functioned to facilitate the health changes that were intended by the programs or services. With this idea in mind, the health promoter should consider the following suggestions when preparing evaluation and assessment plans:

► Seek to develop evaluation strategies, methods, and instruments that reflect an understanding of current theory and practice from the evaluation and research literature.

► Understand that evaluation and assessment processes often are difficult to gain support for, even from the most sophisticated of target groups. Thus, efforts to explain these processes and to involve the target group in evaluation and assessment planning and implementation activities can do much to enhance the successful accomplishment of this component of the HPDP program or service process.

► Evaluation of the HPDP program or service must include culturally relevant measures for assessing the impact of the program or service on the target group.

► Assessment and evaluation methods and questions must be tailored to the educational and linguistic capabilities of the target group.

▶ Evaluation processes must include the participation of the community, and criteria for evaluation should be sought from the community because its members are the ones who know what is important to them.

▶ Recognize that HPDP participants might have limited test-taking abilities and skills. Thus, efforts to design evaluation methods and tools should be matched to the relevant experiences, interests, and needs of the target group.

▶ Wherever possible, provide opportunities for staff members from the community to be trained in evaluation and assessment processes including the implementation of these processes throughout the life of the program or service.

▶ Be sure to set up and use evaluation and assessment reporting mechanisms to ensure that the target community receives feedback on how well the program is functioning to improve the health issue or problem for which it was designed.

REFERENCES

Ishida, D. N., Toomata-Mayer, T. F., & Mayer, J. F. (1996). Samoans. In J. G. Lipson, S. L. Dibble, & P. A. Minarik (Eds.), *Culture and nursing care: A pocket guide*. San Francisco: UCSF Nursing Press.

Mokuau, N., & Tauili'li, P. (1992). Families with Native Hawaiian and Pacific Islander roots. In E. W. Lynch & M. J. Hanson (Eds.), *Developing cross-cultural competence: A guide for working with young children and their families*. Baltimore, MD: Paul H. Brookes.

PART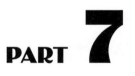

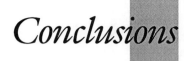

26

The Cultural Assessment Framework

ROBERT M. HUFF
MICHAEL V. KLINE

There are many important factors to be considered in planning programs across cultural groups. Previous chapters sought to highlight and discuss some of the major issues, barriers, and potentialities of multicultural health promotion within five particular population groups and their many and diverse subgroups. Throughout the book, it has been stressed that the practitioner needs to gain knowledge that can be used to tailor health promotion programming that is appropriate to each group's needs. In addition, the practitioner and participants from the target community must be able accurately to assess cultural differences, beliefs, and practices in the contexts of social conditions such as rural/urban, social class, country of origin, language, generational aspects, and historical experiences with the wider society. The importance of cultural assessment never should be underestimated.

Pasick, D'Onofrio, and Otero-Sabogal (1996) discuss the interactions among culture, health behavior, and health promotion and present a framework for *cultural tailoring* in the development of interventions for diverse cultural or ethnic groups. They distinguish between *targeting* of interventions for specific subgroups of the population to ensure exposure of the target group to the intervention and *cultural tailoring,* which is the development of interventions, strategies, messages, and materials that reflect specific cultural characteristics of the population group targeted for intervention. Pasick et al. observe that cultural tailoring provides a way in which to focus more directly on the specific cultural factors including the values, beliefs, and traditions of a particular group that influence behavior related to health and disease. Their framework for cultural tailoring intersects five major components of program planning and implementation. It emphasizes that more cultural tailoring is required at the levels of the behavioral theory being considered for conceptualization of interventions, the intervention design itself, and the implementation plan than at the levels of problem identification and objective setting. Pasick et al. hope that their framework will move researchers and planners to examine old assumptions and to systematically assess the amount of cultural tailoring needed for each phase of the program planning process. Unfortunately, this is not always the case because time, resources, interests, ethnocentric bias, and other related factors can act to mediate the types and amounts of formative needs assessment data that are collected prior to the development of specific intervention strategies. However, awareness of such frameworks can serve to encourage the planner or health promoter to conduct a thorough assessment of the cultural or ethnic population group targeted for intervention with respect to the values, beliefs, attitudes, and traditions directly and indirectly related to the health problem being addressed. It should be noted that the planner also needs to assess the organizational factors that may affect or be affected by cultural differences among the multicultural populations they may serve.

The cultural assessment framework (CAF), developed by the authors and presented in Tables 26.1 to 26.5, provides the practitioner with an assessment approach and a framework for better understanding the similarities and differences between the mainstream culture and the specific cultural or ethnic group targeted for intervention. The framework presented in this chapter evolved out of a variety of planning and cultural assessment models (Andrew & Boyle, 1995; Brownlee, 1978; Clark, 1978; Green & Kreuter, 1991; Leininger, 1995; Lipson & Steiger, 1996; Orque, Block, & Ahumada Monrroy, 1983; Spector, 1996; Tripp-Reimer, Brink, & Saunders, 1984) that seek to provide guidelines for the identification of the major areas that should be considered when assessing individual patients in the clinical setting. These guidelines also have application to the small group, community, and organizational levels of assessment and provide the practitioner with major suggestions pertinent to identifying important demographics, epidemiological factors, cosmology, general and specific cultural characteristics, general and specific health beliefs and practices, environmental and biocultural factors, and organizational variables. To some degree, assessment of these factors should be part of any basic formative evaluation process conducted to determine baseline characteristics of a population being targeted for a health promotion and disease prevention (HPDP) program. These are not, however, always made explicit or included in any type of comprehensive way during the assessment process. There is a need to formally include a cultural assessment as a routine component of any needs assessment process that includes a multicultural population within the target group to be addressed by a program plan.

THE CULTURAL ASSESSMENT FRAMEWORK

The CAF incorporates five primary levels of assessment that should be considered when planning a program for any multicultural population group. Because all planning models include some form of early or formative evaluation to assess demographic, epidemiological, social, and behavioral characteristics of target populations to be served by an HPDP program, the CAF has been organized to overlay and enhance this early assessment process. That is, the categories and associated subcategories of assessment within the framework suggest areas of needed inquiry that are culture specific and should be included in assessment tools such as surveys, focus groups, and other formative evaluation processes. The framework, like similar models, involves asking and answering a planned range of questions at each stage of the assessment process. It assumes, at the outset, that the health promoter or planner has begun to acquire an increased level of cultural competence with respect to the target population with which he or she will be working (e.g., history, culture, language, migration patterns). Interestingly, Andrew and Boyle (1995) suggest that biocultural variations such as the distinctive anatomical and physiological characteristics of the ethnic or cultural group also might be important to the assessment process, although this is not included as a distinct category in the CAF. Rather, questions associated with this area of assessment can be included as part of the general and specific cultural or ethnic group characteristics within the CAF.

The CAF can be applied to address HPDP questions that target individual or family activities in clinical settings as well as those targeted to small group, community, or higher levels of health behavior intervention. The five major levels of assessment for the CAF are as follows:

1. Cultural or ethnic group-specific demographic characteristics
2. Cultural or ethnic group-specific epidemiological and environmental influences
3. General and specific cultural or ethnic group characteristics
4. General and specific health care beliefs and practices
5. Western health care organization and service delivery variables

The CAF is further divided into a number of subcategories with associated assessment questions to provide a more in-depth review of the factors that should be considered when planning HPDP programs or services for multicultural groups. Each of the primary components and subcomponents of the CAF is presented in what follows, with examples where appropriate to highlight the value and importance of each of the assessment levels in the framework.

CULTURAL OR ETHNIC GROUP DEMOGRAPHIC CHARACTERISTICS

The most basic assessment need in most planning models is to determine as accurately as possible what the demographic characteristics of the intended target audience are. In this first level, we are concerned with characteristics related to age, gender, area of residence, education and literacy, religion, language, housing, income, occupation, and related items. The assumption here is that the more we know about these factors, the better we will be at targeting programs that consider these characteristics and issues in the program planning, intervention design, implementation, and evaluation processes. These same issues from a cultural or ethnic group-specific perspective also must be included, as seen in Table 26.1.

As can be seen in this component of the CAF, age and gender factors, social class and social status, education and literacy, language and dialect, religious preferences and practices, income and occupation, patterns of residence and living conditions, and acculturation and assimilation also should be included with any other demographic factors being explored by the health planner.

Age

Age and gender factors need to be considered where there are cultural rules governing issues such as making decisions for the family regarding health care-related matters and food preparation practices. For example, among Samoans, an interaction with a non-Samoan health care provider might involve an elder or the most educated family member to act as the family spokesperson (Ishida, Toomata-Mayer, & Mayer, 1996). Galanti (1991) cites a case in which the paternal grandmother and several older aunts intervened to keep the parents of a sick child from seeing the child until his condition was stabilized in the hospital. This was because they viewed these parents as babies who would not be able to make appropriate decisions regarding the care of their own child. Lynch and Hanson (1992) note that age plays a role in cultural development and observe that by 5 years of age, children have an understanding of their culture of origin. They also recognize that children are much quicker to learn new cultural patterns than are their parents. Thus, beyond the usual reasons for looking at age in a demographic profile, it is important to understand that decision making based on deference to elders who have lived the longest and have more experience with worldly matters may play a major role in how families perceive and use preventive or curative health services. In addition, it is important to determine how the elderly are cared for and what expectations there are for them with respect to self-care, exercise, and other health promotion activities (see Ishida's case study in Chapter 20, this volume). HPDP activities might need to be targeted to or involve the older members of the community in planning and implementation efforts.

Gender

Like age, gender rules within a cultural or ethnic group also need to be assessed. Many cultures have very specific rules and traditional roles prescribed for men and women. For example, among traditional Vietnamese, men are the decision makers and support for the family. Women are expected to prepare all meals, whether they work or not, and to do most of the household chores. Where these roles shift, traditional family relationships often are strained (Farrales, 1996). Gender issues governing modesty, purity, and virginity also are important because many cultural groups highly value and protect these virtues among their women.

TABLE 26.1 Cultural Assessment Framework: Culture-Specific Demographic Characteristics

Assessment Area	*Assessment Questions*
1. Age and gender characteristics	[ ] What are the age and gender distributions of the cultural or ethnic group?
	[ ] What are the cultural or ethnic rules governing behaviors related to age?
	[ ] What are the cultural or ethnic gender rules governing social and other types of interpersonal interactions within and outside family (e.g., how are different genders perceived and treated)? What roles do men and women have with respect to decision making, child rearing and household management, health and disease, medical encounters with Western health care providers, and so on?
2. Social class and status	[ ] What social class and status distinctions exist within the cultural or ethnic group?
	[ ] What are the rules governing social class and status within the cultural or ethnic group?
	[ ] How do these distinctions affect matters of health, illness, and disease?
	[ ] What specific impact does social class and status have on health-promoting or health care-seeking behaviors?
3. Education and literacy	[ ] What is the distribution of formal educational attainment across the cultural or ethnic group?
	[ ] What are the general attitudes toward formal education?
	[ ] What percentage of the cultural or ethnic group can understand, read, and write English?
	[ ] What percentage of the cultural or ethnic group understands, reads, and writes the language or dialect of the culture of origin?
	[ ] How does the cultural or ethnic group learn best?
4. Language and dialect	[ ] What is the primary language of the cultural or ethnic group?
	[ ] What dialect differences exist within the cultural or ethnic group?
	[ ] What language is spoken most often in the home?
	[ ] What are the language preferences with respect to entertainment, education, and information seeking?
	[ ] What words are commonly used by the cultural or ethnic group to describe health, illness, and disease processes?
	[ ] How does the cultural or ethnic group learn best?
5. Religious preferences	[ ] What is the primary religious orientation of the cultural or ethnic group?
	[ ] What variations in religious preferences exist across the cultural or ethnic group?
	[ ] What religious rules govern health and disease practices?
	[ ] What are the primary religious holidays and celebrations of the cultural or ethnic group?
	[ ] What role(s) has the culture's religious leaders played with respect to health and disease, community health action, and so on?
	[ ] Are leaders currently involved in health promotion and disease prevention activities?
6. Occupation and income	[ ] What are the traditional occupations of the cultural or ethnic group?
	[ ] How have these occupations been affected by migration into the United States?
	[ ] How do traditional occupations and changes in these affect health and disease within the cultural or ethnic group?
7. Patterns of residence and living conditions	[ ] What is the typical family size within the cultural or ethnic group?
	[ ] In general, how many families occupy a single-family dwelling?
	[ ] What are the typical physical conditions of housing within the community where the cultural or ethnic group resides?
	[ ] What hygiene and/or environmental health issues or problems related to residence patterns and living conditions affect real or potential health and disease issues?
8. Acculturation and assimilation	[ ] In general, how long has the cultural or ethnic group resided in the United States?
	[ ] What is the distribution of first, second, third, and later generations in the cultural or ethnic group?
	[ ] Is the community in which the cultural or ethnic group resides an open or more insular community?
	[ ] What percentage of the target population works outside the community?
	[ ] How often and with whom does the target population socialize outside the interpersonal and physical boundaries of the community?
	[ ] What percentages of the target population are traditional, marginal, bicultural, and fully acculturated and assimilated into the mainstream culture?

Programs that may require examinations of female patients or participants (e.g., breast examinations, Pap smears) from a male doctor or other health care worker might be frowned on or avoided altogether by these population groups. Mo (1992), reporting on a study conducted among Chinese women in San Francisco, observes that cultural values with respect to modesty and sexuality contributed to less use of breast health services by that group. In addition, she notes that a lack of female physicians and educational materials written in English instead of Chinese also were important barriers. Likewise, the promotion of birth control methods and sexually transmitted disease prevention also might be considered an affront to a cultural group whose religious practices forbid the use of birth control, premarital sex, and the like.

Social Class and Social Status

Social class and status also may be important considerations in a cultural assessment because there are cultural groups in which these factors might serve to help or hinder an HPDP program. Among Samoans, for example, persons perceived as being in positions of authority (e.g., elders, family chiefs, clergy) are given great respect and deference (Ishida et al., 1996). As a result of their status, these individuals might be able to influence health promotion behaviors if they are involved in the planning and execution of HPDP programs (Ishida et al., 1996). Helman (1984) notes that symptoms of illness or disease also might be influenced by one's socioeconomic status. Helman cites an example of backache that was interpreted by members of the highest socioeconomic class as an abnormal symptom, whereas members of the lower socioeconomic class interpreted it as a normal and inevitable part of living. Social class also might play an important role in health care access because, again, those in the lower socioeconomic ranks might be less inclined or able to access HPDP services if these services interfere with or call for them to leave their jobs. The HPDP program planner will need to consider these factors when planning for how and when to deliver HPDP services to the target group.

Literacy

Education and literacy should be considered as major points of interest to the practitioner. Each can play a significant role in whether and how well an HPDP program may be used. That is, how a particular individual or cultural group perceives HPDP might well determine whether target group members avail themselves of the program. If the target group does not have a concept for HPDP, then group members might be much less inclined to accept or even acknowledge the program in their community. Literacy also will be an important factor because many HPDP programs rely on written educational materials and advertising to reinforce concepts and skills they teach and to reach the target audiences with their health promotion messages. Furthermore, Western concepts and examples included within these materials might be completely foreign or counter to the target group's worldview and understanding of health and disease principles and practices.

Language

Although closely related to education and literacy, language or dialect also is an important assessment consideration. That is, what is the preferred language or dialect of the target population? Can its members read this language or dialect if it is presented to them in a written format? Can they speak and read English? Obviously, program materials need to be developed in the preferred language or dialect of the target group and be cross-translated to ensure their accuracy. Materials developed that fail to include dialect differences might result in confusion or indifference on the part of the target group for which they were designed. For example, using Spanish-language materials that have been written in the highest Castillian dialect might not be understood by someone living in a barrio with little education or reading ability. Thus, a program will need to consider how its target group learns best and how best to reach target group members with information about programs in their community. Perhaps an oral approach will have greater impact than will written materials, and perhaps pictures should be considered over words.

Religion

As discussed in numerous places throughout this book, religion and religious preferences are extremely important factors in the lives of many multicultural groups. Knowing how religious views and practices affect the daily lives of target group members including variables such as food practices and taboos, religious observances, dress, and views regarding marriage, family, and sexuality, might well determine how the program is targeted, what can be included with respect to program content, and even on what day(s) a program might be presented. Furthermore, an understanding of how health and disease issues are addressed and taught within the religious cosmology will aid the planner in defining interventions that are more acceptable to the religious heirarchy and the target population itself. It might be possible, as noted earlier, to involve clergy, priests, and other religious leaders in the planning and implementation of the HPDP program.

Occupation and Income

Occupation and income might appear less important than other cultural factors, but they are relevant in that both are connected to socioeconomic factors and epidemiological factors that might be contributing to accidents, illness, and/or disease. For example, occupations that involve high risk such as the fishing industry might place certain population groups in greater jeopardy than they do other groups. A personal observation of Vietnamese fishermen on the West Coast demonstrated to one of the authors (Huff) that attention to the safety of their boats and crew often is a much lower priority than is making the catch and supporting their families. In addition, money to properly outfit their boats is scarce, so this often is a neglected safety factor in their daily occupation. For those population groups in the lower socioeconomic classes, making a living each day often will take priority over matters of health. That is, taking time out to exercise, eat properly, manage their stress, or visit a physician when they are not feeling well might not be in their concept of what it takes to survive. Finding ways in which to incorporate issues of income and occupation might well be one of the more challenging aspects facing the HPDP program planner.

Residence

Closely related to income and occupation are the patterns of residence and the living conditions of the target population. Is the target population living in substandard housing, the inner city, or a rural community? How difficult is it for the target group members to access health services? What perceptions do they have concerning their living conditions with respect to health and disease? For example, are the crime rates excessive, and do they contribute to mental stress within the community? How difficult is it to bring an HPDP program into the community? What options do the target group members have for changing their living conditions? How many people, on average, occupy a single family unit? Are they living as they always have and want to live? As previous experience working in an inner city attested to one of the authors (Huff), the priorities of the target population were not always in line with those of the agencies providing health services to the community. Understanding these factors may help the health planner to develop a more realistic outlook on what is possible and appropriate given the circumstances with which he or she is working.

Acculturation and Assimilation

Acculturation and assimilation are factors that cross all levels of the CAF, and both were covered in some depth by many of the chapters in this book. As noted in Chapter 1, populations immigrating to any new country where the values, beliefs, and ways of life are different from those of their old countries will be required, to some degree, to take on some of the characteristics of the dominant culture if they are to successfully assimilate. As is well known, however, this does not always occur, and the reality is that there will be an acculturation continuum ranging from those who remain completely traditional to those who take on all of the characteristics of the mainstream culture in which they live. Assessment of this process can help the health promoter to determine how best to target his or her program or service to accommodate the values, beliefs, attitudes, and health practices of those whom the health promoter will be serving. That is, for a target group that might be primarily composed of first- and second-generation immigrants, their perceptions of health, disease, and Western health care practices might be sharply divergent. Programs or services that fail to take these differences into consideration might find target population participation to be low or even nonexistent. There are a number of acculturation scales that have been developed and tested, and the reader is encouraged to look at those described or referenced elsewhere in this book.

CULTURE-SPECIFIC EPIDEMIOLOGICAL AND ENVIRONMENTAL INFLUENCES

Environmental and epidemiological factors are generally included in all assessment models, but there is a need for the practitioner to look at these factors in a more focused manner than in the general way these factors normally are considered in an assessment. That is, when morbidity and mortality data are aggregated into larger categories of analysis, specific health issues of many subpopulation groups and their specific health issues can be masked (e.g., Asian or Pacific Islander). In the same way, we also might overlook specific environmental factors such as lead-based paints in older homes, other home hazards (e.g., tubs, stairs, pools), agricultural hazards, alcohol and tobacco advertising, and other associated influences affecting the target group. Table 26.2 identifies some of the most obvious questions that should be considered in the epidemiological and environmental needs assessment.

There are a number of questions that seem worthwhile to explore within this component of the CAF and that can be used to provide a truer picture of the extent of morbidity and mortality rates for the specific cultural or ethnic group being targeted. Admittedly, this is a difficult challenge and may require a significant effort on the part of the health promoter to discover these data. But if the health promoter does not do so, then he or she might miss something very important and target the program efforts inappropriately. The activities required for obtaining data about culturally sanctioned behaviors of a target group also may be challenging but ultimately might prove to be quite enlightening. For example, smoking is a socially sanctioned behavior among many Third World population groups, and one could expect to encounter resistance to smoking cessation programs without some serious preliminary work aimed at reframing how this population group perceives and uses tobacco products. Food preferences, which might include the use of lard or other high-cholesterol foods, could be playing a significant role in the development of chronic disease. Religious preferences and practices might present a problem where programs aimed at reducing sexually transmitted diseases is a concern. Finally, other cultural factors such as a strong value for modesty or a lack of a concept of germ theory might well be contributing factors to the morbidity and mortality issues in the cultural or ethnic group of concern.

GENERAL AND SPECIFIC CULTURAL CHARACTERISTICS

This book has continually advocated the need for the health promoter to become more culturally competent and sensitive to the target group with which he or she

TABLE 26.2 Cultural Assessment Framework: Culture-Specific Epidemiological and Environmental Influences

Assessment Area	Assessment Questions
1. Morbidity, mortality, and disability rates	[ ] What are the leading causes of morbidity in the cultural or ethnic group by age, gender, income, and occupation?
	[ ] What are the leading causes of mortality in the cultural or ethnic group by age, gender, income, and occupation?
	[ ] What are the leading causes of disability in the cultural or ethnic group by age, gender, income, and occupation?
	[ ] What are the immunization rates and levels within the target population?
	[ ] To what specific illnesses or diseases is the cultural or ethnic group most susceptible?
	[ ] What specific culturally sanctioned behaviors (e.g., smoking, alcohol, or other substance use or abuse; violence) may be contributing to the morbidity and mortality rates within the cultural or ethnic group?
	[ ] How do perceptions of quality of life, worldview, and religion influence responses to illness and disease, disease prevention practices, and use of Western health care screening and disease prevention programs and treatment services?
2. Environmental influences	[ ] What types of environmental health hazards can typically be found within the community in which the cultural or ethnic group resides (e.g., toxins, chemicals)?
	[ ] What types of potentially health-damaging advertising (e.g., billboards, signs) can be found within the target community and in what concentrations?
	[ ] How does the community react to these types of advertising?
	[ ] What is the distribution of stores in the community that sell alcoholic products?
	[ ] How many and what types of Westernized fast food resturants exist in the community, and how frequently are they used by the community?
	[ ] What is the general appearance of the community (e.g., clean and safe looking, graffiti strewn, dirty and run down)?
	[ ] What types of people are most often seen on the streets of the community during the day, evening, and night?

is working. This concern is reflected in the third component of the CAF (Table 26.3).

This level of assessment is concerned with a more anthropological evaluation of the cultural or ethnic group under consideration. Of concern are the cosmology; time orientation; perceptions of self and community; social norms, values, and customs; and communication patterns. A thorough cultural assessment must begin with establishing how the group identifies itself with respect to a specific cultural or ethnic tradition. This also will provide a reference point from which to begin this investigation of the group to be targeted for intervention. It also can help ensure that the health promoter is using the correct descriptor when talking about or to the cultural group and can help to identify diversity within the culture being studied. As Seidel, Ball, Dains, and Benedict (1995) observe, within the cultural group there will generally be a variety of populations and subgroups, each of which will manifest a number of shared traits that distinguish its members from the mainstream culture.

TABLE 26.3 Cultural Assessment Framework: General and Specific Cultural Characteristics

Assessment Area	Assessment Questions
1. Cultural or ethnic identity	[ ] How does the target population identify itself with respect to culture or ethnic derivation?
	[ ] What subgroups, if any, exist within the broader cultural or ethnic group?
	[ ] What specific customs and practices govern identification and/or participation in these specific subgroups?
2. Cosmology	[ ] How does the cultural or ethnic group view the world with respect to natural, supernatural, and metaphysical forces?
	[ ] How does the cultural or ethnic group perceive and relate to the mainstream culture in which it is located?
	[ ] How does the cosmology of the cultural or ethnic group affect perceptions of health, disease prevention, illness, death, and dying practices?
	[ ] How does the cultural or ethnic group's cosmology parallel, merge, or conflict with that of the mainstream culture?
3. Time orientation	[ ] What is the general time orientation of the cultural or ethnic group (e.g., past, present, future)?
	[ ] How does the cultural or ethnic group perceive and use time on a daily basis?
	[ ] How does time orientation affect disease prevention, illness, and treatment-seeking behaviors?
4. Perceptions of self	[ ] How is the concept of "self" perceived and described by the cultural or ethnic group?
	[ ] How is individual motivation and determination viewed by the cultural or ethnic group?
	[ ] What impact, if any, do perceptions of self have with respect to disease prevention, illness, treatment seeking, dying, and death practices?
5. Perceptions of community	[ ] How is the concept of community defined by the cultural or ethnic group?
	[ ] How are community gatekeepers defined, described, or identified by the cultural or ethnic group?
	[ ] How are outsiders perceived by the cultural or ethnic group (e.g., Western politicians, medical providers, and educators)?
	[ ] Who, outside of the target population, has entrée to the community gatekeepers?
	[ ] How are mainstream laws, rules, social customs, values, and practices perceived by the cultural or ethnic group?
	[ ] To what degree are the mainstream laws, rules, social customs, values, and practices observed by the cultural or ethnic group?
6. Social norms, values, and customs	[ ] What are the traditional and expected norms, values, and customs related to family and family dynamics (e.g., interpersonal interactions, gender and age roles, decision making and family leadership, dress, food preferences and preparation, child rearing, religious observances, rules and taboos, marriage, sexuality, health and disease practices)?
	[ ] How has acculturation and assimilation into the mainstream culture been affected by traditional norms, values, and customs of the family and culture?
	[ ] What are the traditional and expected norms, values, and customs governing interactions between and among families, community institutions, and the outside world (e.g., the mainstream culture or other cultural or ethnic groups in proximity to the cultural or ethnic group in question)?
	[ ] How do traditional norms, values, and customs merge with, parallel, or conflict with those of the mainstream culture?
7. Communication patterns	[ ] What are the usual and customary communication patterns and practices within the cultural or ethnic group (e.g., the verbal and nonverbal forms of greeting, talking, social interchange, idioms, communication with outsiders)?
	[ ] How does the cultural or ethnic group communicate or expect to be communicated with where matters of health care and health education with folk or traditional healers and Western medical providers are concerned (e.g., the rules of communication and dialogue)?
	[ ] How do the traditional forms of communication in the cultural or ethnic group merge with, parallel, or conflict with those of the mainstream culture?

Cosmology

The cosmology of the cultural or ethnic group also is important to understand because these beliefs can affect behaviors and health practices. For example, some cultural groups, such as the Hmong from Southeast Asia, are highly oriented to the concept of fate, believing that one's life is preordained. Thus, seeking to change what already is established would likely meet with resistance or outright indifference. Certainly, a major question with respect to cosmology would be concerned with whether the cosmology of the group parallels or conflicts with Western beliefs and practices. For the health promoter, understanding these similarities and differences can be helpful in planning programs reflecting, respecting, and working within and between the differing worldviews.

Time Orientation

Time also is an important issue because different cultural groups view and incorporate time-specific activities into their worldviews. Seidel et al. (1995) comment that a present-centered culture (e.g., Hispanic) tends to take each day as it comes and may see the future as unpredictable, a past-oriented worldview (e.g., East Asian) will seek to hold on to traditions that were significant in the past, and a future-oriented group (e.g., dominant American) will likely look to a "better future," thus placing a high value on change. The issue here, then, is about the potential for bringing about change and what the health promoter might need to consider when planning to create health or other social change in the target group.

Perceptions of Self and Community

Perceptions of self and one's relationship to one's community is another important consideration when working with traditional cultural or ethnic groups. That is, in some cultures, such as the dominant American culture, individualism and self-determination are highly valued traits, whereas in other cultural groups these might be frowned on and even discouraged. For example, among traditional Native American, East Asian, and Hispanic populations, group goals take precedence over those of the individual. Thus, efforts to create change in these cultures might need to give consideration to how change interventions can be brought into alignment with group goals so that these interventions can be accepted and adopted by the group as well as promoted by the group to its individual members.

Norms, Values, and Customs

Social norms, values, and customs comprise the next level of assessment. A *cultural norm* is a standard of behavior that is expected by all who represent a cultural or ethnic group. A *value* is a standard that prescribes the relative worth, utility, or importance of a particular belief, custom, or behavior. A *custom* can be defined as a learned and patterned response to a given situation or occasion and may be reflected in dress, language, communications, religion, and other aspects of the cultural or social group. Questions aimed at identifying these aspects of a population group are important because if differences in values, norms, and practices between cultural groups are not identified, then misunderstanding and conflict probably will result. Thus, looking at issues such as who makes the decisions in the family, what the gender roles are, expected marriage and family practices, food preferences and preparation practices, and other family and social dynamic components of the cultural or ethnic group is extremely important. Where these are in conflict with or different from the mainstream culture's views, efforts to work within these frames of reference will be necessary for the health promoter.

Communication Patterns

Like other components of the cultural characteristics assessment, communication patterns should be of great interest to the health planner. This is especially important in the clinical setting where direct contact with a client or patient will necessitate understanding issues such as the rules of greeting, speaking, presenting information, touching, eye contact, and other verbal and nonverbal behaviors. As Brislin and Yoshida (1994) observe, the typical Western medical model is very directive and aimed at getting to the heart of the matter as quickly as possible. This also is reflected in how patient, community, and work site health promotion activities are carried out, that is, getting directly to what the issue is and how best to treat or prevent it with little thought to how these messages will be received, perceived, or acted on. Taking the time to discover how best to address, teach, and work with different cultural groups can make the difference in how HPDP messages and programs are received. Fredericks and Hodge, in Chapter 16 of this volume, discussed the value of "talking circles" as a way in which to educate Native American women about cancer prevention using Native American stories and myths as the entry point for HPDP activities. At a related level, assessing how a given cultural or ethnic group generally acquires health information and what media approaches are the most effective for reaching group members can be extremely valuable to the health promoter or planner. Ramirez, Cousins, Santos, and Supic (1986) devised a simple scale for assessing media and language preferences among Mexican Americans, and similar assessment questions have been incorporated into other acculturation measurement scales (Castro, Cota, & Vega, Chapter 7, this volume; Marin & Gamba, 1996).

GENERAL AND SPECIFIC HEALTH BELIEFS AND PRACTICES

Huff, in Chapter 2 of this volume, presented a discussion of traditional health beliefs and practices that the health promoter or planner should be aware of as he or she designs HPDP interventions for multicultural population groups. Table 26.4 identifies four major assessment areas with associated questions that should be considered when assessing any diverse cultural or ethnic group.

TABLE 26.4 Cultural Assessment Framework: General and Specific Health Beliefs and Practices

Assessment Area	Assessment Questions
1. Explanatory model(s)	[ ] What are the traditional explanations used by the cultural or ethnic group to describe and make sense of health, illness, disease and death?
	[ ] How do these explanations merge with, parallel, or conflict with Western explanatory models?
	[ ] Does the cultural or ethnic group recognize and practice health-promoting behaviors? If so, then what specific health-promoting behaviors are practiced?
2. Response to illness	[ ] What are the usual or traditional responses to a communicable, chronic, or additive illness episode?
	[ ] Who makes the decision(s) within the family regarding health care and treatment seeking for sick family members?
	[ ] What types of traditional healing methods and healers are routinely consulted, and under what conditions are they consulted?
	[ ] What negative consequences, if any, are perceived by the cultural or ethnic group related to the use of traditional healing methods?
	[ ] How are episodes of communicable, chronic, addictive, or mental illness perceived and treated within the family?
	[ ] What is the usual response to illness when traditional treatment approaches fail?
	[ ] In general, who does the cultural or ethnic group consult with or listen to when health-related information is being sought or presented, and how do group members like this information to be given?
3. Western health care and health promotion use	[ ] What are the cultural or ethnic group's perceptons of Western health care practices and services?
	[ ] In what ways, and under what conditions, does the cultural or ethnic group currently use Western health care services?
	[ ] What are the traditional cultural rules governing interaction with a Western health care provider, health educator, or other health care professional in the clinical or community setting?
	[ ] What are the cultural or ethnic group's perceptions about change and change processes with respect to health behavior change recommendations from Western health providers?
	[ ] How are traditional health beliefs and practices mediated by acculturation and assimilation into mainstream society?
	[ ] What seem to be the major barriers to the target population's use of Western health care services?
	[ ] How have past efforts to reach the cultural or ethnic group with Western health care and/or screening and educational services been received? What worked, what did not work, and why?
4. Health behavior practices	[ ] What specific predisposing, enabling, and reinforcing factors are acting to maintain the health issue or problem to be addressed by the program?
	[ ] What specific predisposing, enabling, and reinforcing factors will need to be put in place to help promote the health changes being recommended to the cultural or ethnic group?
	[ ] What specific cultural or ethnic group factors may act to block the effectiveness of the health promotion program to achieve its objectives?

Explanatory Model

This level of assessment begins with a consideration of the explanatory model(s) that is used by the target group to explain and make sense of health and disease issues. As we have seen in the other chapters of this book, significant differences between the cultural or ethnic group model and the Western biomedical model can lead to differences of opinion, lack of adherence to prescribed treatment methods, and lack of involvement in health promotion efforts. Response to illness episodes is another area to be explored because many multicultural groups begin illness interventions by seeking the assistance of a traditional healer or by using traditional medicines that have been acquired in the community, handed down through the family, or suggested by close friends of the family. As noted elsewhere in this book, these traditional health practices often are used in conjunction with Western medical treatments, so determining what traditional measures have been or are likely to be taken can aid the health promoter in determining what interventions or combination of interventions will have the greatest likelihood of acceptance by the target group.

Perceptions

The perceptions of the target group with respect to the Western health care system also may come into play in both the clinical and health promotion settings. For example, if target group members perceive the Western health care facility as a "death house" where family or friends go in alive and come out dead, or as a place that shows little respect for or understanding of their traditional health beliefs and practices, then they will be more likely to avoid contact with this type of facility except under the most dire of circumstances. In addition to these variables, there may be other factors governing the target population's interest in or ability to access the HPDP program or service including barriers such as transportation, distance, hours of availability of the program or service, and language. Perceptions of change also may play a role in the target group's interest in or motivation to access the HPDP program or service. As noted in the earlier discussions of cosmology, time, and perceptions of self and community, for some traditional cultural groups the idea of change is foreign and the probability of resistance is quite high unless attention is paid to cultivating the value of a change and how it can be woven into the fabric of the target group's belief system.

Health Behavior Factors

The identification and role of predisposing, enabling, and reinforcing factors that are contributing to the health problem or issue or that will be brought into play to intervene and promote change also is an important assessment activity (Green & Kreuter, 1991). Here, the focus is on the specific health beliefs and practices that cut across the culture and are supported by other variables within the cultural milieu. For example, there may be specific food preferences and practices such as the use of high-fat foods, little use of fruits and vegetables, or much use of alcohol or tobacco products that might be contributing to the problem. Environmental conditions, including sanitation beliefs and practices or other factors, also might be acting to reinforce the issue or problem. An accurate assessment and educational-behavioral diagnosis is critical to understanding the problem and designing the most appropriate interventions.

WESTERN HEALTH CARE
ORGANIZATION AND ASSESSMENT

The final area of the CAF is concerned with the actual organization and staff who are providing the services to the multicultural group. Although one could make the argument that this area is a separate assessment unto itself, the authors would argue that the way in which the health promotion organization perceives the target group, how it prepares to deliver culturally competent services, and how the actual organizational facility is organized both physically and in its mission and policy documents play as great a role in the assessment process as does looking at those for whom the services are targeted. Table 26.5 presents the organizational assessment areas and associated questions for the reader's consideration.

Cultural Competency and Sensitivity

The first of these areas addresses cultural competence and sensitivity, which was discussed in some detail in Chapter 1. Of concern here are the agency's management and staff perceptions, interest, and motivation at every level to understand, respect, and interact appropriately with the target group. As noted in Chapter 1, a failure to take the steps to begin developing cultural competence within the agency is likely to contribute to interpersonal and communication problems between and among the agency's staff and those they are serving. A number of models have been proposed for how to begin developing cultural competence and sensitivity (Bell & Evans, 1981; Borkan & Neher, 1991; Campinha-Bacote, 1994). However, the first need is to determine, through the assessment process, where agency management and staff are in terms of cultural competence and sensitivity. This can set the scene for in-service and continuing education programming to help the agency better prepare and deliver culturally competent and sensitive care.

Organizational Policy and Mission

An agency's policy and mission statements can provide the impetus for moving its management and staff toward higher levels of culturally competent care and programming. Thus, an examination of current policy and mission statements should be undertaken to ensure that they incorporate a cultural competence philosophy that all can follow. If these features already exist in the policy and mission statements, then an assessment as to how well they are followed would be worthwhile with variables such as direct observation of staff and management interaction between and among themselves; observation of interactions in the clinic, waiting area, educational area, and other areas where the target group and facility staff interact; and observation of materials being given to the target group to determine how the materials are received, perceived, read, and understood as well as whether they are written in a language the target group can read and understand at the appropriate grade or reading level. This assessment also would

TABLE 26.5 Cultural Assessment Framework: Western Health Care Organization and Service Delivery

Assessment Area	Assessment Questions
1. Cultural competence and sensitivity	[ ] How well prepared are the staff and management of the agency to provide culturally competent services to the targeted cultural or ethnic group?
	[ ] How sensitive are agency staff and management to the cultural nuances and needs of the targeted cultural or ethnic group?
	[ ] How well prepared are the health promotion staff and management to provide culturally competent health promotion services to the targeted cultural or ethnic group?
	[ ] How sensitive are the health promotion staff and management to the cultural nuances and needs of the targeted cultural or ethnic group?
	[ ] How much training have all agency staff and management had in cultural competence and sensitivity to multicultural populations being served by them?
	[ ] What additional training in cultural competence and sensitivity is needed by all agency staff and management?
	[ ] How well prepared is the agency to deliver training to staff and management in the areas of cultural competence and sensitivity?
2. Organizational policy and mission	[ ] What written policy and/or mission statements exist pertaining to the provision of culturally competent and sensitive health care and and health promotion services?
	[ ] If policy or mission statements exist, then how well do agency staff and management adhere to these?
	[ ] If no specific policy or mission statements exist, then how might these be developed and implemented in the agency?
3. Facilities and program preparation	[ ] How well organized is the agency's facility with respect to signs, directions, bilingual or bicultural staff, translators, and written materials specific to the multicultural populations to be served by the agency?
	[ ] How well prepared is the program with respect to signs, directions, bilingual or bicultural staff, translators, and written program and educational materials specific to the multicultural populations to be served?
	[ ] What additional preparation will be needed to bring the agency or program on-line, and who will facilitate that process?
4. Evaluation of culturally competent services	[ ] What evaluation processes currently are in place to monitor the delivery and efficacy of the culturally competent and sensitive program or service being provided to the targeted multicultural population group?
	[ ] What additional evaluation processes are needed to monitor delivery and efficacy of this program or service, and who will develop these processes?
	[ ] What staff training is needed to implement evaluation and monitoring of the program or service to be provided?
	[ ] When will monitoring and evaluation processes be carried out, and who will carry them out?
	[ ] How will monitoring and evaluation results be used to improve program or service delivery, and at what points will this take place?

apply to signs within and around the facility and in other locales where services including health promotion programming may be offered.

Performance Evaluation

Perhaps the most critical aspect of the agency's preparation and delivery of culturally competent and sensitive medical treatment and HPDP services is that of evaluation, that is, the need to conduct regular evaluations of management, staff, the target group, and the physical plant to ensure that the highest levels of culturally competent and sensitive care are being provided and that ongoing efforts are being made through in-service and continuing education to keep all agency personnel adequately trained in this area. The authors recognize that this is a tall order, necessitating resources including staff and money, but feel that the benefits of such activity will far outweigh the costs in the long term including litigation to settle disputes that may arise as a result of ignoring cultural differences.

CHAPTER SUMMARY

The need to adequately assess culture-specific variables when planning HPDP programming cannot be stressed enough. As has been repeatedly described throughout this book, there are many approaches that can be taken to assess, plan, implement, and evaluate HPDP programs for multicultural population groups. All of these share common elements including the need to accurately determine what the target population is, what group members' specific health needs and concerns are, what makes group members unique as a cultural or ethnic group, and what special planning efforts will be needed to deliver culturally competent and sensitive services to them.

This chapter has sought to provide a CAF that includes questions the health promoter or planner should consider asking when designing programming for a multicultural population target group. The framework presents five major levels of assessment including culture-specific demographic variables, culture-specific epidemiological and environmental influences, general and specific cultural characteristics, general and specific health beliefs and practices, and Western health care organization and service delivery variables. Each of these levels of assessment can help bring the health practitioner to a higher level of understanding about the cultural or ethnic group with which he or she is working and can help ensure that culturally appropriate, competent, and sensitive HPDP programs or services are planned for group members.

REFERENCES

Andrew, M. M., & Boyle, J. S. (1995). *Transcultural concepts in nursing care* (2nd ed.). Philadelphia: J. B. Lippincott.

Bell, P., & Evans, J. (1981). *Counseling the black client.* Center City, MN: Hazelden Education Materials.

Borkan, J., & Neher, J. (1991). A developmental model of ethnosensitivity in family practice training. *Family Medicine, 23,* 212-217.

Brislin, R. W., & Yoshida, T. (Eds.). (1994). *Improving intercultural interactions: Modules for cross-cultural training programs.* Thousand Oaks, CA: Sage.

Brownlee, A. T. (1978). *Community, culture, and care: A cross-cultural guide for health workers.* St. Louis, MO: C. V. Mosby.

Campinha-Bacote, J. (1994). Cultural competence in psychiatric mental health nursing: A conceptual model. *Nursing Clinics of North America, 29*(1), 1-8.

Clark, A. L. (1978). *Culture, childbearing, health professionals.* Philadelphia: F. A. Davis.

Farrales, S. (1996). Vietnamese. In J. G. Lipson, S. L. Dibble, & P. A. Minarik (Eds.), *Culture and nursing care: A pocket guide*. San Francisco: UCSF Nursing Press.

Galanti, G. A. (1991). *Caring for patients from different cultures: Case studies from American hospitals*. Philadelphia: University of Pennsylvania Press.

Green, L., & Kreuter, M. W. (1991). *Health promotion planning: An educational and environmental approach* (2nd ed.). Mountain View, CA: Mayfield.

Helman, C. (1984). *Culture, health and illness: An introducton for health professionals*. Bristol, UK: John Wright.

Ishida, D. N., & Toomata-Mayer, T. F., & Mayer, J. F. (1996). Samoans. In J. G. Lipson, S. L. Dibble, & P. A. Minarik (Eds.), *Culture and nursing care: A pocket guide*. San Francisco: UCSF Nursing Press.

Leininger, M. (1995). *Transcultural nursing: Concepts, theories, research and practices* (2nd ed.). New York: McGraw-Hill.

Lipson, J. G., & Steiger, N. J. (1996). *Self-care nursing in a multicultural context*. Thousand Oaks, CA: Sage.

Lynch, E., & Hanson, M. (1992). Steps in the right direction: Implications for interventionists. In E. Lynch & M. Hanson (Eds.), *Developing cross-cultural competence: A guide for working with young children and their families*. Baltimore, MD: Paul H. Brookes.

Marin, G., & Gamba, R. (1996). A new measurement of acculturation for Hispanics: The Bidirectional Acculturation Scale for Hispanics (BAS). *Hispanic Journal of Behavioral Sciences, 18,* 297-316.

Mo, B. (1992). Cross-cultural medicine a decade later: Modesty, sexuality, and breast health in Chinese-American women. *Western Journal of Medicine, 9,* 260-264.

Orque, M. S., Block, B., & Ahumada Monrroy, L. S. (1983). *Ethnic nursing care: A multicultural approach*. St. Louis, MO: C. V. Mosby.

Pasick, R. J., D'Onofrio, C. N., & Otero-Sabogal, R. (1996). Similarities and differences across cultures: Questions to inform a third generation for health promotion research. *Health Education Quarterly, 23*(Suppl.), S142-S161.

Ramirez, A. G., Cousins, J. H., Santos, Y., & Supic, J. D. (1986). A media-based acculturation scale for Mexican-Americans: Application to public health programs. *Family and Community Health, 9*(3), 63-71.

Seidel, H. M., Ball, J. W., Dains, J. E., & Benedict, G. W. (1995). *Mosby's guide to physical examination* (3rd ed.). St. Louis, MO: C. V. Mosby.

Spector, R. E. (1996). *Cultural diversity in health and illness* (4th ed.). Stamford, CT: Appleton & Lange.

Tripp-Reimer, T., Brink, P. J., & Saunders, J. M. (1984). Cultural assessment: Content and process. *Nursing Outlook, 32*(2), 78-82.

27

Moving Into the 21st Century

*Final Thoughts About Multicultural
Health Promotion and Disease Prevention*

MICHAEL V. KLINE
ROBERT M. HUFF

The purpose of this book is to highlight the importance of the role of multicultural influences and their effect on health problems, health status, health participation patterns, and health-seeking and health-promoting behaviors. A further intent was to increase the awareness of the health practitioner involved in the planning of health promotion programs that the outcomes of those activities are, to a large extent, shaped by a unique combination of different cultural orientations and influences from target population with which the practitioner is working. The health practitioner also is reminded that his or her own sociocultural orientations can play a role in these outcomes.

Earlier chapters presented health behavior and health promotion planning concepts, theories, and models. Major aspects of culture and cultural diversity among African Americans, Latinos, Native Americans, Asian Americans, and Pacific Islanders also were presented. The concepts of ethnicity, assimilation, and acculturation were described, and the barriers and problems frequently encountered by the health practitioner seeking to design health promotion and disease prevention programs were outlined.

The health promotion practitioner in the future will be confronted with increasing difficulties in accurately defining target populations. This stems from the substantial and growing heterogeneity within groups in terms of culture, racial/ethnic background, social norms, and generational and acculturation differences. The practitioner must be aware of the danger of clumping groups together so as to mask differences including health status. The Chen and Hawks

(1995) study discussed in Chapter 4 exploded the myth of the model healthy Asian American or Pacific Islander. Also, systems that have evolved for purposes of classifying individuals by ethnicity/race have further complicated the accurate definition of target groups. For example, Montes, Eng, and Braithwaite (1995) observe that the term *minority* evolved in 1977 when the Federal Office of Management and Budget established Directive No. 15, which created five designations under which an individual could be identified: Asian or Pacific Islander, black, Hispanic, Native American, and white. Individuals not identified as white were called *minorities*. Working terms and categorizations such as these have become less useful over time to precisely reflect group differences of the various populations in the United States (Montes et al., 1995).

Several chapters were devoted to the demanding and complex topics of health promotion and disease prevention (HPDP) design, implementation, and evaluation aspects in the context of specific cultural settings. Case study chapters were offered with each major section to illustrate and discuss important aspects of application. "Tips" chapters were offered after each major section to help summarize and highlight major points.

The present chapter presents some final thoughts and tries to reinforce some important points and issues raised. These issues undoubtedly will continue to have important implications for the practitioner working in the area of multicultural HPDP in the next millennium.

GROWING MULTICULTURAL DIVERSITY: IMPLICATIONS FOR FUTURE HEALTH PROMOTION AND DISEASE PREVENTION ACTIVITIES

Many groups representing numerous origins and social situations will continue to make up an increasing and significant part of the urban and rural population of the United States—the mainland, islands, reservations, and territories. Overview chapters in each major section of the book provided some information on population growth and trends and examined health problem areas with regard to the five specific population groups covered. That information makes it apparent that, owing to future population trends and disproportionate levels of individual risks of poor health among some population groups, there will be a continuing need to expand HPDP programming efforts within these groups. Some further information is presented in this section to reinforce that contention.

In general, the population of the United States, which numbered nearly 249 million in 1990, is projected to increase by 40 million people by the year 2020 (U.S. Bureau of the Census, 1996). During the 30-year period from 1990 to 2020, projections by the U.S. Bureau of the Census (lowest projection series) anticipate further increases among an already diverse resident population (e.g., a 1.4% increase among African Americans; a 2.3% total increase among the American Indian, Eskimo, and Aleutian Islander populations; a 6% increase among residents of Hispanic origin). Also, if current immigration patterns and policies hold (nearly 1 million people every year could be admitted under a number of classes), then a possible 30 million people could be added between 1990 and 2030, contributing further to the numbers and diversity of the population (U.S. Bureau of the Census, 1996).

The following 1995 census estimates give the health professional an idea of future HPDP programming needs with implications for all population groups: Approximately 51.2% of the U.S. population were women, 7.5% (19.6 million) were under 5 years of age, and those age 65 years or over totaled 33.5 million (13% of the U.S. population; U.S. Bureau of the Census, 1996). At 65 years of age, the average life expectancy in 1993 was projected well into one's 80s (17.3 years). More than one quarter (25.1%) of the total population belonged to ethnic groups other than white. African Americans comprised 12.6% of the total, and individuals of Hispanic origin accounted for 10.3% of the total population (U.S. Bureau of the Census, 1996).

In general, most Americans are seeking and receiving appropriate health care. Most are working and relatively well educated, and most are striving to improve the quality of life for themselves and their families. However, many individuals and families continue to be at higher risk of poor physical, psychological, and/or social health. Regardless of race, ethnicity, citizenship status, employment status, or educational level, each population group has an appreciable number of high-risk mothers and infants, elderly, alcohol and substance abusers, mentally ill, obese, homeless, chronically ill, individuals with AIDS, cigarette smokers, those who work in occupations where their jobs may place them at higher than normal risk, and others in a variety of health risk categories.

There are several basic determinants of health including living conditions, education, nutrition, and protection from environmental hazards. Attainment of these is heavily dependent on jobs and income (Feingold, 1995). Aday (1993) also notes, "Minorities, the poor, and those with less education tend to experience more health problems in general over the course of their lives, based on an array of indicators of need, than do their more socioeconomically advantaged counterparts" (p. 50). Mortality and morbidity rates are higher among poor populations. This observation is all the more significant if one considers that nearly 12% of the white population in the United States lives in poverty. This is much worse for African Americans and Hispanic Americans, as 31% of each group are below the poverty line (U.S. Bureau of the Census, 1996). Furthermore, nearly one third (31.2%) of Native Americans were below the poverty level. The census statistics also disclose that 43.3% of African American children and 41.1% of Hispanic children under 18 years of age live below the poverty level. Furthermore, about 2.2 million African American families and about 1.7 million Hispanic families live below the poverty level (U.S. Bureau of the Census, 1996).

Blane (1995) notes the consistency in the distribution of mortality and morbidity among social groups. "The more advantaged groups, whether expressed in terms of income, education, social class, or ethnicity, tend to have better health than the other members of their societies" (p. 903). Also, data from the National

Health Interview Survey for the years 1978 to 1980 and 1989 to 1991 consistently show that "children in poor families experience a disproportionate burden of health problems, a higher risk of severe illness and chronic conditions, and more limitation of activity than children in more affluent families" (Montgomery, Kiely, & Pappas, 1996, p. 1401). Sorlie, Backlund, and Keller (1995), in their National Longitudinal Mortality Study, observe that within each race group, those identified as being at a higher risk of death are poorer, less educated, employed in service-oriented occupations, or not in the labor force.

MULTICULTURAL HEALTH PROMOTION AND DISEASE PREVENTION: GROWING NEEDS FOR PARTICIPATION AND OWNERSHIP

America is a *multicultural* society, and the American culture is very diverse. Green, in his foreword to this book, noted a major paradox faced by nations, states, communities, and institutions seeking to create multicultural societies, especially where equity is the central value of multiculturalism. There is an effort to maintain a respect for differences while recognizing that differences conspire against equity. Multiculturalism, as it attempts to relate equity to equality, uniformity, and sameness, poses a difficult dilemma. "People cannot be simultaneously different and equal on all counts of living" (p. ix, this volume). It was discussed earlier that some of these dimensions include basic determinants of health such as living conditions, education, nutrition, access to health care, and protection from environmental hazards. It was noted that those who are poor, regardless of race/ethnicity or culture, tend to experience more health problems in general over the course of their lives than do their more socioeconomically advantaged counterparts. A major dilemma always has been how to obtain and increase the involvement of these vulnerable target groups, regardless of ethnicity or culture, in the identification of and response to their health concerns.

It is well recognized that there is a critical need for health care reform in America that makes quality health care services, health promotion services, and disease prevention activities accessible and available to all residents and at the same time helps contain costs. Green and Ottoson (1994) note that a balanced model of community health is needed at each local level and should consist of at least four elements of the health field where interventions could be directed. The first element, human biology, is one that communities in democratic societies can exert very little direct control over other than through genetic counseling. However, there are three other intervention points in a variety of community settings (e.g., health care organizations, work sites, community health programs, schools) where efforts can be directed toward reducing mortality and morbidity: (a) *health protection* (i.e., interventions are directed toward bringing about environmental change through regulatory practices), (b) *health promotion* (i.e., interventions are focused on bringing about lifestyle changes), and (c) *preventive health services* (i.e., interventions are aimed at organizational change and increasing access to health resources within the health care system (Green & Ottoson, 1994). Within these activities conducted at the local levels (health protection, health promotion, and preventive health planning), there is the critical need to obtain the active participation of the target groups who are most vulnerable to health-related problems and conditions that negatively affect their quality of life and that of their families and communities.

There are many ways in which, and reasons why, people become involved and stay involved in multicultural health promotion planning efforts. The challenge, of course, is to be able to identify and initiate appropriate approaches for securing and maintaining involvement. Chapter 4 stressed the importance of identifying the distinct cultural protocols and styles that may lead the practitioner to better recognize where the possible points of securing and maintaining involvement might lie. Community or subgroup participation should occur from the time a problem is first felt but not well defined to the time it is well documented and ultimately serves as a basis for writing objectives, developing strategies, and implementing and evaluating the program. Every health planning and health promotion planning model should recognize the importance of the need for participation.

The principle of participation, discussed in Chapters 3 and 4, is explicit in its recognition that the people—the participants—should have a part in the planning, thus making the situation one in which there is planning *with*, not *for*, the people. Frankish et al., in Chapter 3, observed that when people participate in a program, they feel greater ownership of the program and a sense of "responsibility for and control over promoting changes in their behavior and health status" (p. 61, this volume). Community organization and development approaches are built on the principle of participation, which stresses that an HPDP program is likely to be more successful when the community at risk identifies "its own health concerns, develops its own prevention and intervention programs, and forms a decision-making board to make policy decisions and identify resources for program implementation" (Braithwaite, 1992, p. 327).

THE NEED TO UNDERSTAND THE CONCEPTS OF HEALTH PROMOTION AND DISEASE PREVENTION

Given the trends and projections for the United States noted at the beginning of the chapter, future efforts to plan and implement HPDP program strategies within different multicultural populations will take on greater importance. However, there is a need to acknowledge that the notions of HPDP are conceptually difficult to understand for many participants (including the practitioner). There also is the issue of how to convey adequate understanding in light of differing cultural beliefs and practices concerning health and health behavior change. There is a need for participants to appreciate that putting health promotion programs into place requires time as well as a significant commitment at different levels to provide a range of costly resources and services.

The myriad of definitions and interpretations underlying the concepts can be confusing to the health practitioner and the community members with whom the practitioner will be working. Several earlier chapters provided definitions and discussion concerning the concept of health promotion. These definitions emphasized the importance of conducting a range of HPDP efforts involving a combination of activities at multiple levels of change. For example, at one level, programs may concentrate on facilitating the voluntary acquisition of specific health-related knowledge, attitudes, and practices to achieve behavior related to improving or promoting health where people live and work. Efforts at another level may seek social or environmental changes (supportive structures) in the form of policy changes, regulations, and new or increased organizational arrangements for encouraging, enabling, and reinforcing the practice of certain health-related behaviors (Green & Kreuter, 1991).

The practitioner might find that the most immediate need is to prepare all participants with at least a basic level of conceptual understanding of how the different levels of health promotion strategies and activities can help increase the community's capacity to design and implement effective disease prevention and health programs. It is important that participants recognize that interventions designed to achieve change on only the individual level will not be as effective as those that can achieve change on the community level. Within their own cultural milieu, planning participants need to recognize that any HPDP interventions contemplated must consider the personal experiences, knowledge, health practices, and problem-solving methodologies that are acceptable within the framework of the group or community. They need to understand the basic concepts of predisposing, enabling, and reinforcing factors and their relationship to clearly identifying and building interventions to modify health behaviors or conditions.

Another very important point is that the concept of *disease prevention* needs to be explained to community participants so that they understand its relationship to *health promotion*. The practitioner needs to help participants grasp the differences in the levels of disease prevention activities that might need to be conducted, that is, the primary prevention level (providing specific protection that prevents the onset of the disease itself), the secondary prevention level (providing activities related to early diagnosis and prompt treatment of a disease that is present), and the tertiary level of prevention (activities to minimize disability from existing illness to treatment and rehabilitation efforts). The practitioner, with the help of community planning participants, identifies the most appropriate types of strategies to be used at each prevention level to accomplish overall health promotion goals. Again, these concepts must be put into an appropriate context that considers differing cultural beliefs and practices concerning matters of individual, family, and community health.

CULTURAL ASSESSMENT: A KEY COMPONENT
OF PLANNING HEALTH PROMOTION PROGRAMS
IN MULTICULTURAL POPULATIONS

Gaining knowledge that will enable tailored health promotion programming that is congruent with each group's needs is critical. It requires the practitioner and participants from the target community to accurately assess cultural differences, beliefs, and practices in the contexts of social conditions such as rural/urban, social class, country of origin, language, generational aspects, and historical experiences with the wider society. The challenges of multicultural target group assessment and programming are increased when several culturally diverse groups live within the same community sharing common geographical boundaries. In these situations, it becomes critical to identify group differences and similarities related to specific cultural positions, norms, and practices held within each population and subpopulation. The practitioner will have to be more aware of the need to carry out an accurate assessment of each subgroup's particular or unique set of risk factors and to understand how these should relate to the design and implementation of prevention programs and interventions that will be more congruent with the cultural uniqueness of a community or group. The use of the cultural assessment framework, as described in Chapter 26, can facilitate a more complete assessment of these cultural characteristics.

Huff and Kline, in Chapter 1, discussed *culture* as the repository of devices needed for a group's (or a subgroup's) adaptation that evolves over many generations. A health promotion planning group contemplating the development of health education activities within a first-generation group of immigrants to the United States, regardless of where they came from, needs specific information concerning differences in health-related belief systems and cultural practices. Such issues would be of equal importance if one were assessing differences in program needs related to the second, third, or even fourth generations of the first-generation immigrant. These types of considerations will challenge health promotion programmers for many years to come given current immigration patterns.

Issues of *acculturation* and *assimilation* also become important variables. Although closely related, awareness of these important cultural variables may provide key areas by which to more specifically assess and segment intraethnic groups (Huff & Kline, Chapter 1, this volume; Padilla, 1980). A methodology, such as that developed by Balcazar, Castro, and Krull (1995), can provide the planner with a tool for assessing key factors such as acculturation and educational status in various subgroups of Hispanics. The value of such a tool is that its method can be transferred and used in other ethnic group settings, for example, to help identify information for planning more culturally appropriate cancer risk reduction programs. Huff and Kline, in Chapter 1, and Castro, Cota, and Vega, in Chapter 7, discussed the use and value of these types of assessment tools.

Keogh, Gallimore, and Weisner (1997) stress the need for the practitioner to carefully distinguish ethnicity and culture in educational practice. *Ethnicity,* which was discussed in Chapter 1, has many referents—sense of identity based on common ancestry, national, religious, tribal, linguistic, or cultural origins (Nunnaly & Moy, 1989; Paniagua, 1994); feelings of belonging and continuity through time; shared meanings and traditions; and self-ascribed genealogical and social affiliations including related forms of family and group affect (Keogh et al., 1997). Whereas ethnic identity tends to persist through time, *culture* changes when individuals and groups modify their beliefs and practices to survive and adapt. Although ethnicity and culture are correlated in many ways, the practitioner needs to understand that there are cultural differences among groups with the same ethnic background (Huff & Kline, Chapter 1, this volume). The complexities of health education and health promotion planning are increased when groups share common health-related problems but, owing to culturally unique factors, approach solutions to the problems in different culturally prescribed ways.

One of the dilemmas of a multicultural society is how to effectively take into account issues of cultural or ethnic diversity, particularly in working with, planning, and implementing health promotion programs. The planner must be extremely sensitive to diversity without stereotyping subgroups within the same ethnic or racial groups. For example, Native Americans include many distinct tribal groups with differing cultures and lifestyles, as noted in Chapters 14 and 15 with regard to those individuals and groups in urban settings and those in isolated rural or reservation settings. Keogh et al. (1997) observe that it is imprecise and inaccurate to use identification labels such as *Hispanic, Asian, African American, Native American,* and *Anglo-American* or *Euro-American* as substitute terms for culture. Rather, it is much more precise to use the terms that these different cultural or ethnic groups use to describe themselves.

PROGRAM DIRECTION IN MULTICULTURAL HEALTH PROMOTION

Several chapters in this book dealt specifically with aspects of program assessment, design, implementation, and evaluation in culturally specific settings. Underlying these efforts was an attempt to focus program design in a way that built in a more culturally competent and responsive approach needed for reaching and influencing target group health behavior. Most of the contributors to these chapters agreed that program design and development should intensively capitalize on the strengths of the community in which the participants and program are located (Ashley, Chapter 11, this volume; Castro et al., Chapter 7, this volume; Montes et al., 1995). However, the professional literature is relatively sparse when it comes to agreement on the "best" approach or direction to use when designing effective programs directed at culturally specific ethnic populations or subpopulations. This is a complex issue and is covered here only to the degree that the reader can become aware of at least two different viewpoints concerning program direction.

One school of thought suggests that if a program for a particular ethnic group in the community is organized traditionally (i.e., in terms of the time-tested components of health education program planning such as those discussed in Chapter 4), then with appropriate modification, the program approach should be transferable to other ethnic groups in their specific community settings. However, built into this approach is an intentional separation of factors from their cultural context or setting, even though such a program is focused on changing specific behaviors in the target group (e.g., diet, exercise, periodic screening visits). That is, culture is viewed in more neutral terms but is considered an important factor to be considered as well as other social, psychological, epidemiological, physical, and environmental factors. Montes et al. (1995) observe, "Separation of factors from their cultural context is largely a function of (1) developing programs that can be replicated on a wider scale and (2) the assumption that changes in the cultural context will occur as increasing numbers of people change their behaviors" (p. 248). Program designs that use, for example, the PRECEDE framework use a sequential approach to program planning, starting with the proposition acknowledging that health behaviors are very complex, are multidimensional, and may be influenced by a variety of factors (Gielen & McDonald, 1997). However, within the framework, there is a need to conduct a cultural assessment. Such an assessment can identify important cultural factors of the target group to be taken into consideration with respect to the ultimate educational design of the program. Castro et al., in Chapter 7, and Ashley, in Chapter 11, provided good examples of this type of program approach, even though the respective target group settings were within heavy Hispanic and African American areas.

The second school of thought concerning the direction to be taken in health education and health promotion program design advocates the need to emphasize the cultural aspects of the particular racial/ethnic population for which the program is being planned. In contrast to the first view, this approach acknowledges that there are significant differences in cultural worldviews and norms within each minority group. According to this approach, these differences derive from particular social conditions within urban or rural settings, social class, country of origin, and historical experiences with the larger society. Adherents to this second viewpoint maintain that the practitioner must be able to intensively assess the need for differences in program direction by clearly and sensitively understanding each group's cultural uniqueness. This understanding, it is maintained, can help the programmer to become more knowledgeable about and culturally sensitive to the way in which the specific group defines health problems and needs, how that relates to group members' personal experiences, knowledge required and the context in which that knowledge must be acquired, health practices, and how group members undertake and participate in problem-solving processes that are acceptable within the framework of that group or community.

Marin et al. (1995) believe that, in many instances, if a program is targeted only to the needs of the general population, then it might not be effective in achieving the desired behavioral changes within underserved groups. They also cite the need for health education programs to target and consider the unique conditions experienced by underserved groups owing to their specific cultural characteristics or to the fact that they have been underserved. Aguirre-Molina (1993) observes that mainstream HPDP programs might not work in the Latino community because they are "devoid of cultural competence" (p. 25). She cites instances in which there might be complete disregard for important cultural traits that are specific to Latinos such as the important role the family and other social support systems can play in promoting health and preventing disease. Fredericks and Hodge's "talking circle" health education program, discussed in Chapter 16, is a good example of this second viewpoint because rather than using a well-defined traditional health education planning and intervention model, it was built from the ground up in an attempt to ensure a culturally unique program response. The African-centered model of prevention for African American youths at high risk developed by Nobles and Goddard (1993) is another good example of this second approach and takes an African orientation.

The importance given to culture within this school of thought is "largely a function of (1) developing prevention programs that can be tailored to each community and, hence, may not be transferable and (2) assuming that behavioral change must be sustained through concomitant social change and adaptation to cultural context" (Montes et al., 1995, p. 248).

Regardless of the direction in which the program emphasis focuses, it should be reached through a very intensive process of target group-specific needs assessment and diagnosis. And regardless of which direction program design takes with regard to achieving specific behavior change, there is the need to view the group's cultural uniqueness as it relates to the way in which group members define health problems, how they identify proposed solutions to those problems, how they select types of activities to be initiated, and how favorable behavioral change, once achieved, can be sustained in that population. Those involved in health promotion activities might be hard-pressed to have the range of staff or other resources available that will be able to deal with the needs of each culture in the most appropriate ways. In either case, the practitioner should not adhere rigidly to one approach or the other because the approach should depend on a thorough assessment of the situation and the particular target group. Each approach also requires an explicit recognition of different cultural groups and their diversity, the need for cultural competence, and the need for effective skills in intercultural communications. This topic is discussed in the next section.

ISSUES OF CULTURAL COMPETENCE: PREPARING TO WORK IN MULTICULTURAL POPULATIONS

The health promotion practitioner will increasingly be working in multicultural program settings and will need to possess cultural awareness and knowledge about the target group, cultural skill, and cultural encounter. In short, the practitioner must be culturally competent. Although *cultural competence* was broadly discussed in Chapter 1 and has been alluded to in several sections of this chapter, there is a need to briefly discuss and reinforce the importance of the concept. Cultural competence has been defined as "a set of congruent behaviors, attitudes, and policies that come together in a system, agency, or among professionals and enables that system, agency, or those professionals to work effectively in cross-cultural situations" (Cross, Bazron, Dennis, & Isaacs, 1989, as quoted in Campinha-Bacote, 1994, p. iv). It also has been defined as "a process for effectively working within the cultural context of an individual or community from a diverse cultural or ethic background" (Campinha-Bacote, 1994, pp. 1-2).

The health promotion practitioner who is expected to function in multicultural settings must be aware and accepting of cultural differences, should be culturally knowledgeable about the target group, and should be able to adapt to diverse situations. Kreps and Kunimoto (1994) emphasize that the system in which we work is "a cultural melting pot, comprising individuals from different combinations of national, regional, ethnic, racial, socioeconomic, occupational, generational, and health status cultural orientations" (p. 5). Planning, initiating, and implementing HPDP activities in this complex system of cultural differences and points of view requires great thoughtfulness. If participants are not sensitive to each other's cultural orientations, beliefs, and practices in the variety of possible planning and program scenarios involving different populations, settings, health issues, and level of program focus, then the health promotion processes could be seriously jeopardized.

Brislin and Yoshida (1994) recognized that lack of knowledge concerning health beliefs and practices, as well as competing cultural values, beliefs, and norms among different population groups, can seriously undermine the credibility of the health professional working with these groups and can disrupt the provision of services. It is important to be aware that as the concept currently is employed, it is the responsibility of the health professional to acquire the knowledge and skills needed to work with a specific client, target group, or population. This one-sided situation, it is suggested, encourages only the planner or specific program staff or providers to develop cultural competence and does not place the same requirement on the client, target group, or population. Throughout this book, it has been stressed that effective interaction in planning and program environments cannot take place unless all parties possess mutual respect for the culture and contributions of the others. The notion of cultural competence, particularly in health promotion planning interactions, needs to build on a two-sided partnership with the expectation that individuals need to work together in planning situations or health program settings and that each needs to be aware of the other's cultural values, beliefs, and norms. Each party must be sensitive to its own patterns and styles of interaction with other cultures, particularly as these styles could reflect biases or prejudices that could seriously disrupt the planning process. The planner and the participants must avoid imposing their beliefs, values, and patterns of behavior on another culture (Campinha-Bacote, 1994; Leininger, 1994). Collaboration between the planner and participants is possible only if each understands the other's values, has mutual respect for the agenda to be accomplished, and accepts the other party as integral to the approach to the problem.

MULTICULTURAL HEALTH PROMOTION:
THE ETHICAL DIMENSION

There is a need, in this final section, to briefly consider aspects of the ethical dimension that the practitioner and participants may encounter when working in multicultural health promotion settings. There always have been and always will be many points of view held and espoused by practitioners and participants concerning what should be the "right" methods of assessment, approaches, priorities, and interventions to be used in particular HPDP activities. For example, who should have access to assessment data that are collected? Who should be involved in the interpretation of the information? To what degree should planning information be kept confidential?

When people of different cultures representing a variety of knowledge and skill areas work together, there always will be different points of view about how programs or activities should be implemented, maintained, and evaluated. In reality, these diverse points of view (cultural or otherwise) held by the parties involved ultimately bring creativity, rationality, and progress to the health promotion undertaking. However, when a point of view becomes subject to dispute, it becomes an *issue* to the parties involved. The issue usually arises from the social and cultural values people hold about something that gives meaning and purpose to their lives. Values also provide the means by which the practitioner and participants alike judge or compare the relative worth or the rightness or wrongness of certain ideas, practices, or approaches. Many times, the conflict caused by these issues emanates from differing points of view as to rightness; fair play and justice; respect for one's cultural, personal, or group autonomy; subtle or blatant misrepresentation of one's position or professional skills; and issues of legality. In many instances, the practitioner is told that he or she has an obligation to behave ethically. What does that mean?

Health promotion endeavors are complex because they deliberately focus on making judgments concerning the elimination or modification of some aspect of community health risk or risk behavior of individuals. The practitioner and participants are encouraged to engage in intensive processes of problem identification, select a course of action, and make decisions concerning resource acquisition and use. However, should their desire to enhance personal freedom and self-determination override their desire to modify an environment to shape more healthful behavior? These efforts might involve directing educational interventions at high-risk individuals, families, groups, or whole communities with the intent of facilitating the voluntary acquisition of specific health-related knowledge, attitudes, and practices related to improving or promoting health where people live and work. To what extent can the practitioner impose his or her values on individuals or communities? Is the program or activity designed to further social ends? Whose? Who decides what is a proper social end? The majority? If yes, then what if the majority is wrong? Thus, in an ethical context, any interventions used should seek voluntary behavior and be supported by an informed and consenting public. At another level, health promotion efforts may seek to bring about social or environmental changes (supportive structures) in the form of policy changes, regulations, or new and increased organizational arrangements for encouraging, enabling, and reinforcing the practice of certain health-related behaviors (Green & Kreuter, 1991). Interventions to be used in these instances might be for purposes of fostering economic, political, legal, and organizational changes. The intent of these changes is to support individual or community actions favorable to achieving health behaviors associated with protecting health or lowering risks including the organization and equitable distribution of preventive health care services. All of these levels of change confront the practitioner with complex ethical issues and decisions, especially when the practitioner and the target group have differing cultural beliefs and practices. When change is needed and sought in certain individual or collective health behaviors for reducing risk, ethical issues invariably will be raised concerning what the appropriate actions should be of the people whose health is in question and what the actions should be of community decision makers, health practitioners, teachers, employers, parents, and others who may influence health behaviors, resources, or services in the community. Implied in this process is the element of participation in the design of programs and interventions that are intended, what the changes will be, how they will be affected, and how that will influence them or the target community. What level of participation should be solicited, and should it be voluntary and encouraged?

There are several basic ethical principles that the health promotion practitioner should be concerned about and familiar with. These principles are relevant and provide guidelines or philosophical foundations for practicing ethics. The reader should realize that, at best, the following very complex principles are stated in a very simplistic manner, and the reader is referred to the sources cited. There are at least four basic principles of which the health promotion practitioner should be aware. The first is *respect for people,* which includes allowing them to be free to choose and pursue a course of action (so long as it does no harm to others), being honest in all activities (e.g., complete understanding and consent before people can decide on a course of action), maintaining confidentiality when appropriate, and keeping one's word (Darr, 1991). Is it appropriate to try to persuade people to behave in ways conducive to good health, or do we accept the proposition that it is the right of individuals to do as they please with their own health so long as this does not impinge on the rights of others? The second principle is *nonmalificence.* That is, we should do no harm to others and should not take any intentional risk that could result in doing harm to others. The third is *beneficence,* which requires that one do more than simply doing no harm to others (Butler, 1997) and involves two components: doing all that one can to assist participants but also being able to balance the benefits and risks of the action. Do we then apprise people and communities of the alternatives and the risks of the alternatives? What tactics are to be used? What strategies are appropriate? According to whom? Do the means justify the ends? Who decides this? Who selects the course of action? Should the use of techniques (e.g., fear arousal) that can bring about faster behavior change be used rather than slower educational and organizing methods? The fourth principle is *justice.* This principle implies that "every person should be treated fairly and similarly; norms and rules must be applied to every member of a group consistently and continuously" (Butler 1997, p. 314; see also Beauchamp & Childress, 1989; Darr, 1991; Greenberg & Gold, 1992).

The health promotion practitioner has the awesome responsibility of helping individuals, families, and communities to make health decisions directed toward improving the quality of their lives. It is the health promoter's obligation to pursue this outcome with moral and ethical conduct and at the highest level of professional competence.

FINAL THOUGHTS: THE NEED FOR THE PRACTITIONER TO USE THEORIES, MODELS, AND PRINCIPLES AS GUIDES TO PRACTICE

In too many instances, empirical or pragmatic considerations have guided health promotion program planning and intervention efforts. It becomes rapidly clear to most practitioners that there is no one magic prepackaged HPDP program guaranteed to work in all situations, in all settings, and for all ethnic groups or subgroups. In fact, we are not even quite sure why some programs work or why some of our interventions achieve their desired effects. We do know, however, that each program or intervention design situation requires thought and analysis and that each requires consideration of established guides to practice. There is a need to close the chapter by reminding the reader that throughout this book, he or she has been exposed to an extensive range of subjects, thinking, and approaches that illustrate the richness and scope of health promotion and health education activities in multicultural settings. What has characterized each chapter, particularly the case study chapters and the assessment, design, and evaluation chapters, has been the reliance of the practitioner on frameworks for organizing knowledge and thinking. The frameworks used, whether brand new or traditional, have been derived, over time, from a myriad of health promotion and health education theory, principles, and practice models.

What has made planning and intervention design and selection such a complex task for the practitioner working with specific target groups, settings, and health issues is the overwhelming number of theories, principles, and models that guide health promotion and health education professionals. The usefulness of many is questionable, whereas other frameworks have been well established over time and are of immense value to the field of health promotion. Frankish et al., in Chapter 3, observed that theoretical frameworks can provide program developers "with a perspective from which to organize knowledge and to interpret factors and events" (p. 42, this volume). They discussed the need and rationale for using a theoretical framework; differentiated among theories, models, and principles; and presented many of the dominant theories used in health promotion and health education. Glanz, Lewis, and Rimer (1997) stress that effective intervention designs need to be conducted by the practitioner who understands theories of behavioral change and has the ability to use them skillfully in practice.

Freudenberg et al. (1995) note the confusion between theory and practice and the disconnection among theory, practice, and principles. In an attempt to identify principles that cut across different populations, settings, and strategies, they suggest at least 10 principles that have "informed interventions designed to build the capacity of individuals and communities to promote health and disease" (p. 297). The principles were derived from recent health education practice, and Freudenberg et al. feel that, at best, they constitute a "subjective and preliminary synthesis" and should be viewed as hypotheses requiring further testing. Although with this caveat, these principles provide the health promotion practitioner with tools that encourage rational thinking and selection from among alternative approaches. For example, 4 of the 10 principles that are presented accentuate many of the foundations underlying intervention approaches discussed in several earlier chapters.

Effective health education interventions should be tailored to a specific population within a particular setting; effective interventions involve the participants in planning, implementation, and evaluation; effective interventions integrate efforts aimed at changing individuals, social and physical environments, communities, and policies; and effective interventions build on the strengths found among participants and their communities. (Freudenberg et al., 1995, pp. 297-298)

In the final analysis, there is a need for practitioners to become culturally competent and sensitive to the populations with which they are working and to use current theories, models, and principles of health promotion in their program designs. Given the broad tapestry of cultures that surround us, health promoters must strive to improve on their own individual and collective learning curves through thoughtful, informed, and considerate HPDP programming. This must include reflection on what they see, experience, and feel if they are to gain perspective and skill in working with the diversity of peoples they are encountering in this multicultural world.

REFERENCES

Aday, L. (1993). *At risk in America: The health and health care needs of vulnerable populations in the United States.* San Francisco: Jossey-Bass.

Aguirre-Molina, M.(1993). Health issues panel, health promotion and disease prevention. In U.S. Department of Health and Human Services (Ed.), *One voice, one vision: Recommendations to the Surgeon General to improve Hispanic/Latino health.* Washington, DC: Government Printing Office.

Balcazar, H., Castro, F., & Krull, J. (1995). Cancer risk reduction in Mexican American women: The role of acculturation, education, and health risk factors. *Health Education Quarterly, 22,* 61-84.

Beauchamp, T. L., & Childress, J. F. (1989). *Principles of biomedical ethics.* New York: Oxford University Press.

Blane, D.(1995). Social determinants of health—Socioeconomic status, social class, and ethnicity [editorial]. *American Journal of Public Health, 85,* 903-904.

Braithwaite, R. L. (1992). Coalition partnerships for health promotion and empowerment. In R. L. Braithwaite & S. E. Taylor (Eds.), *Health issues in the black community.* San Francisco: Jossey-Bass.

Brislin, R. W., & Yoshida, T. (Eds.). (1994). *Improving intercultural interactions: Modules for cross-culturalfs training programs.* Thousand Oaks, CA: Sage.

Butler, J. T. (1997). *Principles of health education and health promotion.* Englewood, CO: Morton.

Campinha-Bacote, J. (1994). Cultural competence in psychiatric mental health nursing: A conceptual model. *Nursing Clinics of North America, 29,* 1-8.

Chen, M. S., & Hawks, B. L. (1995). A debunking of the myth of healthy Asian Americans and Pacific Islanders. *American Journal of Health Promotion, 9,* 261-268.

Cross, T. L., Bazron, B. J., Dennis, K. W., & Isaacs, M. R. (1989). *Towards a culturally competent system of care* (Vol. 1). Washington, DC: CASSP Technical Assistance Center, Georgetown University Child Development Center.

Darr, K. (1991). *Ethics in health services management* (2nd ed.). Baltimore, MD: Health Professions Press.

Feingold, E. (1995). The defeat of health care reform: Misplaced mistrust in government. *American Journal of Public Health, 85,* 1619-1622.

Freudenberg, N., Eng, E., Flay, B., Parcel, G., Rogers, T., & Wallerstein, N. (1995). Strengthening individual and community capacity to prevent diseases and promote health: In search of relevant theories and principles. *Health Education Quarterly, 22,* 290-306.

Gielen, A. C., & McDonald, E. M. (1997). The PRECEDE-PROCEED planning model. In K. Glanz, F. M. Lewis, & B. K. Rimer (Eds.), *Health behavior and health education: Theory, research and practice* (2nd ed.). San Francisco: Jossey-Bass.

Glanz, K., Lewis, F. M., & Rimer, B. K. (1997). Linking theory, research, and practice. In K. Glanz, F. M. Lewis, & B. K. Rimer (Eds.), *Health behavior and health education: Theory, research and practice* (2nd ed.). San Francisco: Jossey-Bass.

Green, L. W., & Kreuter, M. W. (1991). *Health promotion planning: An educational and environmental approach.* Mountain View, CA: Mayfield.

Green, L. W., & Ottoson, J. M. (1994). *Community health* (7th ed.). St. Louis, MO: C. V. Mosby.

Greenberg, J., & Gold, R. (1992). *The health education ethics book.* Dubuque, IA: William C. Brown.

Keogh, B. K., Gallimore, R., & Weisner, T. (1997). A sociocultural perspective on learning and learning disabilities. *Learning Disabilities Research and Practice, 12,* 107-113.

Kreps, G. L., & Kunimoto, E. N. (1994). *Effective communication in multicultural health care settings.* Thousand Oaks, CA: Sage.

Leininger, M. (1978). *Transcultural nursing: Concepts, theories and practices.* New York: John Wiley.

Marin, G., Burhansstipanov, L., Connell, C. M., Gielen, A. C., Helitzer-Allen, D., Lorig, K., Moriskey, D. E., Tenney, M., & Thomas, S. (1995). A research agenda for health education among underserved populations. *Health Education Quarterly, 22,* 346-363.

Montes, J. H., Eng, E., & Braithwaite, R. L. (1995). Commentary on minority health as a paradigm shift in the United States. *American Journal of Health Promotion, 9,* 247-250.

Montgomery, L. E., Kiely, J. L., & Pappas, G. (1996). The effects of poverty, race, and family structure on U.S. children's health: Data from the NFUS, 1978 through 1980 and 1989 through 1991. *American Journal of Public Health, 86,* 1401-1405.

Nobles, W. W., & Goddard, L. L. (1993). An African-centered model of prevention for African-American youth at high risk. In L. L. Goddard (Ed.), *An African-centered model of prevention for African-American youth at high risk.* Rockville, MD: U.S. Department of Health and Human Services, Substance Abuse and Mental Health Services Administration.

Nunnally, E., & Moy, C. (1989). *Communication basics for health service professionals.* Newbury Park, CA: Sage.

Padilla, A. M. (1980). *Acculturation: Theory, models and some new findings.* Boulder, CO: Westview.

Paniagua, F. A. (1994). *Assessing and treating culturally diverse clients: A practical guide.* Thousand Oaks, CA: Sage.

Sorlie, P. D., Backlund, E., & Keller, J. B. (1995). U.S. mortality by economic, demographic, and social characteristics: The National Longitudinal Mortality Study. *American Journal of Public Health, 85,* 949-956.

U.S. Bureau of the Census. (1996). *Statistical abstract of the United States: 1995* (Current Population Reports). Washington, DC: Government Printing Office.

Author Index

Subject Index

About the Editors

Robert M. Huff, M.P.H., Ph.D., C.H.E.S., is Associate Professor in the Health Education undergraduate and M.P.H. graduate programs at California State University, Northridge (CSUN). He received his M.P.H. degree in health education from CSUN and his Ph.D. from the University of California, Santa Barbara, in confluent education within the Graduate School of Education. Prior to joining the faculty at CSUN, he was a health education practitioner for Drew University in Los Angeles and later at the Ventura County Public Health Services and Medical Center, where he directed patient education programming for the medical center, organized and managed a teleproduction facility, codeveloped and managed a countywide health promotion center, and consulted on a variety of public health programs including chronic disease prevention, family life education, and AIDS awareness and prevention. He currently teaches both undergraduate and graduate courses that focus on program planning and evaluation, health behavior change, communications and media, cross-cultural issues in health education, and other related courses. He is a consultant on several major projects focused on alcohol, drugs, and violence among college-aged students and a wellness community project focused on youths living in the Ojai Valley of Ventura County, California. He also is an editorial consultant for the *Journal of Drug Education*. His research interests combine his undergraduate training in anthropology with his graduate training in public health education to focus on multicultural health promotion and disease prevention programs in a variety of health care settings.

Michael V. Kline, M.P.H., Dr.P.H., C.H.E.S., is Professor of Community Health Education at California State University, Northridge. He received his M.P.H. degree in public health education and behavioral sciences from the University of California, Berkeley, School of Public Health. He received his Dr.P.H. degree in health administration from the University of California, Los Angeles, School of Public Health. He currently teaches undergraduate and graduate courses involved with training practitioners to design, implement, and evaluate health education programs within a variety of health education settings, population groups, and community organizations. Through the years, he has been actively involved in community organization activities relevant to assisting special populations to plan and organize health programs in their neighborhoods. His most recent work as a behavioral sciences consultant with the Alcohol and Drug Program Administration, Evaluation of Data Management Services, County of Los Angeles Department of Health Services, in the field of alcohol prevention and education has included assisting in the development of data management and information systems for alcohol client tracking activities. He formerly was the director of several alcohol and drug treatment programs in Los Angeles, including the Edgemont House social model program, the Golden State Community Mental Health Center Comprehensive Alcohol Treatment Program, and the Los Angeles County Alcohol Training Consortium. He also has been involved in providing technical consultation and education in the development and evaluation of drinking driver programs. He formerly served as director of public health education at the Orange County (California) Department of Public Health and as district director of health education, Southeast Region, Department of Health Services, County of Los Angeles.

About the Contributors

Mary Ashley, R.N., P.H.N., M.P.H., is Assistant Professor at the Drew University of Medicine and Science in Los Angeles. She has spent the majority of her career working in poor and minority communities. She worked with David Satcher in starting a free clinic in a church basement and has been involved with a variety of health education and health promotion projects throughout the inner city of Los Angeles including programs in hypertension control, cancer, HIV, and other chronic conditions. She currently is director of the Center for Community and Preventive Medicine within the Department of Family Medicine at Drew University.

John Casken, M.P.H., Ph.D., is Assistant Professor in Health Services Administration and Planning at the University of Hawaii School of Public Health. He is director of the school's Educational Opportunities Program and has major responsibility for the recruitment and retention of the school's Native Hawaiian, Pacific Islander, American Indian, and Alaska Native students. He has taught in the Pacific, Saudi Arabia, and Great Britain and has worked on the Pine Ridge Reservation in South Dakota in the Indian Health Service Hospital. He also has taught at Oglala Lakota College in South Dakota.

Felipe G. Castro, M.S.W., Ph.D., is Professor of Clinical Psychology in the Department of Psychology at Arizona State University. He is a nationally known research scientist and leader in the area of Hispanic health research and program development, with expertise in program evaluation and statistical methods. He has served as a consultant to several governmental and community-based organizations and has been extensively involved in research related to drug abuse and the motivational determinants of addiction to drugs. He also was the principal investigator on a study to reduce cancer risks among Hispanic women.

Patricia Chalela, M.P.H., is a Research Associate in the Center for Cancer Control Research at the Baylor College of Medicine. She previously has served as chief of the Department of Preventive Medicine of the Fundacion Oftalmologica de Santander-Clinica Carlos Ardila Lulle, Universidad Autonoma de Bucaramanga, in Bucaramanga, Colombia.

Marya K. Cota, Ph.D., is Director of Behavioral Studies in the Family Practice Residency Program at the Maricopa Medical Center in Phoenix, Arizona. She is a clinical psychologist who has specialized in community and minority psychology. Her areas of research are in ethnic identity and language of Mexican American children and families. She has been a Peace Corps volunteer in Costa Rica and currently is finishing a postdoctoral fellowship.

Bonnie M. Duran, Dr.P.H., is Assistant Professor in the Master of Public Health Program at the University of New Mexico. She teaches theory in the Master of Public Health Program and conducts National Institute of Mental Health and Navajo Nation research projects. For the past 20 years, she has provided training, planning, and evaluation health education services to tribal and urban public health projects in the areas of substance abuse, women's health, HIV, and youth programs.

Eduardo F. Duran, Ph.D., is Director of Chemical Dependency Services at Rehoboth Hospital in Gallup, New Mexico. He is a clinical psychologist who has worked in the field of Native American mental health since 1980. He has directed rural, reservation-based, and urban community mental health treatment and prevention programs in both New Mexico and California.

June Gutierrez English, M.P.H., is Senior Health Educator at Ventura County Public Health Services in Ventura, California. She is a doctoral candidate in medical anthropology at the University of California, Berkeley. Her research interests focus on health care strategies of urban American Indians. Her current health education position is working with Asian American and American Indian communities to involve them in the Breast Cancer Early Detection Program.

C. James Frankish, Ph.D., is Associate Director of the Institute of Health Promotion Research and is Assistant Professor in the Department of Health Care and Epidemiology at the University of British Columbia. He is a registered clinical psychologist with extensive research and clinical experience in employee health and in coping with chronic illness and health behavior change in marginalized groups. He is actively involved in community health and social service organizations.

Larri Fredericks, Ph.D., M.P.H., is Associate Scientist in the Center for American Indian Research and Education at the Western Consortium for Public Health in Berkeley, California. She has a Ph.D. in medical anthropology and an M.P.H. degree and specializes in ethnicity and health. She has significant experience in designing, writing, implementing, and evaluating health care and health education programs for American Indians and Alaska Natives. She also is a consultant to government, academic, and private institutions on American Indian health and education.

Lawrence W. Green, Dr.P.H., is Director of the Institute of Health Promotion Research and is Professor of Health Care and Epidemiology at the University of British Columbia. He has worked for many years as a health educator in local, state, and federal health agencies in California and at the Ford Foundation in Dhaka, East Pakistan, and he served as the first director of the U.S. Office of Health Information and Health Promotion. He has served on the faculties at the University of California, Berkeley, Johns Hopkins University, Harvard University, and the University of Texas and most recently has served as the Kaiser Family Foundation's vice president and director of the Health Promotion Program, which received the Foundation Award of the National Association of Prevention Professionals.

Patti Herring, R.N., Ph.D., affiliated with the Loma Linda University School of Public Health, is Founder/Director of NEET EXPRESSION Inc., a health education drama group composed of African American teenagers in Dallas, Texas. She has worked with teens for more than 15 years and currently is directing research targeting students and their families at risk for chronic disease, domestic violence, and posttraumatic stress.

Felicia Schanche Hodge, Dr.P.H., is Associate Researcher and Associate Adjunct Professor in the School of Public Health and is Director of the Center for American Indian Research and Education at the University of California, Berkeley. She is a Wailaki Indian from Northern California who has been extensively involved in research dealing with cultural sensitivity, cancer, alcohol, tobacco, disabling conditions, and other health care issues of American Indian populations. She has served on a number of organizational boards including the California Teen Nutrition Program, the State of California Breast and Cervical Cancer Advisory Board, the American Indian Child Resource Center board of directors, the Network for Cancer Control Research Among American Indian/ Alaska Native Populations, and the California Pan-Ethnic Health Network. She also is a lecturer in the School of Social Welfare and the director of the American Indian Graduate Program at the University of California, Berkeley.

Joyce W. Hopp, Ph.D., M.P.H, R.N., is Professor of Health Promotion and Education in the School of Public Health and is Dean of the School of Allied Health Professions at Loma Linda University. She has worked internationally and cross-culturally in diverse locations such as the Navajo Reservation in Utah, Saudi Arabia, China, Myanmar, and Tanzania. Her research interests have included school health education and AIDS. She currently is on the editorial board of the *Journal of Allied Health* and serves on the board of the *American Journal of Health Behavior.*

Claire K. Hughes, M.S., R.D., is Chief of the Health Promotion and Education Branch of the Hawaii State Department of Health. She is of Native Hawaiian ancestry and is a graduate of the Kamehameha Schools and Oregon State University. She currently is completing her doctorate at the University of Hawaii and writes a monthly column for *Ka Wai Ola* that focuses on Native Hawaiian culture and past achievements as well as on improving Native Hawaiian health.

Jillian Inouye, Ph.D., R.N., is Associate Professor in and Coordinator of the Graduate Community Mental Health Nursing Program in the School of Nursing at the University of Hawaii. She has a Ph.D. in psychology and is a licensed psychologist who has authored a number of articles and book chapters on Asian Americans and on critical thinking. Her research focus has been in the area of health psychology, Asian health issues, HIV/AIDS, and inquiry-based learning (and consulted in Japan on these topics).

Dianne N. Ishida, Ph.D., R.N., is Associate Professor in the School of Nursing at the University of Hawaii. She has a Ph.D. in anthropology and formerly was the acting director for the International Affairs Office in the School of Nursing. Her research areas have been in culture, learning, and health beliefs and practices among Samoan women in the area of early detection of breast cancer. Her geographic research areas are Pacific and East and Southeast Asia.

Anh Lê, B.A., is Public Health Educator in the Vietnamese Community Health Promotion Project at the University of California, San Francisco. His undergraduate training was in psychology, and his areas of specialization include community health education, youths, policy, and media advocacy. He has worked with Vietnamese youths at Vietnamese-language schools in the San Francisco Bay Area and has produced more than 30 anti-tobacco television advertisements. He was the principal author of the Asian Pacific Islander Tobacco Education Network Policy Statement, which condemned the tobacco industry's marketing tactics in ethnic communities and tobacco exports to Asia. He filed a complaint with the U.S. Federal Trade Commission in 1996 and led a community education campaign that resulted in the FTC's unanimous ruling in June 1998 requiring that tobacco advertisements and sales promotional materials in non-English speaking communities carry the Surgeon General's warnings on smoking translated into the language of the targeted community. He is a contributing author of the *1998 Report of the U.S. Surgeon General–Tobacco Use Among U.S. Racial/Ethnic Minority Groups* and serves on the Vietnamese Tobacco-Free Community Task Force in the Bay Area.

Gregory P. Loos, Ed.D., M.P.H., M.S., is Branch Chief for Training and Educational Systems in the National Institute for Occupational Safety and Health, Centers for Disease Control and Prevention, in Cincinnati, Ohio. He has trained as a learning theorist and public health planner. He has extensive international experience in Southeast Asia and the Pacific Islands, where he was involved in community assessment activities, community health education, and health administration. He has been a special education teacher in K-6 and has been on the faculties of the University of Hawaii and East Stroudsburg University. He also has worked with the Hawaii State Department of Health, the Hawaii State Department of Education, and the Kamehameha Educational Research Institute.

Chris Y. Lovato, Ph.D., is Clinical Associate Professor of Health Care and Epidemiology and is Assistant Director of the Institute of Health Promotion Research at the University of British Columbia. She has served in a variety of educational and research roles including the National Cancer Institute of Canada, the Graduate School of Public Health at San Diego State University, and the University of Texas Health Sciences Center in Houston. In addition, she has been a consultant to the Centers for Disease Control and Prevention and the California Department of Education.

Amelie G. Ramirez, Dr.P.H., is Associate Professor of Medicine and Associate Director of the Center for Cancer Control Research at the Baylor College of Medicine. In addition, she serves as the Associate Director for Community Research for the Cancer Prevention and Health Promotion Program at the San Antonio Cancer Institute in Texas. Her research interests include interventions related to reduction of risk factors for cancer and heart disease as well as prevention of substance abuse in Hispanic and other minority populations.

William J. Shannon, M.A., Ed.D., is Research Associate in the Institute of Health Promotion Research at the University of British Columbia. He has an Ed.D. in education and a master's degree in health education. He has served in a variety of health education roles including director of the Health Education, Communications, and Public Affairs Branch of the British Columbia Ministry of Health and has been involved in many community planning projects focused on issues such as substance abuse, immigrant health needs, heart disease, and other related programs and services.

Lucina Suarez, M.S., Ph.D., is Senior Scientist in the Texas Department of Health. She has worked in the field of epidemiology for more than 20 years. She has been involved in research activities in the areas of occupational health, heart disease, cancer, and disease control research on Hispanic population groups. Her current research efforts are focused on the causes of birth defects in Mexican Americans living on the U.S.–Mexico border.

Santos C. Vega, Ph.D., is Director of the Community Documentation Program in the Hispanic Research Center at Arizona State University. He has more than 25 years of experience creating action research-based programs at various educational levels and with different academic institutions. He has worked extensively in the Hispanic community.

Roberto Villarreal, M.D., M.P.H., is Associate Director in the South Texas Health Research Center within the University of Texas Health Science Center at San Antonio. His main focus on research is based on design, implementation, and outcomes of population-based education and behavioral intervention programs. He also conducts research on population surveys specifically within the Hispanic population on Diabetes, Cancer Prevention and Access to Health Care for minorities. He has more than 15 years of experience in population assessment and community interventions within the US-Mexico border area. His primary interest in medicine is related to clinical outcomes in minority populations.

Gina M. Wingood, Sc.D., M.P.H., is Assistant Professor in the Department of Behavioral Sciences and Health Education, Rollins School of Public Health, at Emory University. Her research focus is on designing, implementing, and evaluating STD/HIV prevention programs for women. She also conducts research on identifying social exposures, such as having a physically abusive partner, that may increase a woman's risk for contracting the HIV virus.

D. William Wood, M.P.H., Ph.D., is Interim Dean and Professor of Public Health, School of Public Health, at the University of Hawai'i. He has served as director of the International Center for Health Promotion and Disease Prevention Research and a senior research investigator for the Hawaii Medical Service Association Foundation. His primary teaching areas are in planning and information systems development and the behavioral sciences as these relate to public health.

About the Editorial Board

Ronald L. Braithwaite, Ph.D., is Associate Professor in the Rollins School of Public Health at Emory University. He has served on the faculties of Virginia Commonwealth University, Hampton University, Howard University, and East Virginia Medical School and has been extensively involved in the African American community. He is widely published, and his research interests are focused on community organization and empowerment for public health practice. He has both national and international experience as a technical adviser, evaluator, and expert panel member on research and evaluation and was a Fulbright Hays Scholar in Ghana and Cameroon, West Africa.

Abel Martinez, M.P.H., C.H.E.S., is Assistant Director of the Binational/Border Health Program, Los Angeles County Department of Health Services. He has worked as a health educator in a variety of community settings and was the department's health education coordinator for 10 years. He has taught and conducted research on a variety of health education and public health topics including *curanderismo,* multicultural health education approaches, culturally associated sources of lead poisoning, and cultural competency. He is past president of the California Conference of Local Directors of Health Education and was selected as the 1997 Health Educator of the Year by the Society for Public Health Education, Southern California chapter.

Kenneth R. McLeroy, Ph.D., is Professor and Chair of the Department of Health Promotion Sciences, College of Public Health, at the University of Oklahoma. He is a very well-known educator, researcher, grantsman, and writer who has been active, and continues to be active, in the Society of Public Health Education and the American Public Health Association. He is significantly involved in state and local organizations and has served as an evaluation consultant on a variety of projects at the federal, state, and local levels. He has been an associate, executive, and guest editor for a variety of professional journals and currently is on the editorial board of *Health Education and Behavior.* His research interests include community capacity building, adolescent pregnancy prevention, and Native American health and disease prevention.

Marjorie Kagawa-Singer, R.N., M.N., Ph.D., is Assistant Professor in the School of Public Health and Asian American Studies Center at the University of California, Los Angeles. She has trained in nursing and has her doctoral degree in anthropology. Her clinical area for the past 30 years has been in oncology, and her research focuses on the discrepancies in physical and mental health care outcomes of ethnic minority populations. She serves on multiple local, state, and national committees involved with issues of ethnicity and health care, and she has taught extensively on issues in cross-cultural health care, cancer, pain, grief and bereavement, end-of-life decision making, and quality-of-life issues. Her current research interests focus on defining and developing standards of cultural competence in health care and investigating the influence of ethnicity on health care decisions.

C. June Strickland, R.N., Ph.D., is Assistant Professor in Psychology and Community Health in the School of Nursing at the University of Washington. She has worked in the Pacific Northwest for 25 years and has concentrated her research efforts on American Indian communities. Her current research is focused on American Indian youth suicide prevention and cancer prevention behaviors of American Indian women. She is regional coordinator for the Fred Hutchinson Cancer Research Center and has served as a director for several clinic- and hospital-based educational departments whose focus was on continuing medical education, staff development, patient education, community education, and related services.